Atlas of Cytopathology and Radiology

Ritu Nayar • Xiaoqi Lin
Ajit S. Paintal • Ramona Gupta
Albert A. Nemcek Jr.
Editors

Atlas of Cytopathology and Radiology

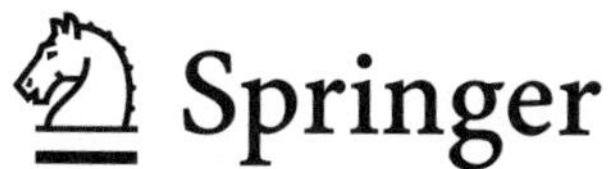

Editors
Ritu Nayar
Northwestern University Feinberg School of Medicine
Northwestern Memorial Hospital
Chicago, IL
USA

Xiaoqi Lin
Northwestern University
Feinberg School of Medicine
Northwestern Memorial Hospital
Chicago, IL
USA

Ajit S. Paintal
Northshore Medical Group
Evanston Hospital
Evanston, IL
USA

Ramona Gupta
Northwestern University Feinberg School of Medicine
Chicago, IL
USA

Albert A. Nemcek Jr.
Northwestern University Feinberg School of Medicine
Chicago, IL
USA

ISBN 978-3-030-24754-6 ISBN 978-3-030-24756-0 (eBook)
https://doi.org/10.1007/978-3-030-24756-0

This Springer imprint is published by the registered company Springer Nature Switzerland AG
The registered company address is: Gewerbestrasse 11, 6330 Cham, Switzerland

To my husband, Rajeev Nayar—the wind beneath my wings.
To my parents, Tilak Raj and Sheila Bhalotra, for their undying encouragement, love, and support.
To my dear sisters, Anju and Sonia.
Ritu Nayar

To my parents, Bingkun Lin and Dr. Guilan Wan, for their emphasis on my education, constant support, and love.
To my beloved wife, Bing Zhu, and son, Jeffrey, for their love, patience, support, and encouragement.
Xiaoqi Lin

To my children, Amrita and Ranjit.
Ajit S. Paintal

To my children, Erich, Rachel, Mitchell, and Grace.
Albert A. Nemcek Jr.

Preface

The diagnostic services—pathology and radiology—are the cornerstone for supporting the delivery of high-quality healthcare by providing timely and accurate diagnosis. In this era of precision medicine, it has become increasingly important for these two services to work collaboratively in supporting our patients and clinical colleagues by informing and communicating the selection and interpretation of appropriate diagnostic tests, as well as obtaining adequate tissue for diagnosis, prognostication, and therapy at initial presentation and, if required, during disease progression/relapse. The importance of access to oncologic imaging and pathology expertise and technologies was highlighted at a recent workshop organized by the National Cancer Policy Forum—*Improving Cancer Diagnosis and Care: Patient Access to Oncologic Imaging and Pathology Expertise and Technologies* [1].

At our large teaching hospital, we are fortunate to have both cytopathology and interventional radiology expertise. Our teams have a close working relationship, with dedicated space for the cytopathology in interventional radiology, where biopsy review and decision-making, with discussion if warranted with the ordering physician, are done on a daily basis. Over the past three decades, we have built a state-of-the-art, collaborative, fine needle aspiration (FNA) and core biopsy service with immediate on-site adequacy evaluation and triage. This joint service provides the majority of primary cancer diagnosis and in advanced stage disease is the only pathology material on which all diagnostic and ancillary testing is done.

We previously published a monograph targeted toward our oncology colleagues, *Cytopathology in Oncology*, with the aim of "demystifying" cytopathology [2]. This current atlas is aimed at practicing cytopathologists and interventional radiologists and trainees in these areas. It is our pleasure to be able to share our experience with the readers of this atlas. We hope you will find it to be a useful reference for your practice.

Ritu Nayar, MD

Professor of Pathology and Medical Education, Northwestern University Feinberg School of Medicine

Vice Chair for Education and Faculty Development, Department of Pathology

Medical Director for Cytopathology, Northwestern Memorial Hospital

Member, Northwestern Robert H. Lurie Comprehensive Cancer Center

Chicago, IL, USA — Ritu Nayar

References

1. Balogh E, Patlak M, Nass SJ. The National Academies of Sciences: Health and Medicine Division. Improving cancer diagnosis and care: patient access to oncologic imaging and pathology expertise and technologies: proceedings of a workshop. Washington, DC: The National Academies Press; September 11, 2018. Available at http://www.nationalacademies.org/hmd/Reports/2018/improving-cancer-diagnosis-and-care-patient-access-to-oncologic-imaging-and-pathology-expertise-and-technologies-proceedings.aspx
2. Nayar R. Preface. Cytopathology in Oncology. Nayar R, ed. Berlin/Heidelberg: Springer-Verlag; 2014. Available at https://link.springer.com/book/10.1007%2F978-3-642-38850-7

Acknowledgments

We would like to acknowledge our physician and staff colleagues along with our residents and fellows at Northwestern Memorial Hospital, with whom we have the privilege of working every day. We are also thankful to the Springer staff—Lee Klein and Lillie Gaurano—for their patience and guidance in the production of this atlas.

Contents

Contributors

Rehan Ali, MD Department of Radiology, Section of Vascular and Interventional Radiology, Northwestern University, Chicago, IL, USA

Ali Al Asadi, BS Department of Radiology, Section of Vascular and Interventional Radiology, Northwestern University, Chicago, IL, USA

Luis Z. Blanco Jr, MD Department of Pathology, Northwestern Memorial Hospital, Northwestern University Feinberg School of Medicine, Chicago, IL, USA

Laura Dean, MD Department of Diagnostic Radiology, Cleveland Clinic, Cleveland, OH, USA

Ahmed Gabr, MD Department of Radiology, Section of Vascular and Interventional Radiology, Northwestern University, Chicago, IL, USA

Juehua Gao, MD, PhD Department of Pathology, Northwestern University, Feinberg School of Medicine, Chicago, IL, USA

Ramona Gupta, MD Northwestern University Feinberg School of Medicine, Chicago, IL, USA

Ali Habib, MD Department of Radiology, Northwestern University, Chicago, IL, USA

Tracey Harbert, MD Cellnetix Pathology, Olympia, WA, USA

Ryan Hickey, MD Department of Radiology, Division of Vascular Interventional Radiology, New York, NY, USA

Steven D. Huffman, MD Aurora St. Luke's Medical Center of Aurora Health Care Metro, Inc., Milwaukee, WI, USA

Xiaoqi Lin, MD, PhD Northwestern University, Feinberg School of Medicine, Northwestern Memorial Hospital, Chicago, IL, USA

Rosewell V. Mackey, MD Department of Radiology, McGaw Medical Center, Northwestern University, Chicago, IL, USA

Khairuddin Memon, MD Department of Radiology, OU Physicians, Oklahoma City, OK, USA

Ronald Mora, MD Department of Radiology, Section of Vascular and Interventional Radiology, Northwestern University, Chicago, IL, USA

Elizabeth Morency, MD Department of Pathology, Northwestern Memorial Hospital, Feinberg School of Medicine, Chicago, IL, USA

Nicholas Morley, MD Department of Radiology, Marshfield Clinic, Marshfield, WI, USA

Ritu Nayar, MD Northwestern University Feinberg School of Medicine, Northwestern Memorial Hospital, Chicago, IL, USA

Albert A. Nemcek Jr. Northwestern University Feinberg School of Medicine, Chicago, IL, USA

Ajit S. Paintal, MD Northshore Medical Group, Evanston Hospital, Evanston, IL, USA

Joseph F. Peevey, MD Department of Anatomic and Clinical Pathology, OSF St. Anthony Medical Center, Rockford, IL, USA

John K. S. S. Philip, MD Department of Pathology, Thomas Health System, South Charleston, WV, USA

Ahsun Riaz, MD Department of Pathology, Northwestern Medicine, Chicago, IL, USA

Jamie Macagba Slade, MD Department of Pathology, Rush Medical College, Chicago, IL, USA

Julianne M. Ubago, MD Department of Pathology, Edward Hospital, Naperville, IL, USA

Brandon A. Umphress, MD Department of Pathology, Northwestern Memorial Hospital, McGaw Medical Center, Chicago, IL, USA

Lilian C. Wang, MD Department of Radiology, Prentice Women's Hospital, Chicago, IL, USA

Ernest F. Wiggins III, MD Department of Radiology, Monmouth Medical Center, Shrewsbury, NJ, USA

Joseph Young, MD Department of Radiology, St. Joseph Health, St. Jude Medical Center, Fullerton, CA, USA

Songlin Zhang, MD, PhD Department of Pathology and Laboratory Medicine, University of Texas McGovern Medical School, Houston, TX, USA

An Introduction to Radiology and Cytopathology Considerations in a Collaborative Biopsy Service

1

Ajit S. Paintal, Ritu Nayar, and Albert A. Nemcek Jr.

Interventional Radiology Fundamentals

Image-guided procurement of tissue or fluid for diagnostic purposes has become one of the most commonly performed procedures in medicine. Although the focus of this Atlas is cytologic analysis of tissue specimens, we would note that cytologic, biochemical, and microbiologic evaluation of fluids obtained in this manner is similarly important, and for the purposes of this text the term "biopsy" will be assumed to cover both settings.

The basic elements of image-guided biopsy are the following: a lesion or organ is identified as amenable and appropriate for biopsy; a method of imaging guidance is chosen; an approach to the lesion or organ is plotted; needle(s) or other devices are used to obtain tissue or fluid; and the material is processed and reviewed.

The target for biopsy is chosen when, on the basis of clinical radiological and/or endoscopic data, the target has potential clinical significance. While this would seem self-evident, it emphasizes that awareness of the imaging appearance of normal variants, pseudolesions, and typically insignificant manifestations of pathology such as focal hepatic steatosis, classic hepatic hemangiomas, and typical adrenal adenomas will minimize performance of unnecessary procedures. Biopsy of normal (or pathologically insignificant) tissues generally results in few complications. However, obtaining normal tissue may lead to the misperception that the operator is "missing" a lesion with biopsy attempts, possibly prompting additional attempts, each with inherent risk. Further, in certain scenarios, biopsy of normal tissue may carry a greater than average risk of complications. It has been suggested, for example, that biopsy of normal pancreas may increase the risk of subsequent pancreatitis [1].

Another consideration in choosing a target for biopsy is that less-invasive methods of obtaining a confident diagnosis are unavailable or unsuccessful. While diagnostic specificity on imaging is often elusive, properly chosen and performed imaging studies can establish a confident diagnosis in many instances. A corollary is that the operator should always evaluate imaging fully to look for the least risky intervention that is likely to obtain an answer (for example, biopsy of a subcutaneous nodule rather than a deep retroperitoneal lymph node).

A question to be answered by both the referring physician and the operator is whether plans for treatment or further investigation are likely to be strongly influenced by the biopsy results. Consider the setting of metastatic disease in a patient with a known primary malignancy. Pathologic analysis of the suspected metastases reinforces the use of potentially hazardous or debilitating therapy when metastatic disease is confirmed, and can alter workup and treatment when another diagnosis is established. Further, decision-making does not necessarily mandate tissue confirmation. Examples would include a patient with strong clinical and biochemical evidence of pheochromocytoma and a large adrenal mass (biopsy of which carries its own significant risks), or a cirrhotic patient with a liver mass with venous invasion, and a markedly elevated alpha-fetoprotein (highly diagnostic of hepatocellular carcinoma without the need for tissue) [2], or a patient who would not be treated regardless of the biopsy results. Image-guided biopsy is also unnecessary for patients who require surgical therapy for emergent clinical conditions caused by suspicious lesions that could be biopsied in the open setting. Progression/relapse of previously confirmed malignancies may require follow up biopsies for molecular testing and considerations for targeted therapy.

There should be both an advantage to imaging guidance and a reasonable chance that tissue or fluid can be obtained

A. S. Paintal (✉)
Northshore Medical Group, Evanston Hospital, Evanston, IL, USA

R. Nayar
Northwestern University Feinberg School of Medicine, Northwestern Memorial Hospital, Chicago, IL, USA

A. A. Nemcek Jr.
Northwestern University Feinberg School of Medicine, Chicago, IL, USA

R. Nayar et al. (eds.), *Atlas of Cytopathology and Radiology*, https://doi.org/10.1007/978-3-030-24756-0_1

from the lesion/organ in question using some form of imaging guidance. For small, non-palpable focal lesions, the likelihood of success depends on many factors, with size becoming important especially at the lower limits of visibility [3, 4].

The literature is replete with studies that have evaluated the risks of percutaneous biopsy procedures [5–7], and in order to proceed with biopsy those risks need to be taken into account, communicated, and prepared for, and if the risks are considered prohibitive the biopsy should not be performed. There is, for example, a low but well-established potential for hemorrhagic complications of biopsy, even in patients with normal hemostasis, regardless of the lesion type or biopsy technique. Basic coagulation studies (international normalized ratio, platelet count) are generally obtained for all but superficial biopsies, with additional studies dependent upon the screening history and initial lab results. However, the correlation between bleeding risk and the results of routine coagulation studies is somewhat tenuous, and a good clinical history regarding bleeding risks should always be obtained [7, 8]. It is rare indeed that a biopsy needs to be performed emergently, and therefore every effort can usually be made to correct significant hemostatic abnormalities. Severe, uncorrectable coagulopathy is generally considered an absolute contraindication to biopsy, while the decision of whether and how to proceed in patients with milder abnormalities will depend on clinical circumstances. Occurrence of a complication during performance of a biopsy often limits the number of needle passes obtainable for biopsy, although in some cases on-site treatment (e.g. chest tube placement for pneumothorax incurred during lung biopsy) may allow the procedure to continue.

The operator also needs to account for the patient's ability to cooperate with the procedure. Biopsies in uncooperative patients are generally more risky and less likely to be successful. A careful pre-procedural explanation of the patient's role in the procedure (e.g. when and how to breath hold) is helpful. Use of local anesthesia is ubiquitous; pharmacologic analgesia and sedation are also useful in most cases, although use of these needs to be balanced against potential oversedation that may make lesion targeting more difficult and increase procedural risks.

Biopsy of specific tissue types, or needle paths through certain tissues, can also increase risks. Appropriate pre-procedural screening and planning can help minimize these risks. As an example, biopsy of lesions that elaborate vasoactive substances—pheochromocytomas, extra-adrenal paragangliomas, and carcinoid tumors—have been associated with severe and sometimes fatal blood pressure swings [9, 10]. When such tumors are suspected on the basis of clinical and/or radiologic findings, targeted biochemical screening should be performed. The operator should, by extension, become familiar with measures for treatment and prevention of such reactions.

Needle track seeding, although generally felt to be rare, almost certainly occurs with increased frequency for certain tumor types. One notable example is hepatocellular carcinoma, for which a meta-analysis estimated a not inconsiderable 2.7% incidence of needle track seeding, with a 0.9% incidence per year [11].

A variety of imaging methods are available for biopsy guidance, the most common currently being ultrasonography (percutaneous or endoscopic) and computed tomography (CT), with modalities such as fluoroscopy and magnetic resonance scanning less frequently used. The method chosen should portray the target well, and ideally allow the safest, technically easiest, and most reliable access. Cost, availability, personal preference/experience, and the potential need for ancillary procedures also enter these considerations. Ultrasound has advantages of real-time needle placement, portability, and relatively low cost; on the other hand, CT will often show lesions better than ultrasound, particularly if gas (as in lung biopsies) is in the path of the needle. Contrast agents may be useful in select CT cases and have begun to be investigated as a technique in ultrasound-guided biopsies (Fig. 1.1) [12]. Although still relatively early in development and not yet widely available, methods using "fusion" imaging (combinations of imaging methods, for example ultrasonography and nuclear medicine) [13] and guidance systems such as electromagnetic tracking [14] are likely to be applied more often in the future. Biopsy should be targeted toward that portion of the tumor most likely to yield diagnostic tissue. For example, lesions with necrotic centers are more profitably biopsied at their periphery, or functional imaging such as positron-emission tomography may direct the operator to more metabolically active portions of the lesion in question that are in turn more likely to yield diagnostic tissue.

In terms of devices used to procure diagnostic material, most are variations of needles, although other options such as biopsy forceps may also be useful. Even the simplest needle design may yield diagnostic material, although various tip alterations—cutting needles, semi-automated and fully automated core devices, and others—have been designed with the aim of improving yield [7]. Although an in-depth discussion is beyond the scope of this chapter, and although these divisions are somewhat arbitrary and subjective, the most basic division of needles is into smaller (around 21 to 26 gauge) devices that typically obtain fragmented tissue or aspirates of separated cells and larger (20 gauge and beyond) devices that obtain more tissue including true "cores" of tissue. Smaller devices are usually less painful for the patient and probably safer, although many studies show differences in complications only at the extreme ranges of needle size. Larger specimens generally translate to higher diagnostic

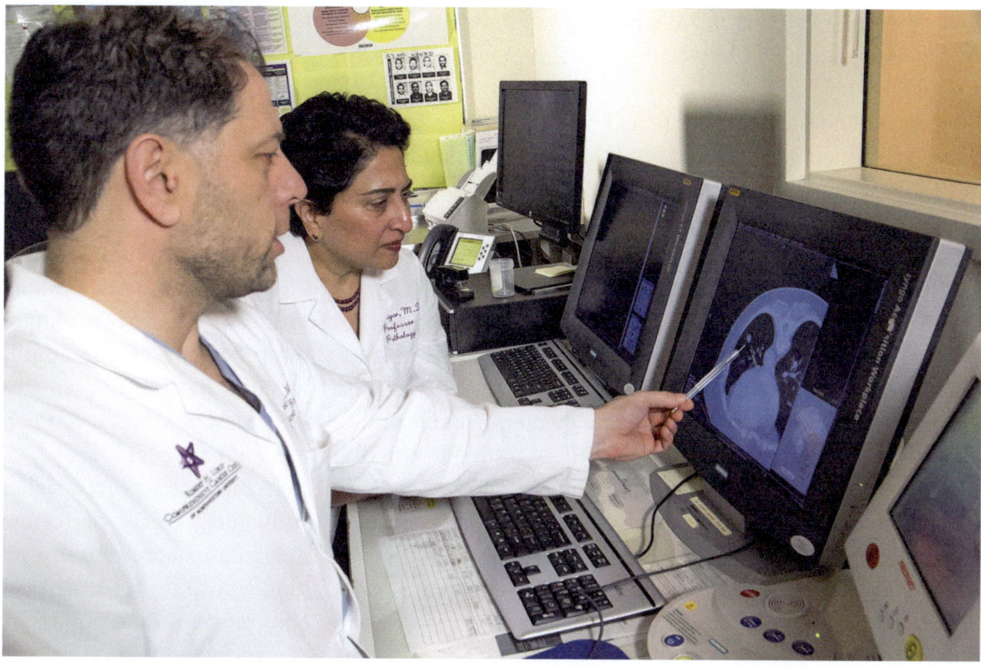

Fig. 1.1 Pathologist and radiologist reviewing patient CT scan in interventional radiology and discussing the case before beginning a lung biopsy procedure

yield, a factor that has become particularly important in recent years given the increasing focus on genomic/molecular analysis of tissue specimens for personalized medicine [15, 16]. Whereas, in the past, the primary goal of biopsy was establishment of a phenotypic diagnosis, requests are now made to characterize tumor genotypes and assess other biomarkers, and to do serial biopsies to assess response to therapy, monitor the progression of disease, and adjust therapy in response to the changing character of tumors. Indeed, this focus on obtaining larger quantities of "high quality" tissue for these purposes has raised a new set of questions applicable to image-guided biopsy that are currently the focus of intensive investigation: How often do we obtain adequate tissue for analysis? What strategies can be used to improve the yield of biopsy for such purposes (needle size, number of passes, presence of an on-site cytopathologist, correlation with functional imaging such as positron-emission tomography scanning)? And what is the cost of these strategies, both in terms of risk to the patient and monetary cost to both patient and society, especially when the benefit may be minimal or unpredictable? Further, will these considerations be rendered obsolete by emerging technologies such as "liquid" biopsy [17]?

Basic Cytopathology

Cytopathology differs from conventional histopathology in regards to specimen preparation, staining techniques, and common applications. Broadly speaking the two most common specimen types are aspiration biopsies and exfoliative specimens. Exfoliative specimens contain cells that have been shed from a surface. These cells may shed spontaneously, as in the case of a pleural effusion, or be removed mechanically, as in the case of a bronchial brushing, bladder washing, or cervical Pap test. These specimens are often prepared by making a direct smear of the specimen. Alternatively, the specimen may be centrifuged directly onto the slide in order to concentrate cellular material.

Fine needle aspiration (FNA) specimens, in contrast, are obtained by inserting a thin needle into an area of abnormal tissue and drawing cellular material into the needle with a combination of capillary action and suction. This material may be then expressed ("squirted") on to a glass slide and smeared or deposited into liquid medium. In contrast to a core biopsy, a macroscopic solid piece of tissue is not obtained in a fine needle aspiration.

Two types of stains are employed in most cytologic specimens. The Diff-Quik stain is commonly used on air-dried specimens and has the advantage of being rapid to perform; specimens can be stained and evaluated in a matter of minutes allowing real time intraprocedural feedback in regards to specimen adequacy and triage (see below). The Diff-Quik stain is excellent at highlighting extracellular material, such as stromal material and mucin as well as cytoplasmic detail. A drawback of this stain is that the combination of air drying and the opaque nuclear dye makes an assessment of fine nuclear detail very difficult.

The Pap stain, in contrast, requires alcohol fixation and a somewhat more complex set of processing steps. As such, this stain is less commonly employed in intraprocedural adequacy assessments ("Rapid Pap"). The main advantage of the Pap stain when combined with alcohol fixation is that it provides excellent nuclear preservation and detail. This fine nuclear detail is vital in the diagnosis of a number of entities including pancreatic adenocarcinoma and papillary thyroid carcinoma.

In addition to using aspirate and exfoliative specimens to generate stained glass slides, cytologic material may also be collected in liquid media. This suspended material can then be used to either create additional slides, including cell blocks, for morphologic examination or for ancillary studies (see below).

There are a number of advantages and disadvantages in performing a fine needle aspiration vis-à-vis a core biopsy. One of the main strengths of a core biopsy is that typically more tissue is obtained. Recovering a greater quantity of tissue with each biopsy pass allows ancillary testing to usually be performed more reliably on core biopsy specimens than on aspirates. In addition, core biopsies are commonly placed directly into a formalin-based fixative and processed to generate formalin-fixed paraffin-embedded tissue (FFPE), the specimen type of choice for many ancillary tests. A final advantage of core biopsy is that an intact piece of tissue is obtained in contrast to the single cells and small groups of cells that are recovered in an aspirate specimen. The ability to examine a larger piece of tissue allows a more precise evaluation of the overall architecture of the tissue.

Fine needle aspirates of superficial lesions have the advantage of typically being less traumatic for patients than core biopsies. Also, they can be performed in a standard examination room and do not require a sterile room. Following the procedure, the patient typically only requires a small bandage for hemostasis. Another advantage of aspirate smears is that aspirate slides, either air dried or fixed in alcohol, provide superior preservation of fine cellular and nuclear detail relative to core biopsies.

A key advantage of FNA specimens is that in many cases, Diff-Quik–stained slides can be prepared and examined intra-procedurally. This allows an assessment of adequacy to be made and potential diagnoses to be communicated to the operator in real time. Using this feedback, material can be triaged appropriately for ancillary studies (microbiology cultures in the case of an inflammatory lesion versus molecular testing in the case of a malignancy, for example). Furthermore, the procedure can be confidently concluded once adequate material has been obtained without the morbidity of superfluous biopsy passes or the potential of an inadequate specimen and a repeat biopsy.

While intra-procedural adequacy assessments are typically most easily performed using aspirate specimens, in many cases core biopsies can be evaluated by tapping, rubbing, crushing, or otherwise exfoliating material from the core biopsies onto a glass slide before the piece of tissue is placed in formalin. The "touch" preparation glass slide can then be Diff-Quik–stained and evaluated in a similar fashion as an aspirate smear. In the case of fibrotic or extremely vascular lesions that do not yield tissue on aspiration, core biopsy with crush preparation provides a useful alternative means to obtain cytologic material, confirm adequacy and triage the tissue during the procedure (Fig. 1.2) [18].

In addition to morphologic assessment, material obtained from core biopsies and aspirate specimens can be used for a variety of ancillary studies. In the current paradigm, many malignancies are evaluated via immunohistochemistry. The general principle behind immunohistochemistry is that by

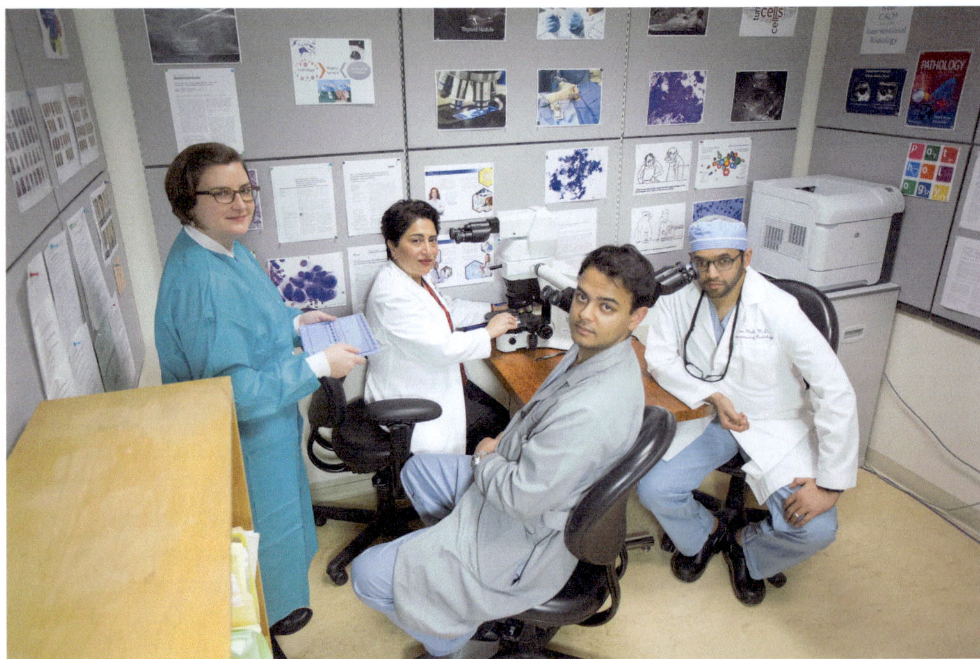

Fig. 1.2 Pathologist/cytotechnologist evaluating a biopsy for adequacy and triage with radiology physicians in interventional radiology

utilizing antibodies directed against various antigens and subsequently labeling these antibodies with a chromogenic reporter that can be visualized microscopically, it is possible to determine if a tumor is expressing a given protein. Knowing which proteins a tumor is making is extremely useful in helping to determine site of origin, lineage of differentiation, as well as predicting response to certain therapies.

Genetic testing has also become important in the management of various malignancies. For certain tumor types, including colonic adenocarcinoma and lung adenocarcinoma, genetic testing is currently the standard of care in cases of metastatic disease in order to determine first-line therapy and eligibility for treatment with targeted agents. While FISH- and PCR-based single-gene tests are still in use, most large institutions currently use multi-gene next-generation sequencing-based assays for the evaluation of solid and hematopoietic tumors when indicated.

In most labs, immunohistochemistry and molecular tests are validated exclusively for use with FFPE tissue. As such, core biopsies are easily utilized for this testing while FNA smears are not. With foresight at the time of the procedure, aspirate material may be collected in liquid medium, embedded in a fibrin clot, and processed in formalin to produce a specimen ("cell block") that is suitable for immunohistochemistry, molecular testing, and a variety of other ancillary tests. Given that molecular and immunohistochemical tests are now mandatory to determine first-line therapy in metastatic non-small cell lung carcinoma and other diseases, we have found it very valuable to triage tissue in multiple containers, which become multiple paraffin blocks, in order to facilitate all of the required testing. Cytologic material from smears and touch preparations can successfully be used for molecular and cytogenetic testing if validated by the laboratory.

In cases in which core biopsies as well as aspirates and touch preparations are procured, it is of value for all material to be reviewed by a single pathologist and a single report issued. This allows for clarity in reporting and also gives the reviewing pathologist the benefit of being able to look at all of the patient's diagnostic material. At our institution we routinely issue integrated cytopathology reports for FNA, touch preparation, core biopsy, and immunohistochemistry.

Radiology–Pathology Coordination

The authors strongly believe that close collaboration is essential between the radiologist performing the biopsy and the cytopathologist. As stated by Leiman [19], "Mutual understanding must exist between the aspirator and the pathologist which, if they collaborate for any length of time, will develop into implicit trust, with better patient care as the outcome". Essential elements of the clinical history and likely considerations based on both clinical data and imaging findings should be communicated. In our opinion, such collaboration is enhanced through immediate assessment by the cytopathologist (either on-site or by telepathology), perhaps even more so in the era of requests for molecular analysis of specimens. The goals of rapid pathologic assessment are to minimize the number of needle passes, potentially adjust approach if necessary, and optimize procurement and handling of material for ancillary studies, and in this way decrease the risk of complications from unneeded sampling while improving diagnostic rates. Interestingly, this practice remains somewhat controversial, with some investigators supportive and others suggesting that it does not influence outcomes [20–22].

Close coordination between the radiology and pathology services is important to ensure that diagnostic material and sufficient tissue for all required ancillary studies is consistently obtained. In an ideal setting, a cytopathologist should be present on-site to evaluate an aspirate smear or touch preparation slide (in the case of a core biopsy) from each biopsy pass and to communicate the findings in real-time to the operator. Alternatively, if the procedure is taking place at a remote location, images can be viewed and evaluated digitally via a number of commercially available systems. If space permits, a multi-headed microscope may be used for the radiologist and pathologist to view aspirate smears or touch preps in tandem with the pathologist. This form of real-time feedback is often of great value to the radiologists by guiding their approach in subsequent biopsy passes and future cases. At our institution, we have a pathologist suite and a laboratory space in the radiology department. Pathology trainees, cytotechnologists, pathology support staff, and attending pathologists work together with their counterparts in radiology on multiple ultrasound-guided and CT-guided on a daily basis, both on site and remotely via telepathology.

Another useful tool to facilitate cooperation between pathology and radiology services is a standing case-based interdisciplinary radiology–pathology conference. The value of this conference is in allowing for an exchange of information between the two specialties and communicating special considerations and techniques. Familiarity on the part of the pathologist with the techniques and considerations in various biopsy modalities along with a similar understanding on the part of the radiologist allows more efficient communication and management of cases.

We have certainly found that having, a dedicated pathologist workspace in radiology with a multi-head microscope, radiologic–pathologic real-time intraprocedural discussion, onboarding orientation of new trainees to the joint biopsy service, presentation and discussion of cases at monthly radiology–pathology conference has further optimized patient care. Additionally this joint service provides excellent training for our residents and fellows, and has resulted in numerous joint publications and national meeting presentations [18, 23–33].

References

1. Mueller PR, Miketic LM, Simeone JF, Silverman SG, Saini S, Wittenberg J, et al. Severe acute pancreatitis after percutaneous biopsy of the pancreas. AJR Am J Roentgenol. 1988;151:493–4.
2. Rastegar RF, Hou D, Harris A, Yoshida E, Lum B, Ho S, et al. Is a liver biopsy necessary? Investigation of a suspected hepatocellular carcinoma: a pictorial essay of hepatocellular carcinoma and the revised American Association for the Study of Liver Disease criteria. Can Assoc Radiol J. 2012;63:329–40.
3. Kim SY, Chung SW. Small musculoskeletal soft-tissue lesions: US-guided core needle biopsy—comparative study of diagnostic yields according to lesion size. Radiology. 2016;278:156–63.
4. Montaudon M, Latrabe V, Pariente A, Corneloup D, Begueret H, Laurent F. Factors influencing accuracy of CT-guided percutaneous biopsies of pulmonary lesions. Eur Radiol. 2004;14:1234–40.
5. Wu CC, Maher MM, Shepard JA. Complications of CT-guided percutaneous needle biopsy of the chest: prevention and management. AJR Am J Roentgenol. 2011;196:W678–82.
6. Klein JS, Zarka MA. Transthoracic needle biopsy: an overview. J Thorac Imaging. 1997;12:232–49.
7. Winter TC, Lee FT Jr, Hinshaw JL. Ultrasound-guided biopsies in the abdomen and pelvis. Ultrasound Q. 2008;24:45–68.
8. Eckman MH, Erban JK, Singh SK, Kao GS. Screening for the risk of bleeding or thrombosis. Ann Intern Med. 2003;138:W15–24.
9. Vanderveen KA, Thompson SM, Callstrom MR, Young WF Jr, Grant CS, Farley DR, et al. Biopsy of pheochromocytomas and paragangliomas: potential for disaster. Surgery. 2009;146:1158–66.
10. Magabe PC, Bloom AL. Sudden death from carcinoid crisis during image-guided biopsy of a lung mass. J Vasc Interv Radiol. 2014;25:484–7.
11. Silva MA, Hegab B, Hyde C, Guo B, Buckels JA, Mirza DF. Needle track seeding following biopsy of liver lesions in the diagnosis of hepatocellular cancer: a systematic review and meta-analysis. Gut. 2008;57:1592–6.
12. Huang DY, Yusuf GT, Daneshi M, Husainy MA, Ramnarine R, Sellars ME, et al. Contrast-enhanced US-guided interventions: improving success rate and avoiding complications using US contrast agents. Radiographics. 2017;37:652–64.
13. Paparo F, Piccazzo R, Cevasco L, Piccardo A, Pinna F, Belli F, et al. Advantages of percutaneous abdominal biopsy under PET-CT/ultrasound fusion imaging guidance: a pictorial essay. Abdom Imaging. 2014;39:1102–13.
14. Hakime A, Barah A, Deschamps F, Farouli G, Joskin J, Tselikas L, et al. Prospective comparison of freehand and electromagnetic needle tracking for US-guided percutaneous liver biopsy. J Vasc Interv Radiol. 2013;24:1682–9.
15. Abi-Jaoudeh N, Duffy AG, Greten TF, Kohn EC, Clark TW, Wood BJ. Personalized oncology in interventional radiology. J Vasc Interv Radiol. 2013;24:1083–92.
16. Marshall D, Laberge JM, Firetag B, Miller T, Kerlan RK. The changing face of percutaneous image-guided biopsy: molecular profiling and genomic analysis in current practice. J Vasc Interv Radiol. 2013;24:1094–103.
17. Diaz LA Jr, Bardelli A. Liquid biopsies: genotyping circulating tumor DNA. J Clin Oncol. 2014;32:579–86.
18. Zhang S, Ivanovic M, Nemcek AA Jr, Defrias DV, Lucas E, Nayar R. Thin core needle biopsy crush preparations in conjunction with fine-needle aspiration for the evaluation of thyroid nodules: a complementary approach. Cancer. 2008;114(6):512–8.
19. Leiman G. My approach to pancreatic fine needle aspiration. J Clin Pathol. 2007;60:43–9.
20. Mohanty SK, Pradhan D, Sharma S, Sharma A, Patnaik N, Feuerman M, et al. Endoscopic ultrasound guided fine-needle aspiration: what variables influence diagnostic yield? Diagn Cytopathol. 2018;46:293–8.
21. Zakowski MF. "…That which we call a rose…": a critical analysis of rapid on-site evaluation. Cancer Cytopathol. 2016;124:857–61.
22. de Koster EJ, Kist JW, Vriens MR, Borel Rinkes IH, Valik GD, de Keizer B. Thyroid ultrasound-guided fine-needle aspiration: the positive influence of on-site adequacy assessment and number of needle passes on diagnostic cytology rate. Acta Cytol. 2016;60:39–45.
23. Lal A, Nemcek AA, Ariga R, Gattuso P, Nayar R. Splenic fine needle aspiration and core biopsy: a review of 49 cases. Acta Cytol. 2003;47(6):951–9.
24. Nayar R, Nemcek A. Microcalcifications in a solitary thyroid nodule. Pathol Case Rev. 2003;8(1):22–5.
25. Rao P, Spies S, Angelos P, Nayar R. The case of the "vanishing" parathyroid adenoma. Pathol Case Rev. 2003;8(1):42–6.
26. Nayar R, Bourtsos E, Lal A, Nemcek A, De Frias VS. Cytomorphology of pancreatic microcystic adenoma (MCA). Cancer Cytopathol. 2004;102(5):288–94.
27. Riaz A, Kulik L, Lewandowski RJ, Ryu RK, Spear GG, Mulcahy MF, et al. Radiologic–pathologic correlation of hepatocellular carcinoma treated with internal radiation using yttrium-90 microspheres. Hepatology. 2009;49(4):1185–93.
28. Riaz A, Kulik L, Lewandowski RJ, Ryu RK, Spear GG, Mulcahy MF, et al. Radiologic-pathologic correlation of hepatocellular carcinoma treated with transarterial chemoembolization. Hepatology. 2009;49(4):1185–93.
29. Oppenheimer J, Kasuganti D, Nayar R, Chrisman H, Lewandowski R, Nemcek A, Ryu R. How to interpret thyroid biopsy results: a three year retrospective interventional radiology experience. Cardiovasc Intervent Radiol. 2010;33(4):800–5.
30. Riaz A, Memon K, Miller FH, Nikolaidis P, Kulik LM, Lewandowski R, et al. Role of the EASL, RECIST, and WHO response guidelines alone or in combination for hepatocellular carcinoma: radiologic–pathologic correlation. J Hepatol. 2011;54(4):695–704.
31. Heller M, Zanocco K, Zydowicz S, Elaraj D, Nayar R, Sturgeon C. Cost-effectiveness analysis of repeat FNA for thyroid biopsies read as atypia of undetermined significance. Surgery. 2012;152(3):423–30.
32. Vouche M, Kulik L, Atassi R, Memon K, Hickey R, Ganger D, et al. Radiological-pathological analysis of WHO, RECIST, EASL, mRECIST and DWI: imaging analysis from a prospective randomized trial of Y90 +/− sorafenib. Hepatology. 2013;58(5):1655–66.
33. Berg N, Gehl J, Vande Haar M, Balco M, Kulesza P. The efficacy of on-site evaluation for identification of transplant pancreas. Acta Cytol. 2013;57(5):443–6.

2 Liver

Xiaoqi Lin, Brandon A. Umphress, Ernest F. Wiggins III, Ramona Gupta, and Albert A. Nemcek Jr.

Introduction

The main indication for fine-needle aspiration (FNA) biopsy of the liver is the diagnosis of localized disease by imaging studies, including hepatocellular carcinoma (HCC) and metastatic neoplasms from either a known or unknown primary tumor. The overall sensitivity, specificity, and accuracy of FNA in the diagnosis of malignant lesions is 92% to 96%, 92% to 100%, and 96%, respectively [1, 2]. Sensitivity of FNA to differentiate HCC from metastatic tumors in the liver is approximately 96%, with a specificity of 100% and a diagnostic accuracy of 97.5% [2]. FNA of benign liver lesions poses an increased diagnostic challenge [3]. Aspiration of cystic lesions, which is less frequently performed, can help in detecting a possible neoplastic origin of the cyst or accompanying microorganisms. As imaging studies have improved, FNA has become less useful for diagnosis of hepatitis and cirrhosis. Moreover, differentiation between cirrhosis and benign hepatocellular lesions (i.e., regenerative nodules) by FNA remains difficult [4].

Complications associated with the performance of liver FNA are rare and are similar to those associated with conventional core biopsies. The most significant is bleeding, which can be associated with severe cirrhosis in patients with coagulopathies [5]. Other complications include infection and risk of tumor seeding along the needle track [6–8].

X. Lin (✉)
Northwestern University, Feinberg School of Medicine, Northwestern Memorial Hospital, Chicago, IL, USA
e-mail: xlin@northwestern.edu

B. A. Umphress
Department of Pathology, Northwestern Memorial Hospital, McGaw Medical Center, Chicago, IL, USA

E. F. Wiggins III
Department of Radiology, Monmouth Medical Center, Shrewsbury, NJ, USA

R. Gupta · A. A. Nemcek Jr.
Northwestern University Feinberg School of Medicine, Chicago, IL, USA

Normal Findings

Benign Hepatocytes

- Account for majority of the cells seen in FNA smears of normal liver.
- Are arranged as single cells, small clusters, or large flat sheets with irregular jagged edges (Fig. 2.1a, b).
- Are polygonal-shaped cells with a low nuclear-to-cytoplasmic (N/C) ratio.
- Have abundant granular cytoplasm. Cytoplasmic vacuoles are seen in both benign and neoplastic cells.
- Have one or two round to oval centrally placed nuclei containing evenly distributed granular chromatin and occasionally prominent nucleoli.

Bile Duct Epithelial Cells

- Typically, flat, monolayered, glandular sheets and occasional acinar structures (Fig. 2.1c, d). However, a picket-fence arrangement of strips of cells can also be observed.
- Cuboidal or columnar cells with high N/C ratios.
- Small, round nuclei with evenly distributed granular chromatin and inconspicuous nucleoli.
- Scant-to-moderate delicate cytoplasm.

Pigments

- Lipofuscin: fine golden, granular pigment, nonrefractile, typically concentrated around nuclei. In modified Giemsa-stained slides lipofuscin shows a blue or greenish color.
- Bile: coarse, globular, nonrefractile and amorphous distributed throughout the cytoplasm or accumulation within the space of Disse. Appears bluish or dark green in modified Giemsa-stained slides.
- Iron/hemosiderin: coarse, brown-black, and refractile in Papanicolaou and modified Giemsa-stained slides.

R. Nayar et al. (eds.), *Atlas of Cytopathology and Radiology*, https://doi.org/10.1007/978-3-030-24756-0_2

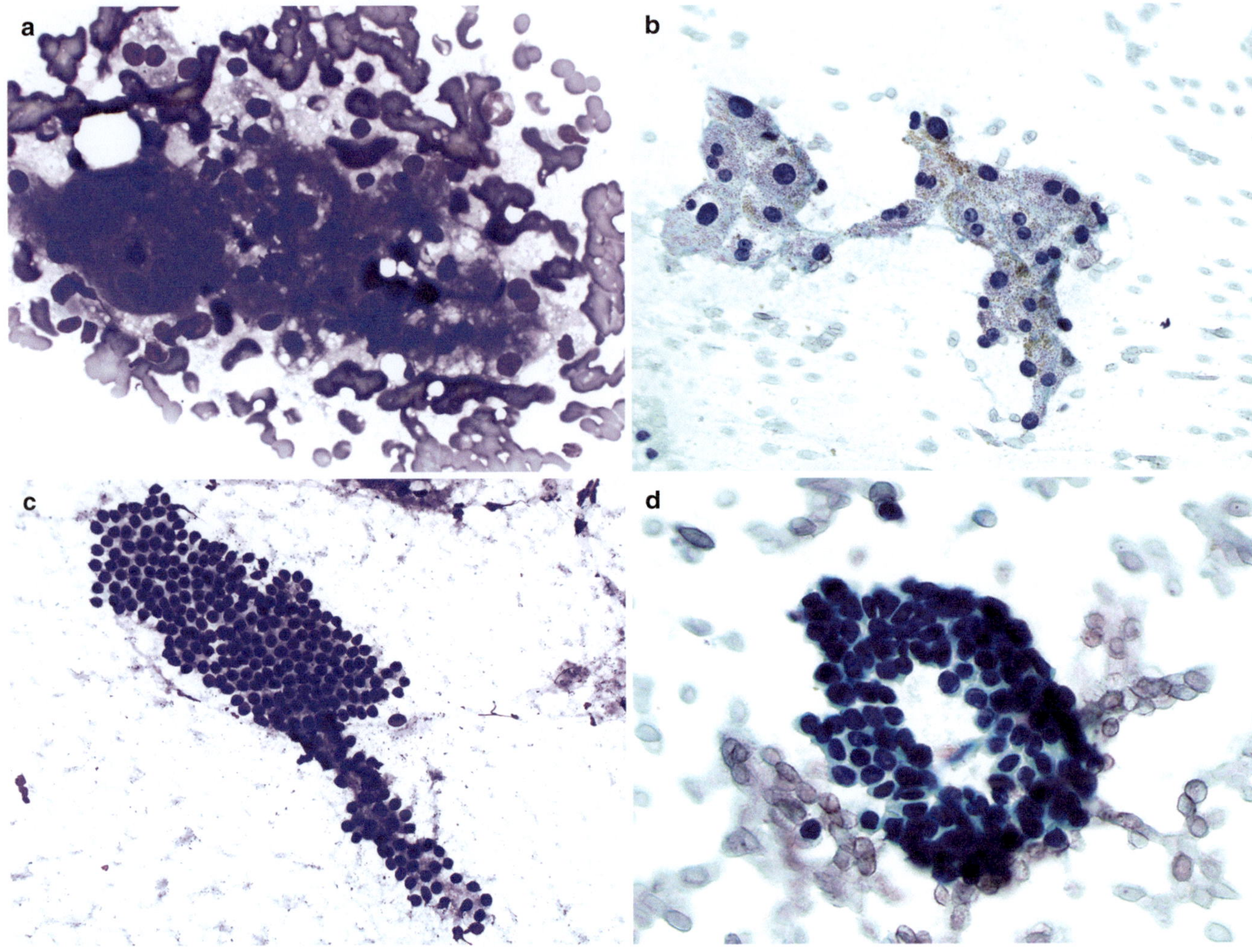

Fig. 2.1 Benign hepatocytes and bile duct epithelial cells. (**a**, **b**) FNA cytology of benign hepatocytes characteristically shows the presence of a monolayer of polygonal cells with abundant granular (occasionally vacuolated) cytoplasm and oval to round nuclei; modified Giemsa stain (**a**) and Papanicolaou stain (**b**), 400×. (**c**, **d**) FNA cytology of bile duct epithelial cells demonstrates the presence of cohesive clusters of cuboidal to columnar cells with small, round, or oval nuclei, smooth nuclear membranes, scant delicate cytoplasm, and high nuclear to cytoplasm ratio; modified Giemsa stain (**c**) and Papanicolaou stain (**d**), 400×

Benign Conditions

Hepatic Cysts

Clinical

- Usually an incidental finding.
- Majority are simple cysts.
- True hepatic cysts are those with an epithelial lining.
- Other etiologies include polycystic liver disease, neoplastic cysts, including intraductal papillary mucinous neoplasms (IPMNs)/intraductal oncocytic papillary neoplasms (IOPNs) [9], hydatid cysts, hepatic abscesses, and ciliated hepatic foregut cysts. The most common cause of hydatid cysts is *Echinococcus granulosus*, while infection related to *Escherichia coli* and *Klebsiella pneumoniae* in the setting of biliary disease can cause abscess formation [10–12].

Radiology

Ultrasound (US)

- Well-circumscribed lesions that are anechoic on ultrasound with a thin wall and posterior acoustic enhancement.

Computed tomography (CT) scan

- These lesions do not enhance and exhibit water attenuation [13, 14].

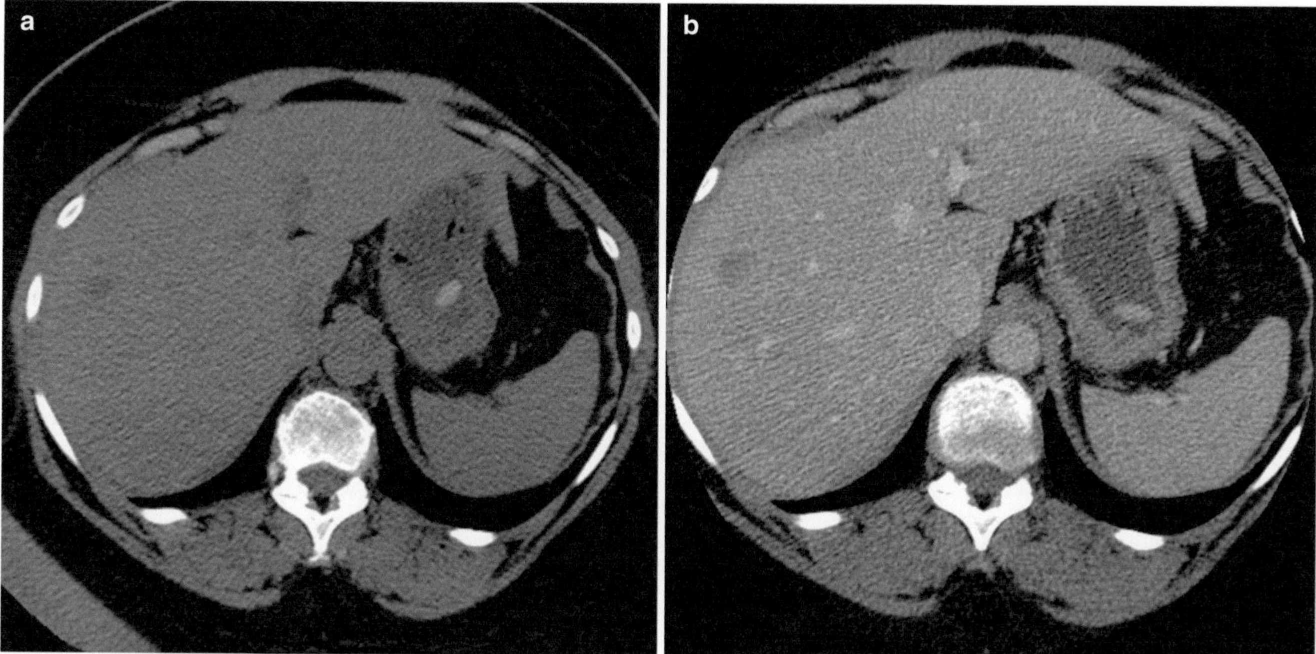

Fig. 2.2 Focal fatty change. (**a**, **b**) Contrast-enhanced CT scan shows a mass-like area of low density

Gross

- Simple cysts: Single, unilocular cysts that are usually subcapsular and range from 2 to 40 cm. Multiple cysts may occur.
- Flat glistening lining.
- Variable amounts of clear, amber, or turbid fluid.

Cytology of FNA or touch preparation of core

- Simple cysts: Proteinaceous material with scattered histiocytes and single or flat nests of bland columnar or cuboidal glandular epithelial cells.
- Rarely calcified debris and squamous metaplastic cells in small clusters are present.
- Intraductal oncocytic papillary neoplasm (IOPN): Nests, three-dimensional or papillary clusters of columnar or cuboidal cells with loss of polarity, uniform nuclei containing even chromatin, and granular or vacuolated cytoplasm [9].

Steatosis

Clinical

- Generally a diffuse process but occasionally irregular or focal [15].
- Steatosis is most commonly associated with alcohol abuse or metabolic syndrome [16].
- In rare instances, hepatic steatosis produces a circumscribed, nodular lesion termed "focal fatty liver change." Focal hepatic fatty change can also be seen in the liver parenchyma surrounding metastatic insulinoma [17], postgastrectomy [17], postpancreaticoduodenectomy [18], hepatocellular adenoma [19], hepatocellular carcinoma [20], and chronic hepatitis C virus infection [21].
- In some cases the nodular fatty infiltrate can be multifocal, mimicking metastases [22].

Radiology

- Diffusely increased echogenicity on US with poor visualization of the hepatic and portal veins [15, 23].
- Decreased attenuation of liver on noncontrast CT as compared to the spleen (normally 8 to 10 Hounsfield units).
- MRI demonstrates diffuse loss of signal intensity on T1 out-of-phase imaging.
- Diffuse or regional in distribution. Focality can mimic a mass lesion (Fig. 2.2a, b).

Cytology of FNA or touch preparation of core

- Benign and/or reactive hepatocytes with small and/or large cytoplasmic fatty vacuoles and vacuolated background (Fig. 2.3a).

Histology of core

- Needle core biopsy shows hepatocytes with vacuolated cytoplasm that are arranged in normal architecture (Fig. 2.3b).

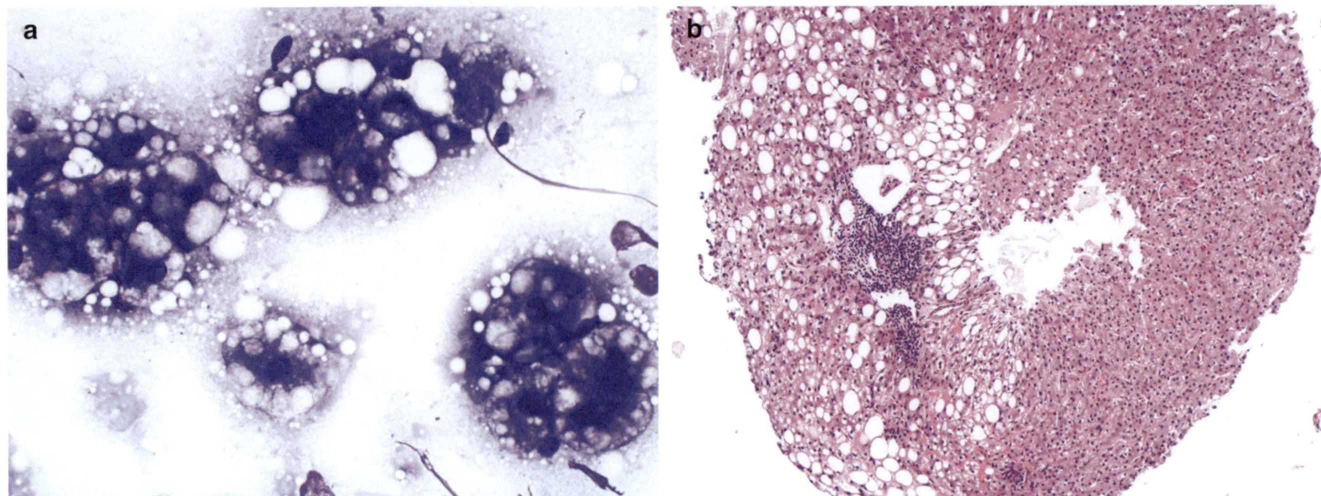

Fig. 2.3 Focal fatty change. (**a**) FNA smears show benign and reactive hepatocytes with vacuolated cytoplasm and vacuolated background; modified Giemsa stain, 600×. (**b**) Needle core biopsy shows benign hepatic parenchyma with focal fatty changes; hematoxylin and eosin stain, 100×

Benign Neoplasms

Hamartoma

Hamartoma: bile duct adenoma or von Meyenburg complexes, small nodules (<1 cm) that can be dispersed throughout the liver. These can be mistaken for adenomas or possibly small metastases. Aspiration may be hypocellular with benign hepatocytes and/or bland bile duct epithelium. Also included in the differential diagnosis is a well-differentiated cholangiocarcinoma [24, 25].

Hemangioma

Clinical

- Most common benign neoplasm of the liver, with a prevalence of 5–20% [26].
- Asymptomatic, and mostly identified incidentally in staging of malignancy.
- FNA of vascular lesions can result in excessive bleeding and in rare instances death; therefore caution should be taken when approaching these lesions [27].

Radiology

US

- Typically, homogeneous and hyperechoic (70%) with sharp margination.
- No Doppler signals.

CT

- Well-circumscribed mass (Fig. 2.4a–c).
- Hypodense on noncontrast images.
- Peripheral, globular enhancement with progressive fill-in on delayed imaging [28].
- Some tumors possibly with rapid filling on arterial phase (flash-filling hemangioma), particularly for smaller lesions.
- The overall diagnostic sensitivity and specificity can range from 75% to 85% and 75% to 100% [29, 30].

Magnetic resonance imaging (MRI)

- Well-defined, round mass with a homogeneous signal.
- T1: Hypo−/isointense.
- T2: Markedly hyperintense, "light bulb" bright lesion.
- T1 postcontrast: Typically peripheral, globular enhancement with progressive fill-in [14].
- Overall, diagnosis of hepatic hemangiomas is highly accurate by MRI [31].

Angiography

- Usually incidental findings on angiography.
- Well-circumscribed mass with irregular, dilated vascular channels and contrast pooling into the venous phase.

Nuclear medicine

- Technetium-99 m-labeled red blood cell scans (Tc99m RBC scan): Initial cold lesion with progressive accumulation of radiotracer on delayed imaging.
- Sulfur colloid examinations: cold defects [11].

Interventional radiology

- Biopsy is rarely required except for atypical lesions or in patients with known malignancies.

Gross

- Usually solitary and less than 4 cm in diameter (Fig. 2.5a).
- Well-circumscribed, spongy, and red-brown lesion.
- Typically subcapsular.

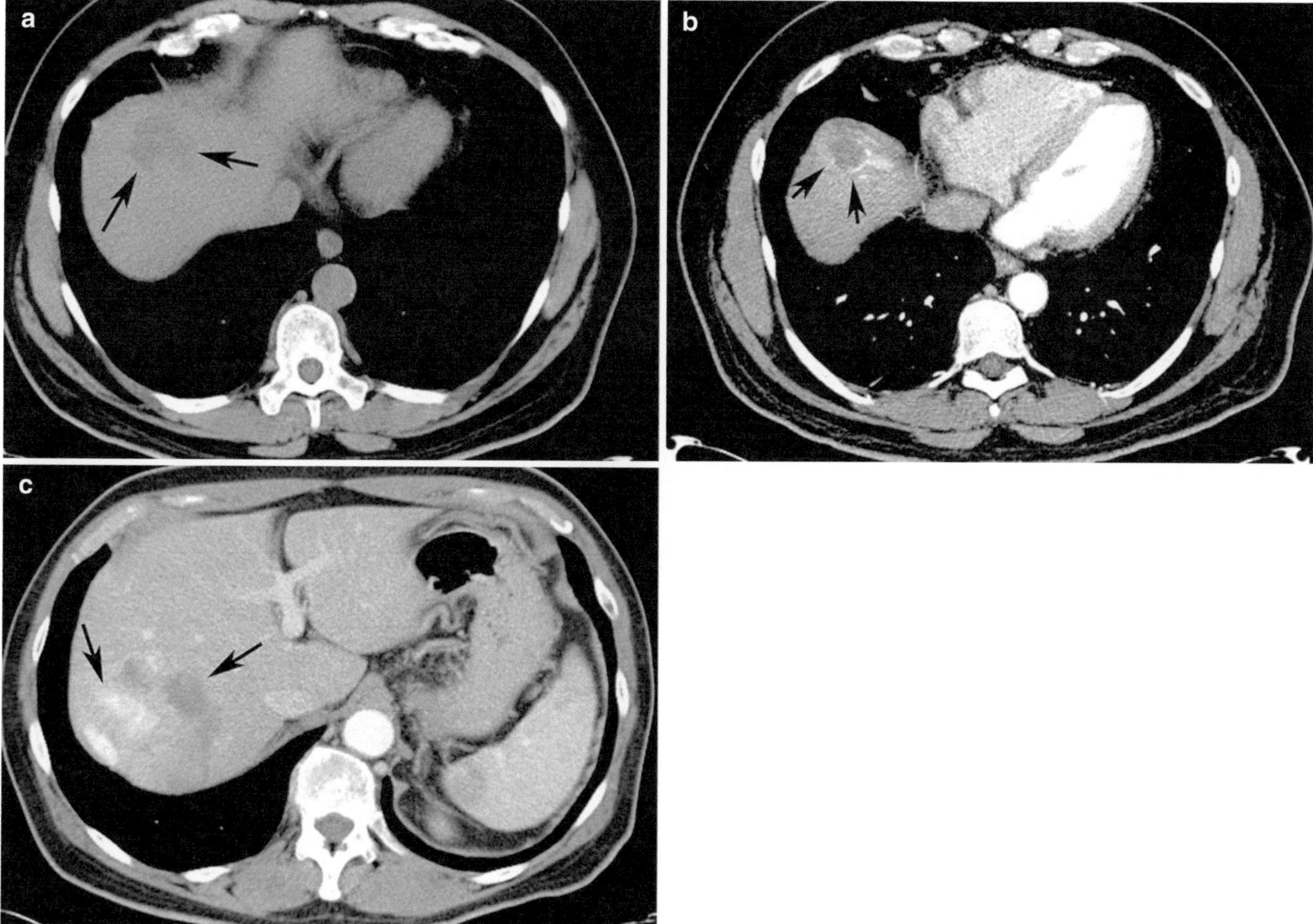

Fig. 2.4 Hemangioma. (**a**) Noncontrast CT shows a hypodense mass in the right lobe of the liver (*arrows*). (**b**) An early arterial phase image shows typical nodular enhancement at the periphery of the right lobe mass (*arrows*). (**c**) Angiography of progressive phase shows enhancement of a hemangioma

Cytology of FNA or touch preparation of core

- The cytologic diagnosis of hemangioma is often one of exclusion.
- Most frequent findings are elongated or plump cells in monolayers — endothelial cells or tissue fragments consisting of fibrous tissue with cellular bland spindle cells (Fig. 2.5b, c) [32, 33].
- The nuclei of endothelial cells follow the shape of the cytoplasm, with finely granular chromatin, inconspicuous to conspicuous single or multiple nucleoli, and occasional longitudinal clefts or grooves [32, 33].
- Occasionally, arborizing capillary vessels are seen.

Histology of core

- Most hepatic hemangiomas are of the cavernous type, composed of a fibrous stroma and wide endothelial-lined channels filled with blood (Fig. 2.5d)

Comments

- The differential diagnosis includes peliosis hepatis (a rare benign condition with dilatation of sinusoidal blood-filled spaces within the liver) [34] and spindle-cell neoplasms [33].
- Side effects of FNA of hepatic hemangioma include fatal hemorrhage, peritonitis, and lymphorrhea [32].

Hepatic Adenoma

Clinical

- True neoplasm.
- Majority occur in young women and are related to oral contraceptive use.
- Liver function tests are usually normal.
- Large, subcapsular tumors are at risk of rupture or hemorrhage.

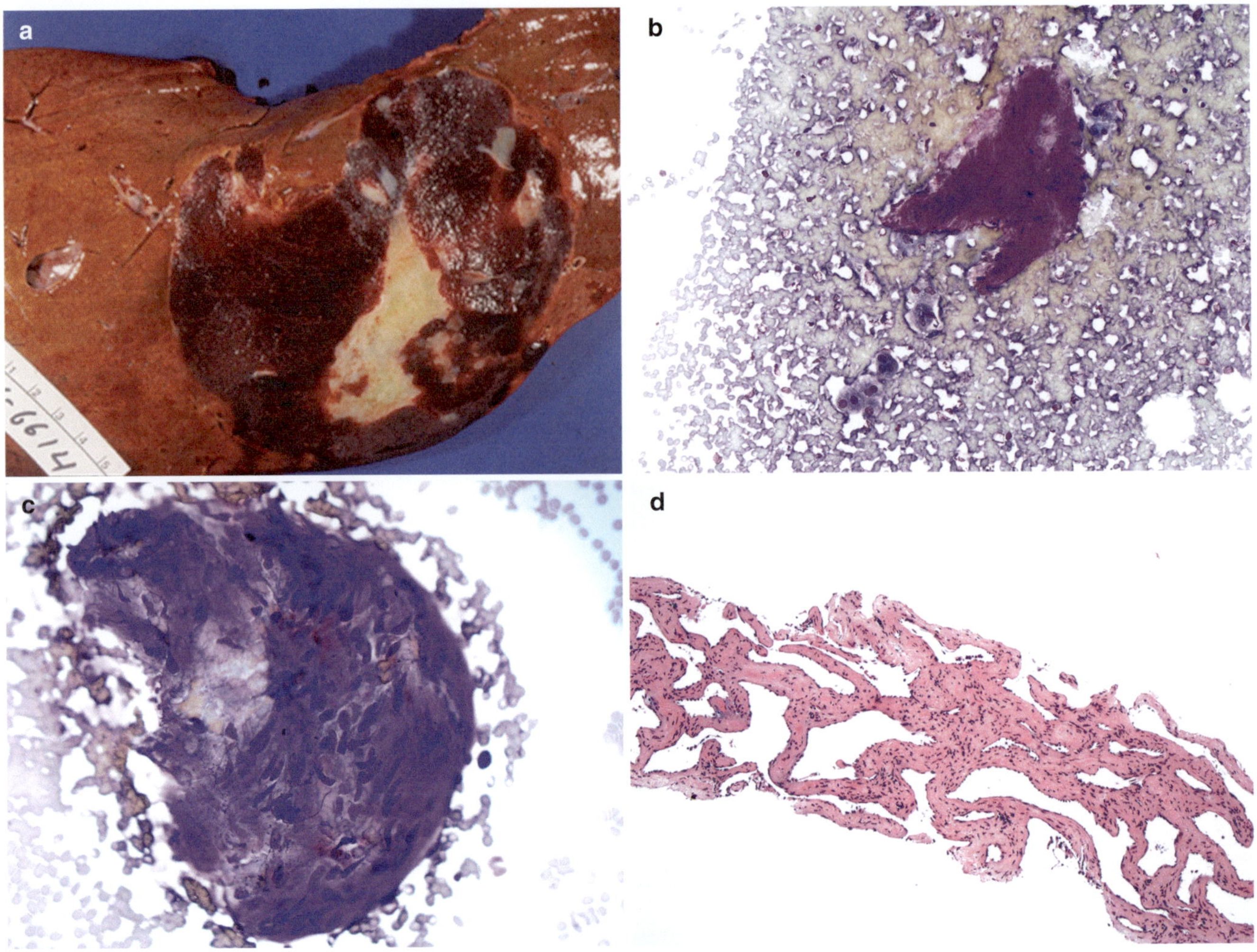

Fig. 2.5 Hemangioma. (**a**) Gross photo shows a well-circumscribed dark red mass with a central scar. (**b**, **c**) FNA shows fibrous tissue containing vessels and spindle cells with ill-defined cytoplasmic borders and fine chromatin; cytology modified Giemsa stain, 400×. (**d**) Needle core biopsy shows an anastomosing dilated vascular proliferation with fibrous stroma; hematoxylin and eosin stain, 100×

Radiology

US

- Hyperechoic appearance, given fat content.

CT

- Arterially-enhancing, well-marginated lesions on contrast-enhanced CT that retain contrast on portal venous phase imaging.
- Variable amount of hemorrhage may be seen.

MRI

- T1: Signal loss out-of-phase imaging caused by intracellular fat content (Fig. 2.6a) [14].

Gross

- Any size, up to 30 cm.
- Solitary, well-defined, partially encapsulated, bulging mass with different color from surrounding liver (yellow to tan or brown) (Fig. 2.7a).

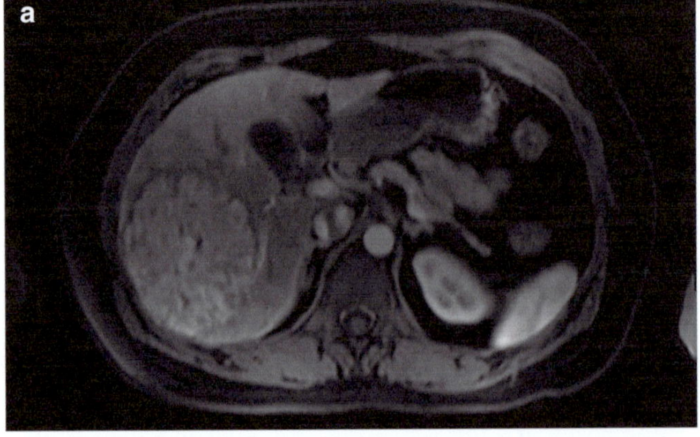

Fig. 2.6 Hepatocellular adenoma. (**a**) T1-weighted arterial phase MRI shows a large complex mass at the caudal aspect of the liver. The complex appearance suggests internal hemorrhage

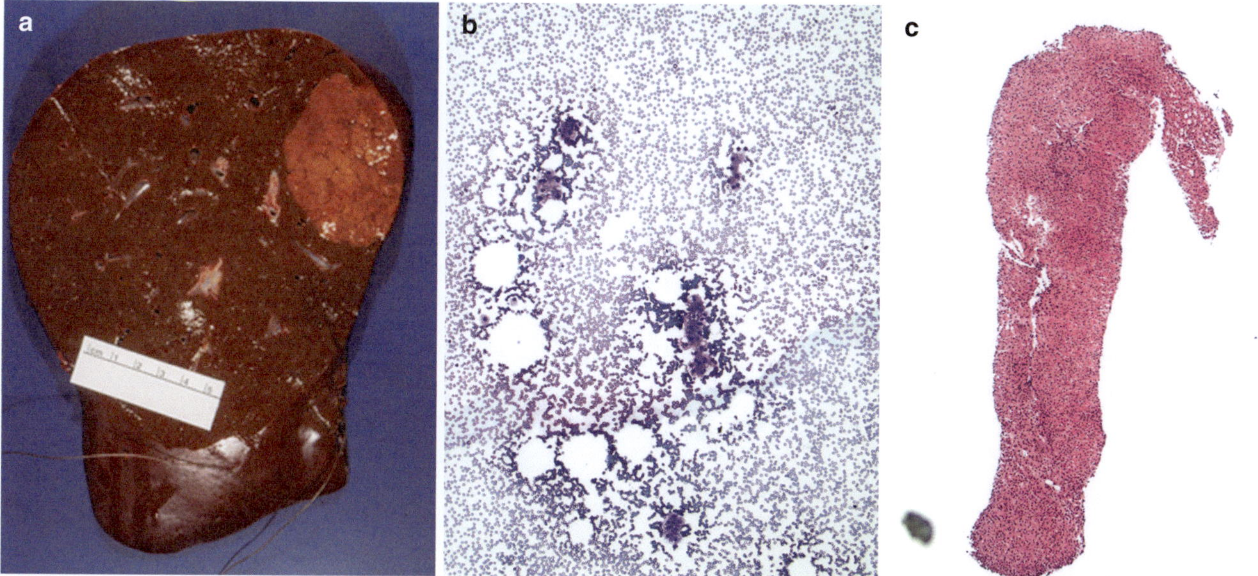

Fig. 2.7 Hepatocellular adenoma. (**a**) Gross photo shows a subcapsular mass with a pale color and delicate irregular borders. (**b**) FNA smears show benign hepatocytes with abundant granular cytoplasm and small round nuclei without bile ductal epithelial cells; modified Giemsa stain, 400×. (**c**) Needle core biopsy shows sheets of benign hepatocytes without portal triads; hematoxylin and eosin stain, 100×

- Often subcapsular.
- Areas of necrosis or hemorrhage frequently present.

Cytology of FNA or touch preparation of core

- Characterized by an abundance of benign-appearing hepatocytes that may show nuclear enlargement and absence of bile ductal cells (Fig. 2.7b).
- Rarely the cytoplasm of hepatocytes in an adenoma may appear paler than normal hepatocytes. Vacuolation is caused by an increased concentration of glycogen or fat.

Histology of core

- Composed of liver parenchyma without portal triads or central veins (Fig. 2.7c).
- Delicate fibrous septa do not contain bile ducts.
- Areas of infarction or hemorrhage are frequently seen.

Differential diagnosis

- Focal nodular hyperplasia: stellate central scar. Portal triads and central veins are present.
- Hamartoma: bile duct adenoma or von Meyenburg complexes, small nodules (<1 cm) that can be dispersed throughout the liver and can be mistaken for adenomas or possibly small metastases. Aspiration may be hypocellular with benign hepatocytes and/or bland bile duct epithelium. Also included in this differential diagnosis is a well-differentiated cholangiocarcinoma [35].
- Well-differentiated hepatocellular carcinoma: thickened hepatic cell plates (>3 cell layers) surrounded by endothelial cells and pseudo-acinar architecture. Tumor cells show minimal nuclear atypia with increased N/C ratio.

Focal Nodular Hyperplasia

Clinical

- Classified as a type of hamartoma.
- Focal nodular hyperplasia (FNH) is comparatively much rarer than other benign lesions (i.e., simple cysts, hemangiomas) [36].
- Can occur in any age group and most common in women in third to fifth decades.
- Usually asymptomatic.

Radiology

US

- Variable appearance on ultrasound, 1/3 hyper-, 1/3 hypo-, and 1/3 isoechoic, well-defined mass.
- Hypoechoic central scar: rarely visualized.

CT

- Isodense on precontrast imaging.
- Rapid arterial enhancement, hyperintense mass upon administration of contrast.
- A hypodense fibrotic central scar is often identified that becomes hyperdense on delayed imaging [37].

MRI

- Homogeneous iso/hypointense mass on T1 with a central scar (Fig. 2.8a, c).
- T2: isointense to liver with a hyperintense central scar. Similar to CT, a rapid, dense enhancement on postcontrast T1 in arterial phase with late enhancement of central scar (Fig. 2.8b) [14].

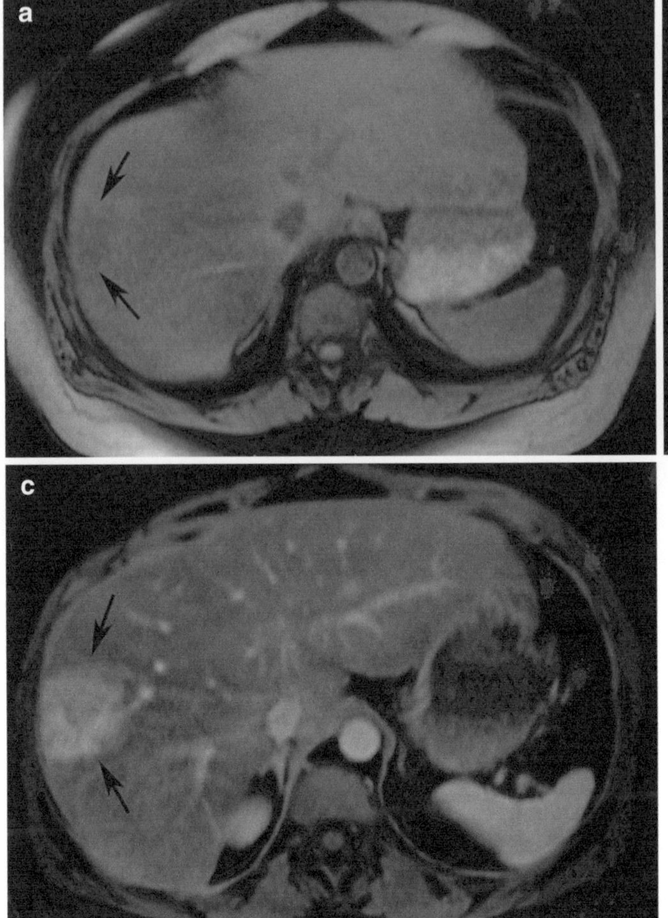

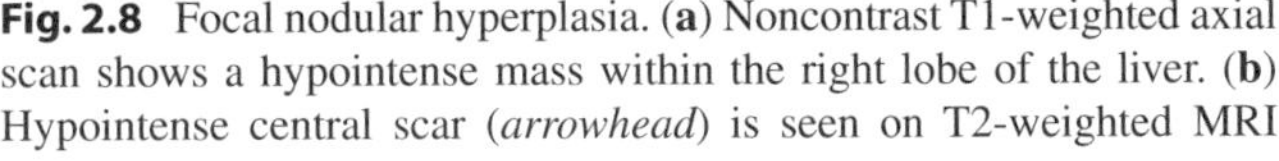

Fig. 2.8 Focal nodular hyperplasia. (**a**) Noncontrast T1-weighted axial scan shows a hypointense mass within the right lobe of the liver. (**b**) Hypointense central scar (*arrowhead*) is seen on T2-weighted MRI within the hyperintense mass (*arrows*). (**c**) Early arterial phase postcontrast T1-weighted MRI shows an intensely enhancing mass (*arrows*) and nonenhancing central scar

Angiography
- Well-defined, hypervascular mass with spoke-wheel pattern.
- Relatively decreased vascularity within central scar.

Nuclear medicine
- Sulfur colloid: 1/3 cold defect, 1/3 normal uptake, and 1/3 increased uptake.

Gross
- Solitary, nonencapsulated, well-circumscribed mass.
- Often subcapsular.
- Generally less than 5 cm; however, any size can occur, with some lesions reaching greater than 10 cm [38].
- Characteristic central stellate scar (Fig. 2.9a).

Cytology of FNA or touch preparation of core
- Difficult to diagnose by means of FNA because cytology resembles normal liver tissue with the presence of abundant benign hepatocytes and bile ductular cells (Fig. 2.9b, c). FNH is a diagnosis made by correlation of clinical-cytologic-radiologic findings.
- Occasionally, stromal material from a central scar or septum will be aspirated.
- Needle placement is crucial in this instance, and US guidance is useful to ensure that the needle tip does not extend beyond the margins of the lesion during sampling.

Histology of core
- Most characteristic histologic features include ductular reaction with varied intensity at the junction of the fibrous septa with the hepatocellular component (Fig. 2.9d) [39].
- Nonclassic variants of FNH (telangiectatic, mixed-hyperplastic, and adenomatous, plus large cell with cytologic atypia), although rare, do exist. These variants usually lack the characteristic central scar but will still contain bile ductular proliferation [38].

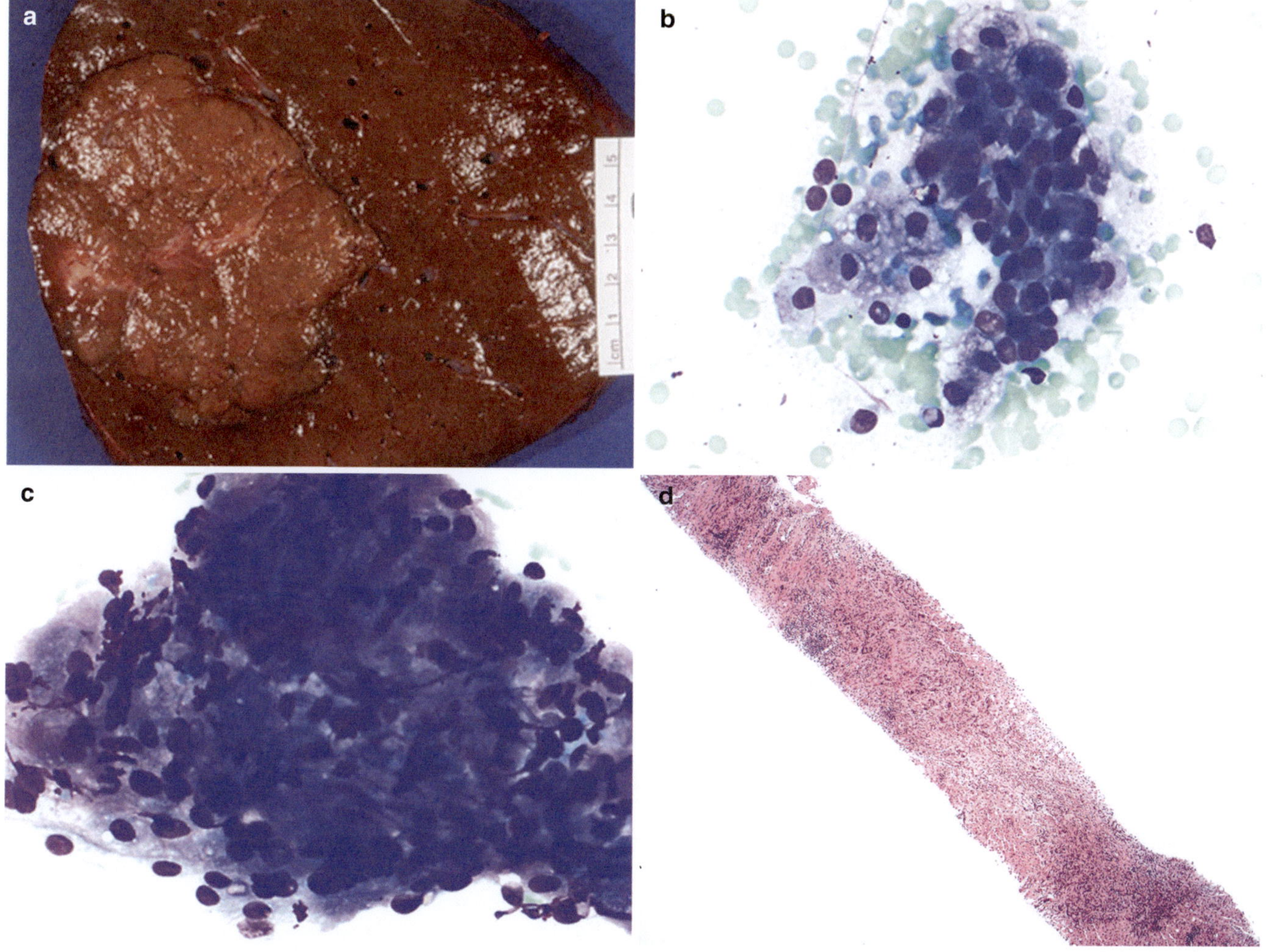

Fig. 2.9 Focal nodular hyperplasia. (**a**) Gross examination of a liver shows a large, smooth, and lobulated lesion. (**b, c**) FNA smears depict benign hepatocytes and bile ductule cells and fibrous stroma containing benign epithelial cells; modified Giemsa stain, 400×. (**d**) Needle core biopsy shows irregular islands of normal hepatocytes and bile ductule cells surrounded by fibrosis. Chronic inflammation is also observed; hematoxylin and eosin stain, 100×

Primary Malignant Neoplasms

Hepatocellular Carcinoma

Clinical

- Major risk factors include but are not limited to cirrhosis, hepatitis B and C, alcohol, or hemochromatosis.
- Other risk factors include aflatoxins, tyrosinemia, and Thorotrast exposure.

Radiology

Extremely diagnostic appearance on CT and MRI.

CT

- Hypodense masses with rapid arterial phase enhancement with delayed "washout" and enhancing rim [40].
- Most commonly a background of cirrhotic morphology and secondary signs of portal hypertension.
- Vascular invasion with portal or hepatic vein tumor thrombus is also frequently identified [40].

MRI

- T1: Hypo- or isointense mass, and well-defined hypodense capsule.
- T2: Mildly hyperintense mass.
- Rapid arterial enhancement on T1 postcontrast imaging with delayed washout and an enhancing rim (Fig. 2.10a, b).
- Detection of HCC by either CT or MRI is superior to US (US detection has a sensitivity of 73–78% in non-surveillance and surveillance settings). MRI has the highest sensitivity [41].

Angiography

- Hypervascular lesions demonstrating enlarged arterial vessels and neovascularity [42].
- Contrast pooling, dense tumor staining, and arteriovenous shunting [42].

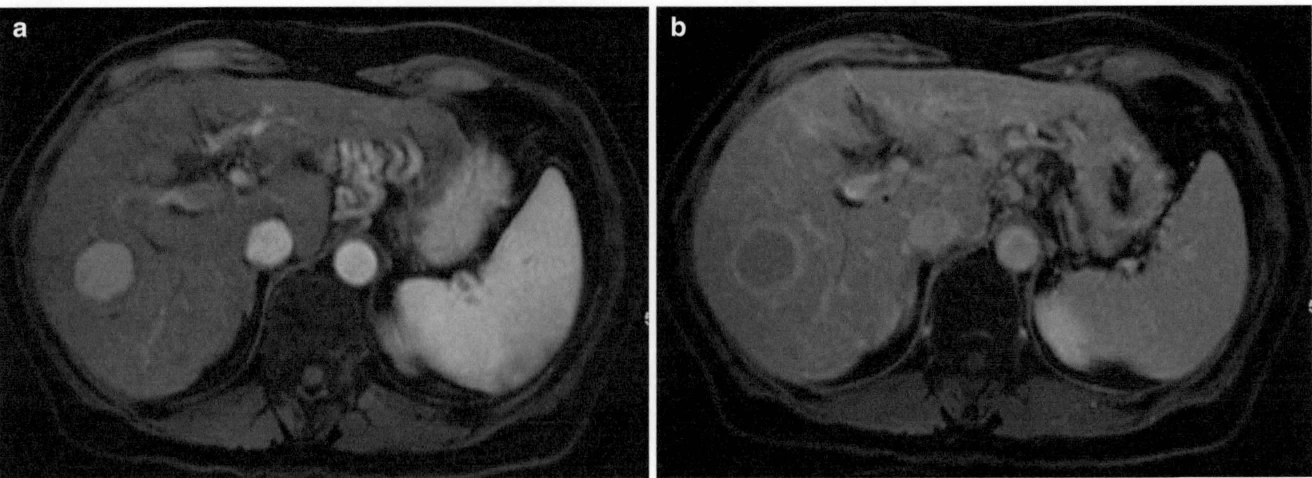

Fig. 2.10 Hepatocellular carcinoma. (**a**) Contrast-enhanced MRI demonstrates a rapidly enhancing lesion on arterial phase imaging. (**b**) On delayed imaging, there is contrast washout and an enhancing rim

- Vascular invasion, portal or hepatic vein tumor thrombus.

Nuclear medicine
- Cold defect on sulfur colloid and hepatobiliary iminodiacetic acid (HIDA) scans.
- Accumulation of radiotracer on gallium scintigraphy.

Interventional radiology
- In some settings, biopsy can be avoided if typical imaging features are present in conjunction with an elevated alpha-fetoprotein level.
- Biopsy should also be avoided in inpatients who are likely to receive a liver transplant in the near future, regardless of biopsy outcome.
- Risk of needle tracking should be taken into account; however, the literature remains somewhat controversial regarding the true risk of tumor seeding following FNA in patients with HCCs [35].

Gross
- Soft, yellow-green, or reddish mass (Fig. 2.11a).
- Solitary, multinodular, and diffuse types.
- Advanced cases often associated with portal vein tumor invasion.

Cytology of FNA or touch preparation of core
- Cytologic diagnosis falls into two main categories:
- Low-grade HCC: well-differentiated and fibrolamellar variant.
- High-grade HCC: moderately and poorly differentiated.

A. **Well-differentiated hepatocellular carcinoma**
   - Cellular specimen consisting of abundant, often uniform polygonal epithelial cells that are arranged in thick trabeculae (≥2 cell thickness) surrounded by endothelial cells or transversing vessels, pseudoglandular architecture, or abundant naked nuclei (Fig. 2.11b, c) [43–45].
   - The tumor cells have decreased-to-moderate granular or vacuolated cytoplasm with intracytoplasmic bile pigment and comparatively uniform, small, eccentric, round to oval nuclei. Cells contain one or multiple conspicuous nucleoli, slightly coarse chromatin, and smooth to slightly irregular thick nuclear membranes [44].
   - Although not always present, the most specific finding of HCCs on aspiration is that of spindled endothelial cells wrapping around groups of hepatocytes. Comparatively, normal liver has a more discohesive appearance [46, 47].
   - Small cell variant of HCC is characteristically composed of numerous small hepatocytes with minimal nuclear atypia and nuclear crowding with reduced cytoplasm; these are grouped together in microacini of five or more cells. Microtrabeculae of one or more cells with irregular thickness and no apparent peripheral endothelium are present [43, 44]. Transversing capillaries can also be seen.
   - Well-differentiated HCCs can often resemble benign entities like hepatic adenoma, regenerative nodules, and FNH, thus making the diagnosis quite challenging.

B. **Poorly differentiated hepatocellular carcinoma**
   - Characterized by the presence of markedly pleomorphic, overtly malignant epithelial cells, present singly and in nests with thick trabeculae surrounded by endothelial cells. Cells can be in three-dimensional

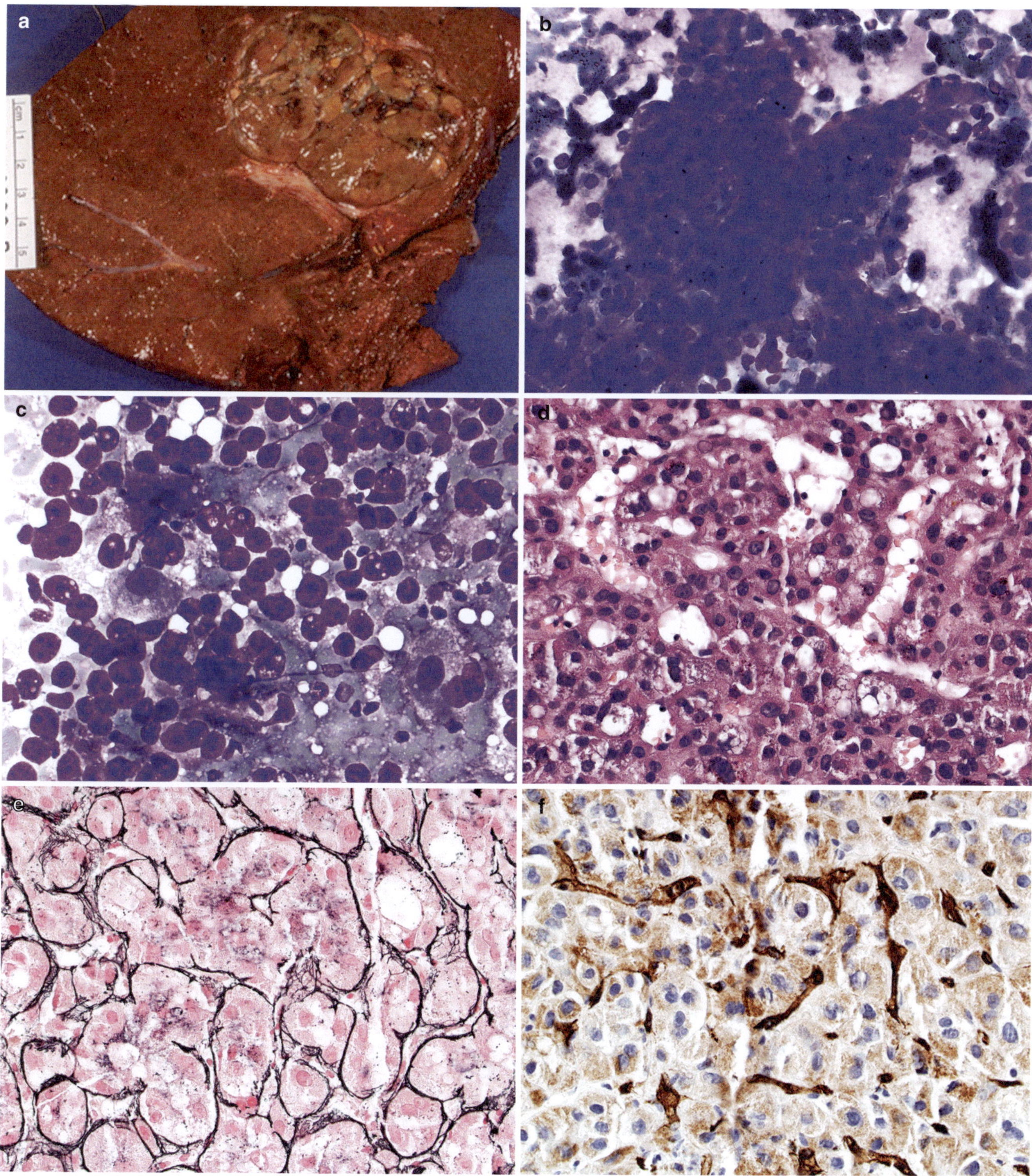

Fig. 2.11 Hepatocellular carcinoma, well differentiated. (**a**) Gross photo shows an irregular shaped, hemorrhagic hepatocellular carcinoma. (**b**, **c**) FNA smears show monolayer or three-dimensional clusters. Malignant hepatocytes are surrounded by endothelial cells with capillaries traversing hepatocellular carcinoma cells (**b**), pseudoglandular formation (**c**), and abundant naked nuclei (**c**); modified Giemsa stain, 600×. (**d**) Core biopsy shows thick cords of well-differentiated hepatocellular carcinoma with greater than three cell thickness and pseudoglands; hematoxylin and eosin stain, 400×. (**e**) Reticulin stain shows thickened trabeculae and pseudoglandular structures, 400×. (**f**) Immunohistochemical stain for CD34 highlights neovascular formation, 400×

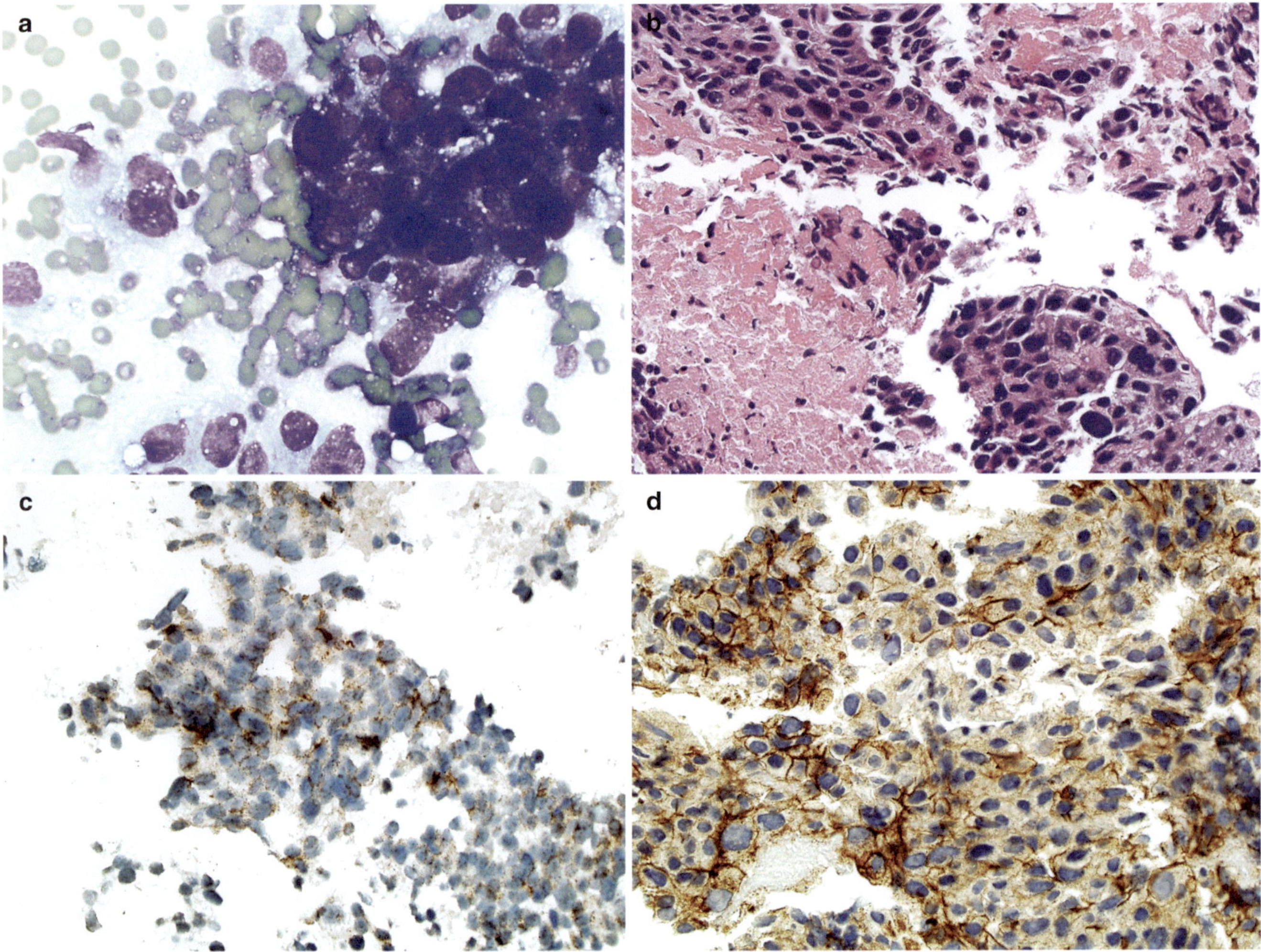

Fig. 2.12 Hepatocellular carcinoma, poorly differentiated. (**a**) FNA smears show single or three-dimensional clusters of pleomorphic polygonal cells that are arranged in a glandular formation, having enlarged nuclei with coarse chromatin. Prominent to macronucleoli, irregular nuclear membranes, and scant-to-moderate delicate cytoplasm with a high nuclear-to-cytoplasmic ratio can be seen; modified Giemsa stain, 600×. (**b**) Needle core biopsy shows sheets of pleomorphic tumor cells with pseudoglandular formation and necrosis; hematoxylin and eosin stain, 400x. (**c**) Tumor cells are positive for Glypican-3, 400×. (**d**) Polyclonal CEA highlights the canalicular pattern commonly seen in hepatocellular carcinoma, 400×

clusters with glandular architecture (Fig. 2.12a) [48]. Numerous naked nuclei with granular background can be seen as a result of the cytoplasmic fragility of malignant cells [45]

- Tumor cells have centrally placed round to oval nuclei containing macronucleoli and unevenly distributed coarse chromatin with irregular nuclear membrane contours. Scant to abundant granular or vacuolated cytoplasm with cytoplasmic hyaline inclusion bodies can be seen [45, 48]. The presence of macronucleoli often suggests malignancy. Intracytoplasmic bile may occur, and apparent hepatic differentiation may be lost.

Histology of core

- A reliable criterion for malignancy is the architectural appearance of thickened trabeculae (>3 cell thickness), nested groups, or sheets of cells (Figs. 2.11d and 2.12b). Pseudoglandular architecture is frequently seen.

Ancillary studies

- Helpful studies include the use of reticulin stain to identify the thickness of hepatocellular trabeculae (Fig. 2.11e). Immunohistochemical stains for HepPar-1, prealbumin, alpha-fetoprotein (AFP) (40%), glypican-3 (Fig. 2.12c) [49], polyclonal carcinoembryonic antigen (CEA) (Fig. 2.12d), CD34 (Fig. 2.11f) [44], CD10, and p53 can also be performed. MOC31 antibody has previously been shown to be helpful in differentiating HCC from metastatic adenocarcinoma because HCC tends to be negative while adenocarcinomas are positive [50].
- Serum levels of AFP higher than 500 ng/mL are highly associated with the presence of HCC; however, not all

tumors are associated with elevated AFP levels (i.e., fibrolamellar variant of HCC).

Diagnostic pitfalls

- Differential diagnosis of poorly differentiated HCC includes metastatic adenocarcinoma, cholangiocarcinoma, squamous cell carcinoma, clear cell renal cell carcinoma, clear cell variant of HCCs, and melanoma. Immunostains are helpful in distinguishing HCCs from metastatic malignant neoplasms.
- Significant variation in nuclear size is often seen in reactive hepatocytes, regenerative and dysplastic nodules, and moderately to poorly differentiated HCCs.
- The transversing vascular pattern is seen in well-differentiated HCCs; however, it can also be seen in other neoplasms, such as renal cell carcinoma.
- The presence of numerous malignant naked nuclei in the FNA smears is a feature occasionally seen in high-grade HCCs. This pattern can be seen in benign liver lesions as a result of mechanical rupture of hepatocytes during smear preparation.

C. **Fibrolamellar variant of hepatocellular carcinoma**

Clinical

- Young adults, 20–40 years old. No gender preference.
- 1–5% of all hepatocellular carcinomas.
- No association with hepatitis B infection, cirrhosis, or metabolic abnormalities.
- Better prognosis than classic HCC with rarely reported metastases [51, 52].

Radiology

US

- Variable echogenicity, central hyperechoic scar.

CT

- Large lobulated heterogeneous mass with an avascular central scar.
- Arterial enhancement in the nonscar portion with enhancement of the central scar on delayed imaging.
- Background liver is normal without evidence of cirrhosis.

MRI

- Dense enhancement in arterial and portal phase imaging [53].
- Hypointense central scar on T1 and T2 with delayed enhancement of central scar [53].

Angiography

- No arteriovenous shunting.
- Avascular central scar.

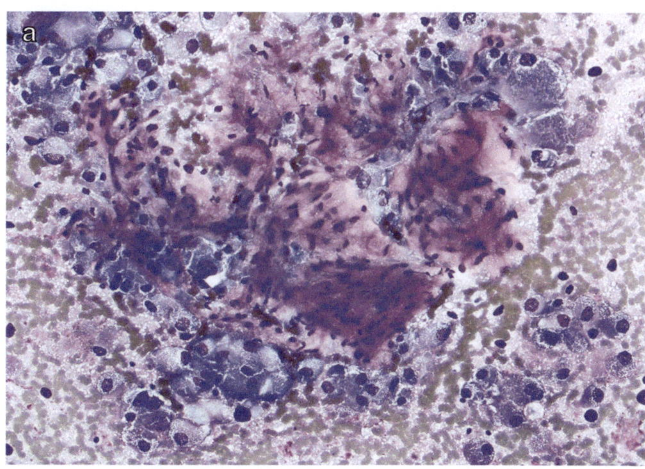

Fig. 2.13 Hepatocellular carcinoma, fibrolamellar variant. (**a**) FNA aspirates show single small nests or trabeculae of large malignant hepatocytes embedded in paucicellular fibrous tissue. The tumor cells have a low nuclear-to-cytoplasmic ratio, abundant dense oxyphilic cytoplasm, and macronucleoli; modified Giemsa stain, 400×

Gross

- Single, large (average 13 cm), hard, cirrhotic, well-circumscribed, bulging, and white-brown tumor.
- Fibrous bands throughout and central stellate scar.

Cytology of FNA or touch preparation of core

- Characterized by the presence of a rather monotonous population of large, discohesive hepatocytes that are separated by fibrous tissue (fibrolamellar pattern) (Fig. 2.13a) [54]. The tumor cells have a low nuclear-to-cytoplasmic ratio, abundant dense oxyphilic cytoplasm, and a large central nucleus frequently containing macronucleoli [54]. Trabecular arrangement of tumor cells surrounded by endothelial cells is not observed, and significant numbers of naked nuclei may be seen [54]. Binucleation and nuclear pseudoinclusions are present in most cases [54].
- Occasionally intracytoplasmic pale bodies and hyaline cytoplasmic bodies can be seen [54].
- Concerning the differential diagnosis, one should consider the sclerosing variant of HCC (SV-HCC). SV-HCC, unlike fibrolamellar HCC, occurs in the setting of chronic liver disease/cirrhosis and lacks lamellar fibrosis, eosinophilic granular cytoplasm, and prominent nucleoli [55].

Comments

- Tumor cells are positive for CK7, CD68, and HepPar-1.

D. **Clear cell variant of hepatocellular carcinoma**

- Presence of loosely cohesive groups and individually scattered malignant cells demonstrating anisonucleo-

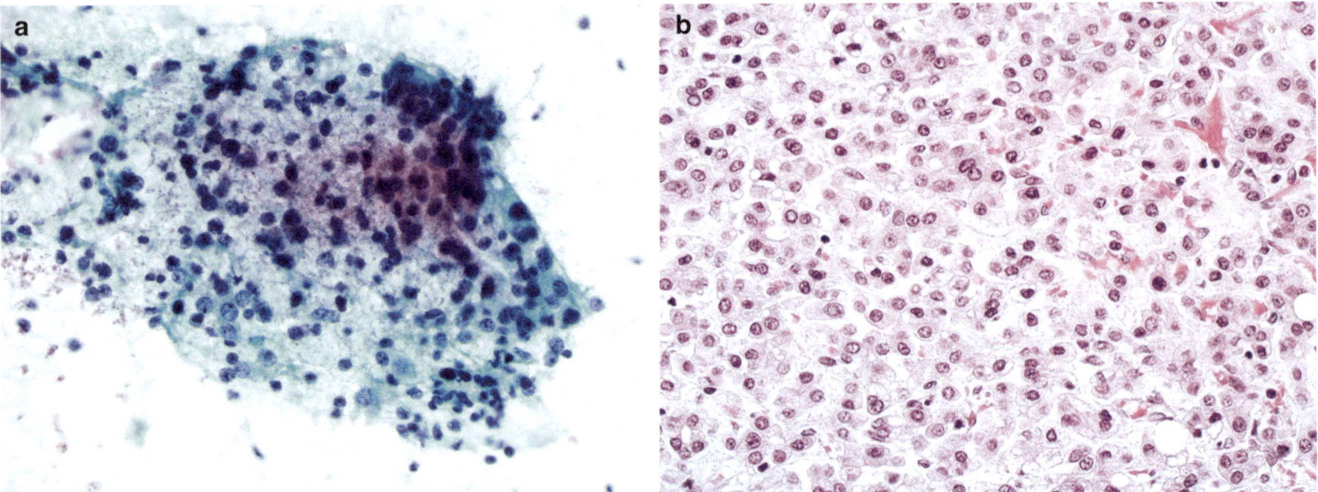

Fig. 2.14 Hepatocellular carcinoma, clear cell variant. (**a**, **b**) FNA smears; Papanicolaou stain, 400× (**a**), and needle core biopsy; hematoxylin and eosin stain, 400× (**b**), show malignant hepatocytes with clear cytoplasm

sis, nuclear hyperchromasia, prominent nucleoli, and abundant finely vacuolated to clear cytoplasm (Fig. 2.14a, b) [56].

- Prognosis similar to that of conventional HCC.
- Differential diagnosis includes metastatic clear cell malignancies to the liver.

Cholangiocarcinoma

Clinical

- Rare primary bile duct carcinoma involving the extrahepatic or intrahepatic ducts.
- Generally arises in a noncirrhotic liver.
- High prevalence in southeast and eastern Asia.
- Usually 60+ years with no gender preference.
- Mean age of 40 years in those with primary sclerosing cholangitis or chronic inflammatory bowel disease.

Radiology

US

- Usually homogeneous hyperechoic mass.
- Biliary dilation common for central lesions but absent for peripheral lesions.

CT

- Irregular and hypodense mass with homogeneous delayed enhancement (10–15 minutes) (Fig. 2.15a–c).
- Enhancement begins from periphery with later filling of the central aspect of the mass with rim washout.
- Hilar lesions may be associated with intrahepatic biliary ductal dilatation.
- Peripheral lesions may be infiltrative or focal. Invasion of hepatic and portal veins is common [57].

MRI

- T1: Hypodense mass.
- T2: Hyperintense periphery with hypointense central fibrosis.
- Marked enhancement on T1 postcontrast imaging.

Nuclear medicine

- Cold defect on sulfur colloid and HIDA scans.
- Gallium uptake.
- Hilar lesions may be associated with intrahepatic biliary ductal dilatation.
- Peripheral lesions may be infiltrative or focal. Invasion of hepatic and portal veins is common [57].
- Intraductal variants can be seen on magnetic resonance cholangiopancreatography (MRCP) or percutaneous transhepatic cholangiography as a polypoid intraluminal filling defect within the common, left, or right hepatic bile ducts.

Gross

- Gray-white cirrhotic mass with finger-likc extensions along major bile ducts and lymphatics (intrahepatic) (Fig. 2.16a).
- Nodular or flat sclerotic lesions with deep penetration into the bile duct wall (extrahepatic).
- Begins at hepatic duct junction and spreads along segments of biliary tree, classically referred to as a "Klatskin tumor."

Cytology of FNA or touch preparation of core

- Pleomorphic cuboidal, columnar, and/or polygonal cells arranged singly or in nests, or clusters with glandular or acinar architecture (Fig. 2.16b).
- Tumor cells with scant to abundant delicate cytoplasm and pleomorphic eccentrically located round or oval nuclei

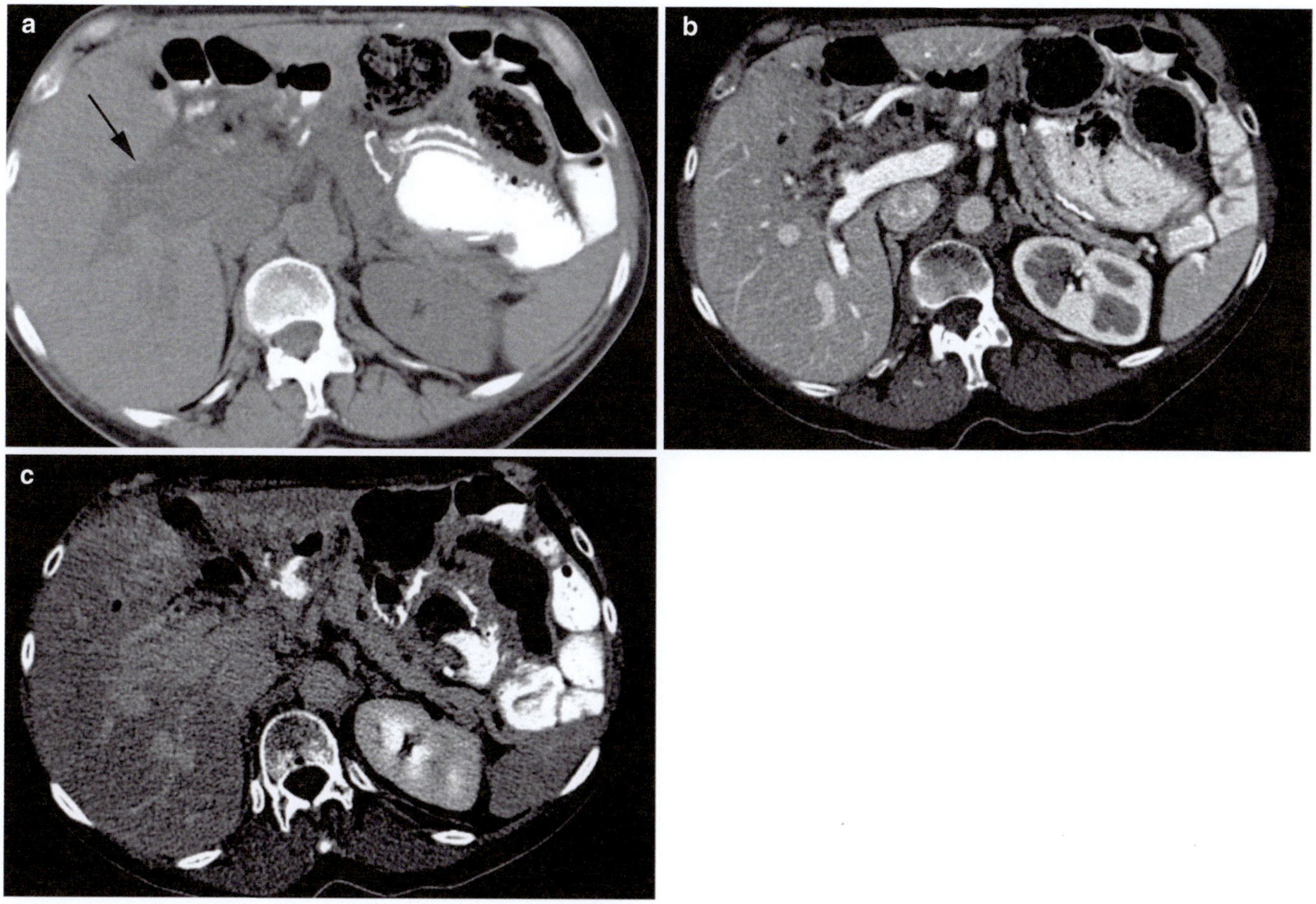

Fig. 2.15 Cholangiocarcinoma. (**a**) Noncontrast CT scan demonstrates a hypodense mass in the periportal region of the liver (*arrow*). (**b**) Early postcontrast CT imaging shows that the mass (*arrow*) enhances but remains relatively hypodense compared to the adjacent enhanced liver. (**c**) Postcontrast CT scan shows delayed progressive enhancement of the abnormal soft tissue (*arrow*)

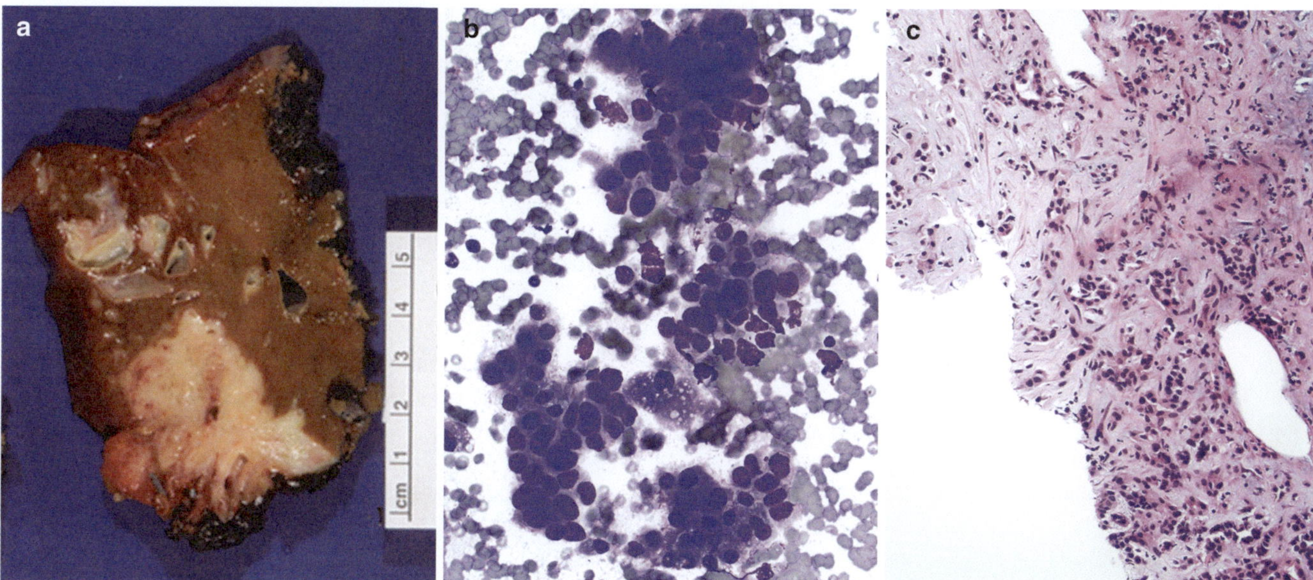

Fig. 2.16 Cholangiocarcinoma. (**a**) Gross section shows a white-tan mass with infiltrating borders. (**b**) FNA smears show cohesive to loosely cohesive clusters of pleomorphic cuboidal to polygonal cells with pleomorphic nuclei containing coarse chromatin and prominent nucleoli. Scant to moderate delicate cytoplasm is present. Glandular architecture is easily observed; modified Giemsa stain, 400×. (**c**) Needle core biopsy shows infiltrating adenocarcinoma cells in a fibrous/desmoplastic stroma; hematoxylin and eosin stain, 100×

containing prominent nucleoli, coarse unevenly distributed chromatin, and irregular nuclear membrane contours.

Histology of core

- Infiltrating glandular cells showing a tubular or acinar growth pattern or singly in fibrous/desmoplastic stroma (Fig. 2.16c).

Ancillary studies and comments

- Immunoreactivity for CK7 and CK19 and possibly for CK20 and CDX-2 is typical. Tumor cells may be positive for mucicarmine stain.
- Cholangiocarcinoma can be multifocal with moderate to poor differentiation mimicking a poorly differentiated HCC or metastasis. Immunohistochemistry can be helpful, as HepPar1 is highly sensitive and specific for HCC in this setting. Differentiation of cholangiocarcinoma from metastatic pancreatic adenocarcinoma may be impossible based on pathology alone [35].
- Differential diagnosis also includes metastatic adenocarcinoma, intraductal papillary neoplasm of the liver [9], and epithelioid hemangioendothelioma [58].

Hepatoblastoma

Clinical

- Most common primary hepatic malignancy in children.
- 70% occur by age 2, and 90% occur by 5 years of age.
- Associated with hemihypertrophy (Beckwith-Wiedemann syndrome), Wilms tumor, glycogen storage disease, and familial colonic polyposis (APC gene, 500× risk).

Radiology

US

- Well-defined mass with heterogeneous echotexture.
- Fibrous bands may have a spoke-wheel appearance.
- Calcifications—posterior acoustic shadowing.
- Right hepatic lobe is usually involved.

CT

- Large, hypodense mass, possibly with calcification.
- Heterogeneous and patchy enhancement.

MRI

- T1: hypointense [59].
- T2: hyperintense, with low-intensity fibrous bands [59].
- Signal may vary with the presence of hemorrhage.
- Marked enhancement.

Gross

- Solitary, nonencapsulated, often large mass measuring up to 25 cm in diameter.
- Usually located in the right lobe.

Cytology of FNA or touch preparation of core

- Cellular specimen composed of polymorphous cells (epithelial, embryonal, and mesenchymal tumor cells) in varying proportions at variable stages of differentiation. Mixed embryonal and fetal subtypes show three-dimensional clusters of neoplastic cells forming straight or branched cords/trabeculae or acinus-like structures. Numerous mitotic figures are present [60].
- Fetal epithelial cells are characterized by cells with abundant granular or clear cytoplasm and a small, rounded nucleus resembling a normal fetal hepatocyte [61]. The chromatin is finely granular, with a single, central nucleolus [61]. Pleomorphism and mitoses are not seen, and the nuclear/cytoplasmic ratio is decreased [61].
- Embryonal cells are cells characterized by small round cells with scant cytoplasm, pleomorphic hyperchromatic nucleus, and an elevated N/C ratio of ≥3/1. Coarse, granular chromatin and 2–4 angulated nucleoli are also present [61]. Mitoses can be seen in these cells (1–4/1000 cells) [61].
- Immature mesenchyme and extramedullary hemapoiesis (77% of cases) may be noted [61, 62].

Histology of core

- Malignant mesenchymal elements may take the form of osteoid.
- Extramedullary hematopoiesis may be present.
- Aggressive tumors may be differentiated from less aggressive ones by immunoreactivity for Survivin molecular biomarker in cancer) and CK19 and negative staining for C-Myc oncogene [63].

Angiosarcoma

Clinical

- Rare primary hepatic tumor.
- May present in a cirrhotic liver; however, classically associated with vinyl chloride or thorium dioxide exposure.
- More commonly presents in older men.

Radiology

CT

- Multiple hypodense masses with a heterogeneous, disorganized enhancement pattern.
- Progressive enhancement on delayed scans.
- Hyperdense areas of fresh hemorrhage.

MRI

- T1: Multiple hypointense nodules with areas of hyperintensity owing to hemorrhage.
- T2: High signal with central areas of low signal [64].

Gross

- Multicentric and diffusely infiltrative mass.
- Gray-white solid nodules with hemorrhagic cavities.

Cytology of FNA or touch preparation of core

- Pleomorphic endothelial cells can be seen subtly interdigitating with hepatocytes or may present singly as compact groups or monolayers. The cells have atypical nuclei with irregular outlines and enlarged nucleoli. The cytoplasm is delicate and may contain intracytoplasmic lumina.
- Poorly differentiated subtypes may mimic adenocarcinomas, germ cell neoplasms, or hepatocellular carcinoma [65].
- When aspirates demonstrate excess blood, vascular lesions should enter into the differential diagnosis (i.e., hemangioma, epithelioid hemangioendothelioma, and angiosarcoma, among others).

Ancillary studies and comments

- Immunoreactivity for CD34, CD31, FLI1, and Factor VIII. Epithelioid variant of angiosarcoma may be positive for CK7 and CK20 [65].
- Differential diagnosis includes metastatic high-grade carcinoma, sarcoma, and hepatic epithelioid hemangioendothelioma [58].

Metastatic Malignant Neoplasms

General

- Metastatic carcinomas account for more than 90% of all malignant hepatic neoplasms. Frequent metastases arise from the colon, pancreas, stomach, breast, and lung with colorectal metastases being the most common.
- Metastatic urothelial carcinoma, melanomas, and sarcomas of variable sites may also occur.

Radiology

- Multiplicity is the most diagnostic feature.
- Lesions can have a heterogeneous appearance on US, CT, and MRI. MRI and contrast enhanced CT are most sensitive for lesion detection.
- Most lesions are best seen on portal venous phase imaging.
- Hypervascular lesions include neuroendocrine carcinoma, melanoma, breast cancer, thyroid carcinoma, and renal cell carcinoma [13].

Metastatic Colonic Carcinoma

Radiology

CT

- Single or multiple with a diffuse, hypodense pattern.
- Enhancement may be seen on postcontrast imaging, suggesting a renal, ovarian, or neuroendocrine primary tumor (Fig. 2.17a).
- Possible presence of calcification on noncontrast CT for mucinous neoplasms or with rare tumors such as osteosarcomas or teratocarcinomas.

US

- Usually hypoechoic and well-circumscribed.
- Hyperechoic metastases suggest colon, thyroid, breast, renal, or melanoma primary.

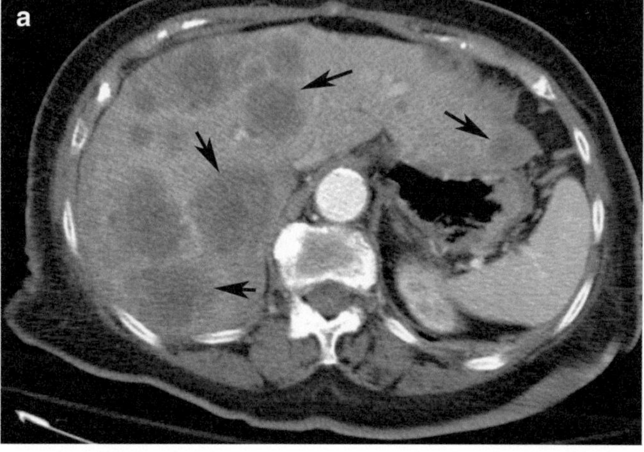

Fig. 2.17 Metastatic colonic adenocarcinoma. (**a**) Postcontrast axial CT scan shows numerous hypodense lesions scattered throughout the liver, several of which are designated by *arrows*

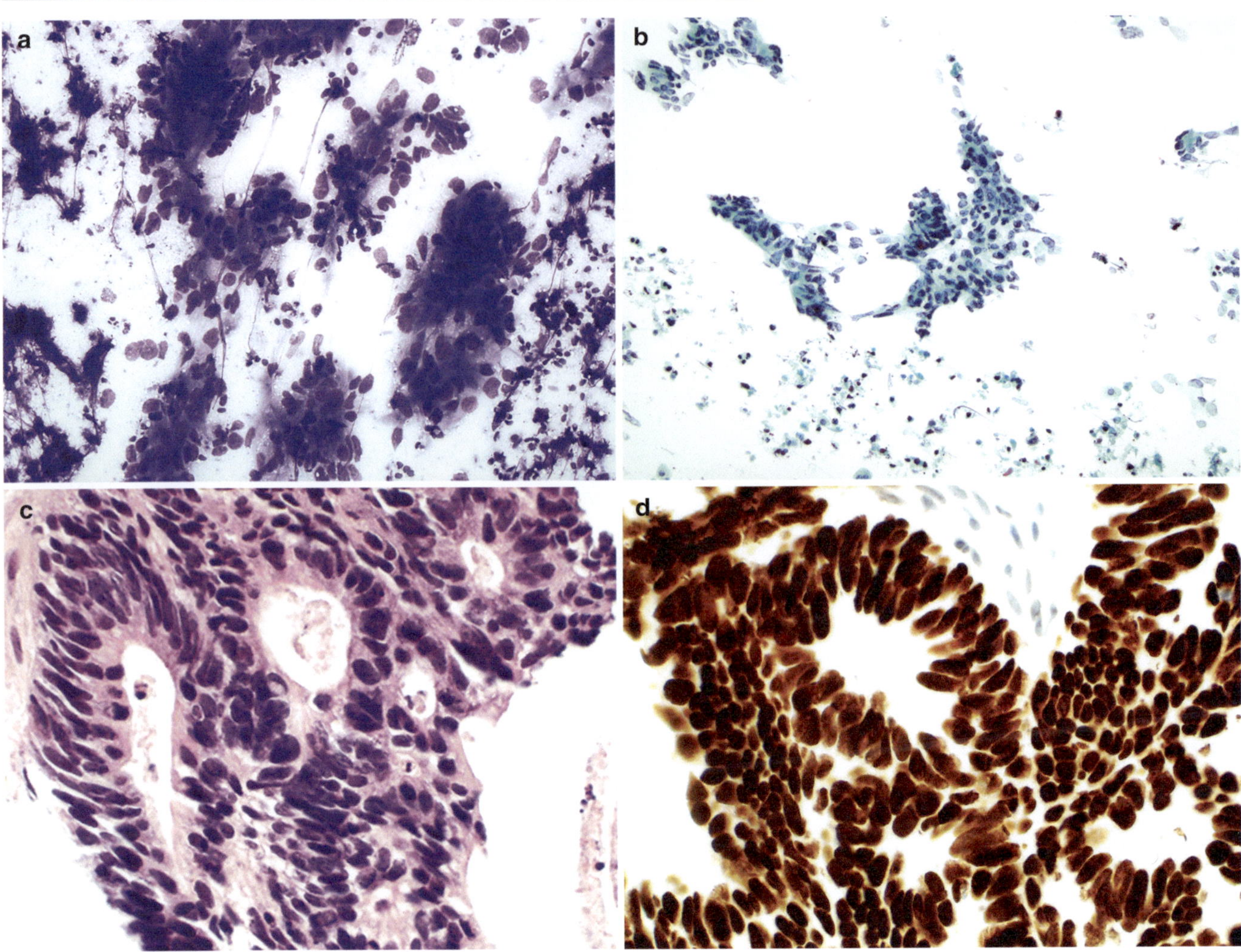

Fig. 2.18 Metastatic colonic adenocarcinoma. (**a**, **b**) FNA smears show loose clusters of columnar cells or polygonal cells that are arranged in palisading, glands, nests, three-dimensional clusters, or singly in the background of necrosis. The tumor cells have elongated or oval nuclei with coarse chromatin or prominent nucleoli, delicate or vacuolated cytoplasm; modified Giemsa stain (**a**) and Papanicolaou stain (**b**), 400×. (**c**) Needle core biopsy shows typical intestinal adenocarcinoma with necrosis; hematoxylin and eosin stain, 600×. (**d**) The tumor cells are positive for CDX-2; 600x

Cytology of FNA or touch preparation of core

- Variably sized clusters of malignant cuboidal or columnar glandular cells arranged in a palisading, tubular, or glandular architecture, with elongated cigar-shaped or oval nuclei containing coarse chromatin and possibly prominent nucleoli (Fig. 2.18a, b). The cytoplasm is delicate or vacuolated. Intracytoplasmic mucin may be seen.
- Dirty necrotic background and extracellular mucin may be present.

Histology of core

- Presence of malignant glands with typical intestinal adenocarcinoma features and abundant "dirty" necrosis are common (Fig. 2.18c).

Ancillary studies

- Immunoreactivity for CDX-2 (Fig. 2.18d) and Cytokeratin 20.

Neuroendocrine Carcinoma

Radiology

US

- Usually hypoechoic and well circumscribed (Fig. 2.19a).

CT

- Enhancement may be seen on postcontrast imaging.
- Intense arterial enhancement with washout on delayed imaging.

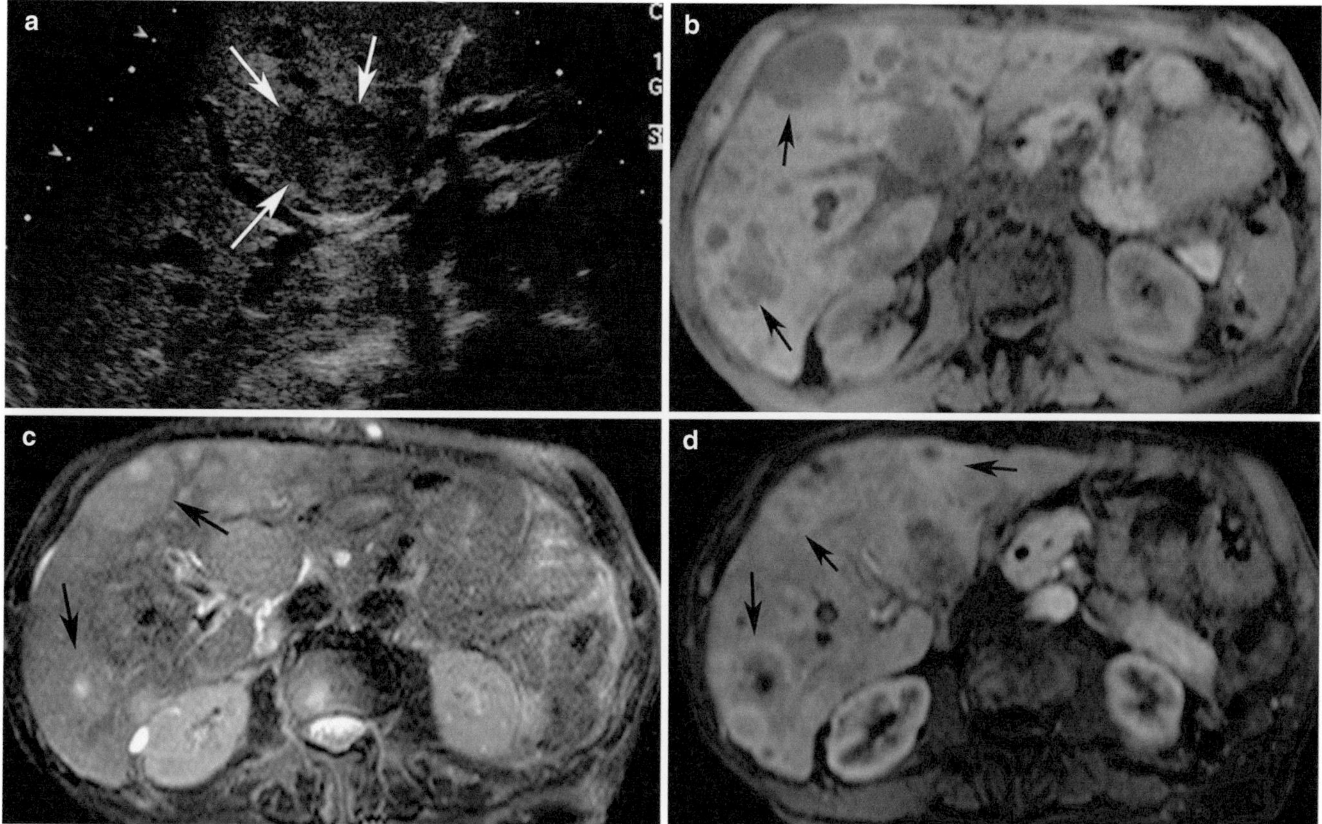

Fig. 2.19 Metastatic neuroendocrine carcinoma. (**a**) Postcontrast axial CT scan shows numerous hypodense lesions scattered throughout the liver, several of which are designated by *arrows*. (**b**) Precontrast T1-weighted MRI scan shows numerous hypointense masses in the liver (*arrows*). (**c**) Precontrast T2-weighted axial MRI scan of the same patient shows mixed iso- and hyperintensity (*arrows*). (**d**) T1-weighted arterial phase MRI postcontrast shows multiple heterogeneously enhancing lesions (*arrows*)

MRI

- T1: Hypointense mass with homogeneous early enhancement on postcontrast (Fig. 2.19b, d).
- T2: Slightly hyperintense (Fig. 2.19c).
- Delayed postcontrast: washout with isodense lesions to liver.

Interventional radiology

- Potential release of vasoactive substances with biopsy of hormonally active tumor.

Cytology of FNA or touch preparation of core

- Polygonal or plasmacytoid cells present singly or as loosely cohesive clusters, cores with variable rosette-like architecture (Fig. 2.20a, b). The tumor cells have eccentrically placed, round, oval, or spindle-shaped nuclei containing stippled ("salt and pepper") chromatin and possible small nucleoli. The cytoplasm may be granular. Large pleomorphic cells with one or multiple nuclei may be seen.

Histology of core

- Tumor cells are present singly, in cores, as trabeculae, and as nests with rosetting or glandular architecture in the background of a fibrous stroma (Fig. 2.20c).
- Immunohistochemical studies should be performed for synaptophysin (Fig. 2.20d), chromogranin, NSE, CD56, Ki-67, CDX-2, and TTF-1 [66]. Immunostains are paramount when the differential diagnosis includes lymphoma.

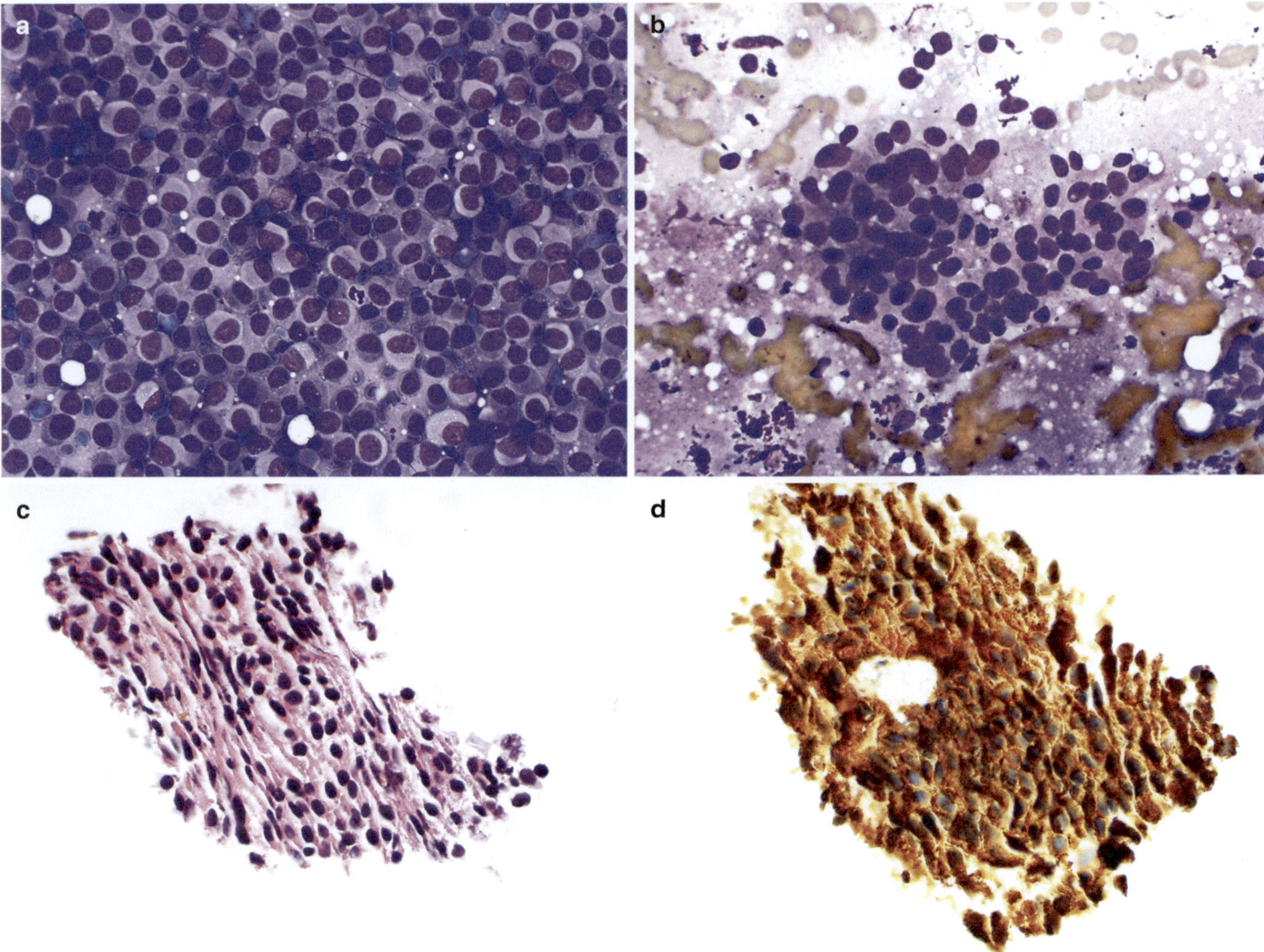

Fig. 2.20 Metastatic neuroendocrine carcinoma. (**a**, **b**) FNA smears show single, loosely cohesive clusters of epithelial cells with rosette formation or naked nuclei. The tumor cells have round to oval nuclei containing stippled chromatin with conspicuous nucleoli and delicate to granular cytoplasm. Some cells show plasmacytoid features; modified Giemsa stain, 600×. (**c**) Needle core biopsy shows sheets or rosettes of epithelial cells; hematoxylin and eosin stain, 400×. (**d**) The tumor cells are positive for synaptophysin; 400×

References

1. Geisinger KR, Stanley MW, Raab SS, Silverman JF, Abati A. Liver. In: Geisinger KR, Stanley MW, Raab SS, Silverman JF, Abati A, editors. Modern cytopathology. London: Churchill Livingstone, Elsevier; 2004. p. 505–42.
2. Nazir RT, Sharif MA, Iqbal M, Amin MS. Diagnostic accuracy of fine needle aspiration cytology in hepatic tumours. J Coll Physicians Surg Pak. 2010;20:373–6.
3. Conrad R, Castelino-Prabhu S, Cobb C, Raza A. Cytopathologic diagnosis of liver mass lesions. J Gastrointest Oncol. 2013;4:53–61.
4. Wee A. Fine-needle aspiration biopsy of hepatocellular carcinoma and related hepatocellular nodular lesions in cirrhosis: controversies, challenges, and expectations. Pathol Res Int. 2011;2011:587936.
5. Wang P, Meng ZQ, Chen Z, Lin JH, Ping B, Wang LF, et al. Diagnostic value and complications of fine needle aspiration for primary liver cancer and its influence on the treatment outcome—a study based on 3011 patients in China. Eur J Surg Oncol. 2008;34:541–6.
6. Livraghi T, Damascelli B, Lombardi C, Spagnoli I. Risk in fine-needle abdominal biopsy. J Clin Ultrasound. 1983;11:77–81.
7. Smith EH. Complications of percutaneous abdominal fine-needle biopsy. Review. Radiology. 1991;178:253–8.
8. Tyagi R, Dey P. Needle tract seeding: an avoidable complication. Diagn Cytopathol. 2014;42:636–40.
9. Jurczyk MF, Zhu B, Villa C, DeFrias D, Lin X. Cytomorphology of intraductal oncocytic papillary neoplasm of the liver. Diagn Cytopathol. 2014;42:895–8.
10. Agarwal PK, Husain N, Singh BN. Cytologic findings in aspirated hydatid fluid. Acta Cytol. 1989;33:652–4.
11. Mettler FA, Guiberteau MJ. Essentials of nuclear medicine imaging. 5th ed. Philadelphia: W.B. Saunders; 2005.
12. Fang CT, Lai SY, Yi WC, Hsueh PR, Liu KL, Chang SC. Klebsiella pneumoniae genotype K1: an emerging pathogen that causes septic ocular or central nervous system complications from pyogenic liver abscess. Clin Infect Dis. 2007;45:284–93.
13. Johnson CD, Schmit GD. Mayo Clinic gastrointestinal imaging review. Rochester: Mayo Clinic; 2005.

14. Horton KM, Bluemke DA, Hruban RH, Soyer P, Fishman EK. CT and MR imaging of benign hepatic and biliary tumors. Radiographics. 1999;19:431–51.
15. Zeppa P, Anniciello A, Vetrani A, Palombini L. Fine needle aspiration biopsy of hepatic focal fatty change. A report of two cases. Acta Cytol. 2002;46:567–70.
16. Anstee QM, McPherson S, Day CP. How big a problem is non-alcoholic fatty liver disease? BMJ. 2011;343:d3897.
17. Takeshita A, Yamamoto K, Fujita A, Hanafusa T, Yasuda E, Shibayama Y. Focal hepatic steatosis surrounding a metastatic insulinoma. Pathol Int. 2008;58:59–63.
18. Tani M, Yamaue H, Oka M, Onishi H, Kinoshita H, Hirabayashi N, et al. Focal fatty liver after pancreaticoduodenectomy: a case report of a rare entity of intrahepatic tumor. Hepato-Gastroenterology. 2002;49:1087–9.
19. Gong L, Su Q, Zhang W, Li AN, Zhu SJ, Feng YM. Liver cell adenoma: a case report with clonal analysis and literature review. World J Gastroenterol. 2006;12:2125–9.
20. Kutami R, Nakashima Y, Nakashima O, Shiota K, Kojiro M. Pathomorphologic study on the mechanism of fatty change in small hepatocellular carcinoma of humans. J Hepatol. 2000;33:282–9.
21. Sookoian S, Castano GO, Burgueno AL, Gianotti TF, Rosselli MS, Pirola CJ. The nuclear receptor PXR gene variants are associated with liver injury in nonalcoholic fatty liver disease. Pharmacogenet Genom. 2010;20:1–8.
22. Tebala GD, Jwad A, Khan AQ, Long E, Sissons G. Multifocal nodular fatty infiltration of the liver: a case report of a challenging diagnostic problem. Am J Case Rep. 2016;17:196–202.
23. Hamer OW, Aguirre DA, Casola G, Lavine JE, Woenckhaus M, Sirlin CB. Fatty liver: imaging patterns and pitfalls. Radiographics. 2006;26:1637–53.
24. Terriff BA, Gibney RG, Scudamore CH. Fatality from fine-needle aspiration biopsy of a hepatic hemangioma. Am J Roentgenol. 1990;154:203–4.
25. Davies R. Haemorrhage after fine-needle aspiration biopsy of an hepatic haemangioma. Med J Aust. 1993;158:364.
26. Reddy KR, Kligerman S, Levi J, Livingstone A, Molina E, Franceschi D, et al. Benign and solid tumors of the liver: relationship to sex, age, size of tumors, and outcome. Am Surg. 2001;67:173–8.
27. Hertzanu Y, Peiser J, Zirkin H. Massive bleeding after fine needle aspiration of liver angiosarcoma. Gastrointest Radiol. 1990;15:43–6.
28. Choi BY, Nguyen MH. The diagnosis and management of benign hepatic tumors. J Clin Gastroenterol. 2005;39:401–12.
29. Trotter JF, Everson GT. Benign focal lesions of the liver. Clin Liver Dis. 2001;5:17–42.
30. Buell JF, Tranchart H, Cannon R, Dagher I. Management of benign hepatic tumors. Surg Clin North Am. 2010;90:719–35.
31. Matos AP, Velloni F, Ramalho M, AlObaidy M, Rajapaksha A, Semelka RC. Focal liver lesions: practical magnetic resonance imaging approach. World J Hepatol. 2015;7:1987–2008.
32. Layfield LJ, Mooney EE, Dodd LG. Not by blood alone: diagnosis of hemangiomas by fine-needle aspiration. Diagn Cytopathol. 1998;19:250–4.
33. Guy CD, Yuan S, Ballo MS. Spindle-cell lesions of the liver: diagnosis by fine-needle aspiration biopsy. Diagn Cytopathol. 2001;25:94–100.
34. Iannaccone R, Federle MP, Brancatelli G, Matsui O, Fishman EK, Narra VR, et al. Peliosis hepatis: spectrum of imaging findings. Am J Roentgenol. 2006;187:W43–52.
35. Chute DJ, Sarti M, Atkins KA. Liver cytology. Cancer Treat Res. 2014;160:83–109.
36. Horta G, Lopez M, Dotte A, Cordero J, Chesta C, Castro A, et al. Benign focal liver lesions detected by computed tomography: review of 1,184 examinations. Rev Med Chil. 2015;143:197–202.
37. Hussain SM, Terkivatan T, Zondervan PE, Lanjouw E, de Rave S, Ijzermans JN, et al. Focal nodular hyperplasia: findings at state-of-the-art MR imaging, US, CT, and pathologic analysis. Radiographics. 2004;24:3–17; discussion, 8–9.
38. Nguyen BN, Flejou JF, Terris B, Belghiti J, Degott C. Focal nodular hyperplasia of the liver: a comprehensive pathologic study of 305 lesions and recognition of new histologic forms. Am J Surg Pathol. 1999;23:1441–54.
39. Makhlouf HR, Abdul-Al HM, Goodman ZD. Diagnosis of focal nodular hyperplasia of the liver by needle biopsy. Hum Pathol. 2005;36:1210–6.
40. Jeong YY, Yim NY, Kang HK. Hepatocellular carcinoma in the cirrhotic liver with helical CT and MRI: imaging spectrum and pitfalls of cirrhosis-related nodules. Am J Roentgenol. 2005;185:1024–32.
41. Chou R, Cuevas C, Fu R, Devine B, Wasson N, Ginsburg A, et al. Imaging techniques for the diagnosis of hepatocellular carcinoma: a systematic review and meta-analysis. Ann Intern Med. 2015;162:697–711.
42. Lewandowski RJ, Sato KT, Atassi B, Ryu RK, Nemcek AA Jr, Kulik L, et al. Radioembolization with 90Y microspheres: angiographic and technical considerations. Cardiovasc Intervent Radiol. 2007;30:571–92.
43. Yang GC, Yang GY, Tao LC. Cytologic features and histologic correlations of microacinar and microtrabecular types of well-differentiated hepatocellular carcinoma in fine-needle aspiration biopsy. Cancer. 2004;102:27–33.
44. Wee A, Nilsson B. Highly well differentiated hepatocellular carcinoma and benign hepatocellular lesions. Can they be distinguished on fine needle aspiration biopsy? Acta Cytol. 2003;47:16–26.
45. Renshaw AA, Haja J, Wilbur DC, Miller TR. Fine-needle aspirates of hepatocellular carcinoma that are misclassified as adenocarcinoma: correlating cytologic features and performance in the College of American Pathologists Nongynecologic Cytology Program. Arch Pathol Lab Med. 2006;130:19–22.
46. Pittman ME, Brunt EM. Anatomic pathology of hepatocellular carcinoma: histopathology using classic and new diagnostic tools. Clin Liver Dis. 2015;19:239–59.
47. Soyuer I, Ekinci C, Kaya M, Genc Y, Bahar K. Diagnosis of hepatocellular carcinoma by fine needle aspiration cytology. Cellular features. Acta Cytol. 2003;47:581–9.
48. Kulesza P, Torbenson M, Sheth S, Erozan YS, Ali SZ. Cytopathologic grading of hepatocellular carcinoma on fine-needle aspiration. Cancer. 2004;102:247–58.
49. Nassar A, Cohen C, Siddiqui MT. Utility of glypican-3 and survivin in differentiating hepatocellular carcinoma from benign and preneoplastic hepatic lesions and metastatic carcinomas in liver fine-needle aspiration biopsies. Diagn Cytopathol. 2009;37:629–35.
50. Porcell AI, De Young BR, Proca DM, Frankel WL. Immunohistochemical analysis of hepatocellular and adenocarcinoma in the liver: MOC31 compares favorably with other putative markers. Mod Pathol. 2000;13:773–8.
51. Crowe A, Knight CS, Jhala D, Bynon SJ, Jhala NC. Diagnosis of metastatic fibrolamellar hepatocellular carcinoma by endoscopic ultrasound-guided fine needle aspiration. Cytojournal. 2011;8:2.
52. Torbenson M. Review of the clinicopathologic features of fibrolamellar carcinoma. Adv Anat Pathol. 2007;14:217–23.
53. Ichikawa T, Federle MP, Grazioli L, Madariaga J, Nalesnik M, Marsh W. Fibrolamellar hepatocellular carcinoma: imaging and pathologic findings in 31 recent cases. Radiology. 1999;213:352–61.
54. Perez-Guillermo M, Masgrau NA, Garcia-Solano J, Sola-Perez J, de Agustin y de Agustin P. Cytologic aspect of fibrolamellar hepatocellular carcinoma in fine-needle aspirates. Diagn Cytopathol. 1999;21:180–7.
55. Sergi CM. Hepatocellular carcinoma, fibrolamellar variant: diagnostic pathologic criteria and molecular pathology update. A primer. Diagnostics (Basel). 2015;6. https://www.ncbi.nlm.nih.

gov/pubmed/?term=Sergi+CM.+Hepatocellular+carcinoma%2C+fibrolamellar+variant%3A
56. Singh HK, Silverman JF, Geisinger KR. Fine-needle aspiration cytomorphology of clear-cell hepatocellular carcinoma. Diagn Cytopathol. 1997;17:306–10.
57. Chung YE, Kim MJ, Park YN, Choi JY, Pyo JY, Kim YC, et al. Varying appearances of cholangiocarcinoma: radiologic-pathologic correlation. Radiographics. 2009;29:683–700.
58. Jurczyk M, Zhu B, Laskin W, Lin X. Pitfalls in the diagnosis of hepatic epithelioid hemangioendothelioma by FNA and needle core biopsy. Diagn Cytopathol. 2014;42:516–20.
59. Rasalkar DD, Chu WC, Cheng FW, Hui SK, Ling SC, Li CK. A pictorial review of imaging of abdominal tumours in adolescence. Pediatr Radiol. 2010;40:1552–61.
60. Weir EG, Ali SZ. Hepatoblastoma: cytomorphologic characteristics in serious cavity fluids. Cancer. 2002;96:267–74.
61. Iyer VK, Kapila K, Agarwala S, Verma K. Fine needle aspiration cytology of hepatoblastoma. Recognition of subtypes on cytomorphology. Acta Cytol. 2005;49:355–64.
62. Viswanathan S, George S, Ramadwar M, Medhi S, Arora B, Kurkure P. Evaluation of pediatric abdominal masses by fine-needle aspiration cytology: a clinicoradiologic approach. Diagn Cytopathol. 2010;38:15–27.
63. Singh V, Manalang M, Singh M, Apte U. A brief report of immunohistochemical markers to identify aggressive hepatoblastoma. Appl Immunohistochem Mol Morphol. 2017:1. https://doi.org/10.1097/PAI.0000000000000492. [Epub ahead of print.].
64. Yu RS, Chen Y, Jiang B, Wang LH, Xu XF. Primary hepatic sarcomas: CT findings. Eur Radiol. 2008;18:2196–205.
65. Lin CF, DeFrias D, Lin X. Epithelioid angiosarcoma: a neoplasm with potential diagnostic challenges. Diagn Cytopathol. 2010;38:154–8.
66. Lin X, Saad RS, Luckasevic TM, Silverman JF, Liu Y. Diagnostic value of CDX-2 and TTF-1 expressions in separating metastatic neuroendocrine neoplasms of unknown origin. Appl Immunohistochem Mol Morphol. 2007;15:407–14.

Lungs, Mediastinum, and Pleura

3

Xiaoqi Lin, Julianne M. Ubago, Rehan Ali, Ali Al Asadi, and Ahsun Riaz

Lungs

Transthoracic and transbronchial fine needle aspiration (FNA) and core biopsies are the main methods used to diagnose mass lesions in the lung parenchyma, pleura, and mediastinum [1, 2], and these techniques can also be used to confirm benign neoplasms, infections, and inflammatory lesions [1–4]. Transthoracic FNA/biopsy is the best method for diagnosing small peripheral lesions [5], while endoscopic ultrasound-guided FNA (EUS FNA) is the preferred method for biopsy of central lesions. FNA biopsy is particularly useful to distinguish between small cell carcinoma and non–small cell carcinoma and is critical to help stage non–small cell lung carcinoma patients. In most cases, the diagnostic benefit of the FNA procedure far outweighs the risk of complications. Therefore, FNA biopsy can significantly impact patient management while avoiding more invasive procedures and unnecessary surgeries.

Transthoracic FNA biopsy has more inherent complications than transbronchial FNA biopsy, especially the risk of pneumothorax. Possible contraindications include bleeding abnormalities (particularly in patients being treated with anticoagulation therapy), uncontrollable cough, poor lung function, severe emphysema, chronic obstructive pulmonary disease, previous pneumonectomy, pulmonary hypertension, and vascular lesions such as arteriovenous malformation [6–8]. Thus, a chest radiograph should be obtained after the procedure, and patients should be observed for several hours afterwards.

X. Lin (✉)
Northwestern University, Feinberg School of Medicine, Northwestern Memorial Hospital, Chicago, IL, USA
e-mail: xlin@northwestern.edu

J. M. Ubago
Department of Pathology, Edward Hospital, Naperville, IL, USA

R. Ali · A. Al Asadi
Department of Radiology, Section of Vascular and Interventional Radiology, Northwestern University, Chicago, IL, USA

A. Riaz
Department of Pathology, Northwestern Medicine, Chicago, IL, USA

Normal Elements

Normal elements along the needle track are often aspirated and admixed with lesional cells. Careful attention should be paid when these normal cells are encountered, especially with the presence of reactive atypia.

- Chest wall tissue may contain skin, fibroadipose tissue, and skeletal muscle.
- Pleural parenchyma contains mesothelial cells. FNA smears show a monolayer of honeycomb sheets of cells. The cells have a small to moderate amount of delicate cytoplasm, well-defined cell borders, prominent spaces between cells (windows) that correspond to long microvilli, and round to oval nuclei with fine, evenly distributed chromatin and small nucleoli. Nuclear grooves may be present. Reactive mesothelial cells often show enlarged nuclei with prominent nucleoli, and can potentially be misinterpreted as being neoplastic cells (Fig. 3.1a).
- Lung parenchyma contains bronchial and bronchiolar cells with or without cilia, mucus cells, goblet cells, alveolar type I and II pneumocytes, and alveolar macrophages. Ciliated and nonciliated bronchial and bronchiolar cells are columnar or cuboidal in shape (Fig. 3.1b). Reserve cells may mimic small-cell carcinoma with nuclear molding, high nucleus to cytoplasm ratio (N/C), and scant cytoplasm but lack other malignant features. Type II pneumocytes are ovoid to columnar in shape; reactive type II pneumocytes can show enlarged nuclei, high N/C ratios, and prominent nucleoli that may be misinterpreted as adenocarcinoma.

R. Nayar et al. (eds.), *Atlas of Cytopathology and Radiology*, https://doi.org/10.1007/978-3-030-24756-0_3

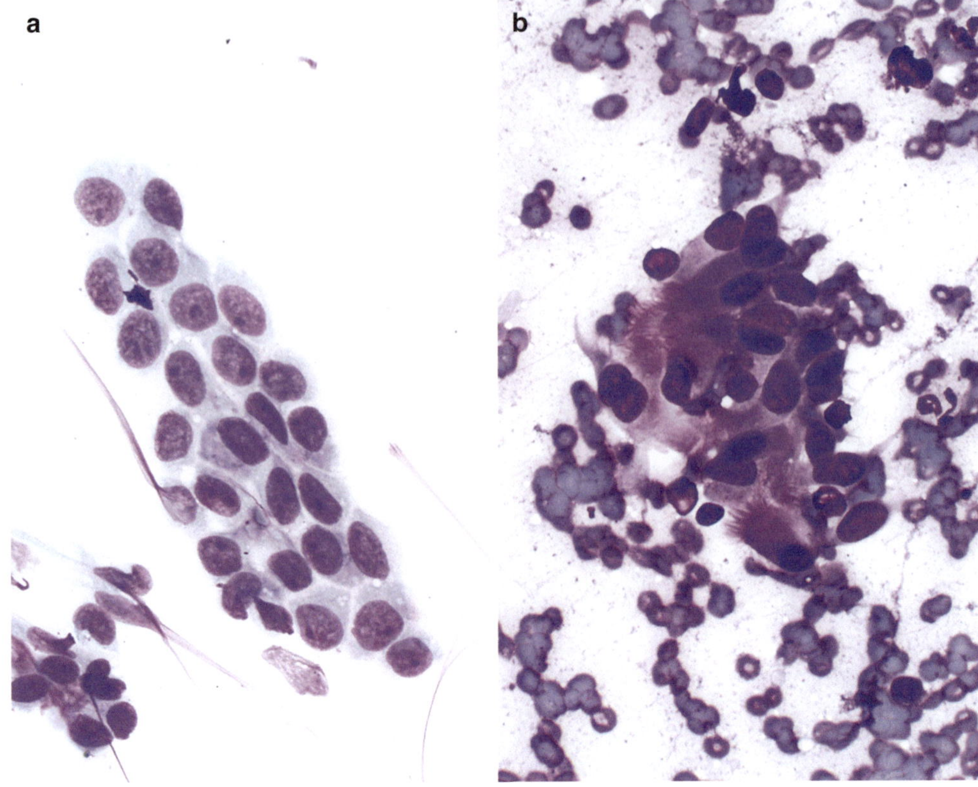

Fig. 3.1 (**a**, **b**) Cytology of benign normal cells. (**a**) Benign mesothelial cells. FNA smears show cohesive, flat, "honeycomb" sheet of cells with nucleoli and "windows" between cells, Diff-Quik stain, 400×. (**b**) Cytology of benign bronchial cells, discohesive and cohesive columnar cells with cilia, Diff-Quik stain, 400×

Benign Lesions

Granuloma

A granuloma is an aggregate of epithelioid histiocytes and may be either caseating or noncaseating, depending on the presence of central necrosis.

Clinical

- Granulomas are common lesions in the lung and mediastinum that may mimic malignancy clinically and radiographically.
- Causes include inflammatory (sarcoidosis, rheumatoid arthritis, Wegener granulomatosis, and eosinophilic pneumonia), infectious (fungi, mycobacteria), malignancies (e.g., Hodgkin lymphoma, squamous cell carcinoma, Langerhans cell histiocytosis), and miscellaneous entities (foreign bodies).
- FNA may be the best initial method for definitive diagnosis if the differential includes granuloma versus malignancy or infectious versus inflammatory causes.

Radiographic Findings

X-ray

- Granulomas on chest radiographs appear as small, round, or oval-shaped nodules with well-defined borders that may be calcified. There are many patterns of calcification that can suggest the nature of the lesion (Fig. 3.2a, b).
- Five patterns of calcification that are likely benign are those with a diffuse, central, laminar, concentric, and popcorn appearance. Stippled and eccentric patterns are two patterns of calcifications that are suspicious for malignancy and require follow up.
- Areas of consolidation, diffuse reticulonodular opacities, pleural effusion, pulmonary artery enlargement, and hilar and mediastinal lymphadenopathy may also be present.

CT Scan

- Granulomas have a variable presentation on CT scans that is associated with the etiology (infectious versus noninfectious). Granulomas with areas of consolidation may be present.
- Other findings may include nodules, areas of scarring, traction bronchiectasis, emphysema, air trapping, pulmonary artery enlargement, and pleural effusion [9].
- Hilar and contiguous mediastinal (paratracheal) lymphadenopathy is common and may be calcified (up to 35%) (Fig. 3.2c–f).

Cytology of FNA or Touch Preparation

- Characteristically shows the presence of syncytial aggregates of epithelioid histiocytes. The epithelioid histiocytes have round or oval elongated, bland nuclei with obvious nucleoli, moderate to abundant cytoplasm, and indistinct cytoplasmic borders (Fig. 3.2g, j). Multinucleated giant

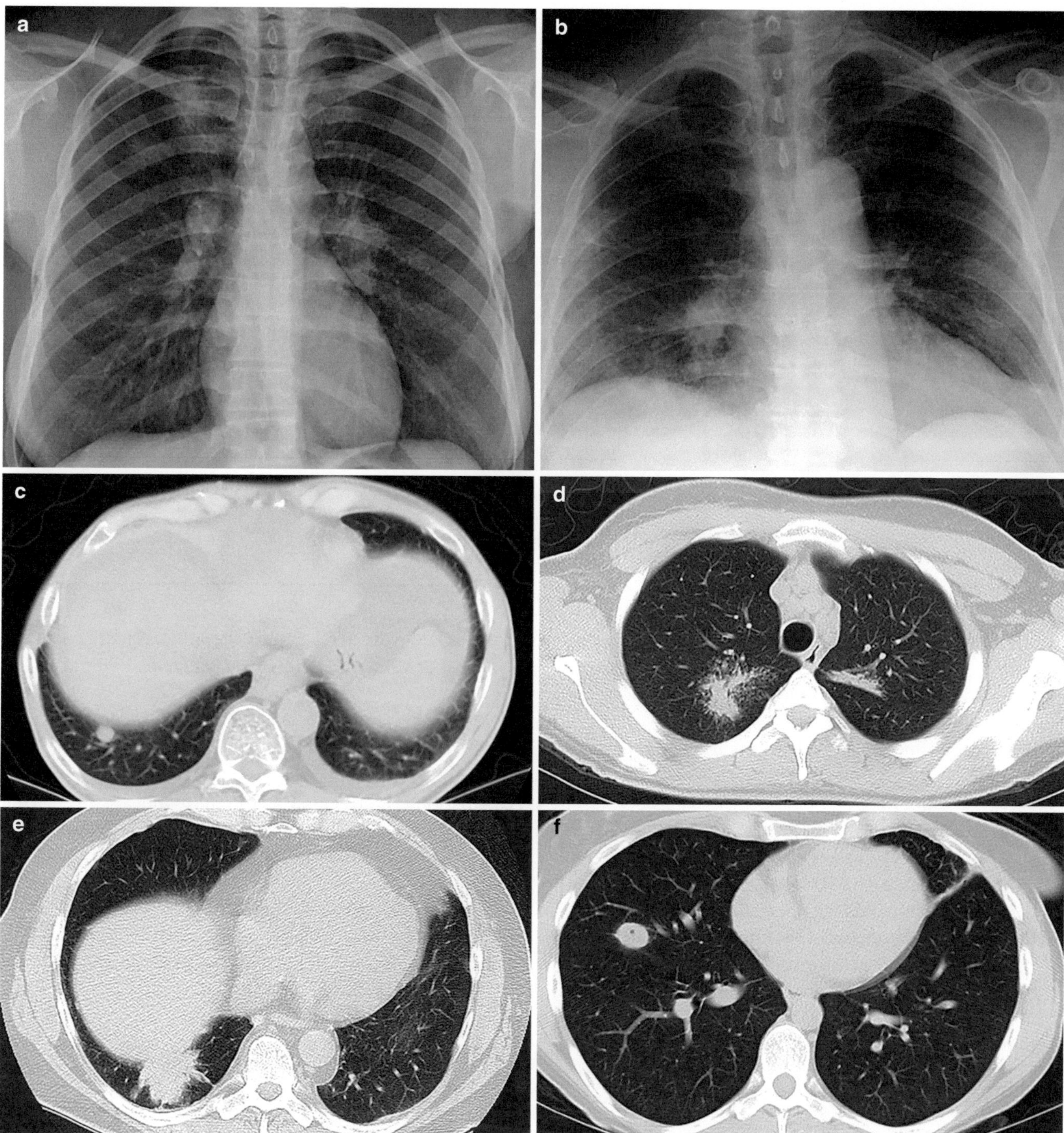

Fig. 3.2 (**a**, **b**) Chest x-ray images of granulomas. (**a**) Anteroposterior view shows a right upper lobe opacity in a patient with sarcoidosis; the same patient as in **d**. (**b**) Anteroposterior view shows a right mid-lung opacity and a right hilar lymph node enlargement; the same patient as in **e**. (**c**–**f**) Chest CT scan images of granulomas. (**c**) A right lower lobe granuloma. (**d**) A right upper lobe density in a patient with sarcoidosis; the same patient as in **a**. (**e**) A right lower lobe mass; the same patient as in **b**. (**f**) A right middle lobe cavitary nodule in a patient with granulomatosis with polyangiitis (Wegener granulomatosis). (**g**–**l**) Cytology and histology of granulomas. (**g**–**i**) Necrotizing granuloma. Diff-Quik-stained smear, 400× (**g**), core histology, hematoxylin and eosin stain, 200× (**h**), and Gomori methenamine silver stain (GMS) shows fungal organisms, 600× (**i**). (**j**–**l**) Noncaseating granuloma. Diff-Quik stained smear, 600× (**j**), core histology, hematoxylin and eosin stain, 400× (**k**) and GMS stain, 400× (**l**)

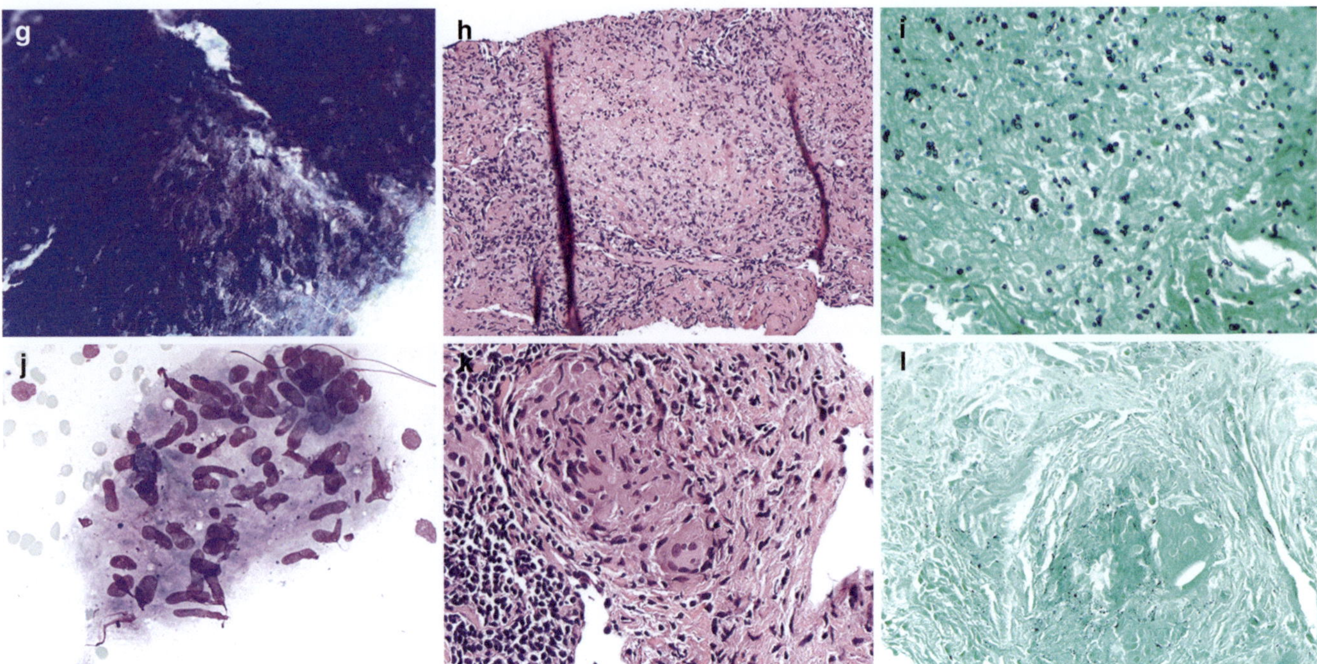

Fig. 3.2 (continued)

cells may be present. Langerhans giant cells are particularly characteristic of tuberculosis.
- Caseating (Fig. 3.2g) and noncaseating granuloma subtyping is possible (Fig. 3.2j).
- Acute or chronic inflammation may also be present.

Histology of Core and Cell Block
- Lung parenchyma with epithelioid histiocytic aggregates with or without necrosis (Fig. 3.2h, k).
- Granulomas often have lymphocytes and possibly neutrophils and eosinophils.
- Fungal or mycobacterial organisms may be seen.
- If the granulomas are associated with malignancy, the malignant tumor cells may be seen as well.

Comments
- The differential diagnosis includes malignancy, infectious etiologies, inflammatory causes, and miscellaneous entities. Adenocarcinoma should be included in the differential diagnosis since epithelioid histiocytic aggregates may mimic adenocarcinoma or squamous carcinoma.
- For a suspected infectious etiology, a core biopsy or an aliquot of FNA can be submitted for culture. FNA can be used to prepare a cell block, for special stains (Fig. 3.2i, l).
- Polarized light is useful for identification of refractory material such as talc.
- Immunohistochemical (IHC) stains for CD68/163 and special stains for lysosomal enzymes are useful to identify histiocytes. IHC stains for epithelial markers (AE1/AE3, CAM5.2) are helpful to exclude carcinoma.

Hamartoma

A hamartoma is a benign neoplasm composed of varying proportions of mesenchymal tissues, typically combined with entrapped respiratory epithelium.

Clinical
- Incidence is 0.25% [10].
- Accounts for about 75% of benign lung tumors.
- Male/female ratio 2:1 to 4:1.
- Peak incidence is in the sixth decade [11].
- Typically present as asymptomatic nodules that are usually less than 4 cm, solitary, well-circumscribed, sometimes calcified, and peripherally located [11].

Radiographic Findings

X-ray
- On chest radiographs, pulmonary hamartomas characteristically appear as well-defined, solitary pulmonary nodules. They may show erratic patterns of calcification, including irregular popcorn and stippled or curvilinear patterns or even a combination of all three. "Popcorn" calcifications are often diagnostic (Fig. 3.3a, b).

CT Scan

- The fundamental appearance of hamartomas on CT scans is similar to those on chest radiographs, but calcifications and fat are better visualized with CT than with radiography (Fig. 3.3c, d).
- The Hounsfield values for fat lie within the range of −50 to −120 HU. Fat is present in 34% to 50% of hamartomatous lesions, and calcifications are seen in 15% to 30% of cases. Calcifications are typically distributed in a clumped distribution throughout the lesion; this pattern is known as popcorn configuration [12].

MRI

- Magnetic resonance imaging (MRI) is not used in the detection or diagnosis of pulmonary hamartomas. However, it is the modality of choice for screening and follow-up of patients with the Carney triad to screen for paragangliomas.
  - On T1, heterogeneous signals, mostly intermediate signals, are present. Foci of high signals represent fat, and low signal foci represent fibrosis or calcifications.
  - On T2, high signals are caused by fat and cartilaginous components, whereas low signals represent fibrotic or calcified material.

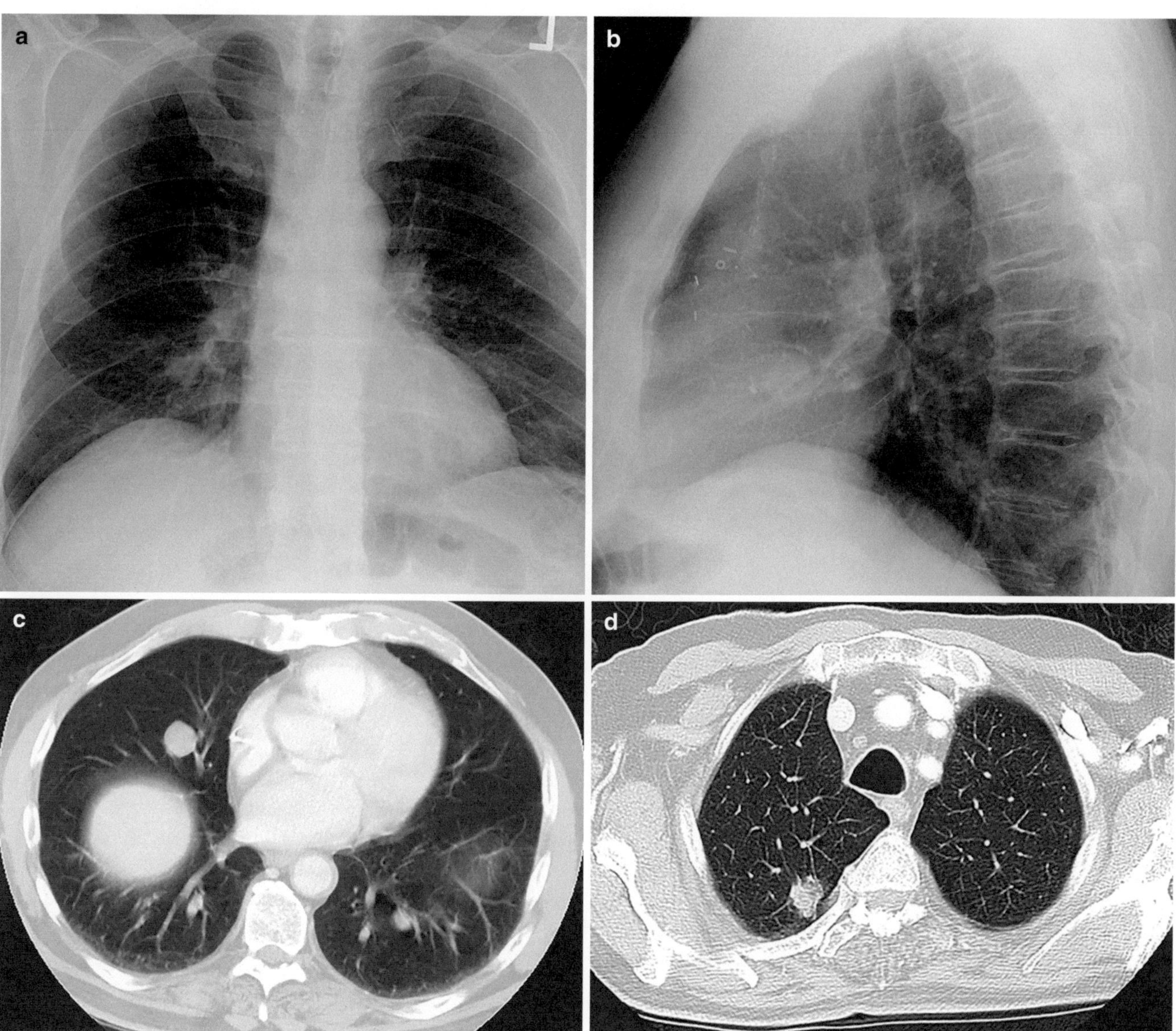

Fig. 3.3 (**a**, **b**) Chest x-ray images of hamartoma. Anteroposterior view (**a**) and lateral view (**b**) show bilateral lower lung nodules; the same patient as in **c**. (**c**, **d**) CT scan images of hamartoma. (**c**) Bilateral lower lung nodules; the same patient as in **a** and **b**. (**d**) A right upper lobe nodule. (**e–h**) Cytology and histology of hamartoma. (**e**) Cytology of immature cartilage, Diff-Quik stain, 400×. (**f**) Cytology of adipose tissue, Diff-Quik stain, 400×. (**g**) Cytology of ciliated bronchial cells, Diff-Quik stain, 400×. (**h**) Histology of core, hematoxylin and eosin stain, 200×

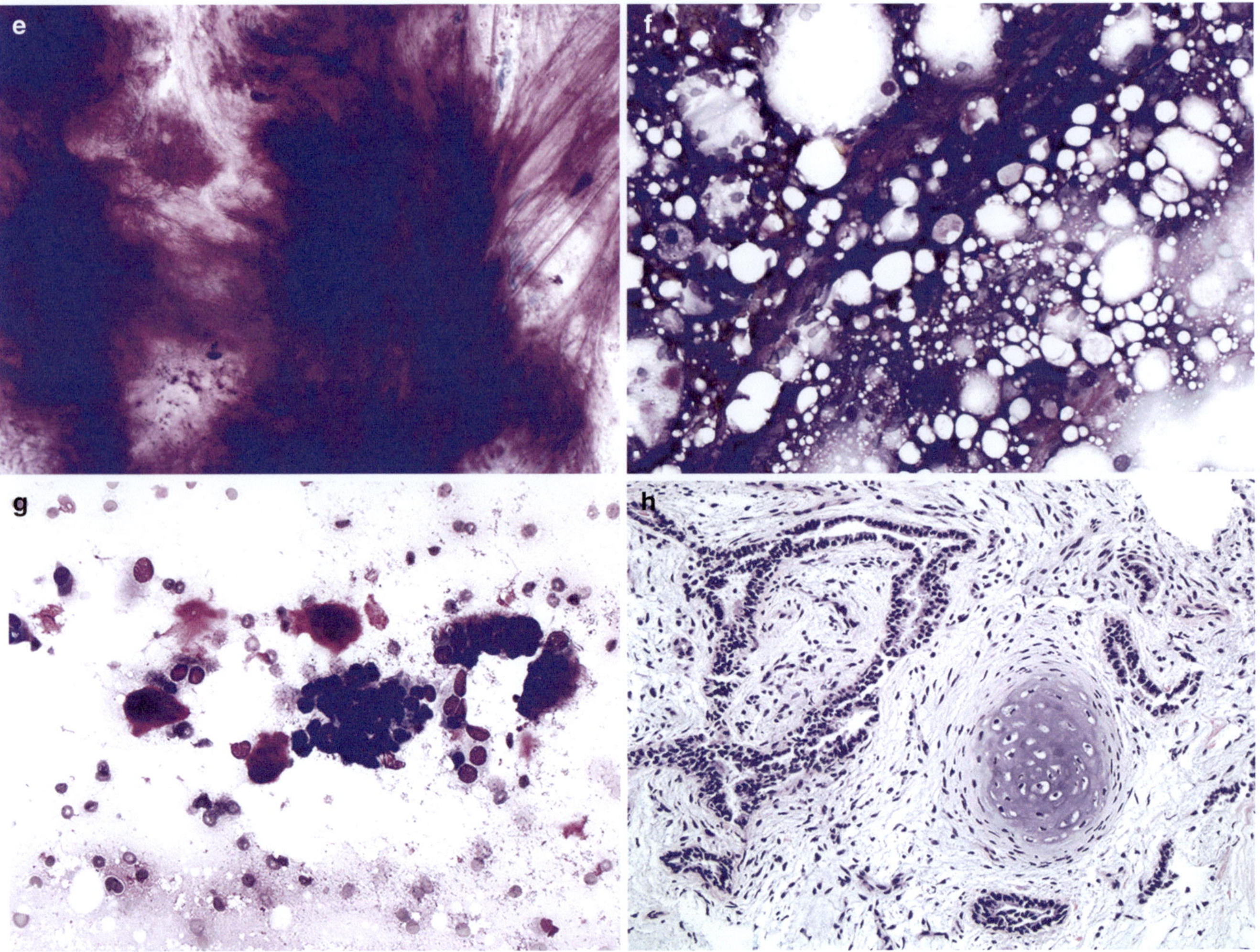

Fig. 3.3 (continued)

- On gadolinium-enhanced T1-weighted axial MRI, heterogeneous enhancement is seen.

PET Images

- Although it is less common, increased avidity may be seen on fluorodeoxyglucose–positron emission tomography (FDG-PET) [13]. Therefore, investigation with PET-CT is confusing, unnecessary, and can contribute to an increased radiation dose.

Cytology of FNA and Touch Preparation

- Characteristically hamartomas show immature fibromyxoid cartilage and/or mature cartilage that is dense, irregular, and homogeneous. The cartilage stains dark blue or purple on Papanicolaou stain and magenta on Diff-Quik stain (Fig. 3.3e).
- Bronchial cells (ciliated and/or nonciliated) and metaplastic cells (possibly with reactive atypia), fat, muscle, fibroconnective tissue, lymphocytes, and histiocytes may be present in variable proportions (Fig. 3.3f, g) in a clean background.

Histology of Core and Cell Block

- Lung parenchyma with a focus composed of a mixture of cartilage, normal bronchial epithelium, and fibroadipose tissue (Fig. 3.3h).

Comments

- The differential diagnosis includes:
  - Malignancy (misinterpreting reactive atypia of bronchial or metaplastic cells) [14].
  - Normal tissue (misinterpreting cartilage, fat, muscle, and bone as from the bronchi and chest wall).
  - Cartilage-producing tumors (teratoma, pulmonary blastoma, pleomorphic adenoma, chondrosarcoma, or osteosarcoma).
  - Connective tissue disease with mucus or basement membrane material (including granulomas, organizing pneumonia, pulmonary infarct, and adenoid cystic carcinoma).
- Hamartoma is a common cause of false positive diagnoses as it may be confused with carcinoid, adenocarcinoma, or

small-cell carcinoma, depending on the components that are present [15].

Inflammatory Myofibroblastic Tumor

Inflammatory myofibroblastic tumor (IMT) is a neoplastic entity thought to be within the broader category of inflammatory pseudotumors. IMTs are composed of collagen, mixed inflammatory cells, and cytologically bland spindle cells showing myofibroblastic differentiation.

Clinical

- IMT occurs at all ages but are most common in patients younger than 40 years [16, 17]. It is the most common endobronchial mesenchymal lesion in childhood.
- It shows no racial or gender predilection [16, 17].
- Most IMTs are asymptomatic, slow-growing, well-circumscribed, and small peripherally located lung masses. Patients with endobronchial lesions complain of bronchial irritation.

Radiographic Findings

X-ray

- IMT of the lung can be detected by chest radiograph, which shows a solitary, well-circumscribed mass or ill-defined, pneumonia-like density. Focal calcifications, coin shadow, multiple nodules, and locally invasive disease have also been reported.

CT Scan

- Chest CT scan is obtained to clarify the extent of disease. IMT usually appears as a single peripheral lobulated mass, predominantly occurring in the lower lobes. However, multiple lesions are seen in approximately 5% of cases. Calcifications can occur and are more common in children. IMT shows heterogeneous enhancement on CT. Rarely, IMT can appear in the upper lobe of the lung and may display homogeneous enhancement on contrast CT [18].

PET Image:

- IMT can also be FDG-avid on PET/CT imaging with high standardized update value (SUV) values. The range of reported SUV values varies from 5 to >35 g/mL. The possible cause for such a high uptake in these benign tumors may be caused by the intense inflammatory infiltrate, as the name implies.

Cytology of FNA and Touch Preparation

- The FNA findings are nonspecific (Fig. 3.4a, b), and the diagnostic accuracy is quite low (42%) [19].
- Characteristically IMTs show myofibroblasts (sometimes forming whorls) and variable proportions of acute and chronic inflammatory cells, multinucleated histiocytes, granulation tissue, and edematous, myxoid, fibrous or hyalinized stroma [19, 20].
- Myofibroblasts appear spindled or stellate, with cellular processes and fibrillary cytoplasm. The nuclei are plump or oval with fine chromatin and one or two nucleoli. Reactive myofibroblasts have enlarged hyperchromatic nuclei and prominent nucleoli. Mitotic figures are few or absent.

Histology of Core and Cell Block

- IMT lesions show inflammatory cells, bland spindle cells, and collagenous stroma (Fig. 3.4c).

Comments

- The differential diagnosis includes:
  - Infection
  - Inflammatory processes, including non-neoplastic inflammatory pseudotumors
  - Plasmacytoma or IgG4-related sclerosing disease [21]
  - Primary or metastatic sarcoma
  - Sarcomatoid carcinoma
  - Melanoma
- Myofibroblasts are positive for vimentin, smooth muscle actin, and rarely desmin [22]. IHC for the ALK-1 is positive in 36–50% of cases (Fig. 3.4d) [21, 23].
- Clonal changes in the ALK gene (chromosome 2p23), including the t(2;5) translocation, are seen in approximately two thirds of cases [23, 24].
- Extrapulmonary sites for IMT include the stomach, liver, pancreas, kidney, soft tissue, bladder, and central nervous system.

Primary Lung Malignancies

Lung cancer is the most common lethal cancer in both men and women [25]. The male/female ratio is 2.7:1 [25], although the frequency is decreasing in men and increasing among women. Most patients with lung cancer are older than 40 years, with a peak incidence around 60 years. Lung cancer is strongly associated with both first- and second-hand smoke [25]. Molecular advances have become increasingly important in determining targeted chemotherapy choices, particularly in cases of lung adenocarcinoma, since the majority of patients with stage III/IV disease are poor surgical candidates [26]. Additionally, FNA cytology plays a critical role in staging cancer patients to determine treatment options, including surgical resection.

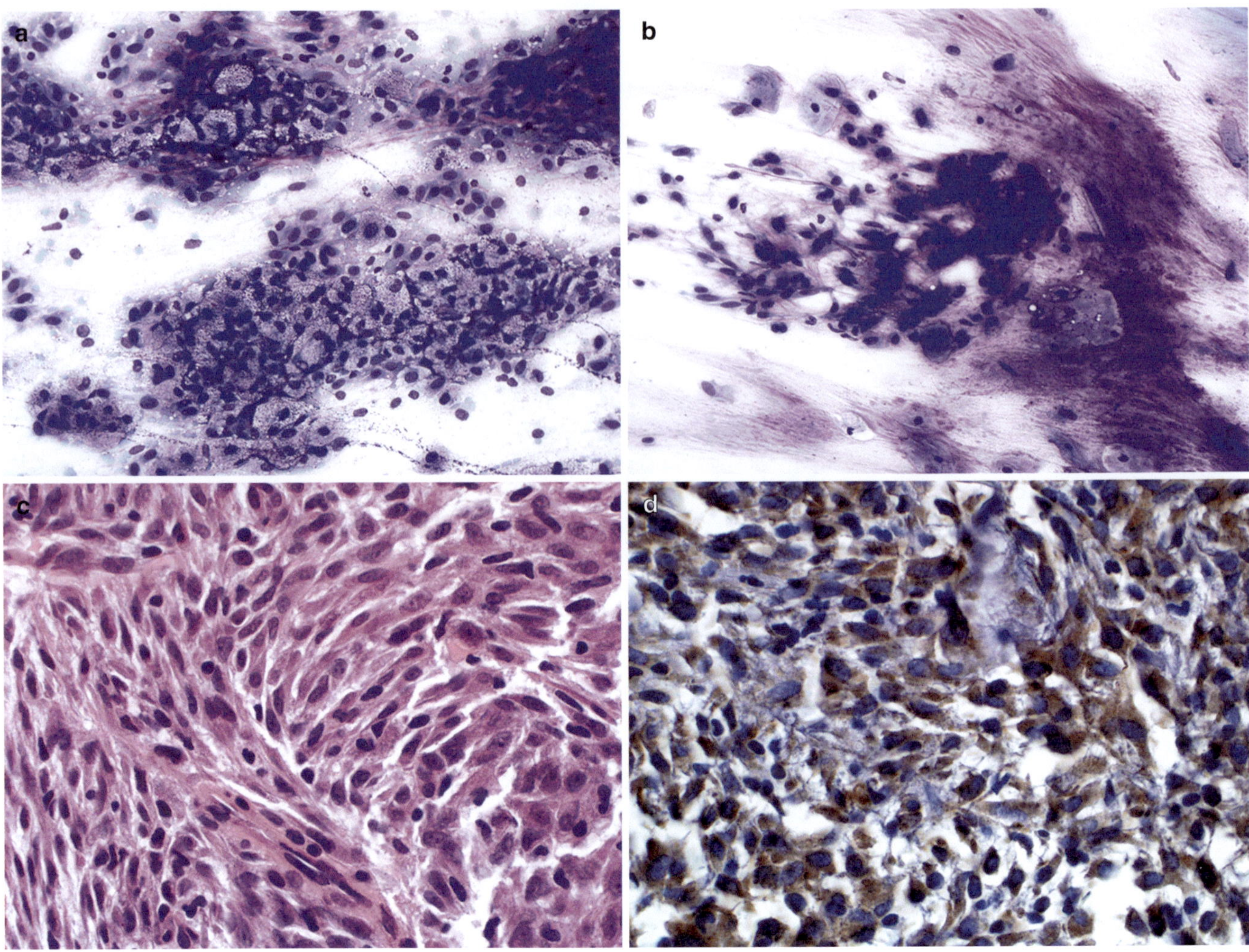

Fig. 3.4 (**a–d**) Cytology and histology of inflammatory myofibroblastic tumor. (**a**, **b**) Cytology, Diff-Quik stain, 200×. (**c**) Histology of core, hematoxylin-and-eosin stain, 600×. (**d**) Immunostain for ALK-1, 600×

Squamous Cell Carcinoma

Squamous cell carcinoma (SCC) is a malignant neoplasm arising from the bronchial epithelium and may show keratinization or intercellular bridges. Squamous cell carcinoma most often presents as keratinizing or nonkeratinizing subtypes, but it may also appear as spindle cell, papillary, clear cell, small cell, basaloid and alveolar space-filling subtypes.

Clinical

- It is the most common lung cancer in men and the second most common in women.
- It is strongly associated with cigarette smoking [25].
- Most cases arise centrally in the mainstem, lobar, or segmental bronchi [27].

Radiographic Findings

While it is not possible to differentiate squamous cell lung cancer from other types of lung cancer on radiography, there are a few classic features that would raise suspicion of a malignant lung lesion.

X-ray

- The diagnostic buoyancy for bronchogenic carcinoma is the greatest when the lesion is at least 8–10 mm.
- The appearance depends on the location of the lesion. Central lesions may appear as a bulky hilum, representing the tumor and local nodal involvement. It may obstruct the bronchus, resulting in lobar collapse. When the right upper lobe is collapsed and a hilar mass is present, this is known as the "Golden S sign." Masses located in the periphery may appear as a rounded or spiculated mass. Cavitation may be interpreted as an air-fluid level (Fig. 3.5a).
- Chest wall invasion is difficult to identify on chest radiography unless there is destruction of the adjacent rib or evidence of tumor growing into the soft tissues superficial to the ribs. Pleural effusion may also be seen.

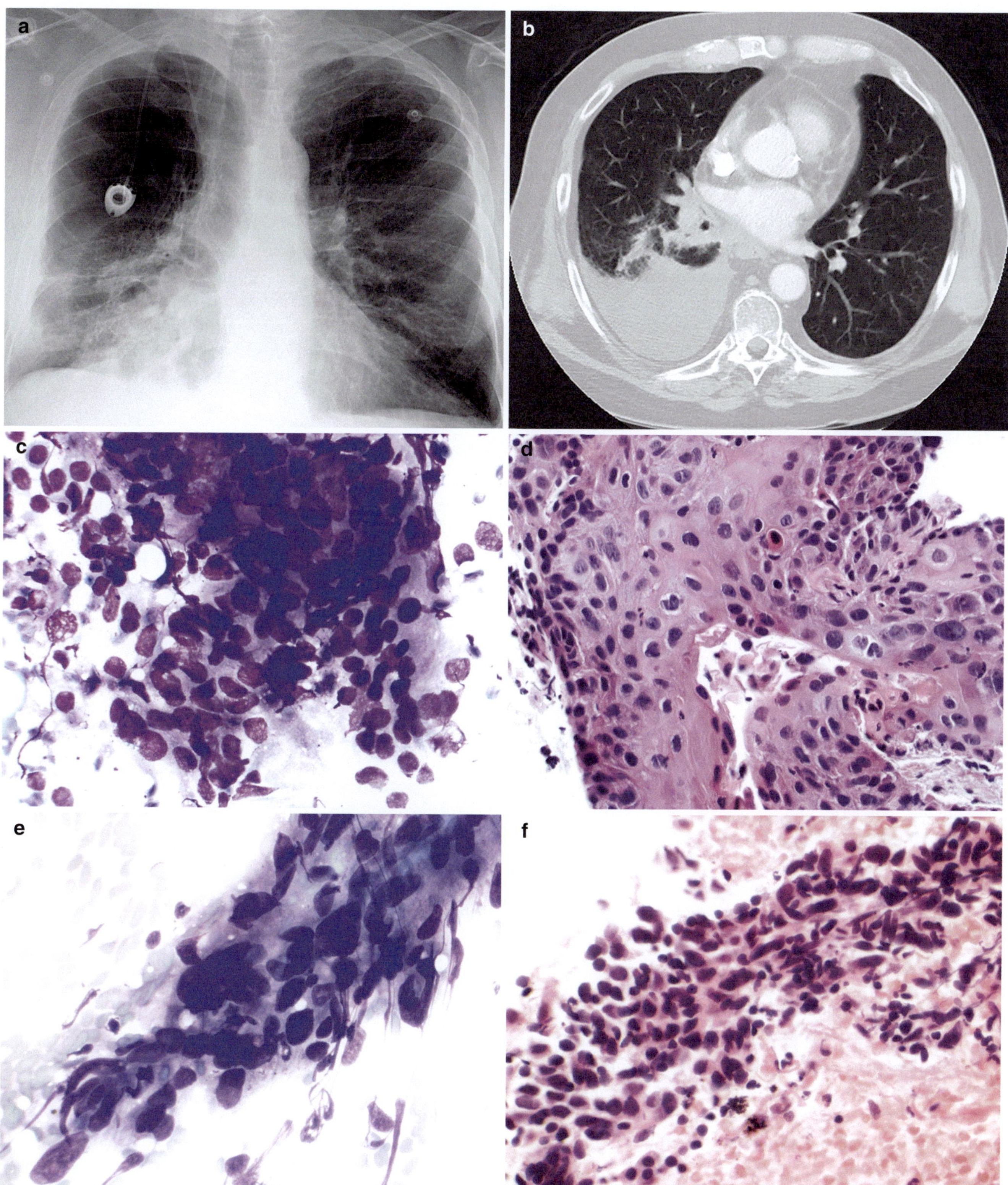

Fig. 3.5 (**a**, **b**) Radiologic images of squamous cell carcinoma. (**a**) Anteroposterior of chest x-ray shows right hilar mass and a bilateral pleural effusion. Chest port is visible. (**b**) CT of chest shows a right hilar mass and bilateral pleural effusion (right-sided greater than left-sided). (**c–f**) Cytology and histology of squamous cell carcinoma. (**c**) Cytology of keratinizing squamous cell carcinoma, Diff-Quik stain, 600×. (**d**) Histology of keratinizing squamous cell carcinoma, hematoxylin and eosin stain, 600×. (**e**), Cytology of nonkeratinizing squamous cell carcinoma. Diff-Quik stain, 600×. (**f**) Histology of nonkeratinizing squamous cell carcinoma, hematoxylin and eosin stain, 600×

CT Scan

CT is the modality of choice for the evaluation of suspected lung cancer. Furthermore, cross-sectional imaging enables staging of the disease and can help in management planning, together with the histologic grading and clinical performance status.

- Central SCC often causes intraluminal obstruction, lung collapse, and/or obstructive pneumonitis. Peripheral SCC may be seen as a solid nodule or mass with or without an irregular border and can also result in obstructive changes such as a mucocele (Fig. 3.5b).
- Cavitation is a common finding in primary lung SCC (seen in up to 82% of cases) and is secondary to tumoral necrosis. It can also be present in metastatic SCC.
- In other instances, SCC may have a central scar with peripheral growth of tumor.

Cytology of FNA and Touch Preparation

Keratinizing Squamous Cell Carcinoma

- Characteristically keratinizing SCC shows single cells or sheets of markedly pleomorphic keratinized cells (Fig. 3.5c). Keratinized cells are often large with a low N/C ratio, pleomorphic nuclei, and distinct cell borders. They commonly show "snake" or "tadpole" forms. The cytoplasm is abundant, dense, or glassy and stains blue or purple on Diff-Quik and yellow/orange on Papanicolaou stain. The cells may contain rings of keratinization around the nucleus or Herxheimer spirals in the cytoplasmic tails [28]. The nuclei are irregularly shaped with coarse, pyknotic, and hyperchromatic nuclei. Nucleoli may also be present. Cells without nuclei (ghost cells) and squamous pearls are also commonly found [28].
- The background is often necrotic. Keratin debris, acute inflammation, and granulomas may be seen.

Non–Keratinizing Squamous Cell Carcinoma

- Characteristically non–keratinizing SCC shows sheets of nonkeratinizing squamous cells (Fig. 3.5e). Tumor cells are comparatively uniform with a high N/C ratio and distinct cell boundaries. The cytoplasm is dense and cyanophilic on Papanicolaou and blue or purple on Diff-Quik stain. The nuclei are centrally located and have irregular nuclear membranes, coarse and hyperchromatic nuclei, and prominent nucleoli.

Histology of Core and Cell Block

- Shows infiltrating nests or sheets of pleomorphic squamous cells with or without cytoplasmic keratinization (Fig. 3.5d, f).

Comment

- The differential diagnosis includes:
  - Poorly-differentiated adenocarcinoma
  - Neuroendocrine carcinoma (large-cell and small-cell carcinoma)
  - Benign reactive changes/reactive mesothelial cells
  - Squamous cell metaplasia
  - Thymoma/thymic carcinoma
- Squamous cells are positive for p63, p40, CK5/6, and K903 and should be negative for TTF-1. The cells are also negative for BerEP4, CK7, and CK20.
- Molecular findings are not well-defined, but future targeted therapy may be directed against *EGFR-1* and CTLA-4 (29). PD-L1 inhibitors are also approved as a first-line therapy in patients with high PD-L1 expression [30].

Adenocarcinoma

Adenocarcinoma is a malignant epithelial neoplasm with glandular differentiation and/or mucin production. Lung adenocarcinoma subtypes include acinar, papillary, lepidic, solid, fetal, mucinous (colloid), mucinous cystic, signet ring, and clear cell variants.

Clinical

- It is the most common type of lung cancer in the United States. It is the most common lung cancer in women and the second most common type in men (40% versus 28%) [25]. The overall incidence of adenocarcinoma is increasing, especially in women [25].
- Adenocarcinoma is the most common type of lung cancer in nonsmokers but may also be associated with cigarette smoking [25].

Radiographic and CT Scan Images of Adenocarcinoma

- Adenocarcinoma may appear as a lung nodule with a rounded or irregular region of increased attenuation. The amount of attenuation can help to further classify the nodules as either ground-glass, subsolid, or solid.
- Adenocarcinoma in situ, minimally invasive adenocarcinoma, and lepidic-predominant invasive adenocarcinoma are often seen as ground-glass nodules or subsolid nodules with a predominant ground-glass component owing to the lepidic growth pattern. While invasive subtypes of adenocarcinoma usually manifest as a solid or subsolid nodule, they can also occasionally be seen as ground-glass nodules (Fig. 3.6a–c).
- Invasive mucinous adenocarcinoma (formerly called mucinous bronchioloalveolar carcinoma) can have a variable appearance and may show air bronchogram, consolidation, or multifocal subsolid nodules or lesions [31].

- There are three distinguishing radiographic patterns for lepidic adenocarcinoma and mucinous adenocarcinoma:
  (a) Single mass or nodular form (~45%)
  (b) Consolidative form (~30%)
  (c) Multinodular form (~25%).
- X-ray
  - Adenocarcinoma with a lepidic pattern and mucinous adenocarcinoma can present as pulmonary nodules, opacities, masses, or clusters of diffuse nodules. The nodular form can be indistinguishable from another adenocarcinoma subtype or inflammatory granuloma on plain film (Fig. 3.6d). They also may show segmental or lobar consolidation with chronic unilateral air-space opacification and air bronchogram
- CT Scan
  - The appearance of lepidic adenocarcinoma on CT depends on its pattern of growth. It may appear as a peripheral nodule (solitary, well circumscribed, or may

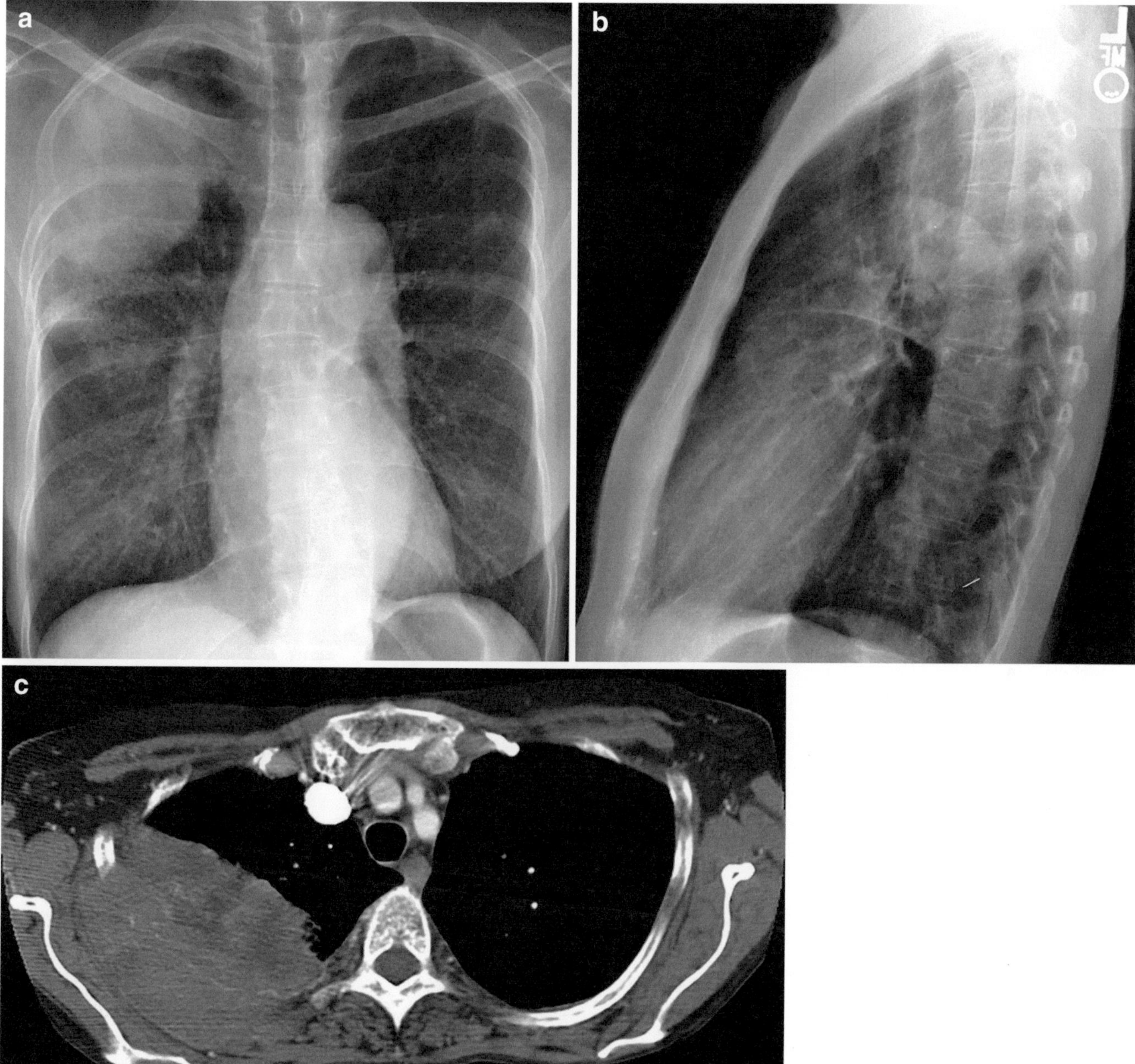

Fig. 3.6 (**a**, **b**) X-ray images of pulmonary adenocarcinoma. (**a**, **b**) Chest radiograph (AP and lateral views) shows a right upper lobe mass. (**c**) CT scan of pulmonary adenocarcinoma shows a right upper lobe mass with soft tissue invading the bones. (**d**, **e**) Radiograph and CT scan of pulmonary adenocarcinoma. (**f–i**) Cytology and histology of pulmonary adenocarcinoma. (**f**) Cytomorphology of touch preparation of needle core, Diff-Quik stain, 600×. (**g**) Histology of core, hematoxylin and eosin stain, 600×. (**h**) Immunostain for TTF-1, 600×. (**i**) Immunostain for napsin A, 600×

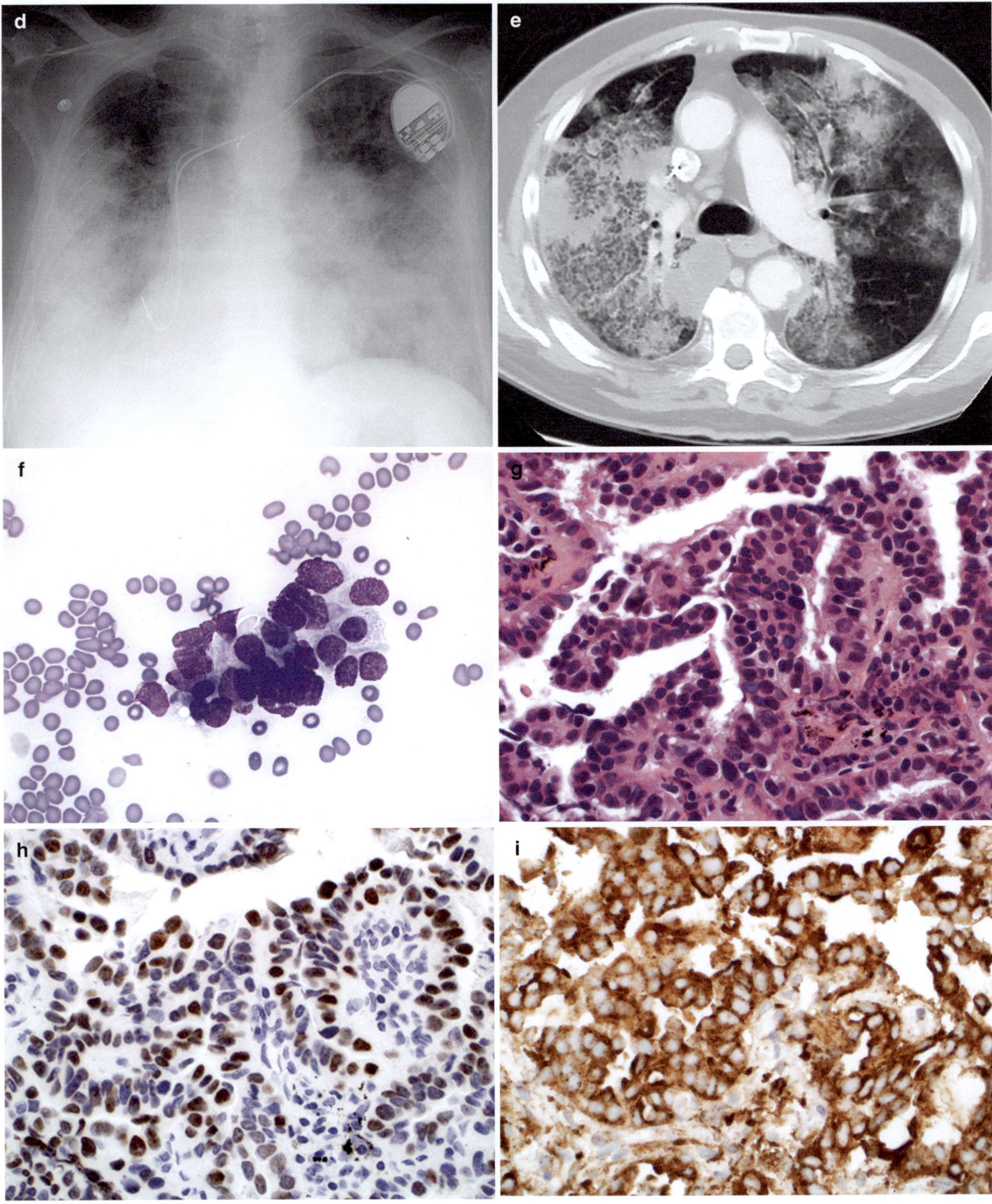

Fig. 3.6 (continued)

be surrounded by a halo of ground-glass opacity, the so-called "Fried Egg Sign"), as a focal area of ground glass with heterogeneous attenuation or as a region of ground glass with or without consolidation (Fig. 3.6e).
  - An air bronchogram may be seen and is known as the "open bronchus sign."
  - Hilar and mediastinal (paratracheal) lymphadenopathy and pleural effusions are uncommon findings.
  - Lepidic adenocarcinoma and mucinous adenocarcinoma are associated with the "CT angiogram sign," referring to vessels that appear prominent during a contrast-enhanced CT as they traverse an airless low attenuation portion of consolidated lung.
- PET Scan
  - Lepidic adenocarcinoma and mucinous adenocarcinoma can be a potential cause of false-negative findings of malignancy on FDG-PET scans and should be interpreted in combination with high-resolution CT findings in suspected cases [32].

Cytology of FNA and Touch Preparation
- The cytomorphology and architecture of tumor cells differ, depending on the subtype of adenocarcinoma.
- Characteristically, glandular differentiation is seen (Fig. 3.6f). The tumor cells appear singly or as three-dimensional disordered clusters of morulae, acini, cell balls with smooth "community" borders, sheets, pseudopapillae, or true papillae with fibrovascular cores.
- The tumor cells are characteristically columnar or cuboidal in shape and exhibit nuclear-cytoplasmic polarity [28]. The amount of cytoplasm is variable and is delicate, granular, or finely vacuolated. They may contain abundant mucin (such as signet ring cells) or intracytoplasmic lumina. The enlarged nuclei are round to oval and may show minimal to significant nuclear membrane irregularity, grooves, and intranuclear cytoplasmic inclusions. The chromatin is open, granular, and unevenly distributed with prominent nucleoli. Binucleation or multinucleation may occur. Cytologic pleomorphism reflects the histologic grade.
- A background of necrosis is often present. Mucus is also present in the background in about 25% of cases [28]. Psammoma bodies may be seen in primary papillary adenocarcinoma or in adenocarcinoma with a lepidic pattern.

Histology of Core and Cell Block
- Adenocarcinoma shows pleomorphic columnar glandular cells that form acini and lepidic, papillary, or solid patterns (Fig. 3.6g).

Comments
- The differential diagnosis includes:
  - Large cell neuroendocrine carcinoma
  - Metastatic adenocarcinoma
  - Nonkeratinizing squamous cell carcinoma
  - Reactive atypia of respiratory epithelial cells
  - Paraganglioma
  - Reactive mesothelial cells
  - Mesothelioma
  - Granuloma
- The tumor cells are positive for TTF-1 (70% to 80%) (Fig. 3.6h) and napsin A (65%) (Fig. 3.6i) [26]. The cells are also positive for CK7 and negative for CK20, CDX-2, and CK5/6. However, mucinous cystadenocarcinoma and some mucinous adenocarcinomas may be positive for CK7, CK20, and CDX-2 and negative for TTF-1 [33].
- Molecular/cytogenetic testing now has a significant predictive role in lung adenocarcinoma as a result of the development of targeted therapies such as *EGFR*, *ALK*, and *ROS1* inhibitors. Thus, testing on FNA or core biopsy material is indicated to determine the presence of mutually exclusive driver mutations for *KRAS*, *EGFR*, and *ALK* gene rearrangements [29, 34, 35]. Additionally, ROS1 rearrangements are present in about 1% of lung adenocarcinomas [36]. PD-L1 inhibitors are also approved as a first-line therapy for patients with high PD-L1 expression [30].

Neuroendocrine Neoplasms of the Lung

Neuroendocrine neoplasms of the lung include carcinoid (typical and atypical carcinoid), large cell neuroendocrine carcinoma, and small cell carcinoma.

Carcinoid Tumor

Carcinoid tumor is characterized by typical growth patterns and cytologic features of tumor cells that suggest neuroendocrine differentiation. It is divided into typical carcinoid (<2 mitoses/2 mm^2 and no necrosis) and atypical carcinoid (2–10 mitoses/2 mm^2 and/or foci of necrosis) [25].

Clinical
- Carcinoid tumors account for approximately 5% of lung tumors.
- The typical carcinoid tumor is most common in middle age (30s–40s) and shows equal gender distribution. It is more common in Caucasians [37].

- Patients rarely develop carcinoid syndrome unless there are widespread metastases [38].
- It is generally considered a low-grade malignancy. Ten to fifteen percent of typical carcinoids metastasize locally and 5–10% metastasize distantly. The most common metastatic site is the liver [25]. In contrast, 40–50% of atypical carcinoids metastasize to regional lymph nodes and beyond. At presentation, approximately 20% of atypical carcinoids are Stage II, 15% Stage III, and 10% Stage IV [39].

Radiographic Findings

X-ray

- On chest radiography, there is either a mass or indirect evidence showing parenchymal changes associated with bronchial obstruction from the mass. Common findings are round or oval opacities with sharp and often notched margins, persistent atelectasis, consolidation secondary to pneumonia, and changes of bronchiectasis and hyperinflation [40].

CT Scan

- High-resolution CT can demonstrate more detailed information about nodules, masses, or suspicious parenchymal changes. Single hilar or perihilar masses are usually well-defined and round or ovoid with eccentric calcification (Fig. 3.7a).
- High-resolution CT can reveal the presence of an air bronchogram within a pulmonary nodule because the majority of carcinoid tumors are intrabronchial. Malignant lesions generally have increased vascularity and show greater enhancement than benign lesions on contrast CT. Carcinoid tumors of the lung often possess some calcifications, although no characteristic pattern is known.
- Peripheral carcinoid tumors may present as solitary lobulated nodules of high attenuation with contrast enhancement, subsegmental airway involvement on thin-section analysis, and be associated with distal hyperlucency, bronchiectasis, or atelectasis.
- Tumors within the bronchi may also be identified.

MRI

- MRI generally provides information similar to that provided by CT. Dynamic MRI may be of use in selected cases.

Cytology of FNA and Touch Preparation

Typical Carcinoid

- Characteristically typical carcinoid shows uniform cells in single and loosely cohesive aggregates arranged in rosettes, acini, flat sheets, or trabeculae (Fig. 3.7b–d) [41]. Conspicuous capillaries and vascularized connective tissue fragments may be seen [42]. There should not be any necrosis present. Crush artifact and mitoses are also uncommon.
- The characteristic tumor cells are plasmacytoid, polygonal, or spindle-shaped. There is minimal to moderate finely granular cytoplasm. The nuclei are centrally located or slightly eccentric and uniformly round to ovoid with smooth nuclear membranes and characteristic "salt-and-pepper" stippled chromatin. Small nucleoli may be present. Occasionally, a few larger atypical cells are present (endocrine atypia), and naked nuclei may be numerous. The spindle cell type may appear somewhat more pleomorphic and may show some nuclear molding.
- Amyloid stroma may be prominent.

Atypical Carcinoid

- The tumor cells often appear larger and more pleomorphic, with a higher nuclear/cytoplasm ratio than typical carcinoids [41]. Nuclei are slightly more hyperchromatic and may have more conspicuous nucleoli.
- Necrosis and/or mitoses are often seen.

Histology of Core and Cell Block

- Uniform small epithelioid cells with round or spindled nuclei containing fine granular chromatin, smooth nuclear membranes, and moderate granular cytoplasm (Fig. 3.7e).
- The tumor cells form trabecular, insular, palisading ribbon, or rosette-like patterns.

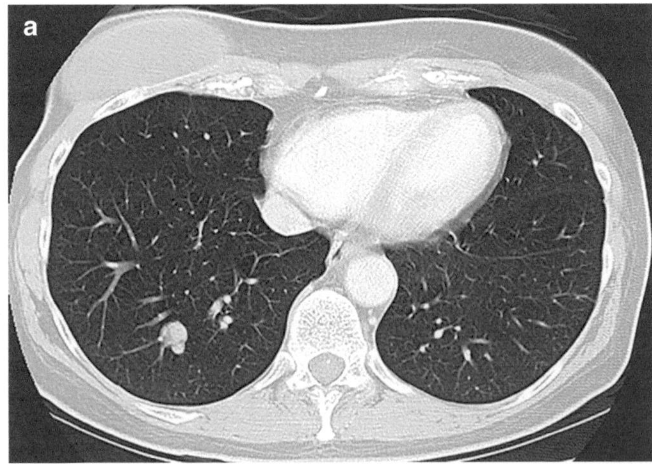

Fig. 3.7 (**a**) CT scan image of carcinoid. CT scan of chest shows a right lower lobe nodule measuring 1.3 cm. (**b–g**) Cytology and histology of carcinoid, typical type. (**b–d**) Cytomorphology of FNA biopsy of a solid lung nodule, Diff-Quik stain (**b**, **c**), 400×, and Papanicolaou stain (**d**), 600×. (**e**) Histology of core, hematoxylin and eosin stain, 600×. (**f**) Immunostain for chromogranin, 400×. (**g**) Immunostain for synaptophysin, 400×

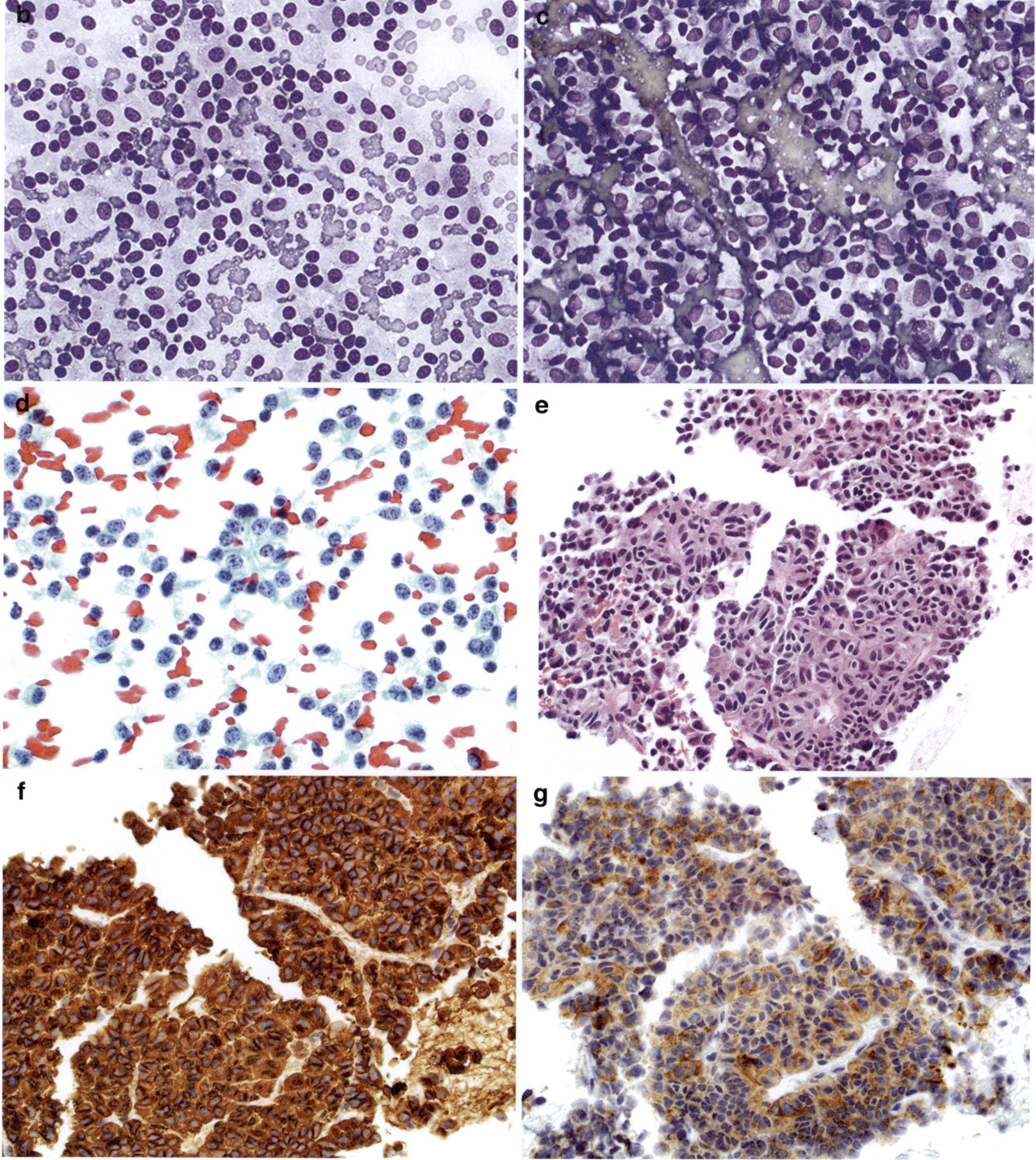

Fig. 3.7 (continued)

Comments

- The differential diagnoses include:
  - Pulmonary tumorlets (<5 mm)
  - Small cell carcinoma
  - Large cell neuroendocrine carcinoma
  - Primary or metastatic adenocarcinoma
  - Paraganglioma
  - Benign bronchial/reserve cells.
- Carcinoid tumors are positive for chromogranin (Fig. 3.7f), synaptophysin (Fig. 3.7g), microtubule-associated protein

2 (MTAP-2), neuron-specific enolase (NSE), CD56, CD57, cytokeratin, and TTF-1 (43%) [43]. Electron microscopy demonstrates desmosomes and dense core neurosecretory granules [44].
- Cellular carcinoid specimens are often a cause overdiagnosis as small cell carcinoma [37].

Small Cell Carcinoma

Small cell carcinoma is a malignant epithelial tumor that is usually centrally located and presents at a high stage. It is strongly associated with cigarette smoking [25].

Clinical

- It accounts for 20% of lung cancer [25].
- The male/female ratio is 4:1, and it is usually diagnosed in the sixth and seventh decades [37].
- It is rapidly growing tumor with a poor prognosis and is commonly associated with paraneoplastic syndromes.

Radiographic Findings

X-ray

- Small cell carcinoma appearance on chest radiography is usually nonspecific. It may be seen as a hilar/perihilar mass with mediastinal widening due to lymph node enlargement. Mediastinal involvement is often the most conspicuous finding, and the primary mass may be subtle.

CT Scan

- On CT imaging, necrosis and hemorrhage are both commonly seen. Rarely, small cell carcinoma presents as a solitary pulmonary nodule. Mediastinal involvement may appear similar to that of lymphoma with numerous enlarged lymph nodes.
- Direct infiltration of adjacent structures is common. Small cell carcinoma of the lung is the most common cause of superior vena cava (SVC) obstruction because of compression, thrombosis, and direct infiltration (Fig. 3.8a) [45].

PET CT Scan

- FDG-PET is a noninvasive method to evaluate mediastinal or distant metastases by detecting areas of high FDG uptake consistent with malignancy. High standardized uptake values are directly correlated with poor prognosis and survival.

Cytology of FNA and Touch Preparation

- FNA biopsy is highly sensitive and specific for the diagnosis of small cell carcinoma.
- Characteristically it shows small to intermediate cells arranged singly, single file, in loosely cohesive syncytial aggregates, and occasionally in rosettes (Fig. 3.8b, c) [41]. The characteristic cells are ovoid or spindled and are two to four times the size of mature lymphocytes. The nuclei are hyperchromatic and have diagnostic nuclear features, including "salt and pepper" stippled chromatin, inconspicuous nucleoli, and nuclear molding. Cellular tangles/nuclear streaming from DNA crush artifact are frequently seen. The cytoplasm is scant and delicate with ill-defined cytoplasmic borders. Perinuclear cytoplasmic inclusions ("blue bodies") are commonly seen. A few larger cells may also be present.
- Necrosis, apoptotic bodies, and mitoses are very common.

Histology of Core and Cell Block

- Nests or sheets of round to spindled small cells with oval nuclei containing stippled chromatin, nuclear molding, and scant cytoplasm (Fig. 3.8d).
- Necrosis, apoptotic figures, and mitotic figures are seen throughout the lesion.

Comments

- The differential diagnosis includes:
  - Large cell neuroendocrine carcinoma
  - Carcinoid
  - Lymphoma (has "lymphoglandular bodies" in the background)
  - Poorly differentiated carcinoma (adenocarcinomas or squamous cell carcinoma)
  - Other small blue cell tumors (Ewing sarcoma, neuroblastoma, rhabdomyosarcoma, Wilms tumor)
  - Benign bronchial epithelial cells/reserve cell hyperplasia
- Small cell carcinoma may be present together with non–small cell carcinoma (usually adenocarcinoma, squamous cell carcinoma, or large cell neuroendocrine carcinoma).
- Small cell carcinoma is positive for neuroendocrine markers, including NSE, neurofilament proteins, chromogranin, synaptophysin, microtubule-associated protein-2 (MTAP-2), Leu-7, and CD56, however these be lost in some cases. It is also positive for TTF-1 (Fig. 3.8e) [43, 46] CK7, and CAM5.2.

Large Cell Carcinoma

Large cell carcinoma is an undifferentiated non–small cell carcinoma that lacks both the cytologic and architectural features of small cell carcinoma as well as glandular or squamous differentiation. This entity includes large cell carcinoma, large cell neuroendocrine carcinoma, combined large cell neuroendocrine carcinoma, basaloid carcinoma, lymphoepithelioma-like carcinoma, clear cell carcinoma, and large cell carcinoma with rhabdoid phenotype.

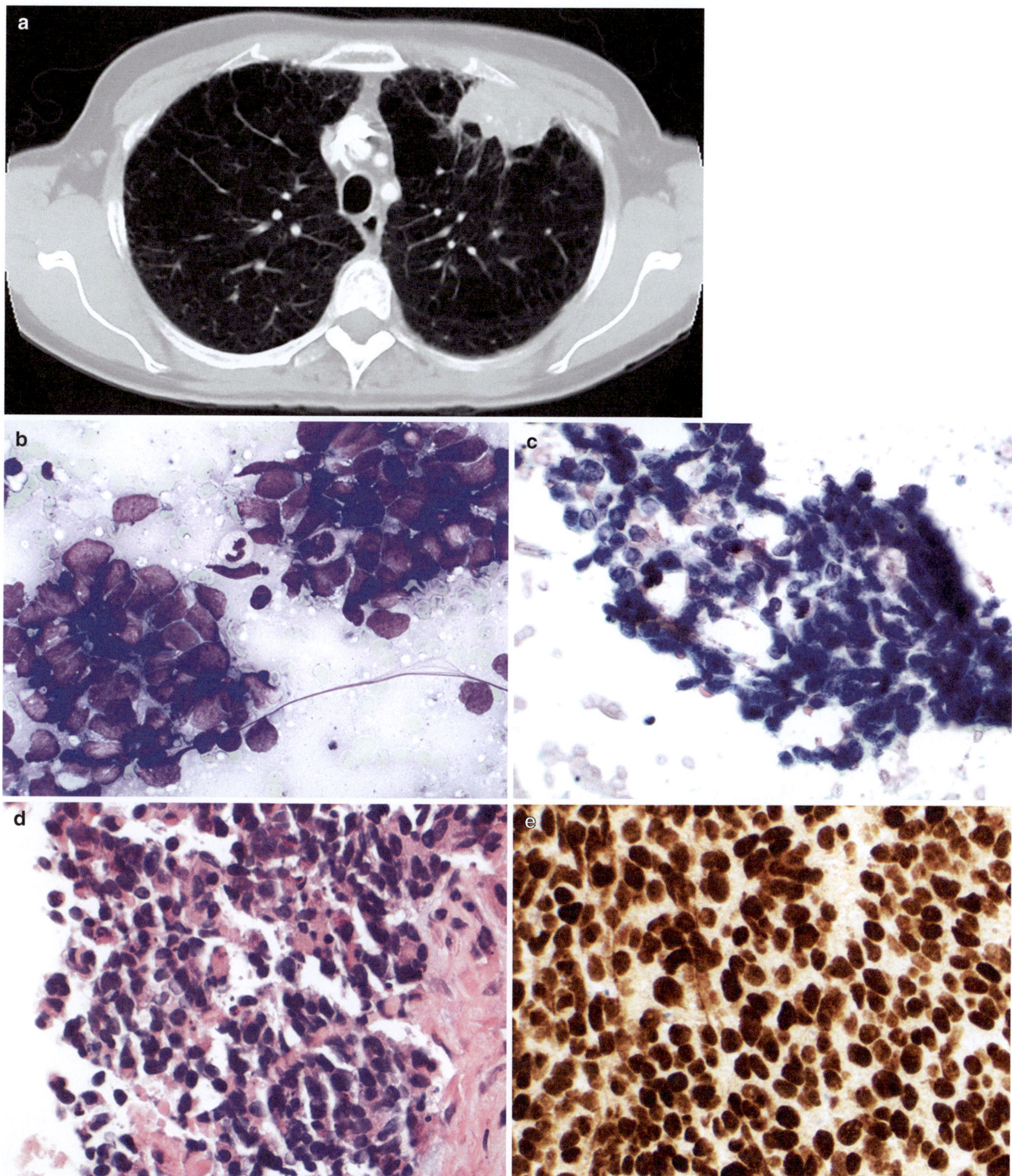

Fig. 3.8 (**a**) Chest CT scan of small cell carcinoma shows a left upper lobe soft tissue mass. (**b–e**) Pathology of small cell carcinoma. (**b, c**) Cytology of biopsy of lung nodule, Diff-Quik stain (**b**) and Papanicolaou stain (**c**), 600×. (**d**) Histology of core, hematoxylin and eosin stain, 600×. (**e**) Immunostain for TTF-1, 400×

Clinical

- Large cell carcinomas account for approximately 9% of all lung cancers [47].
- The average age is approximately 60 years, usually with a male predominance [48, 49]. Only lymphoepithelioma-like carcinoma occurs more frequently in females.
- It is a rapidly growing tumor with a poor prognosis.
- Most cases are related to smoking.
- Most occur in a peripheral location.

Radiographic Findings

A very irregular edge or corona radiata (numerous strands radiating into the surrounding lung) may indicate a bronchogenic carcinoma.

X-ray

- On chest radiograph, large cell carcinoma of the lung presents as a large peripheral mass of solid attenuation with an irregular margin. Focal necrosis can be present. Other characteristics may include rapid growth and early metastasis.

CT Scan

- Large cell carcinoma may present as a peripheral mass or nodule and/or central mass with distal atelectasis. It may be accompanied by mediastinal and hilar lymph node enlargement. The areas of intrinsic lipoid pneumonia and tumor emboli can present as areas of ground-glass opacity surrounding the tumor. Extrathoracic metastases are also a common finding (Fig. 3.9a) [50].

Cytology of FNA and Touch Preparation

- Characteristically large cell carcinoma shows large malignant cells that lack specific differentiation (small cell, squamous, or glandular) (Fig. 3.9b, c). Tumor cells are present singly and in syncytial aggregates. The cytoplasm may range from fine and delicate to granular and dense. The nuclei vary from round to extremely irregular with coarse chromatin. There are prominent nucleoli to macronucleoli. The tumor cells may show perinuclear clearing. The nuclear/cytoplasmic ratio is moderate to high. Mitoses, including abnormal forms, may be frequent and occasional giant multinucleated cells may be seen. If giant multinucleated cells are numerous, giant cell carcinoma should be considered. Necrosis is frequently seen.
- Large cell neuroendocrine carcinoma also shows neuroendocrine features with nuclear palisading and molding; however, these features are distinguished from those of small cell carcinoma by nuclear size, the presence of prominent nucleoli, and the proliferation index (Fig. 3.9b, c) [51].
- Other subtypes:
  - Basaloid carcinoma shows palisading at the periphery of some cellular aggregates.
  - Lymphoepithelioma-like carcinoma shows cohesive flat sheets of malignant cells intimately admixed with abundant small lymphocytes [52]. The tumor cells are spindle-shaped and have solitary large nuclei with large nucleoli.

Histology of Core and Cell Block

- Infiltrating large cells with round nuclei, prominent nucleoli, and moderate to abundant cytoplasm (Fig. 3.9d).
- The tumor cells form nests, trabeculae, rosettes, or peripheral palisading patterns.
- Mitotic figures, apoptotic figures, and necrosis are frequently seen.

Comments

- The differential diagnosis includes:
  - Poorly differentiated squamous cell carcinoma
  - Poorly differentiated adenocarcinoma
  - Giant cell carcinoma
  - Melanoma
- The differential diagnosis of large cell neuroendocrine carcinoma includes atypical carcinoid and basaloid carcinoma.
- The differential diagnosis of basaloid carcinoma includes poorly differentiated squamous cell carcinoma and small cell carcinoma.
- The differential diagnosis of lymphoepithelioma-like carcinoma includes inflammatory pseudotumor, malignant

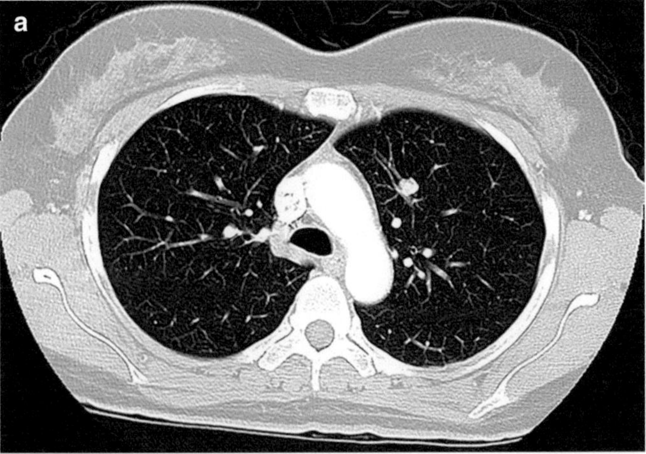

Fig. 3.9 (**a**) Chest CT scan of large cell neuroendocrine carcinoma shows a left upper lobe nodule. (**b–g**) Pathology of large cell neuroendocrine carcinoma. (**b, c**) Cytology of biopsy of lung nodule, Diff-Quik stain (**b**) and Papanicolaou stain (**c**), 600×. (**d**) Histology of core, hematoxylin and eosin stain, 400×. (**e**) Immunostain for TTF-1, 400×. (**f**) Immunostain for chromogranin, 400×. (**g**) Immunostain for synaptophysin, 400×

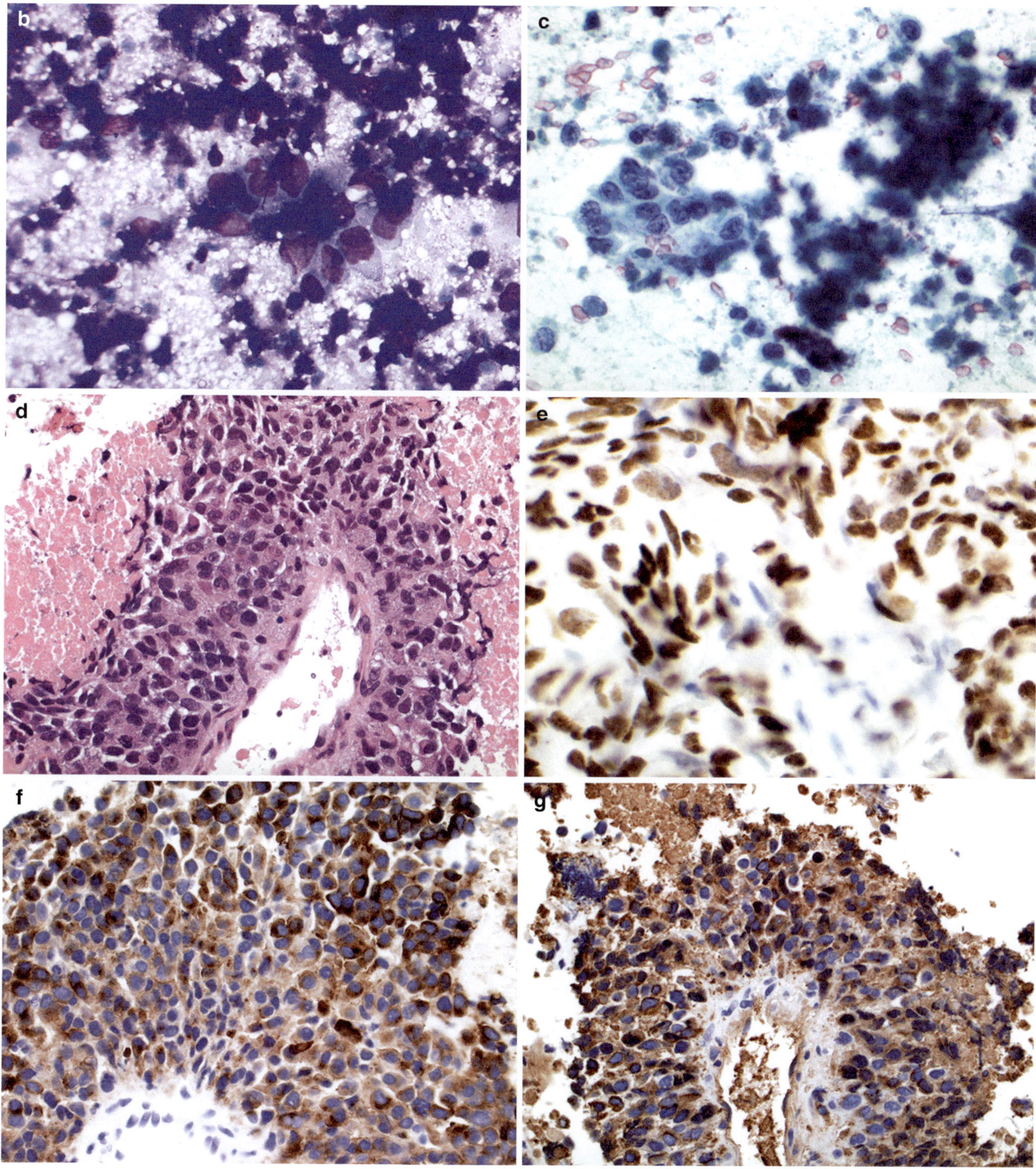

Fig. 3.9 (continued)

lymphoma, and primary lymphoid hyperplasia of the lung.

- The differential diagnosis of clear cell carcinoma includes metastatic renal clear cell carcinoma, squamous cell carcinoma, and adenocarcinoma.
- Large cell neuroendocrine carcinoma is positive for TTF-1 (Fig. 3.9e), chromogranin (Fig. 3.9f), synaptophysin (Fig. 3.9g), NSE, and CD56 [53]. Detection of the BRAF mutation is often used to guide targeted therapy [54].

Mixed Small/Large Cell Neuroendocrine Carcinoma

Mixed neuroendocrine carcinomas are composed of a spectrum of neuroendocrine cells, ranging from typical small cell carcinoma cells to larger cells resembling large cell carcinoma. The nuclei have "salt and pepper" to vesicular chromatin, prominent nucleoli, and variable amounts of slightly cyanophilic to amphophilic cytoplasm on Papanicolaou stain with distinct cytoplasmic cell borders.

Metastatic Malignancy

The lungs are the organs that are most commonly involved by metastatic disease. The most common primary sites of pulmonary metastasis are the colon (32.8%) and breast (28.1%) [55]. Metastatic malignancy should be distinguished from primary lung malignancy.

All new lung nodules in patients with a history of extrapulmonary malignancy should be biopsied for a definitive diagnosis before treatment because of the high frequency of the occurrence of a second primary lung adenocarcinoma (seen in 47.4% of patients). This is critical in determining the appropriate treatment and management for the patient [55]. Overall, 38.5% of patients with primary lung adenocarcinoma have a history of extrapulmonary malignancy. Multiple nodules are not a reliable indicator for metastatic disease. Appropriate immunohistochemical studies. should be performed on cases in which it is difficult to separate the primary malignancy from metastatic tumors.

Mediastinum

Endoscopic ultrasound-guided fine-needle aspiration biopsy (EBUS-FNA) and CT-guided FNA are used to diagnose mediastinal adenopathy of uncertain etiology, including masses, cysts, inflammation, and infection as well as lung cancer staging and upper gastrointestinal cancer staging [2, 56].

Thymoma

Thymoma is a neoplasm arising from or exhibiting differentiation toward thymic epithelial cells. Thymomas are divided into type A (bland spindled to oval epithelial tumor cells with few or no lymphocytes), type B (large polygonal tumor cells with variable numbers of lymphocytes), and type AB (mixture of types A and B). Type B is subclassified into B1, B2, and B3, depending on the number of epithelial tumor cells present and the ratio of epithelial tumor cells to lymphocytes. FNA has a high accuracy rate (86%) [57] and a high positive predictive value (from 69% to 100%) for diagnosis of thymoma [57, 58].

Clinical

- The incidence is 1:15 cases per million [25, 59].
- There is a wide age range (7–89 years), with a peak between 55 and 65 years old; it shows no gender predilection [25].
- It is the most common primary tumor of the anterior mediastinum.

Radiographic Findings

X-ray

- Chest radiographs can vary from subtle mediastinal findings to an obvious mass or widened mediastinum.
- The tumor can be present as a well-defined, lobulated soft tissue density present slightly toward one side of the mediastinum. Calcification can also be seen (Fig. 3.10).

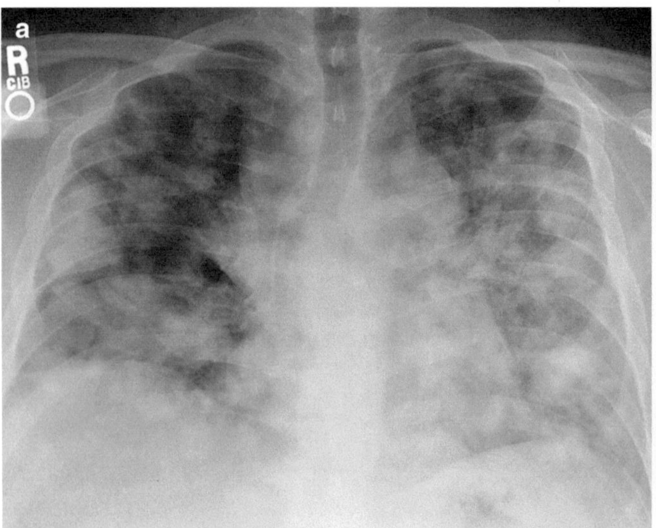

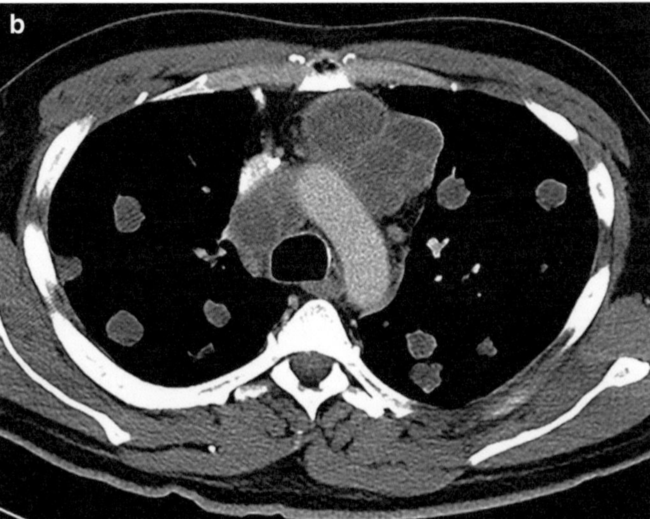

Fig. 3.10 (**a**, **b**) Radiologic images of thymoma. (**a**) Chest x-ray shows multiple bilateral pulmonary nodules. (**b**) Chest CT shows anterior mediastinal mass with multiple pulmonary nodules. (**c**–**h**) Pathology of thymoma. (**c**, **d**) Cytology of thymoma; A (**c**) and B2 (**d**), Diff-Quik stain, 600×. (**e**, **f**) Histology of thymoma; A (**e**) and B2 (**f**), hematoxylin and eosin stain, 600×. (**g**, **h**) Immunostain for p63, A (**g**) and B2 (**h**), 600×

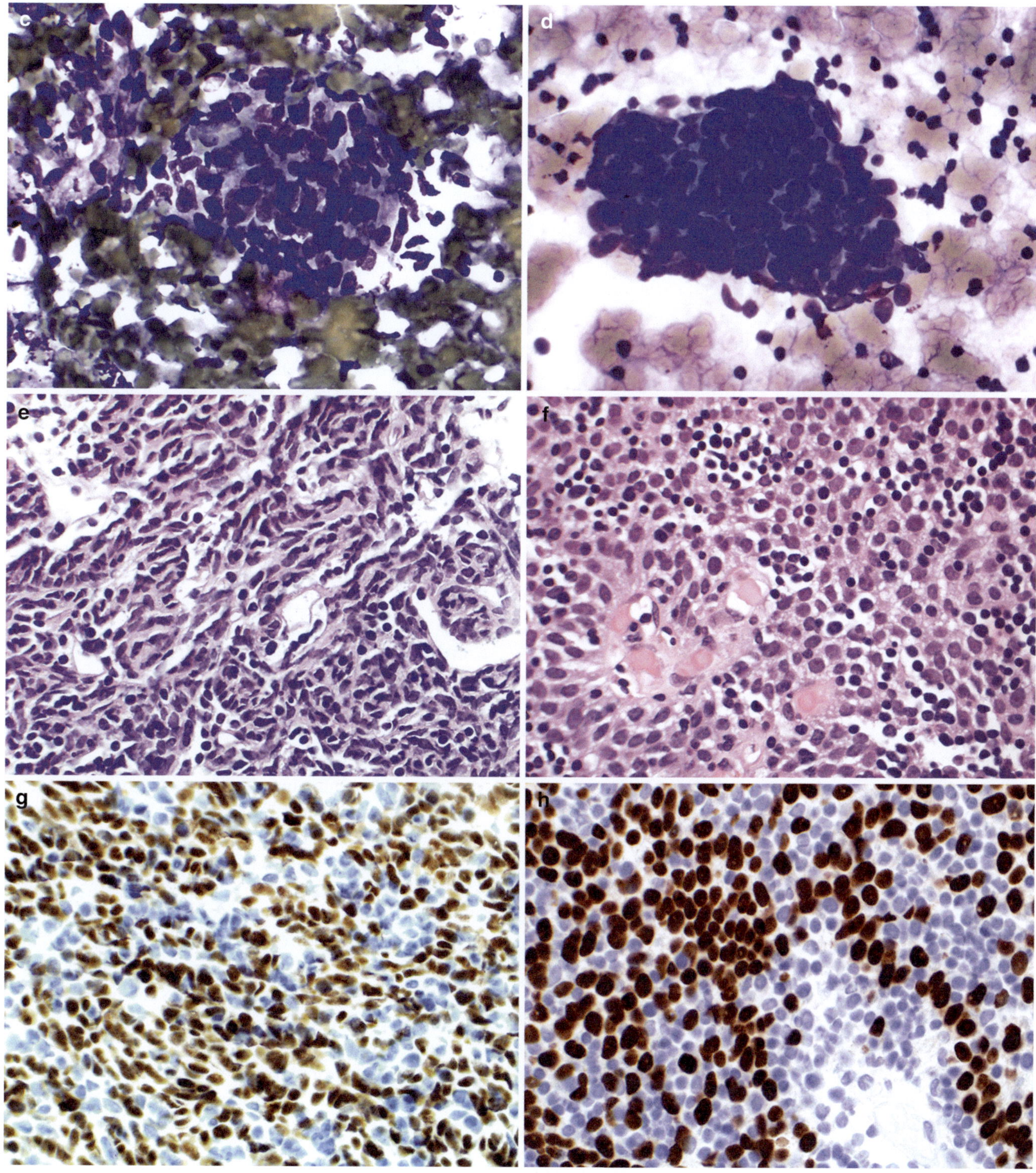

Fig. 3.10 (continued)

CT Scan

CT of the chest with intravenous contrast is typically used to evaluate abnormalities seen on plain radiographs.

- Features that help to differentiate benign thymic epithelial tumors from malignant ones are: (a) larger size and highly aggressive anterior mediastinal mass, (b) areas of necrosis, hemorrhage, calcification, or cyst formation, (c) gross invasion of contiguous mediastinal structures and wide spread involving distant intrathoracic sites, and/or (d) higher incidence of extrathoracic metastases (Fig. 3.10b) [60].

- Increased vascular enhancement, mediastinal lymph node enlargement, and/or pleural seeding on CT scans can also be suggestive of a thymoma.

MRI

MR imaging for an anterior mediastinal mass can be very useful in delineating compression versus invasion. In contrast, MRI can be helpful in posterior mediastinal masses by providing a detailed assessment of the neural foramina or spinal canal [60, 61].

- On T1, isointense to slightly hyperintense signals are seen compared to muscle.
- On T2, heterogeneous signals, slightly higher than muscle, are present. Cystic areas and fibrous septa crossing the mass show a low signal intensity. There is no signal drop (chemical shift) for in/out phase imaging.
- Gadolinium-enhanced T1 imaging shows linear regions of enhancement coursing through the mass, representing fibrous septa [61].

Nuclear Imaging

FDG-PET CT may be useful in differentiating thymic carcinoma from other thymic neoplasms, thymic hyperplasia, and normal physiologic uptake. The standardized uptake value for thymic carcinoma is considered to be significantly greater than that for invasive or noninvasive thymoma. With a standardized uptake value cutoff point of 5.0, thymic carcinoma can be differentiated from thymoma with reasonably high sensitivity (>80%), specificity (>90%), and accuracy (88%).

Cytology of FNA and Touch Preparation

- Characteristically, thymomas show the presence of a dual population of epithelial cells (spindled, round, or polygonal) and lymphocytes in variable proportions [62].
- In type A, spindle cells are present in cohesive groups and rosettes (Fig. 3.10c). The nuclei are elongated and uniform and have granular chromatin and inconspicuous nucleoli [62–64].
- In type B, epithelial cells are present singly, in discohesive small clusters or sheets, and occasionally in rosettes (Fig. 3.10d) [62–65]. There is scant to moderate cytoplasm that appears delicate or dense with indistinct cell borders [64, 65]. The nuclei are bland, round, or oval, and show smooth or slightly irregular contours. They have fine and evenly dispersed granular chromatin and small nucleoli [63, 65]. Mitoses are rare.
- The lymphocytes are predominantly small mature T cells.
- Hassall corpuscles (squamous pearls) are characteristic but infrequently seen and are not necessary for diagnosis. Fibrous fragments from the capsule or septa may also be seen.

Histology of Core and Cell Block

- Type A: Nests of bland spindle cells admixed with small lymphocytes (Fig 3.10e).
- Types B1, B2, and B3: Composed of differing proportions of polygonal epithelioid cells and small lymphocytes. Subclassification of B1, B2 (Fig. 3.10f), and B3 depends on the ratio of epithelioid cells to lymphocytes from predominantly small lymphocytes in B1 to predominantly epithelioid cells in B3. Mild cytologic atypia may be seen in B3.
- Type AB: Admixture of epithelioid cells and spindle cells.

Comments

- The differential diagnosis includes:
  - Thymic hyperplasia
  - Thymic carcinoid
  - Thymic carcinoma
  - Lymphoma (small lymphocytic, follicular, MALToma, lymphoblastic, and Hodgkin)
  - Spindle variant of squamous cell carcinoma
  - Small cell carcinoma
  - Soft tissue and neural tumors
  - Mesothelioma
  - Melanoma
  - Germ cell tumor
- Thymomas have a complex immunohistochemistry pattern, which can overlap with other tumors such as squamous cell carcinoma. The IHC-staining pattern depends on the type of thymona [59].
  - Type A thymoma
    - Spindle tumor cells are positive for p63 (Fig. 3.10g), AE1/AE3, and CK7, are focally positive for BCL-2, CD57, calretinin, and EMA, and are negative for CK20 and CD5. Lymphocytes are positive for CD3 and CD5. Immature T cells may also be present, which are positive for CD1a and CD99 but should make up only a minority of the T-cell population. CD20 B cells are usually absent.
  - Type B thymoma
    - Epithelial cells are positive for p63 (Fig. 3.10h), CD19, AE1/AE3, CK14, and CK18 and are variably positive for CK7. Expression of CD5 and CD20 are also variable, depending on the subtype. Cortical T cells are positive for CD1a, CD4, CD8, CD5, CD99, and TdT.
- When CD57 is strongly positive, it is highly associated with neuromuscular disorders, especially myasthenia gravis [59].

Thymic Carcinoma

Thymic carcinoma (Type C thymoma) is a malignant epithelial tumor with overt cytologic atypia. Thymic carcinomas range from low-grade and well-differentiated to high-grade and poorly differentiated. They are sub-typed according to their differentiation which includes non–keratinizing squamous cell carcinoma, basaloid carcinoma, mucoepidermoid carcinoma, lymphoepithelioma-like carcinoma, sarcomatoid carcinoma, clear cell carcinoma, papillary adenocarcinoma, nonpapillary adenocarcinoma, midline carcinoma with t(15;19) translocation (BRD4/NUTM1 fusion) [66], and undifferentiated carcinoma. Squamous cell carcinoma is the most frequent subtype [67–69].

Clinical

- It is a very rare entity.
- The age range is from 30 to 60 years [69].
- Paraneoplastic syndrome and symptoms are less common than with thymoma.

Cytology of FNA and Touch Preparation

- Characteristically thymic carcinoma shows clearly malignant tumor cells with marked atypia, pleomorphism, enlarged nuclei, coarse chromatin, prominent nucleoli, moderate cytoplasm, and numerous and bizarre mitotic figures (Fig. 3.11a, b). Except for lymphoepithelioma-like carcinoma, thymic carcinoma usually lacks the dual cell populations that are a characteristic of other types of thymomas. Cytomorphology of the tumors varies, depending on the subtype of thymic carcinoma; each is similar to its counterpart in other organs. Necrosis may be seen.

Histology of Core and Cell Block

- Nests or sheets of markedly atypical epithelial cells separated by hypocellular, dense collagen (Fig. 3.11c).

Comment

- The differential diagnosis includes:
  - Thymoma
  - Germ cell tumor
  - Metastatic carcinoma
  - Diffuse large B-cell lymphoma
  - Metastatic sarcoma
  - Mesothelioma

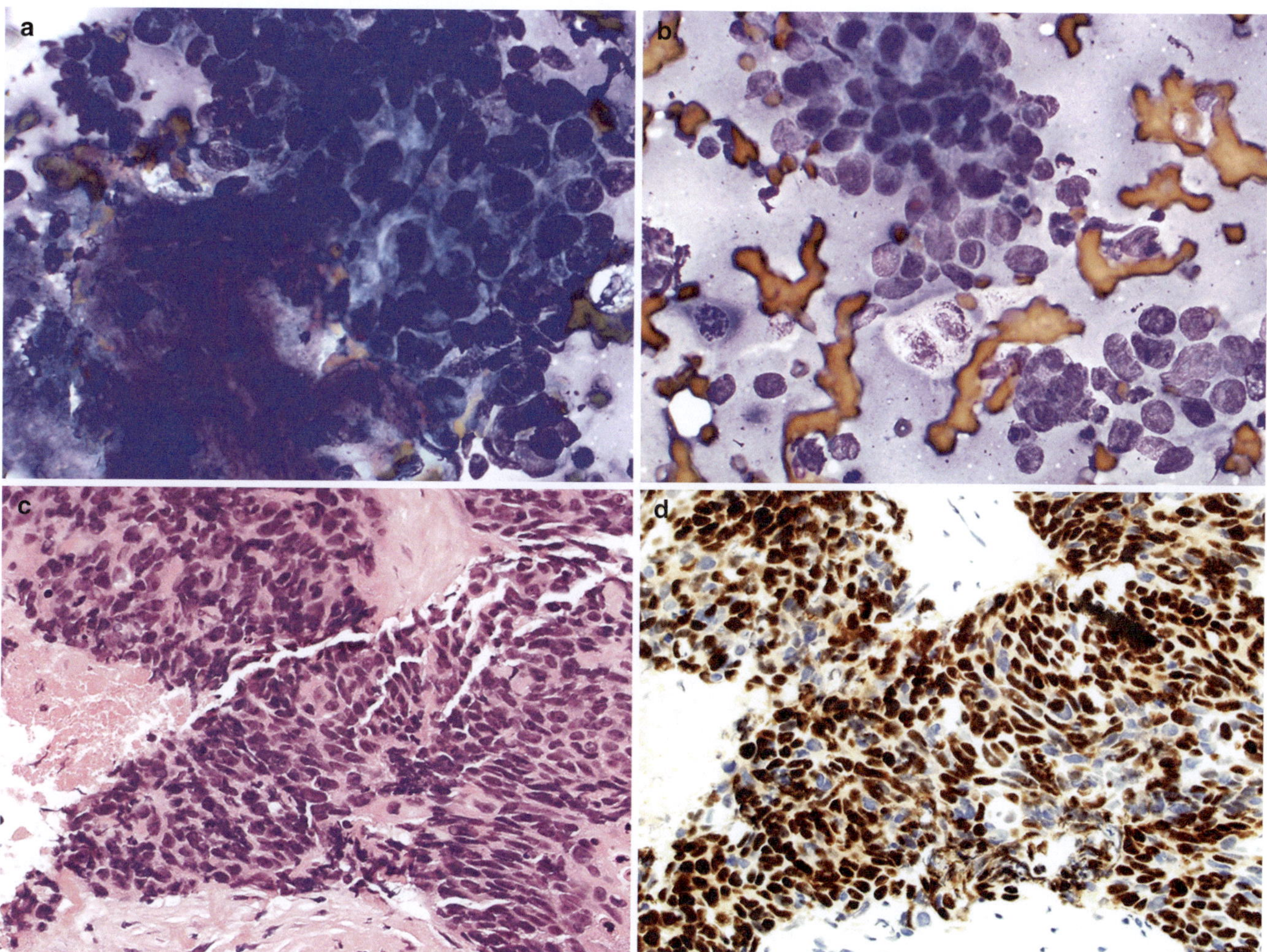

Fig. 3.11 (**a**–**f**) Pathology of thymic carcinoma. (**a**, **b**) Cytology of core touch preparation, Diff-Quik stain, 600×. (**c**) Histology of core, hematoxylin and eosin stain, 600×. (**d**) Immunostain for p63, 600×. (**e**) Immunostain for CD5, 600×. (**f**) Immunostain for CD117, 600×

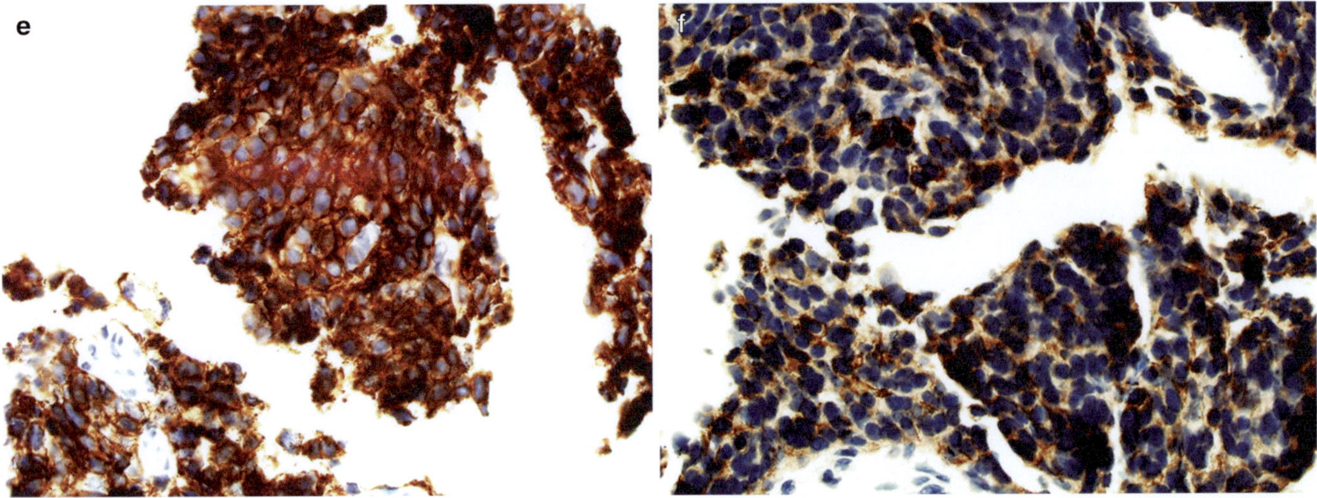

Fig. 3.11 (continued)

- Thymic carcinoma is positive for p63 (Fig. 3.11d), CD5 (Fig. 3.11e), CD117 (Fig. 3.11f), CD56, CK5.6, and CK7.

Thymic Neuroendocrine Tumors

Thymic neuroendocrine tumors are thymic epithelial tumors that are predominantly or exclusively composed of neuroendocrine cells. They are subclassified into typical carcinoid, atypical carcinoid, large cell neuroendocrine carcinoma, and small cell carcinoma. They appear similar to their counterparts arising in the lung and use the same diagnostic criteria [25].

Clinical

- They are rare entities, accounting for 2–5% of thymic epithelial tumors [25].
- The most common variant is atypical carcinoid, and this subtype shows a male predominance [25].

Cytology of FNA and Touch Preparation, and Histology of Core and Cell Block

- The cytomorphology and histology are similar to their counterparts arising in the lung.

Comment

- The differential diagnosis includes:
  - Metastatic neuroendocrine tumors
  - Thymic carcinoma
  - Germ cell tumor
  - Neuroblastoma
  - Lymphoma
  - Adenocarcinoma
  - Squamous cell carcinoma
  - Plasmacytoma
  - Large cell carcinoma

Primary Mediastinal Large B-cell Lymphoma

Primary mediastinal large B-cell lymphoma (PMLBCL) is a type of diffuse large B-cell lymphoma arising in the mediastinum with distinctive clinical, immunophenotypic, and genotypic features [70]. FNA cytology may be useful in the diagnosis, although the sensitivity is only 42% [71].

Clinical

- Most common in the third and fourth decades with a slight female predominance [72].
- Located in anterior/superior aspect of the mediastinum.
- Patients commonly present with superior vena cava syndrome.

Radiographic Findings

X-ray

- The most common features on chest radiographs are multiple nodules, poorly defined opacification with air bronchogram, and mediastinal widening caused by grossly enlarged lymph nodes.
- Less common findings include bilateral airspace consolidation, segmental or lobar atelectasis, and/or pleural effusion (Fig. 3.12a).

CT Scan

- Multiple features may be present on CT, which include: (a) mass or mass-like consolidations (>1 cm) with or without cavitation or bronchogram, (b) masses of pleural origin, (c) nodules <1 cm, (d) alveolar or interstitial infiltrates, (d) peribronchial or perivascular thickening with or without atelectasis, (e) alveolar or interstitial infiltrate (Fig. 3.12b) [73].
- Hilar or mediastinal lymphadenopathy is present and pleural effusion is common.

MRI

- MRI is more accurate in staging mediastinal malignancy, assessing thoracic wall invasion, assessing response to therapy in lymphoma, and assessment of superior vena cava syndrome and other venous obstructions.

Nuclear Imaging

- Lymphomas and thyroid abnormalities may appear as anterior mediastinal masses; therefore, nuclear imaging like technetium-99 m (^{99m}Tc) pertechnetate, iodine-131 (^{131}I), or iodine-123 (^{123}I) may help to confirm or eliminate thyroid tissue as the cause of an anterior mediastinal mass.
- Indium-111 (^{111}In) octreotide and pentetreotide scans may differentiate lymphomas and other mediastinal masses from mediastinal neuroendocrine tumors such as carcinoids.
- Gallium-67 scintigraphy scans are a valuable complement in the detection of viable residual tumor after chemotherapy as well as in the diagnosis of recurrence of lymphoma [74].
- FDG-PET scanning in cases of lymphoma is helpful for the initial diagnosis, diagnosis of recurrent disease, determination of early relapse following chemotherapy, and in long-term remission [74].

Cytology of FNA and Touch Preparation

- Characteristically PMLBCL shows medium to large atypical lymphoid cells. The atypical lymphoid cells vary in size and have large vesicular, hyperchromatic nuclei with irregular or smooth nuclear membranes and scant to moderate amounts of finely vacuolated cytoplasm (Fig. 3.12c) [75, 76]. Lymphoid cells with cleaved or lobulated nuclei may be present [75].
- DNA string artifact, lymphoglandular bodies, and dense fibrous tissue fragments may be seen [75, 76].

Histology and Core and Cell Block

- Fibroconnective tissue infiltrated by large atypical lymphoid cells with prominent nucleoli, irregular nuclear membrane, and small mature-appearing lymphocytes (Fig. 3.12d).

Comments

- The differential diagnosis includes:
  - Thymoma
  - Hodgkin lymphoma
  - Lymphoblastic lymphoma
  - Seminoma/Germ cell tumor
  - Poorly differentiated carcinoma
  - Spindle cell neoplasms [76]
- The tumor cells are usually positive for CD20 (Fig. 3.12f), CD19, CD22, CD79a, and BCL-6 (56–60%) (Fig. 3.12f) and infrequently positive for CD10 (20–25%) and immunoglobulin. CD30 staining is focal and weak. B-cell lymphoma cells are negative for CD3 (Fig. 3.12e).
- Flow cytometry may be useful to detect monoclonal B cells but may demonstrate B cells devoid of surface immunoglobulin expression [75].
- "Gray zone" lymphoma shows clinical and cytologic features that overlap between large B-cell lymphoma and Hodgkin lymphoma, nodular sclerosis subtype [77].

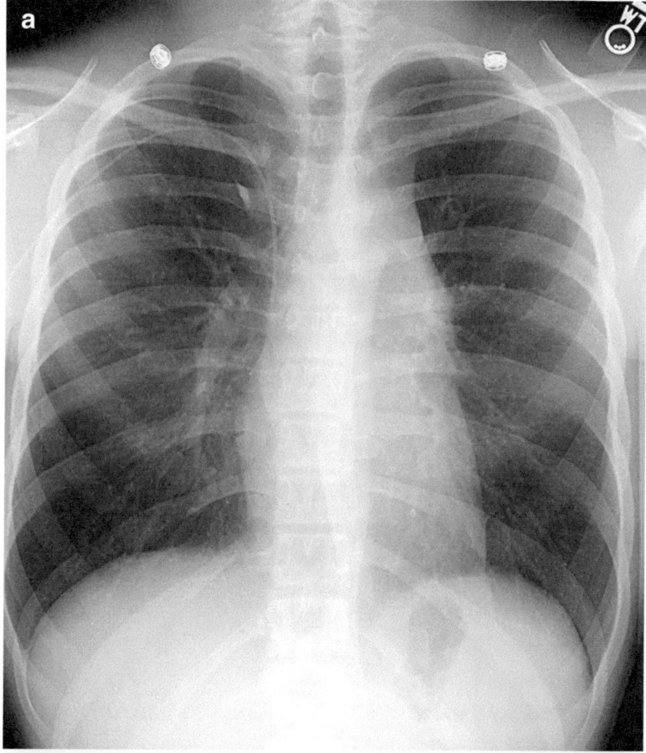

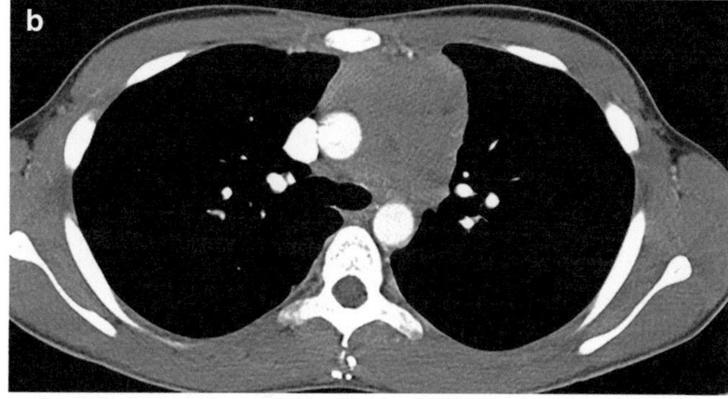

Fig. 3.12 (**a**) X-ray images of mediastinal lymphoma. Anteroposterior x-ray view demonstrates widening of the superior mediastinum. (**b**) Chest CT scan of mediastinal lymphoma shows an anterior mediastinal mass. (**c–f**) Pathology of primary large cell lymphoma. (**c**) Biopsy cytology, Diff-Quik stain, 600×. (**d**) Histology of core, hematoxylin and eosin stain, 600×. (**e**) Immunostain for CD3, 600×. (**f**) Immunostain for CD20, 600×

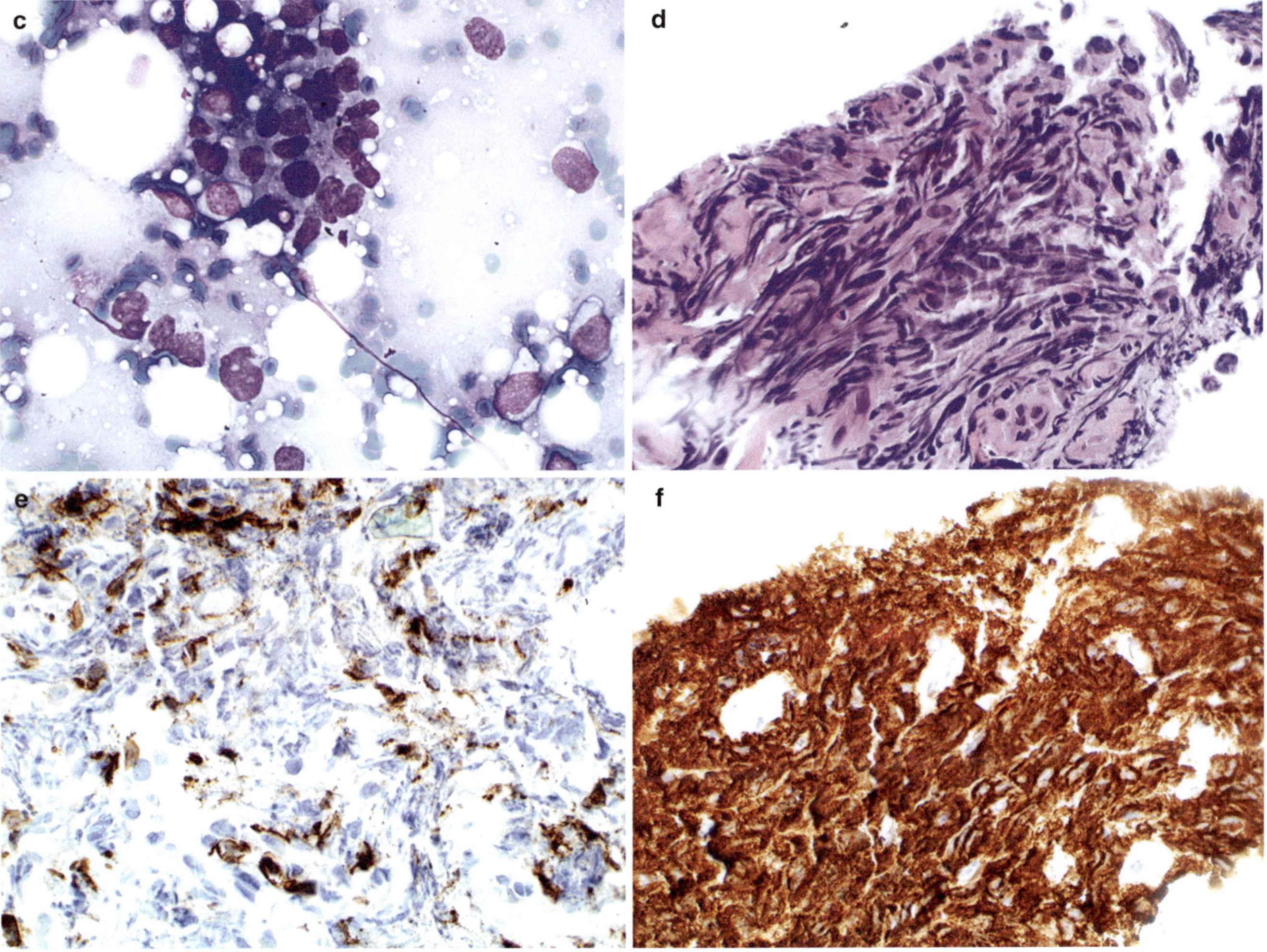

Fig. 3.12 (continued)

Hodgkin Lymphoma of the Mediastinum

Hodgkin lymphoma (HL) is a B-cell neoplasm characterized by large tumor cells scattered among a mixed inflammatory background. It encompasses two entities: classic HL that includes four subtypes (nodular sclerosis, mixed cellularity, lymphocyte-rich and lymphocyte depleted) and nodular lymphocyte predominant HL. The most common subtype of HL in the mediastinum is the nodular sclerosis subtype.

Clinical

- The most common primary mediastinal lymphoma.
- Shows a female predilection.
- There is a bimodal distribution peaking in the second and third decades and again in the seventh decade [78].

Radiographic Findings

X-ray

- On radiography, bilateral, asymmetrical mediastinal adenopathy is the most common presentation (up to 90%), and direct extension of the disease can be detected on chest radiographs. Commonly, perivascular and paratracheal lymph nodes are involved and rarely posterior mediastinal, paracardiac, and/or an internal mammary chain of lymph nodes is involved.
- Chest radiographs demonstrate either a single group with lymph node enlargement or a lobulated appearance resulting from multinodal involvement.
- Lung involvement can produce ill-defined or well-defined unilateral/bilateral nodules that may cavitate. Lung involvement can also appear as consolidation.

- Calcifications are rare in untreated lymphoma. Other findings include pleural effusions and anterior scalloping of vertebrae and skeletal lesions (67% are mixed lytic and sclerotic variety, 10–15% are sclerotic alone, and very few are lytic alone).

Ultrasound

Ultrasonography can help in performing mediastinal biopsies, but it is primarily used for evaluation and biopsies of lesions involving the chest wall. Echocardiography is useful for the detection of clinically undetectable pericardial disease and determination of left ventricular ejection fraction before and after chemotherapy [79].

CT Scan

Contrast-enhanced CT scanning of the thorax, abdomen, and pelvis is performed in all patients.

- The characteristic CT finding for HL is lymph node enlargement, which can be bilateral and may show peribronchial infiltration. Other patterns may include masses, mass-like consolidation, or diffuse interstitial thickening [80].
- Common pulmonary findings are peribronchovascular thickening, small bronchovascular nodules, focal mass-like lesions, airspace consolidation with air bronchogram, and pleural effusion.
- Less common CT findings may include: (a) a discrete or infiltrating thymic mass, (b) mediastinal displacement, compression, and (c) invasion of the vascular structures, pericardium, heart, pleura, lungs, and chest wall.

MRI

MRI is not the primary modality for evaluating HL, but its use is important in the pediatric population to avoid radiation exposure. MRI is useful for assessing chest wall invasion, pericardial involvement, pleural involvement, brachial plexus involvement, spinal cord compression, involvement of the spinal cord and the meninges, involvement of the musculoskeletal system in the chest, cardiac involvement, and involvement of the brachial plexus [81].

- On T1-weighted imaging, tumor involvement can be seen as a relatively homogeneous mass with low signal intensity (similar to that of muscle).
- On T2-weighted imaging, high signal intensity equal to or slightly greater than fat can result from tumoral edema, inflammation, immature fibrosis, granulomatous tissue, or disease recurrence. Dense fibrosis may demonstrate low signal intensity on T2-weighted images.

PET Scan

- HL is FDG-PET-avid in nearly 100% of cases but not reliable for identifying bone marrow involvement. However, use of PET scans is standard practice for staging, restaging, and to document remission/recurrence following therapy [82–84].

Cytology of FNA and Touch Preparations

- Reed-Sternberg cells, Reed-Sternberg variants, and lacunar cells are diagnostic (Fig. 3.13a).
- The background consists of mixed inflammatory cells, including lymphocytes, plasma cells, eosinophils, and histiocytes with or without granulomas.
- Dense fibrous stroma may be seen with the nodular sclerosis subtype.

Histology of Core and Cell Block

- Histology differs, depending on the subtype of HL (*see* Chap. 4 for more details) (Fig. 3.13b).

Comments

- The differential diagnosis includes:
  - Reactive lymph node
  - Large B-cell lymphoma
  - Lymphoblastic lymphoma
  - Thymoma
  - Metastatic carcinoma
- In classic HL, Reed-Sternberg cells and Reed-Sternberg variants are positive for CD15 (85%) (Fig. 3.13c), CD30 (Fig. 3.13d), and rarely for CD20 (20%) [85]. In contrast, in the nonclassic variant, nodular lymphocyte-predominant HL, the lacunar cells are positive for CD20 and EMA and are negative for CD15 and CD30.

Germ Cell Tumors

Clinical

- Although the mediastinum is the most common site of extragonadal germ cell tumors (GCTs), those arising in this location account for only 3–4% of all germ cell tumors. They account for 16% of mediastinal neoplasms in adults and 19–25% of mediastinal neoplasms in children [25]. Thirty-four percent of GCTs are mixed.
- GCTs are more common in males with a wide age range (newborn to 79 years) and a mean age of 24 years [86]. In infancy and early childhood, teratomatous and yolk sac components predominate.
- They are usually located in the anterior mediastinum or near the thymus.
- Elevated β-human chorionic gonadotropin or α-fetoprotein may be found in the serum, depending on the tumor type.

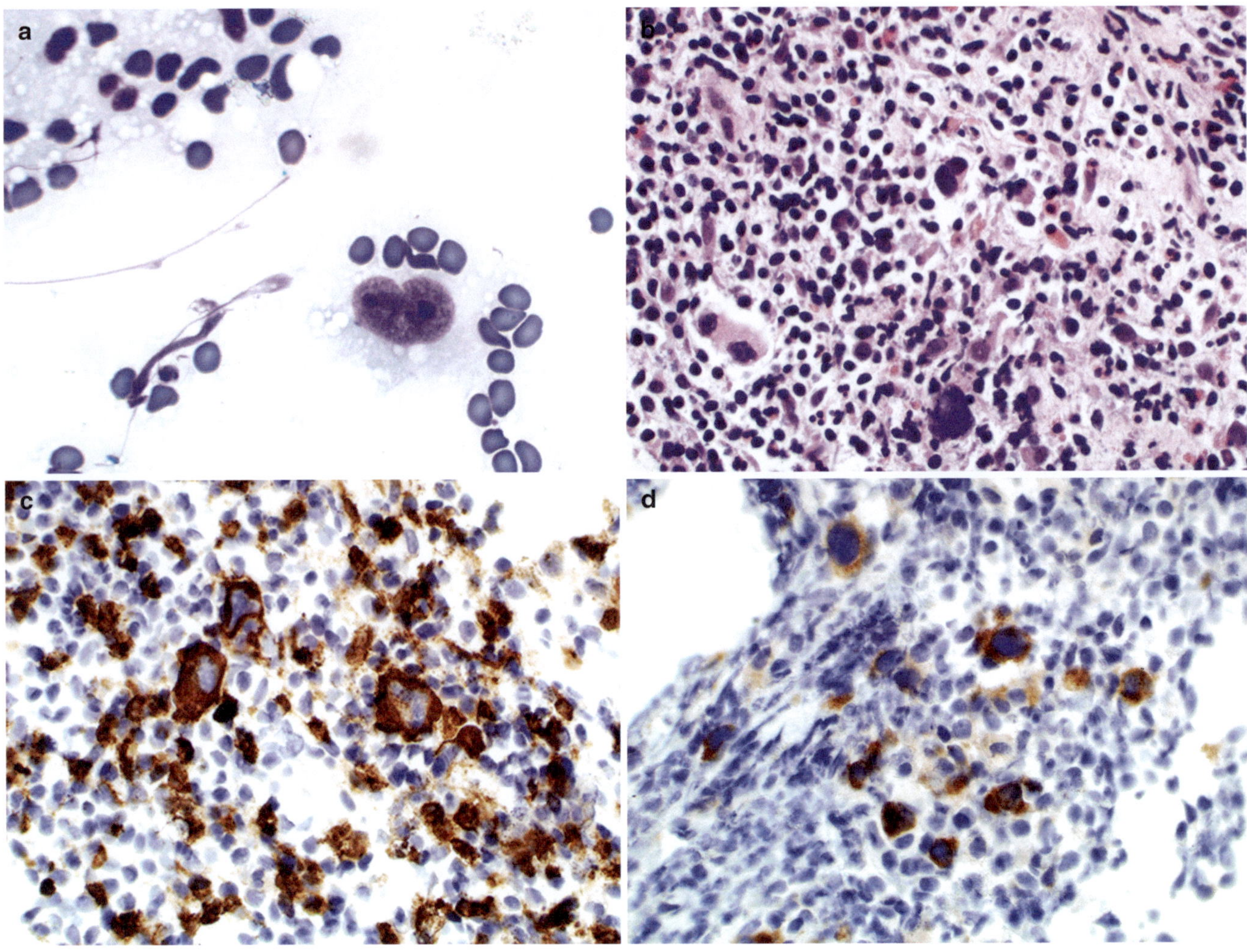

Fig. 3.13 Pathology of Hodgkin lymphoma. (**a**) Biopsy cytology, Diff-Quik stain, 600×. (**b**) Histology of core, hematoxylin and eosin stain, 600×. (**c**) Immunostain for CD15, 600×. (**d**) Immunostain for CD30, 600×

Seminoma

Clinical

- Seminomas are rare in mediastinal GCTs (9–39%)
- They are found almost exclusively in men, usually in the young adult population [87–89].

Cytology of FNA and Touch Preparation

- Characteristically seminomas show a dual cell population consisting of malignant seminoma cells and reactive lymphoid cells with a PAS-positive tigroid background (Fig. 3.14a, b).
- The seminoma cells are loosely cohesive, round to polygonal, and fairly uniform. The nuclei are large, round to oval, centrally located, hyperchromatic or vesicular, and with one or more centrally located prominent nucleoli. The cytoplasm is moderate to abundant, appears clear or vacuolated, and is easily disrupted, resulting in the classic glycogen rich, "tigroid" background.
- Granulomas with multinucleated giant cells and isolated syncytiotrophoblastic giant cells may also be present.

Histology of Core and Cell Block

- Tissue shows sheets, cores, or strands of large round to polygonal tumor cells with central nuclei containing prominent nucleoli and moderate to abundant glycogen-rich cytoplasm (Fig. 3.14b).
- Tumor cells are admixed with small lymphocytes.

Comments

- The differential diagnosis includes:
  - Thymoma/thymic carcinoma
  - Metastatic poorly differentiated carcinoma
  - Primary or metastatic large cell carcinoma
  - Large cell lymphoma
- Tumor cells are positive for OCT3/4, Sal4, CD117, D2-40, and PLAP and are negative for CEA, EMA, and AFP. A special stain for PAS is positive [90, 91].

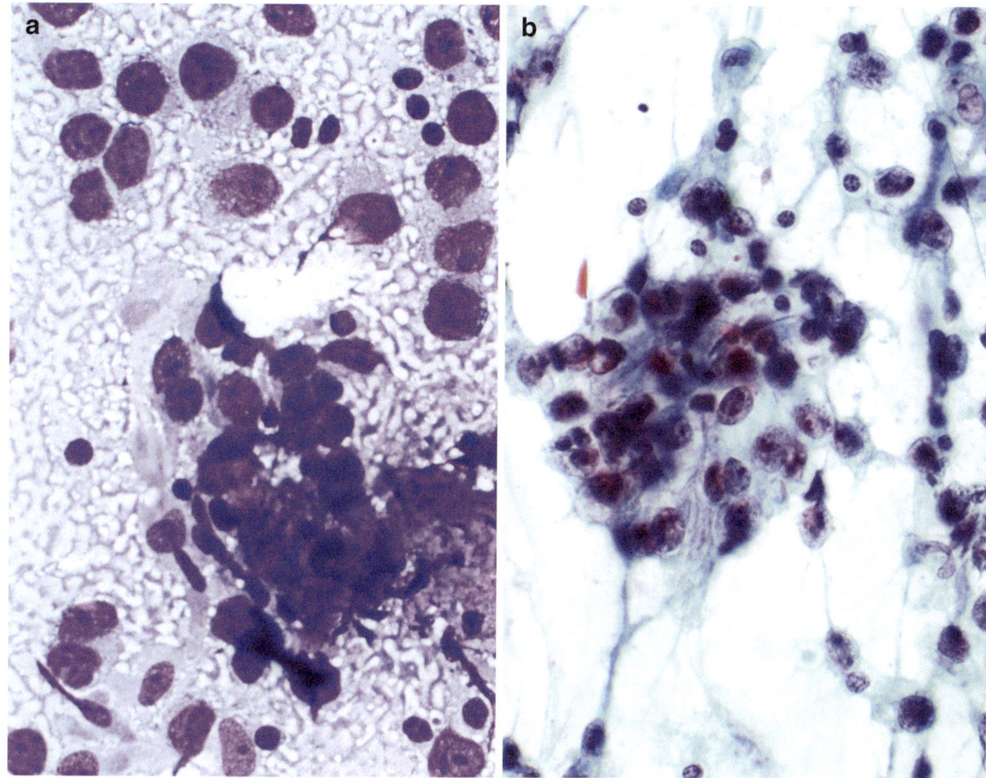

Fig. 3.14 (**a**, **b**) Pathology of seminoma. FNA biopsy cytology, Diff-Quik stain (**a**) and Papanicolaou stain (**b**), 600×

Teratomas

Teratoma is a GCT composed of several types of organoid mature and/or immature somatic tissue types derived from two or three germinal layers (ectoderm, endoderm, and mesoderm). Both mature and immature teratoma variants exist, and it may also be a component of malignant mixed GCTs or somatic-type malignancies (carcinomas and sarcomas).

Clinical

- Teratoma is the most common mediastinal GCT (50–70%) and accounts for 7–9% of all mediastinal tumors [87, 89, 92]. Most (80%) occur in the anterior mediastinum. Immature teratomas are very rare.
- Mature teratomas occur equally in both genders [92]. Immature teratomas occur almost exclusively in males.
- There is a wide age range with a median age in the 20s.
- Mature teratomas are predominantly cystic and may grow very large. Calcifications are common.

Cytology of FNA and Touch Preparation

Mature Teratoma

- The FNA smears can show many types of tissue, including skin and its appendages (e.g., squamous cells, sebaceous cells), neural, and gastrointestinal tissues, including pancreas, smooth muscle, cartilage, and ciliated respiratory cells.
- Immature Teratoma
  - The FNA smears may show both mature and immature tissue types, including embryonic or fetal tissues derived from the various germinal layers. The diagnosis is usually dependent on the presence of fetal brain tissue. Other immature tissue such as immature glands lined by tall columnar epithelial cells, fetal lung, immature cartilage and bone, and rhabdomyoblasts may also be present.
  - Granulomas with foreign body giant cells may be seen.

Histology of Core and Cell Block

- Tissue shows several types of mature as well as immature somatic tissues derived from two to three germinal layers.

Metastatic Malignancy in the Mediastinum

Metastases are the most common mediastinal lesions diagnosed by FNA biopsy [93]. The most common sources of metastases are from the lung, breast, thyroid, and prostate [94, 95]. Other common sources are from the head and neck, kidney, and testis as well as malignant melanoma [93]. The FNA diagnostic features are similar to that seen in their primary tumors.

Miscellaneous

Thyroid and parathyroid normal or abnormal tissue may be present in the mediastinum and may present clinically as a mass or nodule within the mediastinum.

Mediastinal Cysts

Various cysts are commonly found abnormalities within the mediastinum [96]. Most cysts are benign and developmental in origin, although some neoplasms, including malignant tumors, may show cystic change. The FNA biopsy frequently shows poorly preserved cellular debris and fluid and often contains only macrophages or inflammatory cells [96]. Contaminating cells along the needle track, such as mesothelial or respiratory cells, can be misleading. The combination of the clinical, radiologic, and cytologic features allows for a more specific diagnosis.

Developmental Cysts

These include bronchogenic cysts, thymic cysts, parathyroid cysts, thyroid cysts, and meningoceles.

Bronchogenic Cysts

Cytology of FNA and Touch Preparation

- Bronchogenic cysts are more commonly found in the pulmonary parenchyma but also occur in the mediastinum, usually below the carina.
- They are usually unilocular and are often several centimeters in size.
- The FNA biopsy yields clear, mucoid, or opalescent fluid, respiratory-type ciliated columnar cells with ciliocytophoria, and/or squamous metaplastic cells. Cartilage, smooth muscle, bronchial glands, nerves, and focal calcifications may also be found.

Thymic Cyst

Cytology of FNA and Touch Preparation

- Thymic cysts can occur anywhere along the embryologic path from the angle of the jaw in the neck to the mediastinum.
- They are less common than cystic thymoma and may be unilocular or multilocular.
- The characteristic FNA feature is the presence of thymic tissue in the wall of the cyst. The aspirated fluid is either serous or bloody and frequently contains cholesterol crystals.
- The cells lining the cyst may be squamous or columnar.
- Pseudoepitheliomatous hyperplasia and very rarely squamous cell carcinoma may occur in thymic cysts.

Neoplastic Cysts

Cytology of FNA and Touch Preparation

- Many tumors in the mediastinum are either primarily cystic or have a cystic component. These include the thymoma, lymphoma, seminoma, teratoma, nerve sheath tumors, and lymphangioma.
  Pleura

Mesothelioma

Mesothelioma is a tumor derived from mesothelial cells [97]. It is subclassified into diffuse malignant mesothelioma (epithelioid, sarcomatoid, desmoplastic, and biphasic mesothelioma), well-differentiated papillary mesothelioma, localized malignant mesothelioma, and adenomatoid tumor.

Clinical

- Usually diagnosed in adults but can rarely occur in children or even infants. The male-to-female ratio is greater than 9:1 [25].
- There is a strong association with asbestos exposure.
- Pleural effusions are found in approximately 80% of patients [98].

Radiographic Findings

X-ray

- Chest radiographs are of limited utility and are nonspecific. They may demonstrate a pleural opacity that extends around the lung, encasing it. Reduction in volume of the affected hemithorax is a common finding, shifting the mediastinum toward the affected side [99].
- Rib destruction, extension beyond the lateral and anterior margins of the chest wall, mediastinal lymph node enlargement, and pleural effusion may also be seen (Fig. 3.15a).

CT Scan

CT is the most commonly used modality for the assessment of mesothelioma and is able to stage the disease accurately in most patients.

- Mesothelioma appears as a soft tissue attenuated nodular mass that spreads along pleural surfaces, including into pleural fissures and often creating a pleural rind.
- Because of its predilection for direct invasion of adjacent structures and frequent metastases to the contralateral lung and local nodes, there may be extrapleural

fat plane changes caused by infiltration and/or direct extension into bone or muscle (Fig. 3.15b).

- Calcifications (engulfed calcified pleural plaques) and pleural or pericardial effusions can also be seen.

MRI

MRI, although not routinely used, may have a role in refining the staging and better delineating the extent of the disease in surgical candidates, especially when evaluating the chest wall and diaphragm for invasion.

- On T1- and T2-weighted imaging, isointense to slightly hyperintense signals compared to muscle are seen.
- Gadolinium-enhanced imaging shows enhancement.

PET Image

FDG-PET can help in differentiating malignant mesothelioma from asbestos-related benign pleural disease. PET is also helpful in evaluating for recurrence of malignant mesothelioma, post-therapy response, and scattered bony metastases.

- Malignant mesothelioma is often moderately to markedly FDG-avid, whereas benign disease is not.

Epithelioid Malignant Mesothelioma

Cytology of FNA and Touch Preparation

- Characteristically has a heterogeneous appearance with some cases showing the presence of single, loosely cohesive clusters while others show cohesive sheets, papillae, and balls of bland to malignant-appearing epithelioid cells or cells with mesothelial features (Fig. 3.15c). The cells are round or polygonal with well-defined cell borders. The cytoplasm varies from scant to abundant and from dense and squamoid to delicate and vacuolated. The nuclei are round to oval and are centrally or eccentrically located. They have fine to coarse chromatin and single or multiple nucleoli and may show prominent nucleoli. Binucleation or multinucleation is common.
- Mesothelial cell "windows" are often seen.
- Psammoma bodies and asbestos bodies may be seen [100].

Histology of Core and Cell Block

- Shows fibroconnective tissue infiltrated with single, nests, papillae, or acini of pleomorphic epithelioid mesothelial cells (Fig. 3.15d).

Comments

- The differential diagnosis includes:
  - Reactive mesothelial cell hyperplasia
  - Adenocarcinoma
  - Large cell carcinoma
  - Melanoma
- Immunohistochemical stains may be helpful in differentiating mesothelioma from carcinoma and reactive mesothelial cell hyperplasia. Mesothelioma is positive for calretinin (Fig. 3.15e), WT-1 (Fig. 3.15f), CK5/6 (Fig. 3.15g), D2-40 (Fig. 3.15h), and thrombomodulin, all

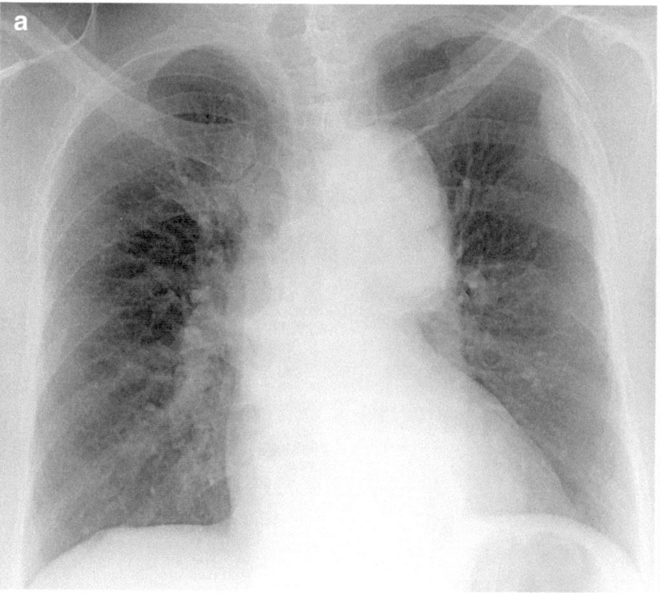

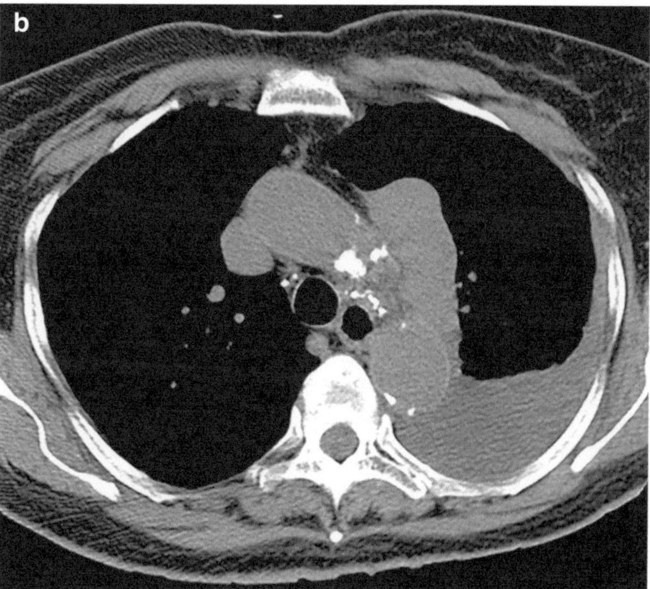

Fig. 3.15 (**a**, **b**) Radiologic images of malignant mesothelioma. (**a**) Chest x-ray demonstrates left pleural thickening. (**b**) Chest CT scan shows left lateral pleural thickening with a left-sided pleural effusion. (**c**–**h**) Pathology of mesothelioma. (**c**) Biopsy cytology, Diff-Quik stain, 600×. (**d**) Histology of core, hematoxylin and eosin stain, 600×. (**e**) Immunostain for calretinin, 600×. (**f**) Immunostain for WT-1, 600×. (**g**) Immunostain for CK5/6, 600×. (**h**) Immunostain for D2-40, 600×

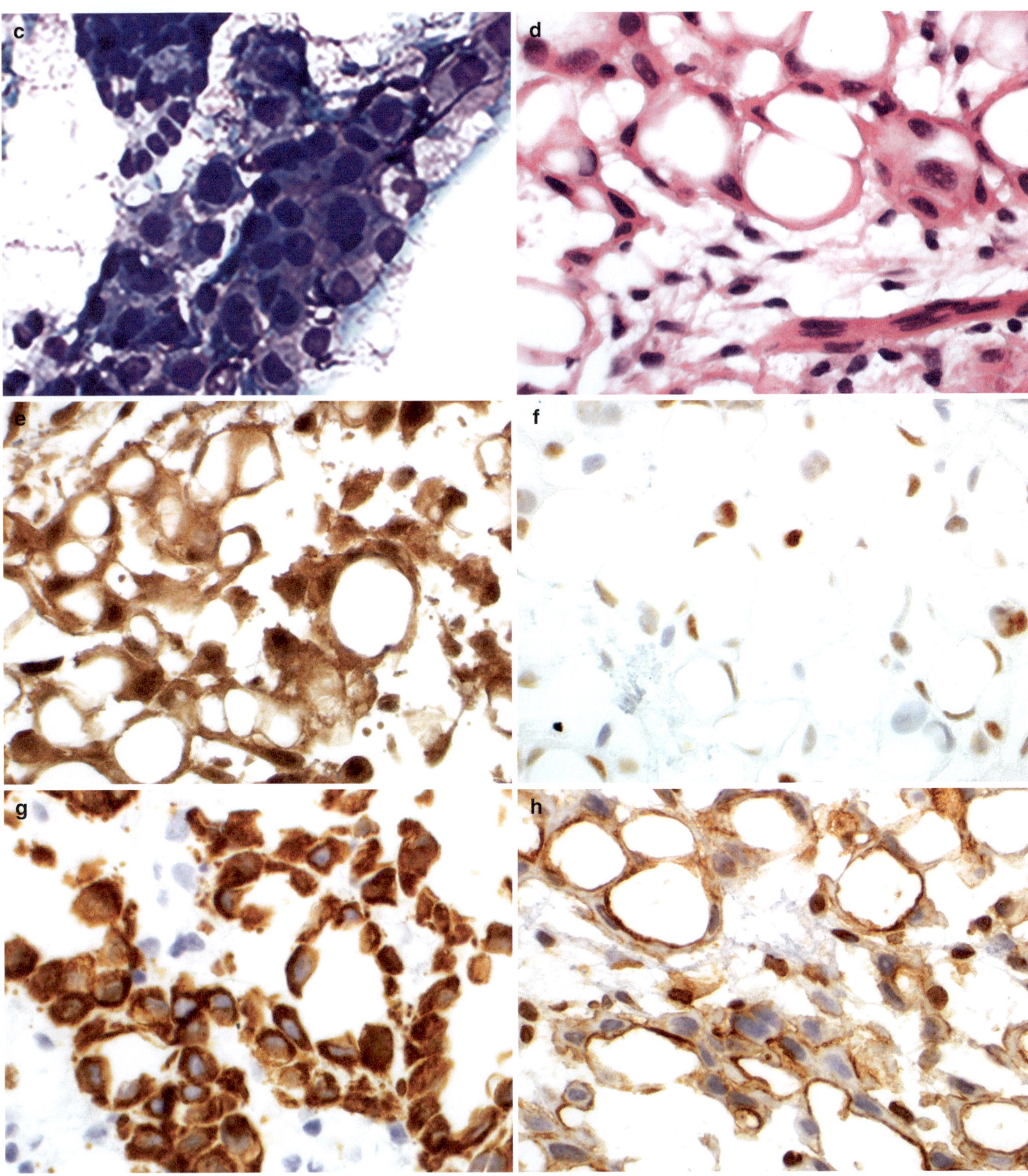

Fig. 3.15 (continued)

of which help to differentiate it from adenocarcinomas [101]. Mesothelioma is also positive for GLUT1 and IMP3 and shows loss of BAP1 and homozygous deletion of p16 by FISH, which can help to distinguish it from reactive mesothelial cells [102, 103].
- Electron microscopy shows long, slender microvilli.

Sarcomatoid Mesothelioma

Cytology of FNA and Touch Preparation
- Characteristically shows single or loose clusters of spindle cells. The spindle cells have a moderate amount of delicate cytoplasm. The nuclei are relatively large, oval to spindled, and variably pleomorphic. They have coarse, hyperchromatic chromatin with small nucleoli. Naked nuclei may be conspicuous [100]. Mitoses and necrosis are commonly seen.

Histology of Core and Cell Block
- Shows fibroconnective tissue infiltrated by markedly pleomorphic spindle cells.

Comments
- The differential diagnosis includes:
  - Chronic pleuritis with reactive inflammatory fibrosis
  - Primary and metastatic sarcomas
  - Spindle cell melanoma
  - Squamous cell carcinoma
  - Sarcomatoid carcinoma of the lung.
- Sarcomatoid mesothelioma cells are positive for cytokeratin, vimentin, actin, desmin, S-100, and calretinin.

Desmoplastic Mesothelioma

Cytology of FNA and Touch Preparation
- The specimen often shows sparse cellularity that may appear inadequate for evaluation, but closer inspection reveals rare atypical spindle cells.

Histology of Core and Cell Block
- Shows paucicellular, dense fibroconnective tissue infiltrated with atypical cells.

Comments
- The differential diagnosis includes:
  - Pleural plaque
  - Sarcomatoid mesothelioma
- Clinical correlation, imaging studies, and IHC stains are important in ruling out other entities in the differential diagnosis.

Biphasic Malignant Mesothelioma

Cytology of FNA and Touch Preparation
- Accounts for 30% of malignant mesotheliomas
- FNA smears are composed of both atypical epithelioid mesothelial cells as well as spindled mesothelial cells

Histology of Core and Cell Block
- Must contain at least 10% of both epithelioid and sarcomatoid mesothelial components.
- IHC stains and electron microscopy are often helpful with the differential diagnosis.

Comments
- The diagnosis of mesothelioma on effusion cytology, FNA, and small biopsy specimens has been controversial; however we have shown that this is possible to do on these specimens with adequate clinical/radiologic correlation and ancillary studies employed. However, subtyping of histologic type of mesothelioma is more difficult on limited tissue [104–106].

References

1. Smolle-Juettner FM, Woltsche M, Roeger G, Gabor S, Fladerer H, Popper H. Is preoperative percutaneous fine-needle aspiration cytology of intrathoracic lesions advisable in resectable patients? Eur J Cardiothorac Surg. 1996;10:1047–50; discussion, 51.
2. Walsh PR, Williams DB. Mediastinal adenopathy: finding the answer with endoscopic ultrasound-guided fine-needle aspiration biopsy. Intern Med J. 2005;35:392–8.
3. Naryshkin S, Young NA. Respiratory cytology: a review of non-neoplastic mimics of malignancy. Diagn Cytopathol. 1993;9:89–97.
4. Fraser RS. Transthoracic needle aspiration. The benign diagnosis. Arch Pathol Lab Med. 1991;115:751–61.
5. Sinner WN. Transthoracic needle biopsy of small peripheral malignant lung lesions. Investig Radiol. 1973;8:305–14.
6. Morkve O, Skaarland E, Myking A, Stangeland L, Gulsvik A. Transthoracic fine-needle aspiration guided by fluoroscopy: validity and complications with 19 operators. Respiration. 1988;53:239–45.
7. Perlmutt LM, Johnston WW, Dunnick NR. Percutaneous transthoracic needle aspiration: a review. Am J Roentgenol. 1989;152:451–5.
8. Tao LC, Sanders DE, Weisbrod GL, Ho CS, Wilson S. Value and limitations of transthoracic and transabdominal fine-needle aspiration cytology in clinical practice. Diagn Cytopathol. 1986;2:271–6.
9. Godoy MC, Vos PM, Cooperberg PL, Lydell CP, Phillips P, Muller NL. Chest radiographic and CT manifestations of chronic granulomatous disease in adults. Am J Roentgenol. 2008;191:1570–5.
10. Koutras P, Urschel HC Jr, Paulson DL. Hamartoma of the lung. J Thorac Cardiovasc Surg. 1971;61:768–76.
11. van den Bosch JM, Wagenaar SS, Corrin B, Elbers JR, Knaepen PJ, Westermann CJ. Mesenchymoma of the lung (so called hamartoma): a review of 154 parenchymal and endobronchial cases. Thorax. 1987;42:790–3.

12. Chai JL, Patz EF Jr. CT of the lung: patterns of calcification and other high-attenuation abnormalities. Am J Roentgenol. 1994;162:1063–6.
13. Klein JS, Braff S. Imaging evaluation of the solitary pulmonary nodule. Clin Chest Med. 2008;29:15–38.
14. Mitchell ML, King DE, Bonfiglio TA, Patten SF Jr. Pulmonary fine needle aspiration cytopathology. A five-year correlation study. Acta Cytol. 1984;28:72–6.
15. Hughes JH, Young NA, Wilbur DC, Renshaw AA, Mody DR, Cytopathology Resource Committee CoAP. Fine-needle aspiration of pulmonary hamartoma: a common source of false-positive diagnoses in the College of American Pathologists Interlaboratory Comparison Program in Nongynecologic Cytology. Arch Pathol Lab Med. 2005;129:19–22.
16. Gal AA, Koss MN, McCarthy WF, Hochholzer L. Prognostic factors in pulmonary fibrohistiocytic lesions. Cancer. 1994;73:1817–24.
17. Souid AK, Ziemba MC, Dubansky AS, Mazur M, Oliphant M, Thomas FD, et al. Inflammatory myofibroblastic tumor in children. Cancer. 1993;72:2042–8.
18. Pavithran K, Manoj P, Vidhyadharan G, Shanmughasundaram P. Inflammatory myofibroblastic tumor of the lung: unusual imaging findings. World J Nucl Med. 2013;12:126–8.
19. Hosler GA, Steinberg DM, Sheth S, Hamper UM, Erozan YS, Ali SZ. Inflammatory pseudotumor: a diagnostic dilemma in cytopathology. Diagn Cytopathol. 2004;31:267–70.
20. Machicao CN, Sorensen K, Abdul-Karim FW, Somrak TM. Transthoracic needle aspiration biopsy in inflammatory pseudotumors of the lung. Diagn Cytopathol. 1989;5:400–3.
21. Yamamoto H, Yamaguchi H, Aishima S, Oda Y, Kohashi K, Oshiro Y, et al. Inflammatory myofibroblastic tumor versus IgG4-related sclerosing disease and inflammatory pseudotumor: a comparative clinicopathologic study. Am J Surg Pathol. 2009;33:1330–40.
22. Barbareschi M, Ferrero S, Aldovini D, Leonardi E, Colombetti V, Carboni N, et al. Inflammatory pseudotumour of the lung. Immunohistochemical analysis on four new cases. Histol Histopathol. 1990;5:205–11.
23. Coffin CM, Patel A, Perkins S, Elenitoba-Johnson KS, Perlman E, Griffin CA. ALK1 and p80 expression and chromosomal rearrangements involving 2p23 in inflammatory myofibroblastic tumor. Mod Pathol. 2001;14:569–76.
24. Cools J, Wlodarska I, Somers R, Mentens N, Pedeutour F, Maes B, et al. Identification of novel fusion partners of ALK, the anaplastic lymphoma kinase, in anaplastic large-cell lymphoma and inflammatory myofibroblastic tumor. Genes Chromosomes Cancer. 2002;34:354–62.
25. Travis WD, Brambilla E, Burke AP, Max A, Nicholson AG. WHO classification of tumours of the lung, pleura, thymus and heart. Lyon: IARC Press; 2015.
26. Stoll LM, Johnson MW, Gabrielson E, Askin F, Clark DP, Li QK. The utility of napsin-A in the identification of primary and metastatic lung adenocarcinoma among cytologically poorly differentiated carcinomas. Cancer Cytopathol. 2010;118:441–9.
27. Tomashefski JF Jr, Connors AF Jr, Rosenthal ES, Hsiue IL. Peripheral vs central squamous cell carcinoma of the lung. A comparison of clinical features, histopathology, and survival. Arch Pathol Lab Med. 1990;114:468–74.
28. Zusman-Harach SB, Harach HR, Gibbs AR. Cytological features of non-small cell carcinomas of the lung in fine needle aspirates. J Clin Pathol. 1991;44:997–1002.
29. VanderLaan PA. Molecular markers: implications for cytopathology and specimen collection. Cancer Cytopathol. 2015;123:454–60.
30. Mino-Kenudson M. Programmed death-ligand 1 immunohistochemistry testing for non-small cell lung cancer in practice. Cancer Cytopathol. 2017;125:521–8.
31. Austin JH, Garg K, Aberle D, Yankelevitz D, Kuriyama K, Lee HJ, et al. Radiologic implications of the 2011 classification of adenocarcinoma of the lung. Radiology. 2013;266:62–71.
32. Higashi K, Ueda Y, Seki H, Yuasa K, Oguchi M, Noguchi T, et al. Fluorine-18-FDG PET imaging is negative in bronchioloalveolar lung carcinoma. J Nucl Med. 1998;39:1016–20.
33. Silverman JF, Zhu B, Liu Y, Lin X. Distinctive immunohistochemical profile of mucinous cystic neoplasms of pancreas, ovary and lung. Histol Histopathol. 2009;24:77–82.
34. Coley SM, Crapanzano JP, Saqi A. FNA, core biopsy, or both for the diagnosis of lung carcinoma: obtaining sufficient tissue for a specific diagnosis and molecular testing. Cancer Cytopathol. 2015;123:318–26.
35. Cai G, Wong R, Chhieng D, Levy GH, Gettinger SN, Herbst RS, et al. Identification of EGFR mutation, KRAS mutation, and ALK gene rearrangement in cytological specimens of primary and metastatic lung adenocarcinoma. Cancer Cytopathol. 2013;121:500–7.
36. Gainor JF, Shaw AT. Novel targets in non-small cell lung cancer: ROS1 and RET fusions. Oncologist. 2013;18:865–75.
37. Stoll LM, Johnson MW, Burroughs F, Li QK. Cytologic diagnosis and differential diagnosis of lung carcinoid tumors: a retrospective study of 63 cases with histologic correlation. Cancer Cytopathol. 2010;118:457–67.
38. Fink G, Krelbaum T, Yellin A, Bendayan D, Saute M, Glazer M, et al. Pulmonary carcinoid: presentation, diagnosis, and outcome in 142 cases in Israel and review of 640 cases from the literature. Chest. 2001;119:1647–51.
39. Beasley MB, Thunnissen FB, Brambilla E, Hasleton P, Steele R, Hammar SP, et al. Pulmonary atypical carcinoid: predictors of survival in 106 cases. Hum Pathol. 2000;31:1255–65.
40. Nessi R, Basso Ricci P, Basso Ricci S, Bosco M, Blanc M, Uslenghi C. Bronchial carcinoid tumors: radiologic observations in 49 cases. J Thorac Imaging. 1991;6:47–53.
41. Szyfelbein WM, Ross JS. Carcinoids, atypical carcinoids, and small-cell carcinomas of the lung: differential diagnosis of fine-needle aspiration biopsy specimens. Diagn Cytopathol. 1988;4:1–8.
42. Mitchell ML, Parker FP. Capillaries. A cytologic feature of pulmonary carcinoid tumors. Acta Cytol. 1991;35:183–5.
43. Lin X, Saad RS, Luckasevic TM, Silverman JF, Liu Y. Diagnostic value of CDX-2 and TTF-1 expressions in separating metastatic neuroendocrine neoplasms of unknown origin. Appl Immunohistochem Mol Morphol. 2007;15:407–14.
44. Warren WH, Memoli VA, Gould VE. Immunohistochemical and ultrastructural analysis of bronchopulmonary neuroendocrine neoplasms. II. Well-differentiated neuroendocrine carcinomas. Ultrastruct Pathol. 1984;7:185–99.
45. Chong S, Lee KS, Chung MJ, Han J, Kwon OJ, Kim TS. Neuroendocrine tumors of the lung: clinical, pathologic, and imaging findings. Radiographics. 2006;26:41–57; discussion, 58.
46. Lin X, Deng C, Tung T, Liu Y, Silverman JF. Diagnostic value of transcriptional factors and differential cytokeratins in separating primary pulmonary from metastatic mucinous cystadenocarcinoma. Mod Pathol. 2005;18(Suppl 1):315A.
47. Travis WD, Travis LB, Devesa SS. Lung cancer. Cancer. 1995;75(1 Suppl):191–202.
48. Haraldsson BT, Langberg H, Aagaard P, Zuurmond AM, van El B, Degroot J, et al. Corticosteroids reduce the tensile strength of isolated collagen fascicles. Am J Sports Med. 2006;34:1992–7.
49. Moro D, Brichon PY, Brambilla E, Veale D, Labat F, Brambilla C. Basaloid bronchial carcinoma. A histologic group with a poor prognosis. Cancer. 1994;73:2734–9.
50. Jung KJ, Lee KS, Han J, Kwon OJ, Kim J, Shim YM, et al. Large cell neuroendocrine carcinoma of the lung: clinical, CT, and pathologic findings in 11 patients. J Thorac Imaging. 2001;16:156–62.

51. Yang YJ, Steele CT, Ou XL, Snyder KP, Kohman LJ. Diagnosis of high-grade pulmonary neuroendocrine carcinoma by fine-needle aspiration biopsy: nonsmall-cell or small-cell type? Diagn Cytopathol. 2001;25:292–300.
52. Chow LT, Chow WH, Tsui WM, Chan SK, Lee JC. Fine-needle aspiration cytologic diagnosis of lymphoepithelioma-like carcinoma of the lung. Report of two cases with immunohistochemical study. Am J Clin Pathol. 1995;103:35–40.
53. Hiroshima K, Iyoda A, Shida T, Shibuya K, Iizasa T, Kishi H, et al. Distinction of pulmonary large cell neuroendocrine carcinoma from small cell lung carcinoma: a morphological, immunohistochemical, and molecular analysis. Mod Pathol. 2006;19:1358–68.
54. Chae Y, Tamragouri K, Chung J, Lin X, Miller V, Ali S, et al. Large cell neuroendocrine carcinoma of lung: a focused analysis of BRAF alterations and a case report of a BRAF non-V600 mutated tumor responding to targeted therapy. JCO Precis Oncol. 2018;2:1–12.
55. Zhu B, Dalal S, Kamp DW, Lin X. Warranting investigation of primary lung adenocarcinoma in patients with an extrapulmonary malignancy and lung nodules due to high frequency. Am J Clin Pathol. 2014;141:429–36.
56. Yu CJ, Yang PC, Chang DB, Wu HD, Lee LN, Lee YC, et al. Evaluation of ultrasonically guided biopsies of mediastinal masses. Chest. 1991;100:399–405.
57. Shin HJ, Katz RL. Thymic neoplasia as represented by fine needle aspiration biopsy of anterior mediastinal masses. A practical approach to the differential diagnosis. Acta Cytol. 1998;42:855–64.
58. Chhieng DC, Rose D, Ludwig ME, Zakowski MF. Cytology of thymomas: emphasis on morphology and correlation with histologic subtypes. Cancer. 2000;90:24–32.
59. Alexiev BA, Drachenberg CB, Burke AP. Thymomas: a cytological and immunohistochemical study, with emphasis on lymphoid and neuroendocrine markers. Diagn Pathol. 2007;2:13.
60. Takahashi K, Al-Janabi NJ. Computed tomography and magnetic resonance imaging of mediastinal tumors. J Magn Reson Imaging. 2010;32:1325–39.
61. Sakai F, Sone S, Kiyono K, Kawai T, Maruyama A, Ueda H, et al. MR imaging of thymoma: radiologic-pathologic correlation. Am J Roentgenol. 1992;158:751–6.
62. Ali SZ, Erozan YS. Thymoma. Cytopathologic features and differential diagnosis on fine needle aspiration. Acta Cytol. 1998;42:845–54.
63. Marino M, Muller-Hermelink HK. Thymoma and thymic carcinoma. Relation of thymoma epithelial cells to the cortical and medullary differentiation of thymus. Virchows Arch A Pathol Anat Histopathol. 1985;407:119–49.
64. Tao LC, Pearson FG, Cooper JD, Sanders DE, Weisbrod G, Donat EE. Cytopathology of thymoma. Acta Cytol. 1984;28:165–70.
65. Wakely PE Jr. Fine needle aspiration in the diagnosis of thymic epithelial neoplasms. Hematol Oncol Clin North Am. 2008;22:433–42.
66. Zhu B, Laskin W, Chen Y, French CA, Cameron MJ, Nayar R, et al. NUT midline carcinoma: a neoplasm with diagnostic challenges in cytology. Cytopathology. 2011;22:414–7.
67. Chalabreysse L, Roy P, Cordier JF, Loire R, Gamondes JP, Thivolet-Bejui F. Correlation of the WHO schema for the classification of thymic epithelial neoplasms with prognosis: a retrospective study of 90 tumors. Am J Surg Pathol. 2002;26:1605–11.
68. Okumura M, Miyoshi S, Fujii Y, Takeuchi Y, Shiono H, Inoue M, et al. Clinical and functional significance of WHO classification on human thymic epithelial neoplasms: a study of 146 consecutive tumors. Am J Surg Pathol. 2001;25:103–10.
69. Moran CA, Suster S. Thymic carcinoma: current concepts and histologic features. Hematol Oncol Clin North Am. 2008;22: 393–407.
70. Klapper W, Jaffe ES, Gaulard HNL, Gascoyne R, Moller P, et al. Primary mediastinal large B-cell lymphoma. In: Travis WD, Brambilla E, Burke AP, Marx A, Nicholson AG, editors. WHO classification of tumors of the lung, pleura, thymus and heart. Lyon: IARC Press; 2015. p. 267–9.
71. Hughes JH, Katz RL, Fonseca GA, Cabanillas FF. Fine-needle aspiration cytology of mediastinal non-Hodgkin's nonlymphoblastic lymphoma. Cancer. 1998;84:26–35.
72. Cazals-Hatem D, Lepage E, Brice P, Ferrant A, d'Agay MF, Baumelou E, et al. Primary mediastinal large B-cell lymphoma. A clinicopathologic study of 141 cases compared with 916 nonmediastinal large B-cell lymphomas, a GELA ("Groupe d'Etude des Lymphomes de l'Adulte") study. Am J Surg Pathol. 1996;20:877–88.
73. Lewis ER, Caskey CI, Fishman EK. Lymphoma of the lung: CT findings in 31 patients. Am J Roentgenol. 1991;156:711–4.
74. Divgi C. Imaging: staging and evaluation of lymphoma using nuclear medicine. Semin Oncol. 2005;32(Suppl 1):S11–8.
75. Hoda RS, Picklesimer L, Green KM, Self S. Fine-needle aspiration of a primary mediastinal large B-cell lymphoma: a case report with cytologic, histologic, and flow cytometric considerations. Diagn Cytopathol. 2005;32:370–3.
76. Silverman JF, Raab SS, Park HK. Fine-needle aspiration cytology of primary large-cell lymphoma of the mediastinum: cytomorphologic findings with potential pitfalls in diagnosis. Diagn Cytopathol. 1993;9:209–14; discussion, 14–5
77. Dunleavy K, Grant C, Eberle FC, Pittaluga S, Jaffe ES, Wilson WH. Gray zone lymphoma: better treated like Hodgkin lymphoma or mediastinal large B-cell lymphoma? Curr Hematol Malig Rep. 2012;7:241–7.
78. Shenoy P, Maggioncalda A, Malik N, Flowers CR. Incidence patterns and outcomes for Hodgkin lymphoma patients in the United States. Adv Hematol. 2011;2011:725219.
79. Saito T, Kobayashi H, Sugama Y, Tamaki S, Kawai T, Kitamura S. Ultrasonically guided needle biopsy in the diagnosis of mediastinal masses. Am Rev Respir Dis. 1988;138:679–84.
80. Guermazi A, Brice P, de Kerviler EE, Ferme C, Hennequin C, Meignin V, et al. Extranodal Hodgkin disease: spectrum of disease. Radiographics. 2001;21:161–79.
81. Uehara M, Takahashi J, Hirabayashi H, Kitahara J, Kamijyo T, Ebara S, et al. Hodgkin's disease of the thoracic vertebrae. Spine J. 2013;13:e59–63.
82. Evens AM, Kostakoglu L. The role of FDG-PET in defining prognosis of Hodgkin lymphoma for early-stage disease. Hematology ASH Educ Program. 2014;2014:135–43.
83. Zijlstra JM. PET-CT: reliable cornerstone for Hodgkin lymphoma treatment? Blood. 2016;127:1521–2.
84. Kasamon YL, Wahl RL. FDG PET and risk-adapted therapy in Hodgkin's and non-Hodgkin's lymphoma. Curr Opin Oncol. 2008;20:206–19.
85. von Wasielewski R, Mengel M, Fischer R, Hansmann ML, Hubner K, Franklin J, et al. Classical Hodgkin's disease. Clinical impact of the immunophenotype. Am J Pathol. 1997;151:1123–30.
86. Liu TZ, Zhang DS, Liang Y, Zhou NN, Gao HF, Liu KJ, et al. Treatment strategies and prognostic factors of patients with primary germ cell tumors in the mediastinum. J Cancer Res Clin Oncol. 2011;137:1607–12.
87. Takeda S, Miyoshi S, Ohta M, Minami M, Masaoka A, Matsuda H. Primary germ cell tumors in the mediastinum: a 50-year experience at a single Japanese institution. Cancer. 2003;97:367–76.
88. Moran CA, Suster S, Przygodzki RM, Koss MN. Primary germ cell tumors of the mediastinum: II. Mediastinal seminomas—a clinicopathologic and immunohistochemical study of 120 cases. Cancer. 1997;80:691–8.
89. Moran CA, Suster S. Primary germ cell tumors of the mediastinum: I. Analysis of 322 cases with special

emphasis on teratomatous lesions and a proposal for histopathologic classification and clinical staging. Cancer. 1997;80:681–90.
90. Gopalan A, Dhall D, Olgac S, Fine SW, Korkola JE, Houldsworth J, et al. Testicular mixed germ cell tumors: a morphological and immunohistochemical study using stem cell markers, OCT3/4, SOX2 and GDF3, with emphasis on morphologically difficult-to-classify areas. Mod Pathol. 2009;22:1066–74.
91. Lau SK, Weiss LM, Chu PG. D2-40 immunohistochemistry in the differential diagnosis of seminoma and embryonal carcinoma: a comparative immunohistochemical study with KIT (CD117) and CD30. Mod Pathol. 2007;20:320–5.
92. Lewis BD, Hurt RD, Payne WS, Farrow GM, Knapp RH, Muhm JR. Benign teratomas of the mediastinum. J Thorac Cardiovasc Surg. 1983;86:727–31.
93. Linder J, Olsen GA, Johnston WW. Fine-needle aspiration biopsy of the mediastinum. Am J Med. 1986;81:1005–8.
94. Lindell MM, Doubleday LC, von Eschenbach AC, Libshitz HI. Mediastinal metastases from prostatic carcinoma. J Urol. 1982;128:331–4.
95. McLoud TC, Kalisher L, Stark P, Greene R. Intrathoracic lymph node metastases from extrathoracic neoplasms. Am J Roentgenol. 1978;131:403–7.
96. Rice TW. Benign neoplasms and cysts of the mediastinum. Semin Thorac Cardiovasc Surg. 1992;4:25–33.
97. Rosario CM, Lin X, Kamp DW. Mesothelioma – update on diagnostic strategies. Clin Pulm Med. 2012;19:282–8.
98. Sterrett GF, Whitaker D, Shilkin KB, Walters MN. Fine needle aspiration cytology of malignant mesothelioma. Acta Cytol. 1987;31:185–93.
99. Wang ZJ, Reddy GP, Gotway MB, Higgins CB, Jablons DM, Ramaswamy M, et al. Malignant pleural mesothelioma: evaluation with CT, MR imaging, and PET. Radiographics. 2004;24:105–19.
100. Tao LC. Aspiration biopsy cytology of mesothelioma. Diagn Cytopathol. 1989;5:14–21.
101. Ordonez NG. Application of immunohistochemistry in the diagnosis of epithelioid mesothelioma: a review and update. Hum Pathol. 2013;44:1–19.
102. Cigognetti M, Lonardi S, Fisogni S, Balzarini P, Pellegrini V, Tironi A, et al. BAP1 (BRCA1-associated protein 1) is a highly specific marker for differentiating mesothelioma from reactive mesothelial proliferations. Mod Pathol. 2015;28:1043–57.
103. Lee AF, Gown AM, Churg A. IMP3 and GLUT-1 immunohistochemistry for distinguishing benign from malignant mesothelial proliferations. Am J Surg Pathol. 2013;37:421–6.
104. Paintal A, Raparia K, Nayar R. Cytomorphologic findings of malignant mesothelioma in FNA biopsies and touch preps of core biopsies. Diagn Cytopathol. 2016;44(1):14–9.
105. Paintal A, Raparia K, Zakowski MF, Nayar R. The diagnosis of malignant mesothelioma in effusion cytology: a reappraisal and results of a multi-institution survey. Cancer Cytopathol. 2013;121(12):703–7.
106. Paintal A. The evolving role of effusion cytology in the diagnosis of malignant mesothelioma. Cytopathology. 2015;26(3):137–8. https://doi.org/10.1111/cyt.12252.

Lymph Nodes and Spleen

4

Xiaoqi Lin, Juehua Gao, John K. S. S. Philip, Rosewell V. Mackey, Rehan Ali, and Ahsun Riaz

The main indication for fine needle aspiration (FNA) and core needle biopsy (CNB) of lymph nodes or spleen is to rule out metastatic disease of either a known or unknown primary for staging or for local or diffuse lymphadenopathy in order to exclude lymphoma. We describe the radiographic features, cytomorphology of FNA or touch preparation of the cores, histology of CNB, immunohistochemical stains, flow cytometry, and molecular studies of common hematopoietic lesions and non-neoplastic lesions as well as metastatic malignancy.

Lymph Node

Introduction

The main indication for fine needle aspiration (FNA) and core needle biopsy (CNB) of lymph nodes is to rule out metastatic disease of either a known or unknown primary for staging or for local or diffuse lymphadenopathy in order to exclude lymphoma. Although FNA or CNB of the spleen may cause bleeding, we do sometimes perform FNA and CNB targeting splenic lesions. FNA cellblock and CNB can be used for histologic examination, special stains, immunohistochemical stains, and cytogenetic and molecular studies. Either an FNA aliquot or CNB can be submitted for flow cytometry. Complications associated with the performance of lymph node FNA and/or CNB are relatively few. These include hemorrhage or infection and rare cases of tumor seeding along the needle track.

X. Lin (✉)
Northwestern University, Feinberg School of Medicine, Northwestern Memorial Hospital, Chicago, IL, USA
e-mail: xlin@northwestern.edu

J. Gao
Department of Pathology, Northwestern University, Feinberg School of Medicine, Chicago, IL, USA

John K. S. S. Philip
Department of Pathology, Thomas Health System, South Charleston, WV, USA

R. V. Mackey
Department of Radiology, McGaw Medical Center, Northwestern University, Chicago, IL, USA

R. Ali
Department of Radiology, Section of Vascular and Interventional Radiology, Northwestern University, Chicago, IL, USA

A. Riaz
Department of Pathology, Northwestern Medicine, Chicago, IL, USA

Normal Findings

Normal lymph nodes are usually painless, smaller than 1 cm, and mobile and have smooth contours.

Cytology of FNA and Touch Preparation

- Polymorphous population of lymphoid cells (predominantly small mature lymphocytes), scattered immunoblasts, plasma cells, histiocytes, and lymphohistiocytic aggregates (germinal center) (Fig. 4.1a, b).

Histology of Core

- The core contains three regions: the cortex, paracortex, and medulla (Fig. 4.1c, d).
- The cortex contains B-cell rich primary and secondary follicles.
- The paracortex is predominantly composed of T cells.
- The medulla is composed of sinuses surrounded by plasma cells.

Reactive/Non-neoplastic Conditions

Reactive lymph node enlargement is often used synonymously with reactive lymphadenopathy to indicate benign, reversible enlargement of lymph nodes in response to an antigen stimulus, which may be acute or chronic, localized or generalized.

R. Nayar et al. (eds.), *Atlas of Cytopathology and Radiology*, https://doi.org/10.1007/978-3-030-24756-0_4

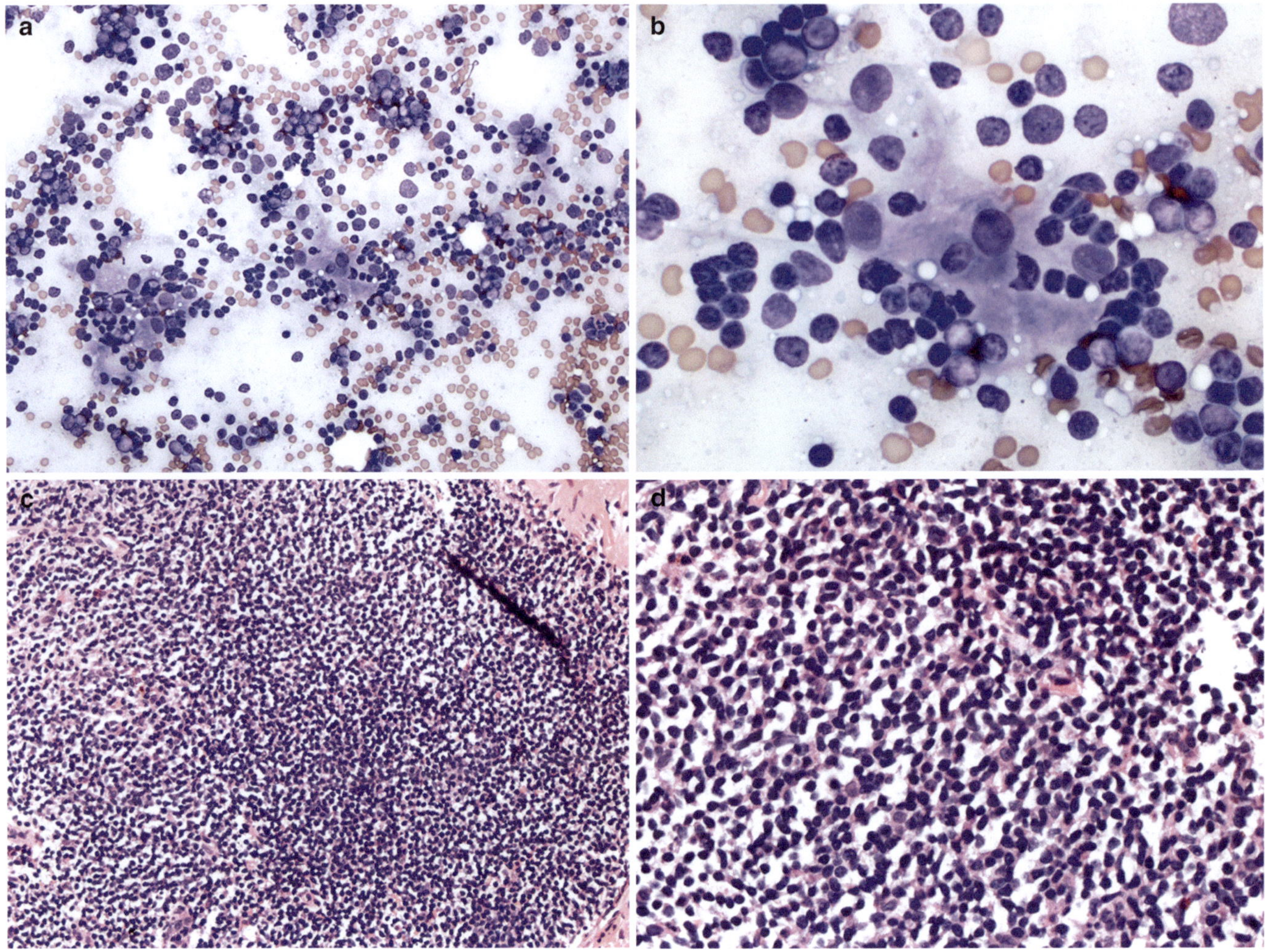

Fig. 4.1 Pathology of normal lymph node. (**a**, **b**) Biopsy cytology, Diff-Quik stain, 200× and 400×. (**c**, **d**) Histology of core, hematoxylin and eosin stain, 200× and 400×

General Radiologic Features of Reactive Lymph Nodes

- Reactive lymph nodes have a wide size range up to 1.5 cm in adults and up to 2 cm or greater in children. Size is a relatively poor predictor of benignity when considered alone.
- The long-to-short axis ratio is also used to evaluate enlarged nodes when an underlying malignancy is known or suspected [1].
- Multiple imaging modalities are used for the assessment and characterization of lymph nodes, each with their unique advantages and disadvantages.
- Computed Tomography (CT) Scan
  - Contrast-enhanced CT shows enlarged lymph nodes with a variable appearance that can be homogeneously solid or hypodense with peripheral enhancement (Fig. 4.2a).
  - Perinodal tissue may show associated inflammatory changes as in Kikuchi disease [2].
- Positron Emission Tomography (PET) CT Scan
  - Findings are nonspecific with avid fludeoxyglucose (FDG) uptake in enlarged lymph nodes (Fig. 4.2b) [3].
  - Reactive adenopathy demonstrates mild F-18 FDG uptake with avid uptake seen in cases of active granulomatous disease.
- Ultrasound (US)
  - Assess size, shape, echotexture, vascularity, contour, hilum, the presence of calcifications, and long to short axis ratio. Enlarged lymph nodes are hypoechoic, homogeneous with an echogenic hilum, a nonspecific finding.
  - Reactive lymph nodes demonstrate sharp margins with a hypoechoic uniformly thick peripheral parenchyma, an echogenic central hilum, and no or central hilar vascularization of low impedance (Fig. 4.2c).

- Irregular margins and absence of hilum or hypoechoic center can be seen in some reactive lymphadenopathies [4].
- Benign lymph nodes have a lower stiffness on US elastography compared to malignant lymph nodes [5].
- Power Doppler assessment reveals prominent vascularity of the perihilar cortex and hilum in Kikuchi disease [6].

- Magnetic Resonance Imaging (MRI)
  - Involved nodes show peripheral enhancement with nonenhancing central areas that are not hyperintense on T2-weighted imaging.
  - Low to intermediate homogeneous signal intensity on T1-weighted imaging and intermediate to high homogeneous signal intensity on T2-weighted imaging.
  - On contrast enhanced MRI, there are variable enhancement patterns, with mild homogeneous enhancement being the most common. Linear central enhancement on T1-weighted contrast-enhanced images favors a benign node [7].
  - Diffusion-weighted imaging with apparent diffusion coefficient (ADC) mapping is a new promising technique that can differentiate benign from malignant lymph nodes [8]. Benign reactive lymph nodes tend to have higher ADC values than neoplastic nodes [9].

Acute Lymphadenitis

Acute lymphadenitis is defined as enlarged, inflamed, and tender lymph node(s) developed over days, often caused by infectious organisms, most frequently bacteria.

Clinical

- Usually the involved lymph nodes are tender, warm, and red.
- Most often caused by infection with various microorganisms.
- Noninfectious causes are less common but may include connective tissue disorders, medication, Kawasaki disease, and Kikuchi disease.

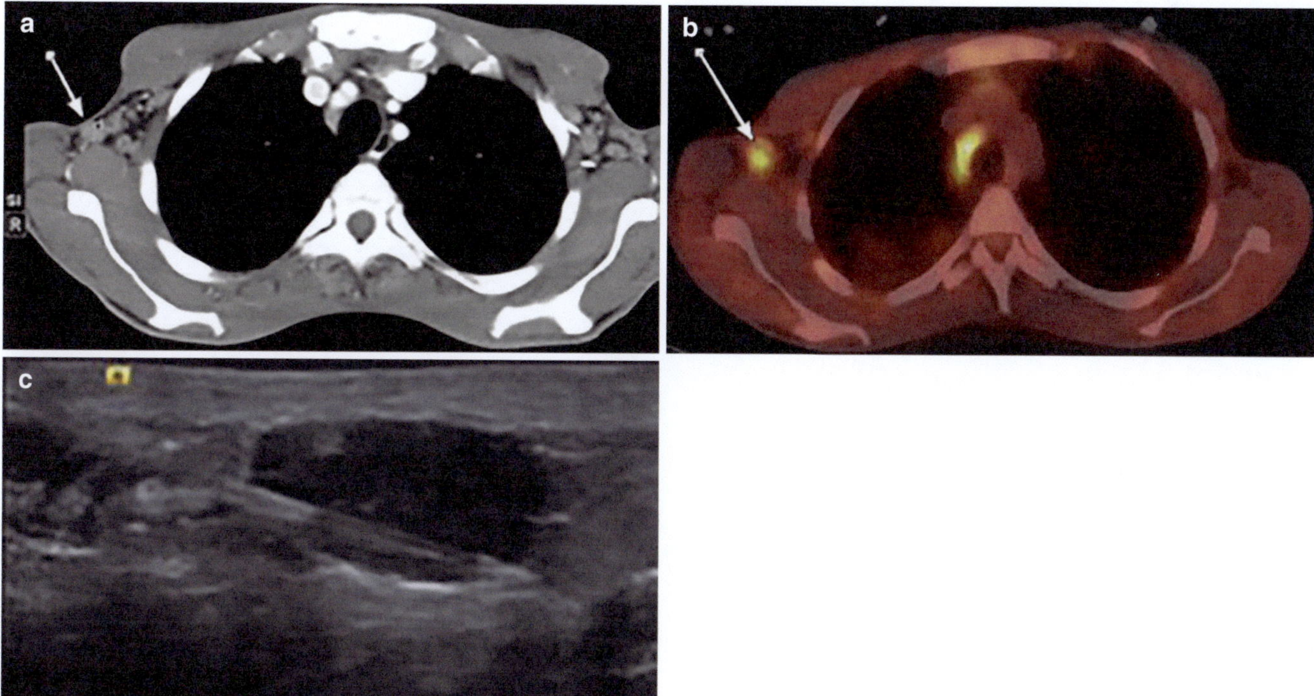

Fig. 4.2 (**a**, **b**) Radiologic images of reactive lymphadenopathy. (**a**) CECT demonstrates a homogeneous enlarged lymph node. (**b**) F-18 FDG PET/CT demonstrates focally increased metabolic activity involving right axillary lymph node corresponding to the CECT. (**c**) Gray scale US at the time of biopsy shows a hypoechoic, oval-shaped lymph node with an echogenic hilum. (**d**, **e**) Acute lymphadenopathy. (**d**) Cytomorphology of FNA of a lymph node with necrosis; Diff-Quik stain, 600×; (**e**) FNA cell block, Gram stain, 600×. (**f**, **g**) Reactive lymphadenopathy. Cytology of FNA of a reactive lymph node; Diff-Quik stain (**f**) and Papanicolaou stain (**g**), 200×. (**h**, **i**) Granulomatous lymphadenitis. Cytology of FNA of an enlarged lymph node; Diff-Quik stain (**h**) and Papanicolaou stain (**i**), 600×

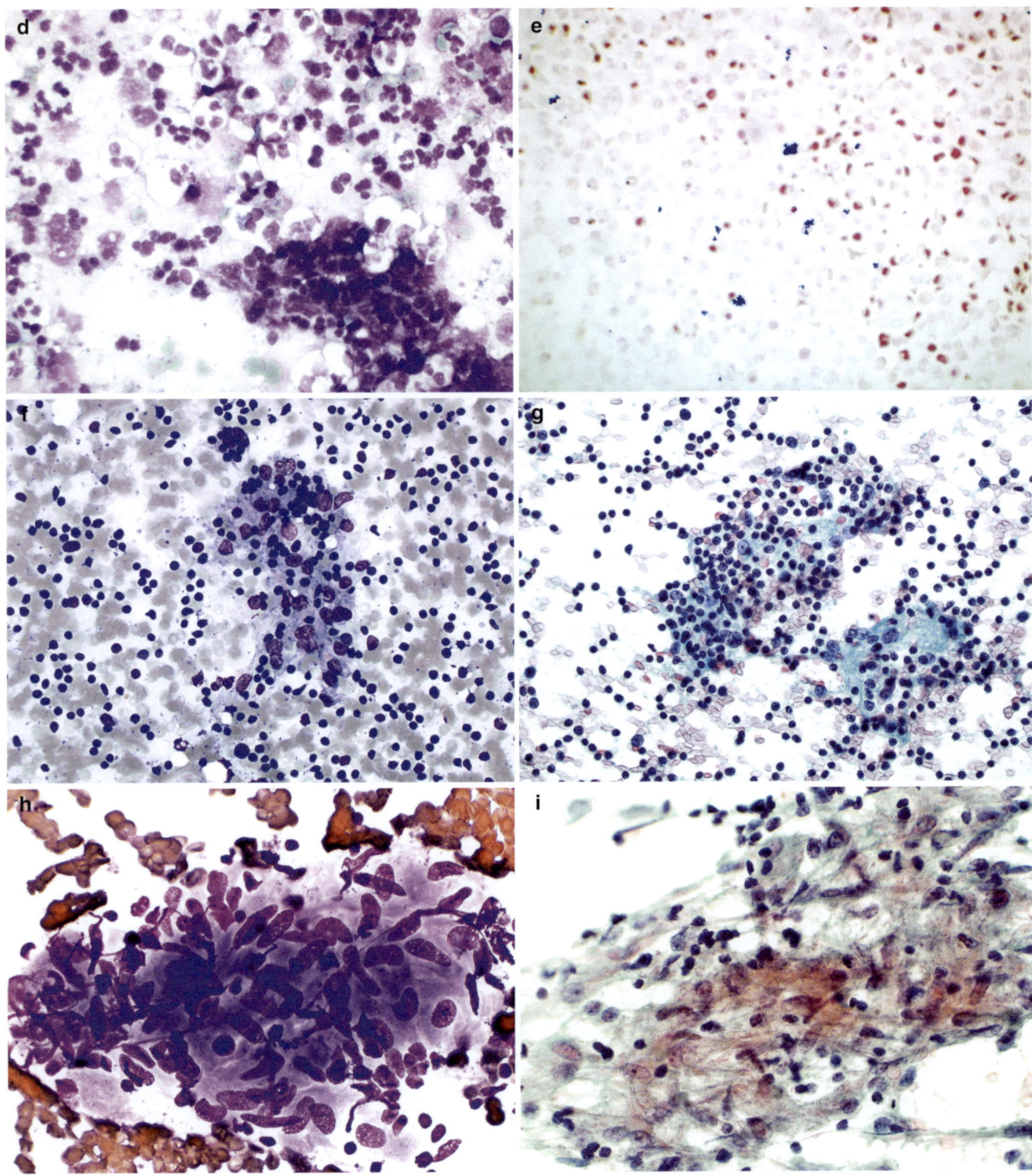

Fig. 4.2 (continued)

Cytology of FNA and Touch Preparation

- Not frequently biopsied.
- Findings are similar to those of an abscess, including neutrophils, other inflammatory cells, and necrotic debris (Fig. 4.2d).

Histology of Core

- Core biopsies are infrequently obtained in this setting.
- Lymphoid tissue with focal acute inflammation and necrosis.

Comments

- **Differential Diagnosis**
  - Reactive atypia can mimic malignancy, such as lymphoma or metastatic malignancy.
  - Metastatic malignancies to a lymph node may undergo cystic degeneration and mimic a reactive lymph node, particularly squamous cell carcinoma or thyroid papillary carcinoma.
- **Ancillary Studies**
  - Some microorganisms are more readily identified on Diff-Quik or Papanicolaou stain on the smears. Special stains (Gomori methenamine silver stain (GMS), periodic acid Schiff stain (PAS), acid-fast bacilli smear (AFB), and Gram stain) (Fig. 4.2e) can be performed on FNA smears, cell blocks, or cores.
  - Culture of the aspirated material is the most useful ancillary test in this setting. Molecular studies including polymerase chain reaction (PCR) are more sensitive and specific for microorganisms.

Chronic Lymphadenitis

Chronic lymphadenitis is defined as enlarged, inflamed, and tender lymph node(s) developed over weeks or months, attributable to an infectious or noninfectious etiology.

Clinical

- One of the most common processes encountered in FNA biopsy of lymph nodes.
- Moderately enlarged, nontender lymph nodes.
- Single node or single group of nodes involved.
- Often have a history of regional infection preceding lymph node enlargement or represent lymph node involvement of a systematic disease.

Cytology of FNA and Touch Preparation

- Polymorphous population of lymphocytes, predominantly small lymphocytes, admixed with lymphohistiocytic fragments (germinal centers), immunoblasts, reactive lymphocytes, and tingible body macrophages (Fig. 4.2f, g).

Histology of Core

There are four major patterns. However, they are often difficult to appreciate in small core biopsies.

- Follicular hyperplasia: Enlarged germinal center with tingible body macrophages.
- Paracortical hyperplasia: Increase in paracortex and decrease in size of germinal centers.
- Sinus histiocytosis: Dilated sinuses with increased histiocytes.
- Mixed reactions: Show mixture of above patterns.

Granulomatous Lymphadenitis

Granulomatous lymphadenitis is defined as the presence of granulomas in the lymph nodes, which is associated with a variety of disorders or infections.

Clinical

- Possibly associated with infection, immune disorders, and malignancies, for example, Hodgkin lymphoma (HL), T-cell lymphoma, germ cell tumor, and some carcinomas.
- Distinct infections with specific patterns of granulomatous inflammation [10].
  - Epithelioid granulomatous lymphadenitis
    - With necrosis: Mycobacterial and fungal infections.
    - Without necrosis: Sarcoidosis, Crohn disease.
  - Suppurative granulomatous lymphadenitis: Cat scratch disease (*Bartonella henselae*), lymphogranuloma venereum (*Chlamydia trachomatis*), tularemia (*Francisella tularensis*), and others.

Cytology of FNA and Touch Preparation

- Epithelioid histiocytic aggregates, lymphocytes, and multinucleated giant cells, with or without necrosis (Fig. 4.2h, i).

Histology of Core

- Nodular aggregates of epithelioid histiocytes with or without multinucleated giant cells.
- Classified as suppurative, noncaseating, or caseating granulomas with different disease associations.

Comments

- Special stains for microorganisms should be ordered.

Tumors of the Lymphoid Tissue

Lymphoid malignancies may involve lymph nodes.

General FNA Characteristics of Lymphoid Malignancies

- Highly cellular specimen consisting of discohesive atypical lymphoid cells, unless lymphoma with associated sclerosis.
- Presence of lymphoglandular bodies.
- FNA cytologic features vary, depending on the type of lymphoma, ranging from a monotonous population to a polymorphous population of cells and from small to large size.

Non-Hodgkin Lymphoma (NHL)

Precursor B/T-Cell Neoplasm

Lymphoblastic lymphoma (LBL) is defined as tissue involvement by precursor

T- or B-cells, representing the same disease process as lymphoblastic leukemia.

Clinical

- Approximately 90% of LBLs arise from T-cells (T-LBL), and another 10% are from B-cells (B-LBL).
- T-LBLs commonly present as bulky anterior mediastinal masses in young males, whereas B-LBLs most commonly involve the skin, lymph nodes, bone, and soft tissue.

Cytology of FNA and Touch Preparation

- B- and T-LBLs are indistinguishable by morphology.
- They are dispersed small to intermediate sized cells.
- The cells show round to variably irregular nuclear contours, open fine chromatin, multiple small nucleoli, and scant cytoplasm. Some of the cells show coarse azurophilic granules and vacuolation in the cytoplasm (Fig. 4.3a, b).
- Mitotic figures are usually numerous.

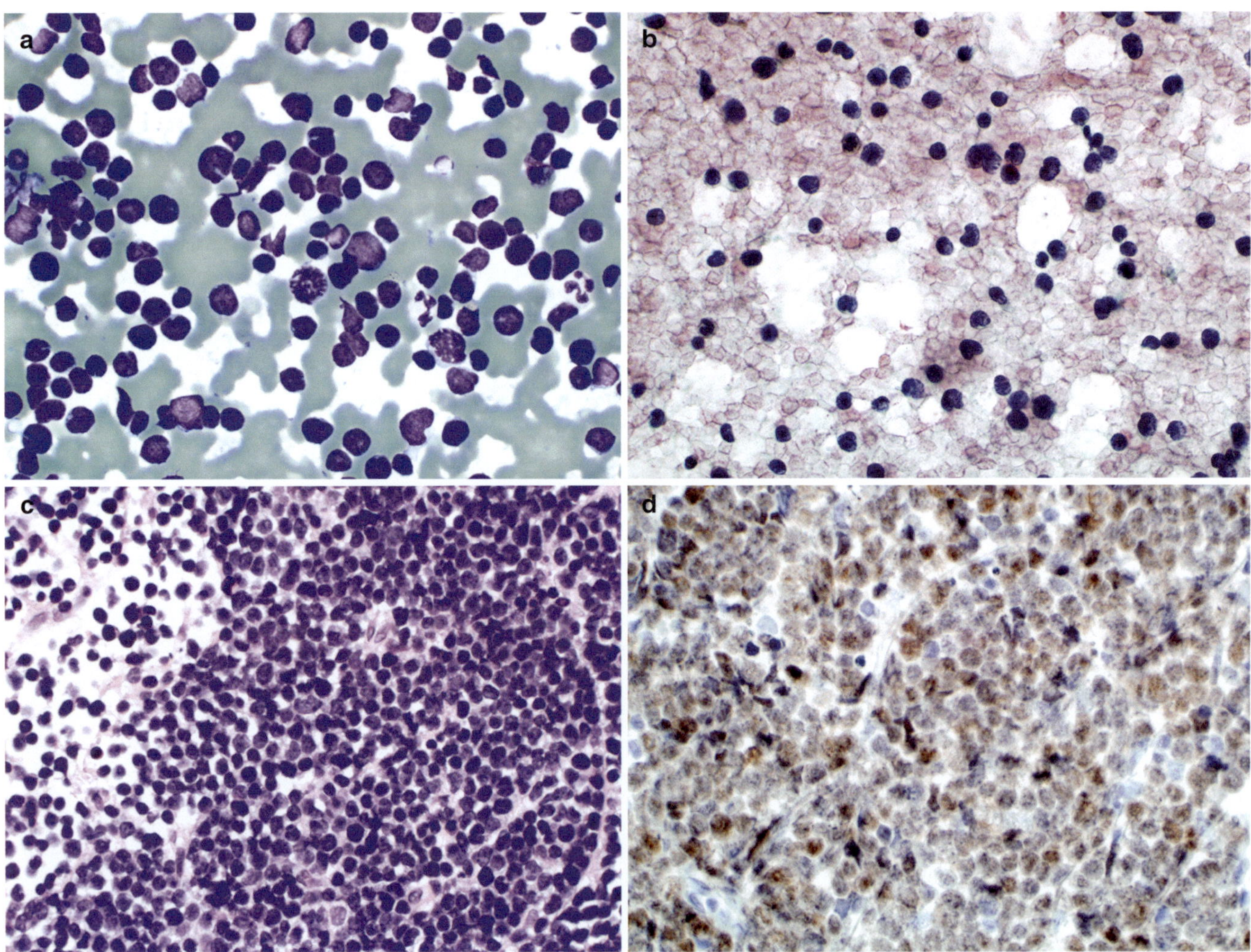

Fig. 4.3 Pathology of lymphoblastic lymphoma (T cell). (**a**, **b**) Cytomorphology of FNA of a lymph node in a patient with lymphoblastic lymphoma; Diff-Quik stain (**a**) and Papanicolaou stain (**b**), 600×. (**c**) Histolomorphology of needle core, hemotoxylin and eosin stain, 600×. (**d**) Immunostain for TdT, 600×

Histology of Core

- Effaced architecture by diffuse medium-sized cells, as described previously.
- The lymphoma has a high proliferation index and may reveal a "starry-sky" appearance with frequent tingible-body macrophages (Fig. 4.3c).

Comments

- **Differential Diagnosis**
  - Includes myeloid sarcoma, Burkitt lymphoma, blastoid variant of mantle cell lymphoma, thymoma, and thymic tissue.
- **Ancillary Studies**
  - CD34, terminal deoxynucleotidyl transferase (TDT) (Fig. 4.3d), and CD1a (for T-lineage) expression are used to define immaturity in LBLs.
  - B-LBLs express CD10, CD19, CD22, CD34, CD79a, and PAX-5. T-LBLs are positive for CD3.

Mature B-Cell Neoplasms

Chronic Lymphocytic Leukemia (CLL)/Small Lymphocytic Lymphoma (SLL)

CLL/SLL are B-cell neoplasms, composed of small monoclonal B lymphocytes in the peripheral blood, bone marrow, spleen, and lymph nodes.

Clinical

- CLL/SLL account for 6.7% of NHLs in biopsies.
- More common in the elderly with a median age of diagnosis at 65 years; rarely diagnosed before 40 years of age [11].
- More common in men, with a male: female ratio of 1.5–2:1.
- Most are asymptomatic, but some may present with generalized lymphadenopathy, hepatosplenomegaly, and systemic symptoms like fatigue and weight loss.
- Bone marrow and/or peripheral blood are usually involved in CLL.
- They may or may not have a monoclonal gammopathy and autoimmune cytopenias.
- Indolent course, unless transformation to a higher-grade lymphoma (Richter transformation).
- Prototypic small mature B-cell lymphoma.

Radiography

X-ray

- Intrathoracic lymphadenopathy is a nonspecific finding, as there is thickening of mediastinal lines and stripes, loss of normal mediastinal contours, or mediastinal widening.

CT Scan

- CT is the modality of choice to establish baseline disease and to monitor disease progression.
- Contrast-enhanced CT (CECT) demonstrates diffuse generalized lymphadenopathy with homogeneous enhancement and loss of the normal central fatty hilum (Fig. 4.4a, b).
- Splenomegaly and hepatomegaly can be seen without focal masses or lesions.
- Pulmonary consolidative or ground-glass opacities are the dominant findings in cases of pulmonary parenchymal involvement [12]. There may be associated pleural effusion in cases of central lymphatic obstruction, pleural invasion, or infection.

PET/CT

- Nonspecific findings with increased F-18 FDG uptake in cases of Richter transformation [13].
- There is variable and often little to no FDG uptake.
- High standardized uptake value (SUV) max is associated with a poor prognosis [14].

MRI

- As with other bone marrow infiltrative diseases, MRI demonstrates diffuse low bone marrow T1 signal indicative of leukemic infiltration.

Gross

- Enlarged, tan lymph nodes with a fleshy texture.
- Larger masses may represent a matted group of nodes.

Cytology of FNA and Touch Preparation

- Highly cellular aspirate consisting of dispersed monotonous small lymphocytes that are only slightly larger than normal lymphocytes.
- Cells with a thin rim of pale cytoplasm, round nuclei showing regular to slightly irregular nuclear membranes, hyperchromatic clumped chromatin, and inconspicuous nucleoli are characteristic (Fig. 4.4c, d).
- Few large cells (prolymphocytes and paraimmunoblasts) may show prominent nucleoli.

Histology of Core

- Lymph node with effaced architecture secondary to the diffuse proliferation of small round lymphocytes with scant cytoplasm, regular to slightly irregular nuclear membrane, clumped chromatin, and inconspicuous nucleoli.
- Pseudofollicular pattern with proliferation centers consisting of larger cells (prolymphocytes and paraimmunoblasts) in a background of small lymphocytes.

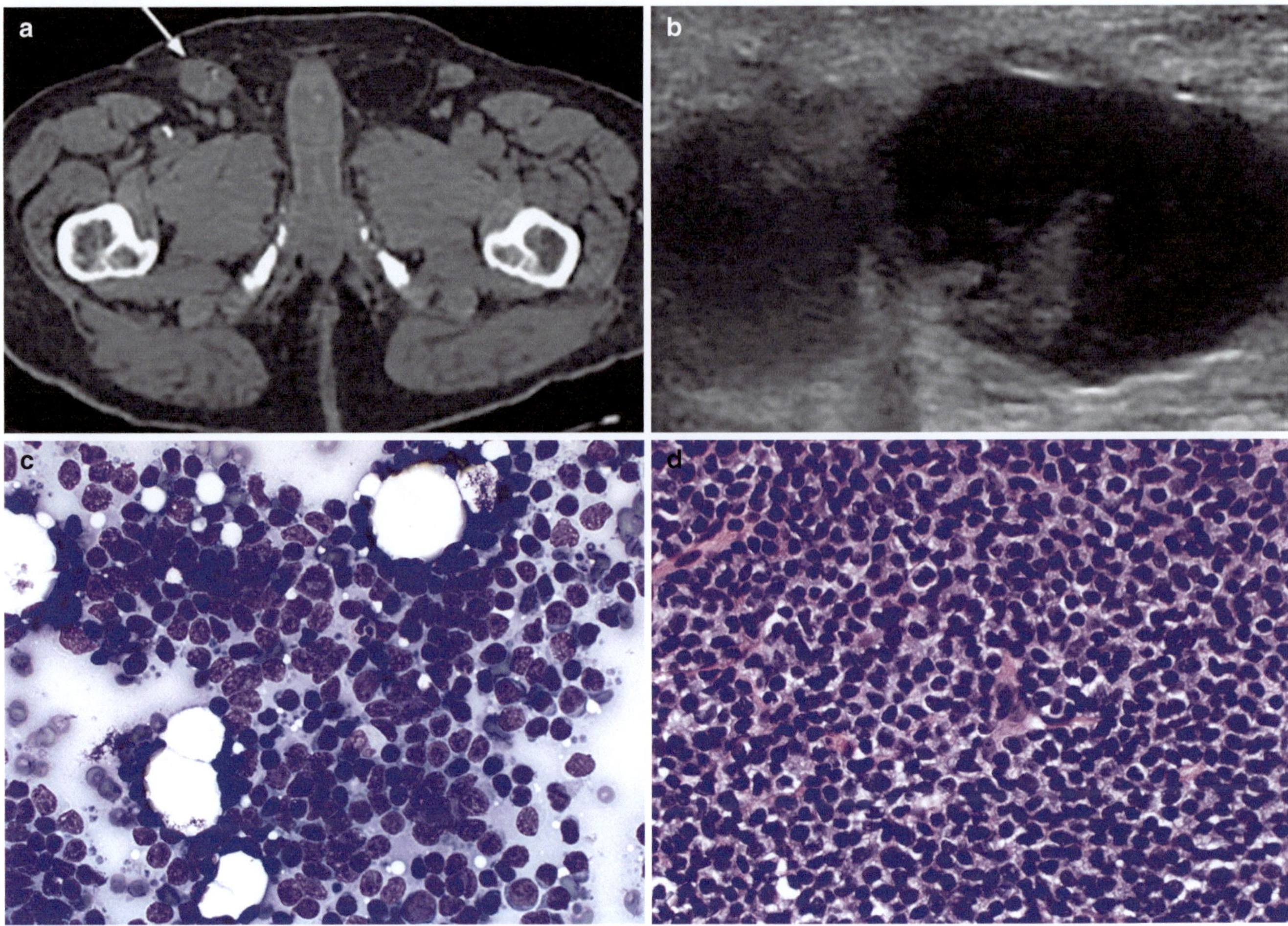

Fig. 4.4 (**a**, **b**) Radiologic images of small lymphocytic lymphoma (SLL)/chronic lymphocytic leukemia (CLL). (**a**) Noncontrast CT scan shows an enlarged bilateral inguinal lymph node, right greater than left. There was also extensive mesenteric lymphadenopathy. (**b**) Gray scale US demonstrates a round hypoechoic lymph node with a suspicious morphology at the time of biopsy. (**c**, **d**) Pathology of SLL/CLL. (**c**) Cytomorphology of FNA of a lymph node in a patient with CLL/SLL; Diff-Quik stain, 600×. Histology of needle core, hematoxylin and eosin stain, 600×

Comments

- **Differential Diagnosis**
  - Includes mantle cell lymphoma, hairy cell leukemia, follicular lymphoma, and lymphoplasmacytic lymphoma.
- **Ancillary Studies**
  - Flow cytometry and immunocytochemistry are highly recommended in patients over the age of 45 with lymphadenopathy, especially if it is generalized.
  - Assessment of clonality can be performed by numerous approaches: molecular analysis of clonal gene rearrangement, immunohistochemistry to assess immunoglobulin expression (kappa to lambda ratio), and flow cytometry can also detect a clonal population of cells.
  - Immunophenotype: CD19+, CD5+, and CD 23+, weak expression of CD20, and surface immunoglobin light chains and CD10 negative [15].
- **Prognostic factors**:
  - Poor prognosis: ZAP-70, CD38 expression; deletion of 11q, 17p, 6q; rapid lymphocyte doubling time in the peripheral blood <12 months; elevated serum thymidine kinase, CD23, and beta 2 microglobulin.
  - Good prognosis: isolated deletion of 13q.

Follicular Lymphoma

Follicular lymphoma is a B-cell neoplasm composed of follicular center B-cells (centrocytes and centroblasts) with at least a partial follicular pattern.

Clinical

- Second most common lymphoma worldwide after diffuse large B-cell lymphoma; comprises 20% of all lymphomas with the highest incidence in the United States and Western Europe.

- Affects predominantly adults, with a median age of diagnosis in the sixth decade [16].
- Male:female ratio of 1:1.7 [16].
- Most patients present with generalized lymphadenopathy, even though they may be asymptomatic.
- Prognosis depends on histologic grading (grades 1 and 2 indolent, grade 3 aggressive) and the Follicular Lymphoma International Prognostic Index (FLIPI). Grade 3 is a more aggressive disease; however, it has the potential for cure. In contrast, grade 1 and 2 follicular lymphoma are more indolent but incurable.

Radiography

Ultrasound Image

- Mediastinal, paratracheal, and hilar lymphadenopathy (Fig. 4.5a).

CT Scan

- The modality of choice for the assessment of non-FDG avid lymphoma and radiotherapy planning.
- Lymph node enlargement is greater than 1 cm in short axis.
- There may be scattered mediastinal, supraclavicular, and axillary lymphadenopathy that may wax and wane over time without complete resolution.
- Histologic transformation of follicular lymphoma to diffuse large B-cell lymphoma (DLBCL) is marked by rapid progression of lymphadenopathy and infiltration of uncommon extranodal sites [17].

PET/CT

- PET/CT is superior to CT for initial staging of disease, interim evaluation, and at the end of treatment in FDG avid non-Hodgkin lymphoma.
- There is increase FDG uptake of involved lymph nodes in non-Hodgkin lymphoma.
- Follicular lymphoma is typically FDG avid on FDG PET/CT despite being one of the most common indolent non-Hodgkin lymphoma subtypes [18].

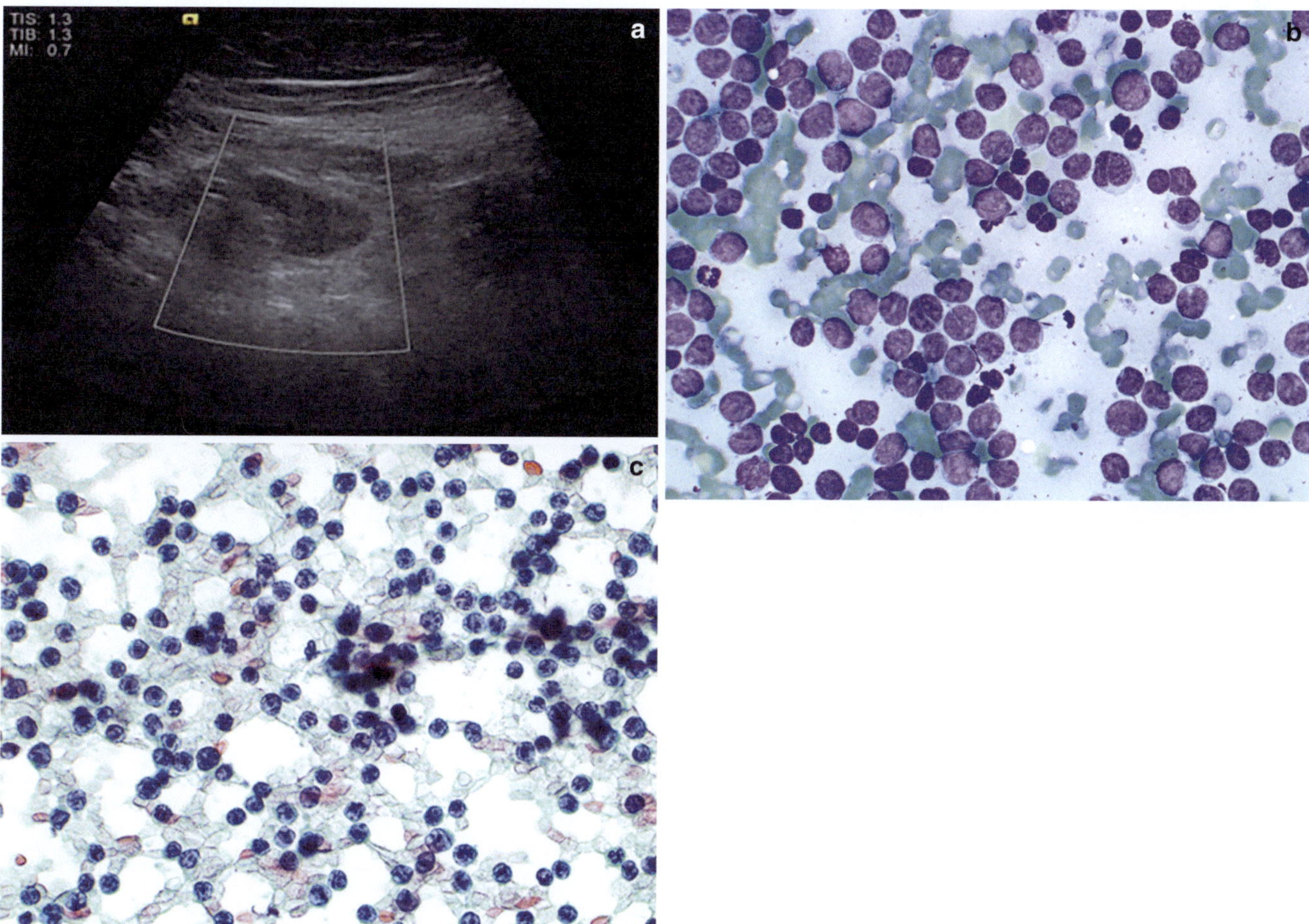

Fig. 4.5 (**a**) US image of follicular lymphoma. Color US image of a nodal pelvic mass at the time of biopsy with biopsy-proven follicular lymphoma. (**b**, **c**) Pathology of follicular lymphoma. Cytomorphology of FNA of a lymph node in a patient with follicular lymphoma; Diff-Quik stain and Papanicolaou stain, 600×

MRI

- The modality of choice for assessment of central nervous system and cardiac involvement.
- Involved lymph nodes demonstrate a homogeneous signal on T1-weighted imaging and a heterogeneous signal owing to nodal necrosis on T2 and contrast-enhanced T1-weighted sequences [17].

Cytology of FNA and Touch Preparation

- Cellular smears consist of varying proportions of follicular center cells, centrocytes, and centroblasts, depending upon the grade.
- Centrocytes are small to medium-sized cells with scant cytoplasm, cleaved nuclei, and inconspicuous nucleoli.
- Centroblasts show large round or slightly irregular nuclei with basophilic cytoplasm and small nucleoli. The cytology of grade 3 follicular lymphoma is essentially that of diffuse large B-cell lymphoma, which is composed of large lymphoid cells with enlarged nuclei, irregular nuclear membranes, prominent nucleoli, hyperchromatic or vesicular chromatin, and moderate amounts of bluish cytoplasm (Fig. 4.5b, c).
- Lack of normal range of maturation and rare or absent tingible body macrophages.

Histology of Core

- Lymph node architecture effaced by a follicular or diffuse proliferation of atypical centrocytes and centroblasts.
- Distinction between grades 1 and 2 and grade 3 may not always be possible on core biopsy specimens.
- Histologic grading is based upon the number of centrocytes per high power field (HPF). Grades 1 and 2 (<15/HPF), grade 3 (>15/HPF). An adequate core is often necessary to confirm the diagnosis and for grading purposes.

Comments

- **Differential Diagnosis**
  - Reactive follicular hyperplasia
  - Mantle cell lymphoma
  - Small lymphocytic lymphoma (SLL/CLL).
  - Diffuse large B-cell lymphoma
- **Ancillary Studies**
  - Assessment of clonality with flow cytometry.
  - Majority of follicular lymphomas have t(14;18), *BCL2/IgH* rearrangement, which results in the overexpression of BCL2 protein [19, 20].
  - Immunophenotype: CD19+, CD20+, CD5–, CD 23–, CD10+, BCL2+, and BCL6+.

Nodal Marginal Zone B-Cell Lymphoma

Nodal marginal zone B-cell lymphoma is a nodal neoplasm consisting of B cells growing in a marginal zone pattern without evidence of extranodal or splenic involvement.

Clinical

- Median age of diagnosis is 60 years old.
- Usually present as asymptomatic generalized or localized peripheral lymphadenopathy.

Cytology of FNA and Touch Preparation

- Cells showing lymphoplasmacytic features and monocytoid B cells may be present in varying proportions, along with plasma cells and sometimes immunoblasts (Fig. 4.6).

Histology of Core and Touch Preparation

- A heterogeneous population of B lymphocytes, predominantly composed of small- to medium-sized cells with heterogeneous nuclear morphologies.

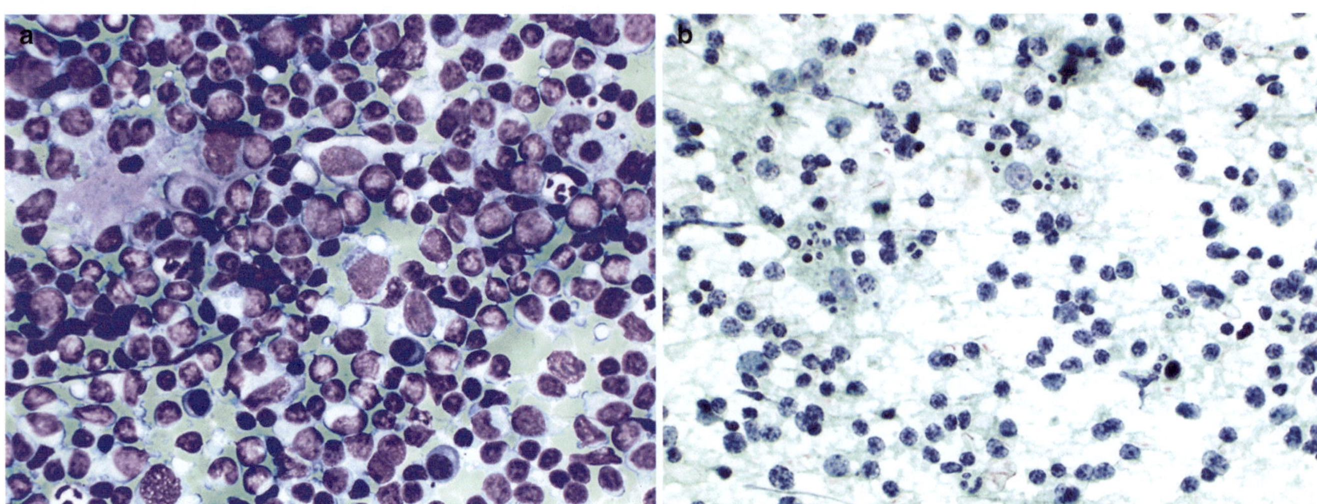

Fig. 4.6 Pathology of marginal zone lymphoma. Cytomorphology of FNA of a lymph node in a patient with marginal zone lymphoma; Diff-Quik stain and Papanicolaou stain, 600×

Comments

- **Differential diagnosis:**
  - Reactive lymph node
  - Extranodal marginal zone lymphoma
  - Follicular lymphoma
  - Mantle cell lymphoma
  - Small lymphocytic lymphoma
  - Lymphoplasmacytic lymphoma
- **Ancillary Studies**
  - Positive: CD20, CD19, CD43, and BCL2.
  - Negative: CD5, CD10, CD23, BCL6, and cyclin D1.

Extranodal Marginal Zone B-Cell Lymphoma (MALT Lymphoma)

Extranodal marginal zone B-cell lymphoma is composed of morphologically heterogeneous small B cells, including small lymphocytes, monocytoid lymphocytes, or lymphocytes with centrocyte-like morphology.

Clinical

- Accounts for 5% of all B-cell lymphomas and at least 50% of primary gastric lymphomas [11, 21].
- Occurs in adults with a median age of 61 years and has a slight female predominance.
- Association with previous *H. pylori* infection in the development of primary gastric lymphoma [22].
- One of the most indolent lymphomas.
- Transformation to diffuse large B-cell lymphoma results in a significantly lower survival rate.

Cytology of FNA and Touch Preparation

- Show discohesive monotonous or polymorphic lymphoid cells with monocytoid or plasmacytoid features. No lymphohistiocytic aggregates (germinal center) present.

Histology of Core

- Fragments of lymphoid tissue consisting of small lymphocytes, marginal zone (centrocyte-like) B cells, monocytoid B cells, and plasmacytoid cells as well as less frequent large activated cells.

Comments

- **Differential Diagnosis**
  - Reactive hyperplasia
  - Other small B-cell lymphomas
- **Ancillary Studies**
  - Immunophenotype: CD19+, CD20+, CD5–, CD10–, CD 23–, and CD43+ (50% of cases) [23].
  - Molecular evidence of monoclonality detected by PCR.
  - Fluorescence in situ hybridization (FISH) detection of t(11;18) [24].

Mantle Cell Lymphoma

Mantle cell lymphoma is a B-cell neoplasm composed of monomorphic small-to-medium sized lymphocytes with irregular nuclear contours and characterized by *CCND1* translocation.

Clinical

- Accounts for 3–10% of non-Hodgkin lymphomas.
- Occurs in older adults with a median age of 60 years with a male predominance (male:female ratio of >2:1).
- Presents with generalized lymphadenopathy, hepatosplenomegaly, extranodal or bone marrow involvement, and less commonly peripheral blood involvement.
- Relatively aggressive clinical behavior with a poor response to conventional therapeutic regimens.
- Proliferative activity is the most important prognostic parameter.

Cytology of FNA and Touch Preparation

- Monomorphic medium-sized lymphocytes with irregular nuclear membranes, prominent nucleoli, and scant cytoplasm (Fig. 4.7a, b).

Histology of Core

- Lymph node architecture effaced by vaguely nodular, diffuse, or mantle zone proliferation of monomorphic small-to-medium sized lymphocytes (Fig. 4.7C).
- The cells resemble centrocytes with irregular nuclear contours, dispersed chromatin, and inconspicuous nucleoli.
- Cells resembling centroblasts, immunoblasts, or paraimmunoblasts and proliferation centers are absent
- Morphologic variants:
  - Blastoid variant (cells resemble lymphoblasts with high mitotic rate) and pleomorphic variant (pleomorphic large cells with prominent nucleoli) behave aggressively.
  - Small cell variant mimics small lymphocytic lymphoma.

Comments

- **Differential Diagnosis**
  - Chronic lymphocytic leukemia/small lymphocytic lymphoma (CLL/SLL).
  - CD5+ marginal zone lymphoma.
  - Diffuse large B-cell lymphoma (pleomorphic variant).
  - B-lymphoblastic leukemia (blastoid variant).
- **Ancillary Studies**
  - Monotypic surface or cytoplasmic immunoglobulin detected by flow cytometry.
  - Clonal rearranged immunoglobulin heavy or light chains detected by PCR.
  - Immunophenotype: CD19+, CD20+, CD5+, FMC7+, CD10–, CD 23+, BCL6-, cyclin D1+, and SOX11+ [25, 26].
  - Characteristic genetic alteration t(11;14), *CCND1/IgH* rearrangement. Immunostain for cyclin D1 (Fig. 4.7d).

Diffuse Large B-Cell Lymphoma

Diffuse large B-cell lymphoma is a neoplasm of large B-lymphoid cells with a diffuse growth pattern.

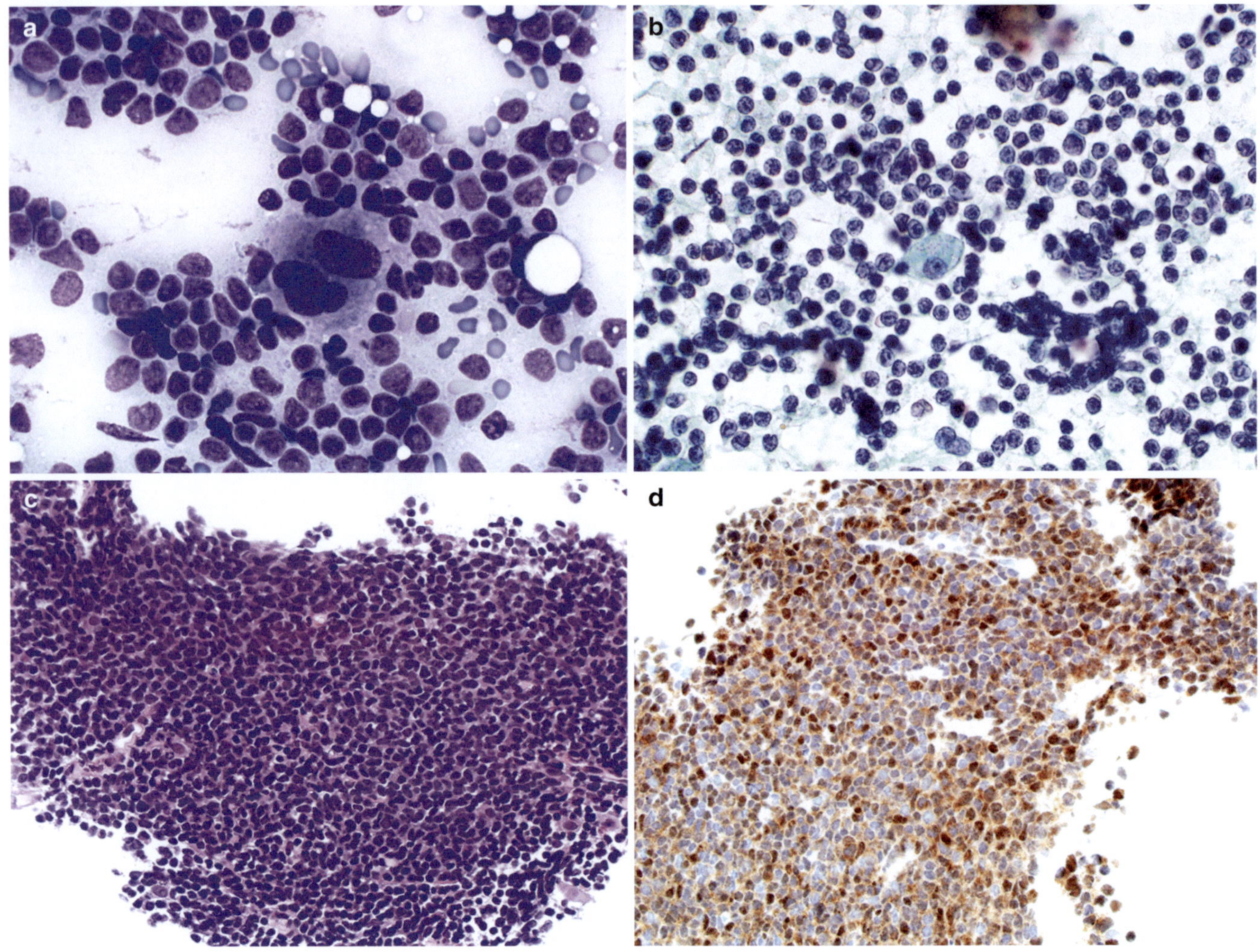

Fig. 4.7 Pathology of mantle cell lymphoma. (**a**, **b**) Cytomorphology of FNA of a lymph node in a patient with mental cell lymphoma; Diff-Quik stain (**a**) and Papanicolaou stain (**b**), 600×. (**c**) Histology of needle core, hematoxylin and eosin stain, 600×. (**d**) Immunostain for cyclin D1, 600×

Clinical

- Most common NHL; accounts for 25–30% of adult lymphomas in Western countries.
- Median age of patients is seventh decade, but it can occur in any age group.
- Most patients have no underlying risk factors, but a minority of patients are immunodeficient.
- Rare cases are associated with chronic inflammation and irritation.
- Most cases arise de novo; however, some cases are from transformation of a low-grade B-cell lymphoma.
- Patients present with rapidly enlarging lymph nodes or tissue masses.

Radiography

- General radiography findings include mediastinal and hilar adenopathy, a nonspecific initial finding that warrants further evaluation with contrast-enhanced CT.

Ultrasound

- Ultrasound findings show typical features that favor malignancy.
- Increased peripheral vascularity, loss of central fatty hilum, round morphology, heterogeneous echotexture, eccentric thickening of the cortex, and ill-defined capsular margins [4, 27].

CT Scan

- In most cases, contrast-enhanced CT is the imaging modality of choice for assessment of non-FDG avid NHL and radiotherapy planning.
- Contrast-enhanced CT demonstrates lymphadenopathy, which is the most common finding with lymph node size greater than 1.0 cm in the short axis (Fig. 4.8a, b).
- Hypodense nodes in DLBCL are usually indicative of cystic changes or necrosis. Location of lymphadenopathy within the chest includes perivascular and paratracheal

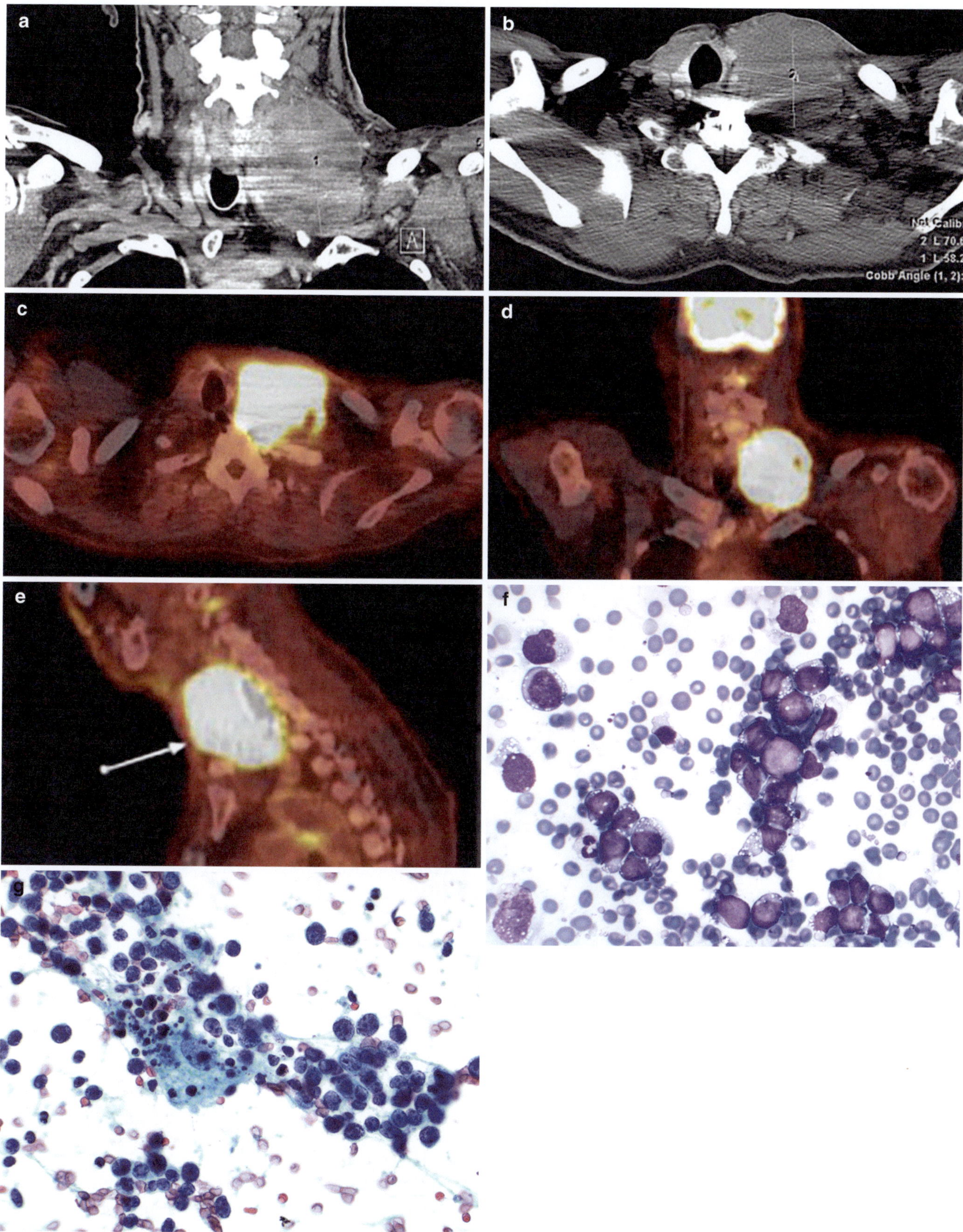

Fig. 4.8 (**a–e**) Radiography of diffuse large B-cell lymphoma. (**a**, **b**) CECT axial (**a**) and coronal (**b**) images demonstrate a large 5.8 × 7.1 × 8.9 cm soft-tissue mass in the left supraclavicular region extending into the left thoracic inlet encasing the left subclavian vein in a patient with biopsy-proven DLBCL. (**c–e**) F-18 FDG PET/CT axial (**c**), coronal (**d**), and (**e**) sagittal images demonstrate a large hypermetabolic lymph node mass with its origin in the left supraclavicular space, extending into the neck and the superior mediastinum (Deauville Score). (**f**, **g**) Pathology of diffuse large B-cell lymphoma. Cytomorphology of FNA of a lymph node; Diff-Quik stain (**f**) and Papanicolaou stain (**g**), 600×

(75%), subcarinal (30%), hilar (20%), posterior mediastinal, paracardiac (10%), retrocrural (20%), paravertebral, and para-aortic nodal stations [28].

PET CT Scan

- The imaging modality of choice to evaluate FDG-avid non-Hodgkin lymphoma.
- Intense FDG-avid lymphadenopathy is usually seen with DLBCL (Fig. 4.8c–e).
- PET/CT is useful to assess the response of lymphoma to treatment and is superior to CT in the initial staging, post-treatment evaluation, and end of treatment evaluation [29].

MRI

- As with most lymphomas, MRI is the modality of choice for assessment of central nervous system and cardiac involvement, with findings similar to those of follicular lymphoma.

Cytology of FNA and Touch Preparation

- Cellular smears consist of discohesive medium-to-large centroblasts and/or immunoblasts.
- Centroblasts are medium-to-large cells with scant to moderate cytoplasm, central round to ovoid nuclei, smooth nuclear contours, vesicular chromatin, and two to four nucleoli located close to the nuclear border.
- Immunoblasts are larger than centroblasts with prominent central nucleoli and a moderate amount of bluish cytoplasm, with frequent vacuolation.
- The anaplastic variant is composed of large pleomorphic cells (Fig. 4.8f, g).

Histology of Core

- Diffuse proliferation of large lymphoid cells with total or partially effaced architecture.
- Large lymphoid cells with nuclear size equal to or exceeding that of normal macrophage nuclei or more than twice the normal lymphocyte.
- Morphologic variants: centroblastic, immunoblastic, and anaplastic variants.

Comments

- **Differential Diagnosis**
  - Nonhematologic malignancies (carcinoma, melanoma, seminoma).
  - Anaplastic large cell lymphoma
  - Lymphoblastic lymphoma
  - High grade B-cell lymphoma with *MYC* and *BCL2* or *BCL6* rearrangements
  - Burkitt lymphoma
  - Mantle cell lymphoma, blastoid and pleomorphic variant
  - NK/T cell lymphoma
  - Myeloid sarcoma
- **Ancillary Studies**
  - Monotypic surface or cytoplasmic immunoglobulin by flow cytometry.
  - Clonally rearranged immunoglobulin heavy or light chains.
  - Immunophenotype: CD19+, CD20+, CD5+ (~10%), CD10+ (~40%), BCL6+ (~60%).
  - Classified into germinal center B-cell type (CD10+ and CD10-, BCL6+, MUM1-) and activated B-cell-like type (CD10-, BCL6- and CD10-, BCL6+, MUM1+) by immunohistochemistry based on Hans algorithm [30]; this is highly concordant with gene expression profile [31].
  - MYC gene rearrangement is seen in ~10%, *BCL6* rearrangement in ~30%, and *BCL2* rearrangement in ~20% [32–34].
  - Double hit with both *MYC* and *BCL2* rearrangement or *MYC* and *BCL6* rearrangement should be classified as high-grade B-cell lymphoma with specific rearrangements
  - Double expresser with both MYC (>40%) and BCL2 (>50%) expression by immunohistochemistry.

Burkitt Lymphoma

Burkitt lymphoma is a B-cell lymphoma composed of medium-sized lymphoid cells with characteristic *MYC* translocation and an extremely short doubling time.

Clinical

- Highly aggressive lymphoid neoplasm, often present at extranodal sites or as leukemia.
- Three clinical variants: endemic (affects children in equatorial Africa, usually present as abdominal or jaw mass), sporadic (mainly affects children and young adults throughout the world, usually extranodal), and immunodeficiency-associated (seen in association with HIV and most commonly involves lymph nodes, bone marrow, and CNS).

Cytology of FNA and Touch Preparation

- Comparatively uniform medium-sized lymphoid cells with round nuclei, granular chromatin, multiple small prominent nucleoli, and variable dense blue cytoplasm with small cytoplasmic vacuoles (Fig. 4.9a).
- Mitotic figures, apoptotic figures, tingible body macrophages, and necrosis are readily seen.

Histology of Core

- Lymph node architecture is effaced by the proliferation of a diffuse monotonous population of medium-sized lymphoid cells (Fig. 4.9b).
- High proliferation fraction with numerous mitoses, abundant apoptotic debris, necrosis, and tingible body macrophages imparting a starry sky pattern.

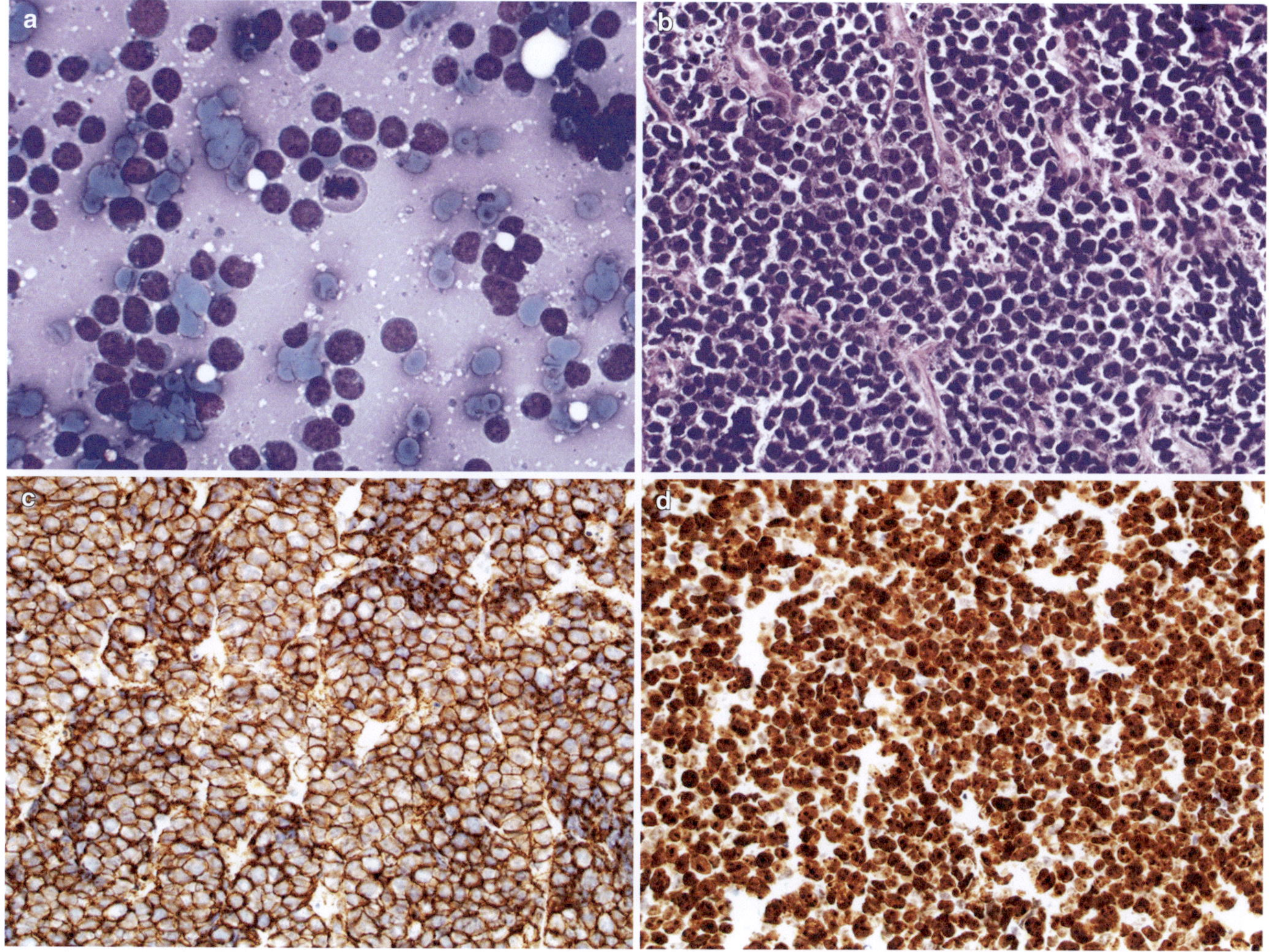

Fig. 4.9 Pathology of Burkitt lymphoma. (**a**) Cytomorphology of FNA of a lymph node; Diff-Quik stain, 600×. (**b**) Histology of needle core, hematoxylin and eosin stain, 400×. (**c**, **d**) Immunostains for CD20 (**c**) and Ki-67 (**d**), 400×

Comments

- **Differential Diagnosis**
  - Diffuse large B-cell lymphoma
  - High grade B-cell lymphoma
  - Lymphoblastic lymphoma
  - Mantle cell lymphoma, blastoid type
  - Myeloid sarcoma
- **Ancillary Studies**
  - Monotypic surface or cytoplasmic immunoglobulin by flow cytometry.
  - Clonally rearranged immunoglobulin heavy or light chains.
  - Immunophenotype: CD19+, CD20+ (Fig. 4.9c), CD10+, BCL6+, CD5-, CD23-, cyclin
  - D1-, TdT-, BCL2- or weakly positive, and Ki67 >95% (Fig. 4.9d).
  - Characteristic genetic abnormalities: *MYC* rearrangement to immunoglobulin partners, t(8;14) or variant t(2;8) or t(8;22), mostly as simple karyotypes.

Plasma Cell Neoplasm

Plasma cell neoplasms are composed of clonally expanded plasma cells (immunoglobulin secreting terminally differentiated B cells).

Clinical

- Plasma cell neoplasms include plasma cell myeloma, plasmacytoma, monoclonal gammopathy of unknown significance, and immunoglobulin deposition diseases.
- Most commonly originates as bone marrow tumors, with occasional occurrence in extramedullary sites, including lymph nodes.
- Most common hematolymphoid malignancy in African Americans.
- Rare before the age of 40.
- Clinical work-up includes CBC with differential count, chemistry panel, serum protein electrophoresis, immunofixation, and bone survey.

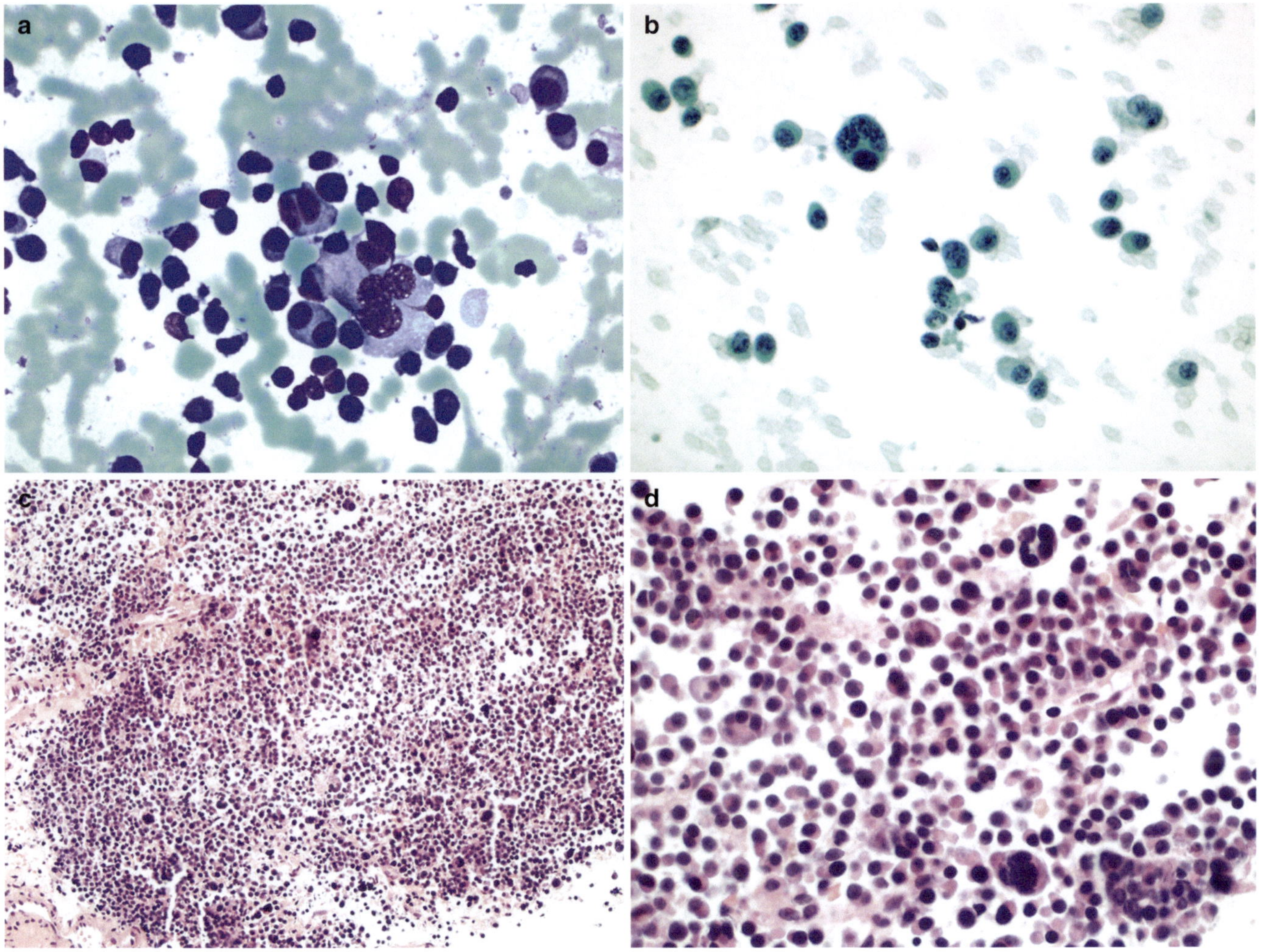

Fig. 4.10 Pathology of plasmacytoma. (**a**, **b**) Cytomorphology of FNA, Diff-Quik stain (**a**) and Papanicolaou stain (**b**), 600×. (**c**, **d**) Histology of needle core, hematoxylin and eosin stain, 200× (**c**) and 600× (**d**)

- Patients with plasma cell myeloma may have multiple organ impairments causing anemia, pathologic bone fractures, renal failure, amyloidosis, repeated infections, and hypercalcemia [35].

Cytology of FNA and Touch Preparation
- Cellular specimen consisting of discohesive plasma cells, the majority of which are normal-appearing and mature; the minority are more immature or atypical (Fig. 4.10a, b).
- Binucleated forms are common in plasma cell neoplasms. Multinucleated, giant, and bizarre cells that are unrecognizable as plasma cells can also be present (Fig. 4.10a, b, d).
- Dutcher bodies and intranuclear immunoglobulin inclusions identified in plasma cells are an indicator of malignancy.

Histology of Core
- Sheets of plasma cells, often mature-appearing but may be poorly differentiated with plasmablastic or anaplastic morphology (Fig. 4.10c, d).

Comments
- **Differential Diagnosis**
  - Lymphoplasmacytic lymphoma
  - Marginal zone lymphoma
  - Plasmablastic lymphoma
  - Reactive plasmacytosis
  - Metastatic melanoma
  - Metastatic adenocarcinoma
- **Ancillary Studies**
  - Assessment of clonality by flow cytometry, immunocytochemistry, or molecular diagnostics.

Lymphoplasmacytic Lymphoma (LPL)

Lymphoplasmacytic lymphoma is composed of small B lymphocytes, plasmacytoid lymphocytes, and plasma cells.

Clinical

- Uncommon mature B-cell lymphoma that usually involves the bone marrow and sometimes the spleen and lymph nodes.

- Often associated with IgM monoclonal gammopathy (Waldenstrom macroglobulinemia).
- Patients present with symptoms related to tumor infiltration (lymphadenopathy, organomegaly, cytopenia) or monoclonal protein production (hyperviscosity, neuropathy).

Cytology of FNA and Touch Preparation

- Cytology is similar to that of CLL/SLL except that it displays a fuller range of B-cell maturation with the addition of plasmacytoid cells, plasma cells, and occasional blasts.

Histology of Core

- Monotonous proliferation of small lymphocytes, plasma cells, and plasmacytoid lymphocytes.
- Plasmacytoid cells with Dutcher bodies, increased mast cells, and hemosiderin deposition may be seen.

Comments

- **Differential Diagnosis**
  - Other small B-cell lymphoid neoplasms with plasmacytic differentiation: marginal zone lymphoma, CLLs/SLLs, follicular lymphoma, and plasma cell neoplasm.
- **Ancillary Studies**
  - Lymphocytes: strong surface and cytoplasmic Ig+, CD19+, CD20+, CD79a+. Occasionally CD5+, CD23+, and rarely CD10+.
  - Plasma cells are positive for CD138 and CD38. Serum protein electrophoresis (SPEP) shows IgM monoclonal gammopathy in cases with Waldenstrom macroglobulinemia.
  - *MYD88* mutation is highly associated with LPL but is not entirely specific and has been reported in other B-cell neoplasms with a much lower frequency [36, 37].

Mature T-Cell and NK-Cell Neoplasms

Peripheral T-Cell Lymphoma, Not Otherwise Specified (NOS)

Peripheral T-cell lymphoma (PTCL) is a heterogeneous group of nodal or extranodal mature T-cell lymphomas that do not fit into any of the defined mature T-cell lymphomas.

Clinical

- PTCL, NOS is the most common subtype of PTCL in Western countries.
- It is more common in males, with a median age at diagnosis of 60 years [38, 39].
- Patients present with generalized lymphadenopathy with or without extranodal disease, hepatosplenomegaly, and bone marrow involvement [39].

Cytology of FNA and Touch Preparation

- Heterogeneous appearance, composed of atypical medium to large cells with exuberant benign inflammatory reaction in the background that may mimic a reactive lymph node.
- Occasionally, monomorphous proliferation of small, medium, or large atypical cells may be seen.
- Nuclei are often indented with convolutions.

Histology of Core

- Effaced normal architecture with paracortical or diffuse infiltrate.
- Broad morphologic spectrum from polymorphous to monomorphous proliferation of variably sized atypical lymphocytes.
- An inflammatory background of small lymphocytes, eosinophils, plasma cells, and epithelioid histiocytes is often present.

Comments

- **Differential Diagnosis**
  - Angioimmunoblastic T-cell lymphoma
  - Anaplastic large cell lymphoma
  - Hodgkin lymphoma
  - T-cell/histiocyte rich large B-cell lymphoma
- **Ancillary Studies**
  - Immunophenotype: Tumor cells variably express T-cell–associated antigens (CD3+/−, CD2+/−, CD5+/−, and CD7−/+) and are generally negative for B-cell–associated antigens.
  - Most cases express alpha/beta T-cell receptors, while a minority express gamma/delta T-cell receptors.
  - Clonal T-cell receptor (TCR) gene rearrangements.

Adult T-Cell Leukemia/Lymphoma

Adult T-cell leukemia/lymphoma (ATLL) is peripheral T-cell lymphoma composed of pleomorphic lymphoid cells and associated with HTLV-1 infection.

Clinical

- Uncommon lymphoid neoplasm associated with human T-lymphotropic virus, type I (HTLV-I) infection.

- Affects people who live in or originate from endemic areas (Japan, Caribbean, central Africa, and Iran).
- Risk of ATLL following infection with HTLV-I in endemic areas is 4–5%, usually after a latent period of several decades [40].
- Clinical variants: acute, lymphomatous, chronic, and smoldering.

Cytology of FNA and Touch Preparation

- Cellular smears composed of pleomorphic intermediate-to-large lymphocytes with marked nuclear membrane irregularities, coarse clumped chromatin, and prominent nucleoli.
- Giant cells with multilobulated nuclei (floret-like), prominent nucleoli, and deeply basophilic cytoplasm with occasional vacuoles are characteristic.

Histology of Core

- Several morphologic variants exist, with a variable appearance.
- Majority of cases show diffuse effacement by pleomorphic, medium- to large-sized lymphocytes with marked nuclear irregularity and coarsely clumped chromatin.

Comments

- **Differential Diagnosis**
  - Anaplastic large-cell lymphoma
  - Peripheral T-cell lymphoma
  - Angioimmunoblastic T-cell lymphoma
  - HTLV1-associated lymphadenitis
- **Ancillary Studies**
  - Immunophenotype: CC25+, CD2+, CD4+, CD52+, CD5+, dim CD3+, and CD7-. Most cases are CD4+ and CD8-; rare cases are CD4-/CD8+ or CD4+/CD8 + .
  - Detection of serologic antibodies to HTLV-I by enzyme-linked immunosorbent assay (ELISA).
  - PCR-based testing to detect proviral DNA in tumor cells.
  - Clonal T-cell receptor gene rearrangement.

Anaplastic Large Cell Lymphoma

Anaplastic large cell lymphoma (ALCL) is characterized by large anaplastic lymphoid cells that express CD30, with or without expression of anaplastic lymphoma kinase (ALK).

Clinical

- One of the most common forms of peripheral T-cell lymphoma.
- Male predominance with a bimodal age distribution, with peaks in childhood/young adulthood and again in late adulthood.
- ALK+ ALCL patients are younger than patients with ALK- ALCL and other T-cell lymphomas.
- ALK- ALCL tumors have a prognosis that is inferior to that of ALK+ ALCL. Among ALK- ALCL, *DUSP22* rearrangement (30%) is associated with favorable outcomes, and *TP63* rearrangement (8%) is associated with aggressive clinical behavior and poor outcomes.
- Present with painless lymphadenopathy and/or extranodal disease in any site
- Majority have systemic symptoms.

Cytology of FNA and Touch Preparation

- Cellular specimen consisting of large, pleomorphic, discohesive lymphocytes with irregular nuclei, prominent nucleoli, and moderate to abundant cytoplasm that may contain cytoplasmic vacuoles (Fig. 4.11a).
- Some of the cells show horseshoe-shaped (hallmark cells) or donut-shaped nuclei. Multinucleation may be seen.

Histology of Core

- Large pleomorphic cells grow in solid cohesive sheets, especially within sinuses and interfollicular areas (Fig. 4.11b).
- The cells show one or several nuclei, prominent nucleoli, and abundant eosinophilic or amphophilic cytoplasm.

Comments

- **Differential Diagnosis**
  - Diffuse large B-cell lymphoma
  - Hodgkin lymphoma
  - Peripheral T-cell lymphoma, NOS
  - Metastatic carcinoma
- **Ancillary Studies**
  - CD30+ (Fig. 4.11c), CD45+/−, variable positivity for one or more T-cell markers, negative for B-cell surface markers (CD19, CD20 (Fig. 4.11d), CD22), EMA+, TIA1+, granzyme B+, and perforin+.
  - ALK protein expression in ALK+ ALCL.
  - Clonal T-cell receptor gene rearrangement (60% of cases).
  - Rare cases of null cell type are negative for all lineage markers, with or without clonal T-cell receptor gene rearrangement.
  - Rearrangement of *ALK* by FISH, most frequent t(2;5), *NPM/ALK* (70–75%).
  - FISH for *DUSP22* rearrangement in ALK- ALCL.

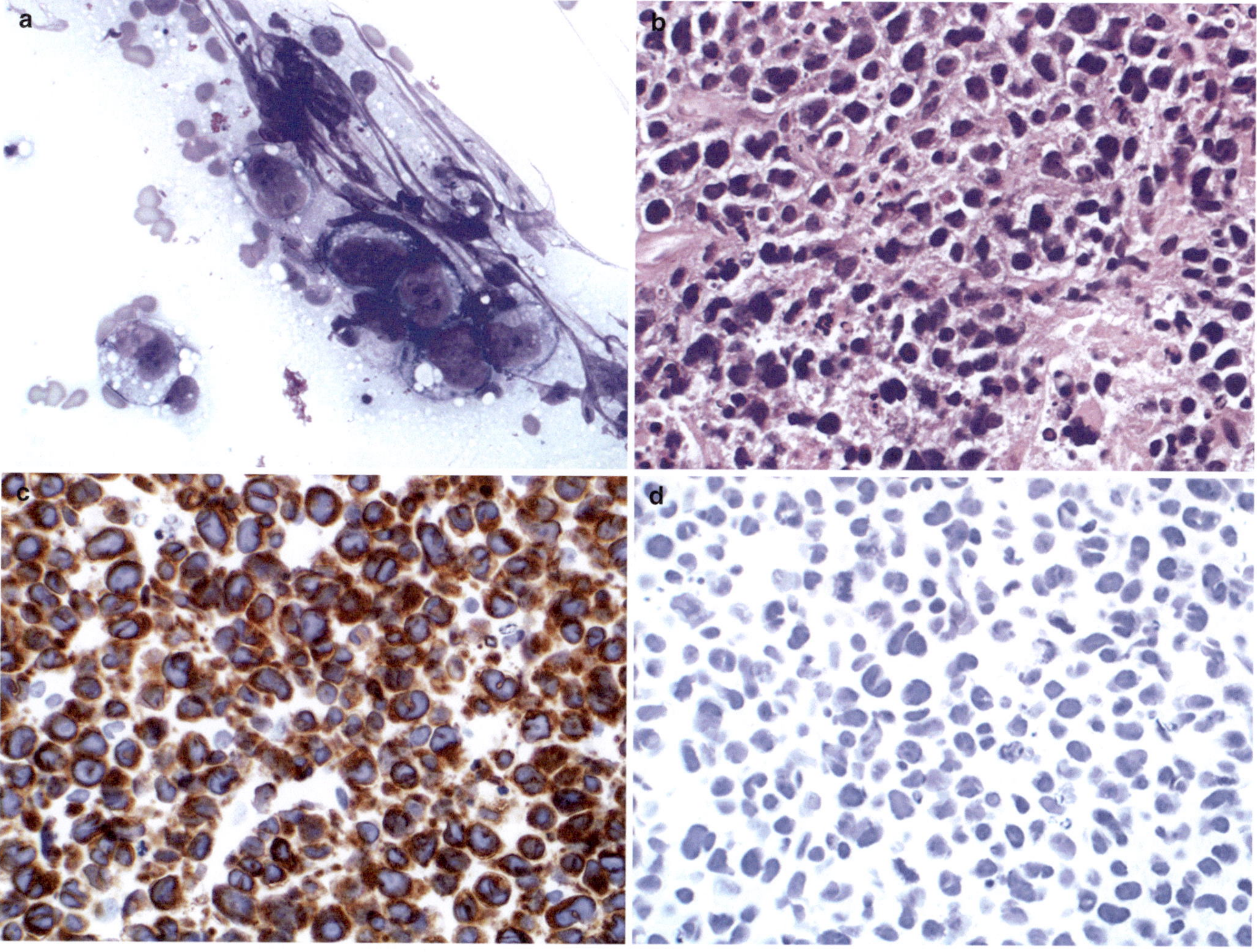

Fig. 4.11 Pathology of anaplastic T-cell lymphoma. (**a**) Cytomorphology of FNA of a lymph node; Diff-Quik stain, 600×. (**b**) Histology of needle core, hematoxylin and eosin stain, 600×. (**c**, **d**) Immunostains for CD30 (**c**) and CD20 (**d**) 600×

Angioimmunoblastic T-Cell Lymphoma

Angioimmunoblastic T-cell lymphoma is a peripheral T-cell neoplasm characterized by systemic symptoms, a polymorphous infiltrate, and a prominent proliferation of high endothelial venules and follicular dendritic cells.

Clinical

- Affects older adults with a peak incidence in sixth and seventh decades.
- Patients present with acute onset of systemic illness, including generalized lymphadenopathy, hepatosplenomegaly, B symptoms, rash, and effusion/ascites.
- Laboratory abnormalities are common: elevated lactic acid dehydrogenase (LDH) and erythrocyte sedimentation rate (ESR), polyclonal hypergammaglobulinemia, hypoalbuminemia, positive Coombs test, cytopenias.
- May be associated with autoimmune diseases, including hemolytic anemia, vasculitis, polyarthritis, rheumatoid arthritis, and cryoglobulinemia.

Cytology of FNA and Touch Preparation

- Heterogeneous population of small, medium, and large irregular lymphoid cells.
- Reactive background composed of small round lymphocytes, eosinophils, plasma cells, dendritic cells, and epithelioid and nonepithelioid histiocytes.

Histology of Core

- Effaced lymph node architecture with perinodal infiltration and sparing of sinuses.
- Polymorphic infiltrate of lymphocytes, granulocytes, plasma cells, immunoblasts, and T cells with abundant clear cytoplasm.
- Proliferation of arborizing high endothelial venules and follicular dendritic cells.
- Paracortical expansion by abnormal infiltrate may not be readily appreciated on small core biopsy.

Comments

- **Differential Diagnosis**
  - Peripheral T-cell lymphoma, NOS.
  - Classic Hodgkin lymphoma (CHL).
  - T-cell/histiocyte-rich large B-cell lymphoma.
  - Epstein Barr virus (EBV)-positive diffuse large B-cell lymphoma.
- **Ancillary Studies – Immunophenotype:**
  - Tumor cells express pan T-cell antigens (CD3, CD2, and CD5) and almost always CD4 and coexpress CD10, CXCL13, PD-1, ICOS and BCL-6; expanded follicular dendritic cell networks by CD21, CD23, and CD35. **EBV is detected in many cases and is more common in B cells** [41, 42].
  - Frequently associated with mutations in the genes *TET2, IDH2, RHOA,* and *DNMT3A* [43].
  - Clonal T-cell receptor genes rearrangement (75% to 90%) and clonal immunoglobulin heavy chains rearrangement (25%) [44, 45].

Hodgkin Lymphoma

Hodgkin lymphoma (HL) is divided into nodular lymphocyte-predominant Hodgkin lymphoma (NLPHL) and classic Hodgkin lymphoma (CHL).

Nodular Lymphocyte-Predominant Hodgkin Lymphoma (NLPHL)

NLPHL is a germinal center B-cell neoplasm characterized by a nodular or nodular and diffuse proliferation of scattered multilobulated large neoplastic cells called popcorn cells or lymphocyte-predominant (LP) cells in a background of B-cell–rich lymphoid follicles.

Clinical

- Can occur at any age, with a peak incidence at the fourth decade. Men are affected 2.4 times more commonly than women.
- Present with early stage disease, with longstanding isolated lymphadenopathy, nonbulky disease, and absence of B symptoms.
- Bone marrow involvement is uncommon. Patients with marrow involvement have tumors that are difficult to distinguish from T-cell/histiocyte–rich large B-cell lymphoma.

Cytology of FNA and Touch Preparation

- Scattered lymphocyte-predominant cells (LP or popcorn cells) are seen in a background of numerous polymorphous lymphocytes.
- The LP cells are large cells with multilobulated nuclei and multiple nucleoli. Large lymphocytic aggregates may also be seen.

Histology of Core

- Nodular or nodular and diffuse growth pattern; may be difficult to appreciate in a core biopsy.
- Variable number of scattered LP cells with multilobulated nuclei and prominent nucleoli admixed with polymorphous lymphocytes and histiocytes.

Comments

- **Differential Diagnosis**
  - Progressive transformation of germinal centers (PTGCs)
  - T cell/histiocyte-rich large B-cell lymphoma
  - Lymphocyte-rich classic HL
- **Ancillary Studies**
  - Immunophenotype of LP cells: CD45+, BCL6+, CD20+, CD79a+, CD15-, and CD30-.
  - Background cells consisting of scattered small B cells, a wreath of CD3+/CD57+ T cells surrounding LP cells, and meshwork of CD21+ or CD23+ follicular dendritic cells.

Classic Hodgkin Lymphoma

CHL is composed of mononuclear Hodgkin cells and multinucleated Reed-Sternberg cells in an admixture of non-neoplastic inflammatory cells.

Clinical

- CHL accounts for approximately 10% of all lymphomas.
- Bimodal age distribution, adolescents/young adults, and 60-to-70-year olds.
- Histologic variants: Nodular sclerosis, mixed cellularity, lymphocyte-rich, and lymphocyte depleted Classic HL.
- Usually present with painless localized peripheral lymphadenopathy.

Radiography

CT Scan

- Cervical lymphadenopathy on CECT often presents as a soft-tissue mass or discretely enlarged lymph nodes with variable enhancement (Fig. 4.12a).
- Lymph node necrosis is very rare both before and after treatment and appears as a central area of low attenuation [46].

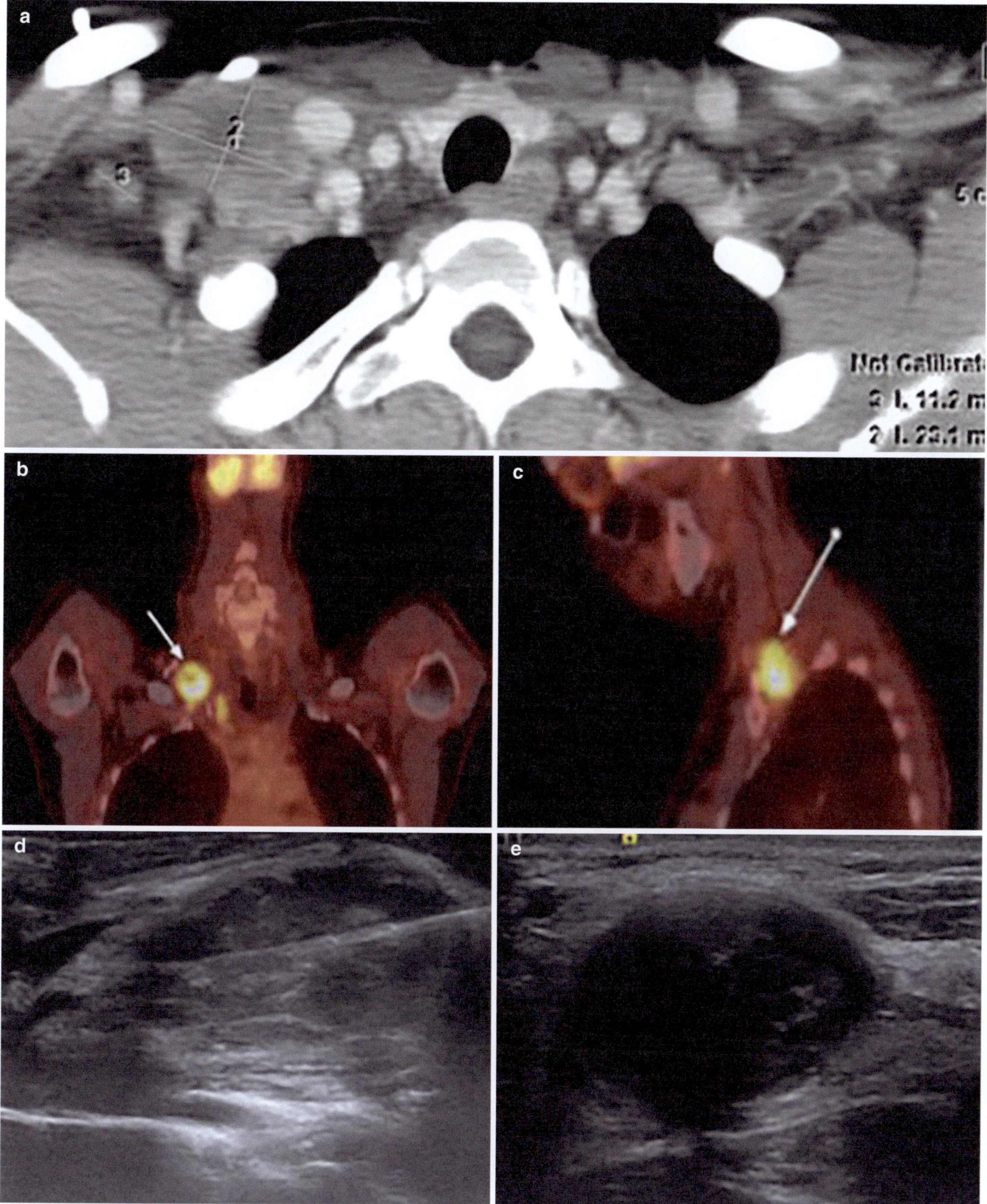

Fig. 4.12 (**a**–**e**) Radiography of HL. (**a**) CECT axial image demonstrates a large conglomerate mass of lymph nodes in the right level 4 and right supraclavicular region, causing a mass effect on the adjacent right internal jugular vein, which corresponds to the FDG PET/CT images in a patient with biopsy-proven HL. (**b**, **c**) F-18 FDG PET/CT coronal (**b**) and sagittal (**c**) images demonstrate large hypermetabolic mass in the right supraclavicular region corresponding to the findings seen on the CECT in a patient with HL. (**d**, **e**) Gray scale US images show a round hypoechoic left supraclavicular nodal mass with suspicious morphology at the time of biopsy with pathology consistent with HL. (**f**, **g**) Biopsy cytology of HL. Cytomorphology of FNA of a lymph node; Diff-Quik stain 600×

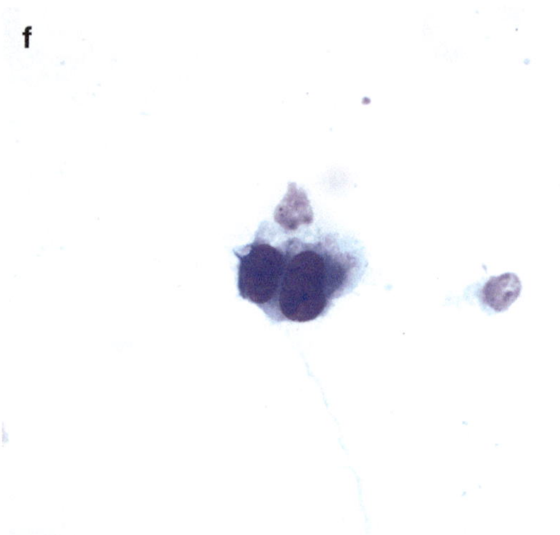

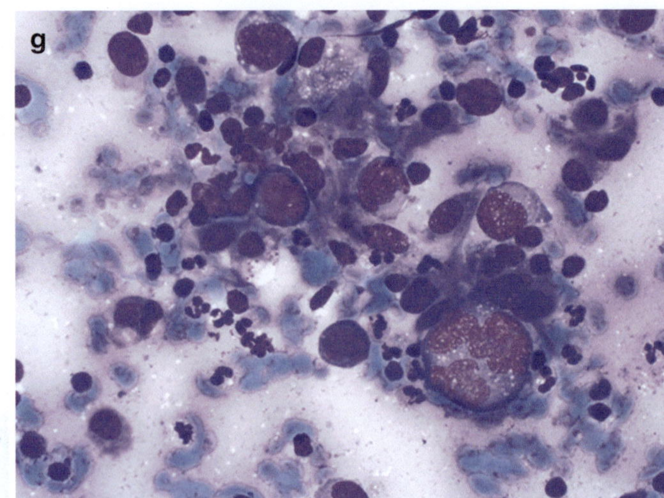

Fig. 4.12 (continued)

- CT may show findings similar to those of inflammatory adenopathy, and tissue sampling is often required for diagnosis [46].
- Pulmonary involvement occurs in 40% of patients with HL, usually as multiple pulmonary nodules or masses with poorly or well-defined borders on CT. There may be associated air bronchograms or central cavitation.
- Endobronchial lesions with postobstructive volume loss. Hilar adenopathy with or without mediastinal adenopathy may be the only finding seen on chest CT [47].
- On CECT lymphomatous involvement of the spleen may appear as homogeneous splenomegaly alone or as solitary or multiple nonenhancing, low attenuation masses [46].

PET CT scan

- The modality of choice to evaluate FDG-avid HL (Fig. 4.12b, c).
- There is intense FDG-avid lymphadenopathy and variable uptake with pulmonary HL [48].
- Bone marrow involvement can be seen as focal bone marrow uptake, which eliminates the need for biopsy [48].

MRI

- The preferred modality to assess central nervous system vascular or cardiac involvement of HL.
- The lymphadenopathy demonstrates low-to-intermediate signal intensity on T1-weighted images and intermediate-to-high signal intensity relative to surrounding muscle on T2-weighted images.
- On contrast-enhanced T1-weighted images, there may be variable enhancement of lymph nodes.
- MRI is also useful to assess lower cervical lymphadenopathy that is incompletely assessed on CT owing to beam-hardening artifacts, often from the shoulder girdles [46].
- Spleen lymphomatous infiltration has T1 and T2 relaxation times similar to those of normal splenic parenchyma. However, on T2-weighted images, infiltration may have a spotted appearance as a result of associated fibrosis, edema, hemorrhage, or necrosis. Gadolinium-enhanced sequences are more sensitive for the evaluation of splenic lymphoma [49].

Ultrasound

- Malignant lymph nodes are hypoechoic with a round morphology with a tendency to aggregate. There may be sharp margins and nodal reticulation (Fig. 4.12d, e).
- On power Doppler US, there may be vessel truncation or distortion of the vascularity in lymphomatous nodes with increased flow peripherally and centrally.
- Power Doppler can also be useful in monitoring response to treatment. A reduction in vessel signal on color Doppler indicates not only a favorable response but also a prolonged disease remission [50]. A change in size over times indicates a favorable response to treatment.
- Splenic involvement can present with homogeneous splenomegaly, solitary or multiple nodular lesions that are hypoechoic relative to the normal splenic parenchyma [46].

Cytology of FNA and Touch Preparation

- Generally cellular specimens consisting of scattered Reed-Sternberg cells in a background of numerous polymorphous lymphoid cells as well as possibly eosinophils.
- RS cells are large cells with round, bean-shaped or indented nucleus/nuclei with one or more macronucleoli (Fig. 4.12f, g).
- Granulomas may be seen.

Histology of Core

- Architecture is effaced with variable numbers of Reed-Sternberg cells in a background of polymorphous lymphocytes, histiocytes, and eosinophils.
- The neoplastic cells can be very few in a background of cellular infiltrate.

Comments

- **Differential Diagnosis**
  - Anaplastic large cell lymphoma
  - Nodular lymphocyte–predominant HL
  - Diffuse large B-cell lymphoma
- **Ancillary Studies**
  - Reed-Sternberg cells of classic HL: CD30+, CD15+/–, CD20 (negative to weak), PAX5 (weak).
  - EBV may be found in nodular sclerosis HL (infrequent), lymphocyte-rich HL (40%), mixed cellularity HL (70%), and lymphocyte-depleted HL (100%) [51].

Histiocytic and Dendritic Neoplasms

Histiocytic Sarcoma

Histiocytic sarcoma is a malignant tumor with morphologic and immunophenotypic features of mature tissue histiocytes.

Clinical

- Rare tumor affecting lymphoid or extranodal tissue.
- Most cases occur in adults with a median age of 52 years.
- Can occur as an isolated disease or in the context of other hematologic neoplasms that are often clonally related [52, 53].
- Commonly presents with symptoms caused by unifocal or multifocal extranodal tumors.

Cytology of FNA and Touch Preparation

- Very pleomorphic multinucleated cells with multilobed nuclei.
- Morphologically similar to high-grade large cell lymphomas.

Histology of Core

- Diffuse proliferation of large cells.
- May have focal areas of spindling (sarcomatoid morphology).
- Admixed with variable number of inflammatory cells, including neutrophils, small lymphocytes, plasma cells, benign histiocytes, and eosinophils.

Comments

- **Differential Diagnosis**
  - Other histiocytic and dendritic cell neoplasm
  - Anaplastic large cell lymphoma
  - Diffuse large B-cell lymphoma
  - **Hemophagocytic lymphohistiocytosis**
  - Metastatic carcinoma
  - Metastatic melanoma
- **Ancillary Studies**
  - Immunohistochemistry is essential in making the diagnosis.
  - The tumor cells express one of the histiocytic markers CD163, CD68 (KP1 and PGM1), and lysozyme.
  - No expression of Langerhans cells (CD1a, langerin), follicular dendritic cell (CD21 and CD35), and myeloid (CD33, CD13 and myeloperoxidase) markers.

Langerhans Cell Histiocytosis

Langerhans cell histiocytosis is a clonal neoplastic proliferation of Langerhans cells.

Clinical

- Diagnosed in all age groups, but is most common in children.
- More common in males, with a male:female ratio of 3.7:1.
- Disease can be localized to a single site, multiple sites in a single system, or more disseminated involving multiple systems [54, 55].

Cytology of FNA and Touch Separation

- Langerhans cells admixed with eosinophils, neutrophils, histiocytes, and small lymphocytes.
- Langerhans cells are large ovoid cells with folded bean-shaped nuclei, inconspicuous nucleoli, and abundant eosinophilic cytoplasm (Fig. 4.13a).

Histology of Core

- Heterogeneous collection of Langerhans cells with eosinophils, neutrophils, small lymphocytes, and histiocytes (Fig. 4.13b).

Comments

- **Ancillary Studies**
  - Langerhans cells express S100 (Fig. 4.13c), CD1a (Fig. 4.13d), and CD207 (langerin).
  - *BRAF* V600E mutations are described in Langerhans cell histiocytosis (LCH) [56, 57].
  - Birbeck granules are intracytoplasmic rod-shaped organelles with central striation, giving the appearance of a "tennis racket" under electron microscopy.

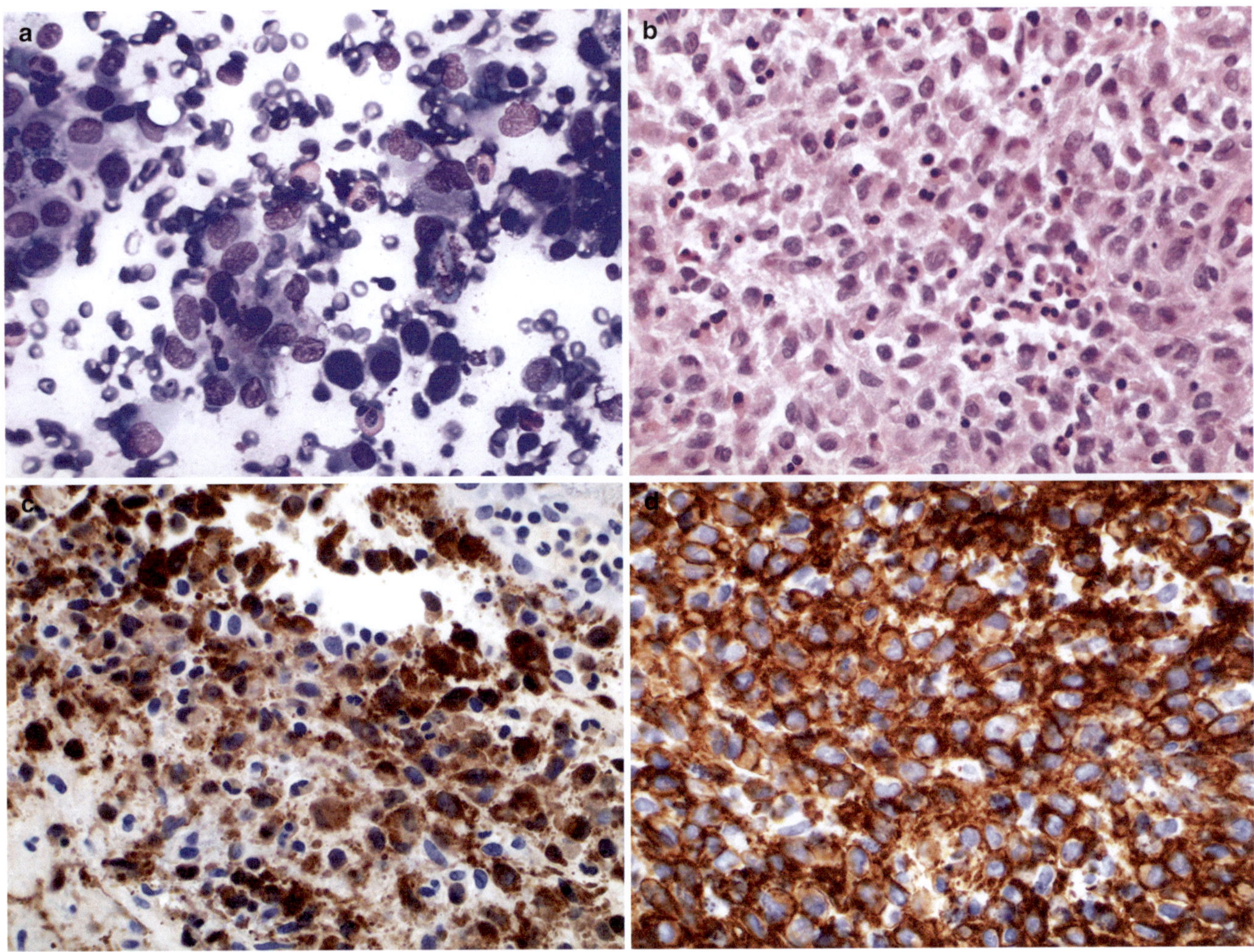

Fig. 4.13 Biopsy pathology of Langerhans cell histiocytosis. (**a**) Cytomorphology of FNA of a lymph node; Diff-Quik stain, 600×. (**b**) Histology of needle core, hematoxylin and eosin stain, 600×. (**c, d**) Immunostains for S100 (**c**) and CD1a (**d**) 600×

Langerhans Cell Sarcoma

Langerhans cell sarcoma is a high-grade neoplasm with overt cytologic atypia and Langerhans cell phenotype.

Clinical

- Very rare tumor affecting lymphoid or extranodal tissue.
- Almost all reported cases occurred in adults.

Cytology of FNA and Touch Preparation

- Pleomorphic cells, some showing abundant cytoplasm and nuclear grooves suggestive of Langerhans cell origin.

Histology of Core

- Pleomorphic tumor with overt malignant cytologic atypia and high mitotic rate.
- Some cells may have complex grooves
- Rare eosinophils may be present.

Comments

- **Ancillary Studies**
  - Immunophenotype is identical to LCH; the tumor cells express markers of Langerhans cells CD1a, S100, and CD207 (langerin).
  - Birbeck granules are present by electron microscopy.

Immunodeficiency-Associated Lymphoproliferative Disorders

Post-transplant Immunodeficiency-Associated Lymphoproliferative Disorders

Clinical

- Lymphoid and/or plasmacytic proliferations in the setting of post-transplantation, primary immune deficiency, iatrogenic medication, or immunosuppression secondary to HIV infection.
- Majority are related to the presence of EBV.

- Four general types of post-transplant lymphoproliferative disorder (PTLD): early lesions (plasmacytic hyperplasia and infectious mononucleosis-like PTLD), polymorphic PTLD, monomorphic PTLD, Classic HL-like PTLD.

Cytology of FNA and Touch Preparation

- Early lesions show polymorphous lymphocytes.
- Later, they may resemble one of the B- or T-lymphomas described above or Classic HL.

Histology of Core

- Early lesion demonstrates preserved architecture of the involved tissue with polyclonal B-cell or plasma cell proliferation.
- Polymorphic PTLD demonstrates effacement of tissue architecture by a pleomorphic lymphoid infiltrate that does not fulfill the criteria for one of the B-cell or T/NK-cell lymphomas recognized in immunocompetent patients.
- Monomorphic PTLD demonstrates effacement of the normal tissue architecture by a lymphoid infiltrate that fulfills the criteria for one of the B-cell or T/NK-cell lymphomas recognized in immunocompetent patients.
- Classic HL-like PTLD demonstrates effacement of the normal tissue architecture by a minority of neoplastic cells (Reed-Sternberg cells and their variants) in an inflammatory background, fulfilling the criteria required for the diagnosis of Classic HL.

Comments

- **Differential Diagnosis**
  - Polymorphic PTLD may have features similar to those of infection.
  - PTLD involving the allograft may morphologically resemble graft rejection.
- **Ancillary Studies**
  - Mono- or oligoclonal lymphoid cell populations by immunoglobulin light chain expression and antigen receptor gene rearrangements.
  - Presence of EBV infection in many cells by in situ hybridization for EBV RNA (EBER).

Other Immunodeficiency-Associated Lymphoproliferative Disorders (Primary Immune Disorders/Iatrogenic/AIDS)

Clinical

- Lymphoid proliferation in other immune deficiency states shows a spectrum similar to that of PTLD from reactive hyperplasia, polymorphous lymphoid infiltrates, to frank lymphoma.
- HIV-associated lymphomas also occurring in immunocompetent patients: Burkitt lymphoma, diffuse large B-cell lymphoma, and HL; more specific HIV-associated lymphoma: primary effusion lymphoma, and plasmablastic lymphoma.
- The diagnosis of primary immune disorder could be established because of other manifestations.
- Iatrogenic immunodeficiency-associated lymphoproliferative disorders are often seen in patients who received immunosuppressive agents, including methotrexate and/or anti-tumor necrosis factor (TNF) therapy.

Extramedullary Hematopoiesis

Extramedullary hematopoiesis refers to hematopoiesis occurring outside of the bone marrow.

Clinical

- Small foci of extramedullary hematopoiesis can be seen in the lymph nodes of infants and children.
- In adults, it may be associated with hemorrhage, infection, severe inflammation, and chronic myeloproliferative disorders.

Cytology of FNA and Touch Preparation

- Usually two or three cell lineages are present in extramedullary hematopoiesis.

Histology of Core

- Lymphoid tissue with bone marrow components.

Comments

- **Differential Diagnosis**
  - Should be distinguished from inflammatory infiltrates and myeloid sarcoma

Malignant Neoplasms: Secondary Involvement

Lymph nodes are involved by the patient's prior malignancy.

General

Clinical

- A number of non-hematolymphoid malignancies metastasize to the lymph nodes and may mimic high-grade lymphomas.
- The commonest of these are metastatic carcinomas and melanomas.

- Sarcomas and germ cell tumors also infrequently metastasize.
- Sarcomas that more commonly involve lymph nodes include synovial sarcoma, epithelioid sarcoma, angiosarcoma, rhabdomyosarcoma, and Kaposi sarcoma.

Radiography

- Metastatic melanoma is used as an example for the radiographic findings.

Metastatic Melanoma

Metastatic melanoma may originate from known or occult malignant melanoma, has variable morphology, and involves lymph nodes in 75% of cases [58]. The first nodes to be involved are usually regional lymph nodes with contiguous spread through lymphatic chains [59]. In general, lymph nodes that demonstrate interval enlargement in size or change in morphology are highly suspicious imaging findings for metastatic involvement, especially in cases of known malignant melanoma. There is considerable overlap with imaging features of metastatic melanoma and lymphoma.

Radiography

CT Scan

- Lymph node metastases not accessible to clinical examination or ultrasound evaluation are imaged on CT.
- Appears on the scan as enhancing nodes with irregular margins and loss of fatty hilum. In some cases, there may be associated peripheral enhancement with areas of necrosis and hemorrhage (Fig. 4.14a) [60].

Nuclear Medicine Imaging

- PET CT scan includes increased FDG avidity in most sites of melanoma metastasis (Fig. 4.14b).
- PET often shows metastases to atypical sites that may be difficult to detect on CT alone [58]. However, PET/CT has a limited role in stage I or stage II disease and is unlikely to detect microscopic nodal disease in normal-sized lymph nodes [61].

MRI

- Hyperintense to liver owing to melanin content, which can also be seen with other primary malignancies with high fat content or that are prone to hemorrhage.
- Lesions on T2-weighted images are hyperintense, similar to other primary malignancies.
- On postcontrast T1-weighted images, hyperenhancement may be seen in the arterial phase and is most conspicuous on the portal venous phase.

Ultrasound

- Nonspecific with superficial lymph nodes appearing as oval or rounded nodes without echogenic hilum and focal cortical hyperplasia with irregular borders (Fig. 4.14c, d) [62].

Cytology of FNA and Touch Preparation

- Varied morphology, depending on the type of metastasis.
- Cohesive clusters of cells admixed with lymphocytes.
- Based on origin, tumor cells may show cytoplasmic keratin (squamous cell carcinoma), intracytoplasmic mucin (adenocarcinoma), or intracytoplasmic pigment (black melanin pigment in melanoma) (Fig. 4.14e).
- Melanoma cells are usually dispersed and appear plasmacytoid or spindle-shaped.
- Sarcoma cells usually appear spindle-shaped or pleomorphic and occasionally epithelioid.

Histology of Core

- Predominantly distributed in sinusoids in earlier stages (Fig. 4.14f).
- May form glands (adenocarcinoma).
- The tumor may replace the lymph node in later stages; thus lymphocytes may not be seen on FNA/CNB.

Comments

- **Ancillary Studies**
  - Carcinomas: cytokeratin +, CD45 negative.
  - Melanoma: S100 (Fig. 4.14g), SOX10, Melan A (Fig. 4.14h), and HMB-45 positive.
  - Germ cell tumors: SALL4+.

Leukemic Involvement

Clinical

- Extramedullary disease of acute myeloid leukemia may involve lymph nodes.
- Careful review of the patient's history and correlation with other findings in the blood and bone marrow are needed.
- Precursor B- or T-cell lymphoblastic leukemia/lymphoma may present with lymphadenopathy or tissue masses.
- Evaluation often includes both immunohistochemistry and flow cytometry.

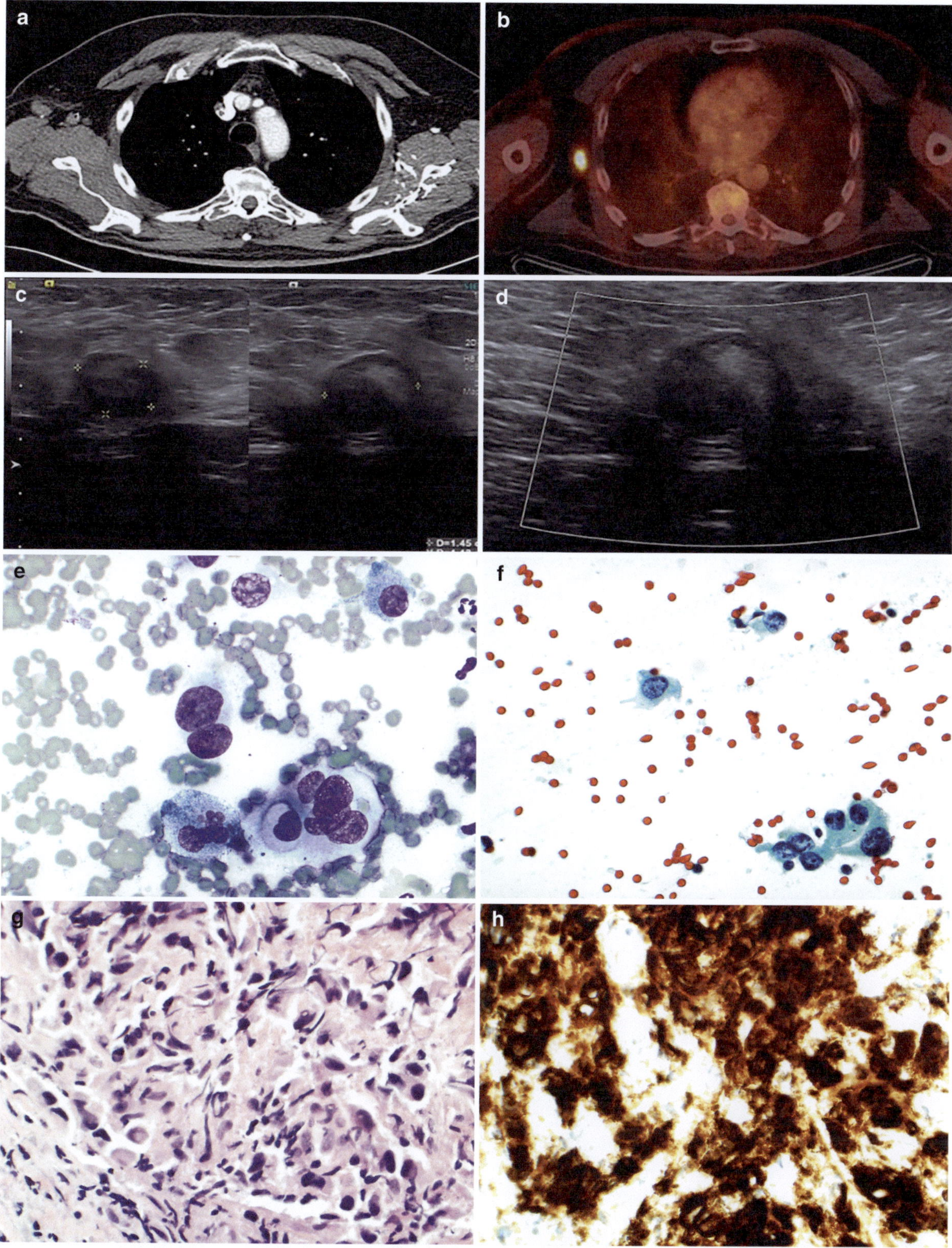

Fig. 4.14 (**a–d**) Radiography of metastatic melanoma. (**a**) Axial CECT at the level of the aortic arch demonstrates enlarged right axillary lymph nodes. (**b**) F-18 FDG PET/CT of the patient demonstrates hypermetabolic lymph nodes. (**c**) Longitudinal gray scale ultrasound of right axilla demonstrates a round lymph node. (**d**) Transverse color Doppler ultrasound demonstrates a hypoechoic round right axillary lymph node with suspicious morphology without central vascularity at the time of biopsy. (**e–h**) Biopsy pathology of metastatic melanoma. (**e**, **f**) Cytomorphology of FNA of a lymph node; Diff-Quik stain (**e**), Papanicolaou stain (**f**), 600×. (**g**) Histology of needle core, hematoxylin and eosin stain, 600×. (**h**) Immunostains for melan A, 600×

Spleen

The main indication for FNA of the spleen is the diagnosis of a mass lesion, either a metastatic focus or one of the rare primary solitary splenic lesions. Cystic lesions of the spleen are rarely aspirated. They may be aspirated to exclude the possibility of a neoplastic origin of the cyst.

Complications associated with the performance of splenic FNA include hemorrhage caused by a tear in the splenic capsule and pneumothorax, less common than in conventional core biopsies. One large multicenter study reported an overall accuracy rate of 91%, an incidence of major complications of 1%, and similar yields of FNA specimens compared to core biopsy material [63].

Normal Findings of Spleen

Radiography

Ultrasound

- On gray scale US, a normal spleen demonstrates a homogeneous echotexture similar to that of the liver and may be slightly more hyperechoic or isoechoic relative to the liver [64].

CT

- On non-enhanced CT (NECT), a normal spleen is approximately 5–10 Hounsfield units lower than the liver with a crescent-shaped morphology (Fig. 4.15a) [65].
- There is a variable enhancement pattern on contrast-enhanced CT (CECT) that depends on the phase in which the images are obtained.
- On the arterial phase, there is a heterogeneous enhancement pattern, described as a moiré pattern of enhancement that can be mistaken for pathologies such as splenic laceration or contusion.
- On venous or delayed-phase CT, the spleen should demonstrate homogeneous enhancement, which is optimal for assessing the parenchyma [66].

MRI

- A normal spleen on contrast-enhanced MRI demonstrates similar enhancement characteristics to CECT with a heterogeneous enhancement pattern on the arterial phase and a homogeneous enhancement on venous or delayed phase imaging.
- On T1-weighted images, the normal MR signal intensity of the spleen is less than that of the hepatic parenchyma and slightly greater than that of muscle (Fig. 4.15b, c) [65].

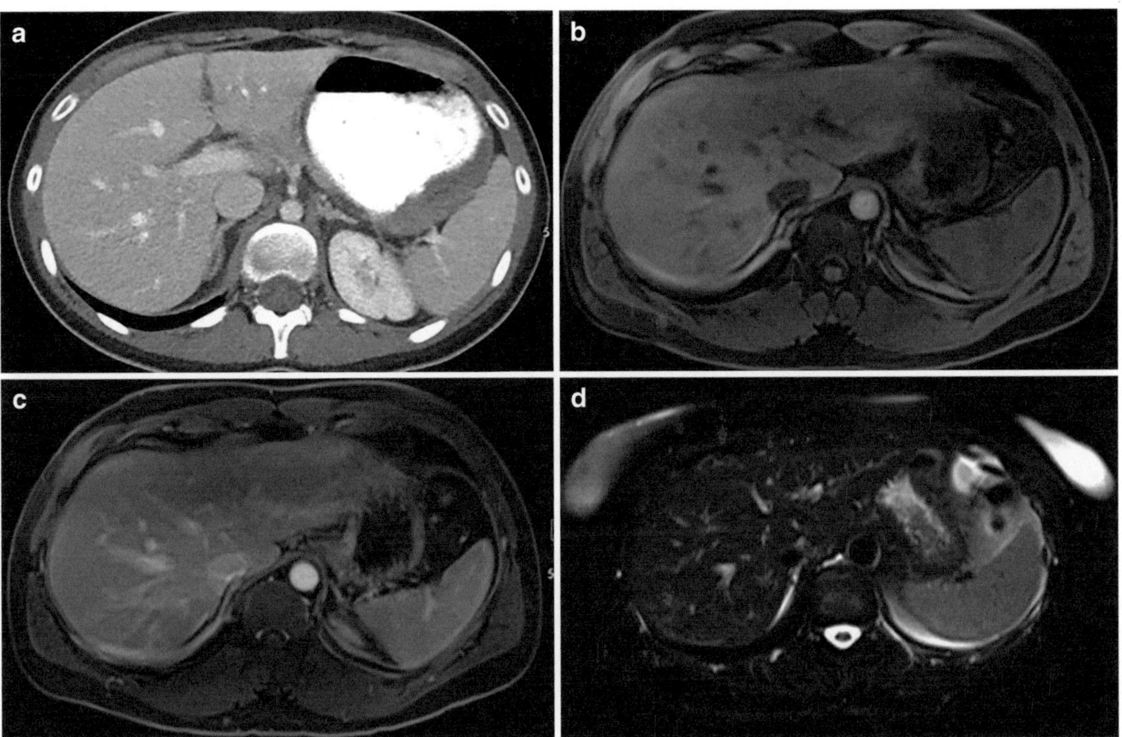

Fig. 4.15 Radiography of normal spleen. (**a**) Axial CECT through the level of the celiac plexus shows normal density of the spleen compared to the liver with a homogeneous enhancement pattern on delayed phase. (**b**) Axial volumetric interpolated breath-hold examination (VIBE) with FS noncontrast T1-weighted MRI shows diffuse homogeneous low signal intensity compared to the liver, which is seen in the absence of pathology. (**c**) Axial volumetric interpolated VIBE with fat-suppressed postcontrast T1-weighted image of the same patient shows an isointense to slightly hyperintense signal of the spleen relative to the liver. (**d**) Axial T2 fat-suppressed MRI demonstrates higher signal intensity of the spleen on T2-weighted image than the liver, which is seen in the absence of splenic pathology

- Higher signal intensity is seen on T2-weighted images, appearing brighter than that of the liver (Fig. 4.15d) [65].

Cytology of FNA and Touch Preparation

- The aspirated material is similar to that of a normal lymph node; however, a branching capillary network along with numerous histiocytes may be aspirated.

Histology of Core

- Splenic parenchyma consists of white pulp, red pulp, and an ill-defined intervening marginal zone.
- White pulp consists of lymphatic nodules made up of a polymorphous population of B and T lymphocytes. In younger people, prominent germinal centers are present. In patients with acquired immunodeficiency syndrome (AIDS), the white pulp may be markedly diminished.
- Red pulp surrounds the lymphatic nodules and consists of a meshwork of venous sinuses surrounded by a thin cord of small lymphocytes and macrophages.

Inflammatory Processes

Reactive Follicular Hyperplasia and Diffuse Lymphoid Hyperplasia

Cytology of FNA and Touch Preparation

- Cytomorphology similar to that of reactive lymph nodes.

Abscess Formation

Abscess can be seen in uncommon infections that are usually secondary to seeding from some other site of infection such as endocarditis.

Cytology of FNA and Touch Preparation

- Numerous degenerated neutrophils, macrophages, and necrosis.
- Microorganisms may be identified.

Comments

- **Ancillary Studies**
  - Aliquot of FNA/core can be sent for culture and molecular studies to detect microorganisms and sensitivity to antibiotics.

Granulomatous Inflammation

Clinical

- The clinical presentation and pathology are the same as that described above for lymph nodes. Splenic involvement by sarcoidosis has been reported in up to 40–60% of patients [67, 68].
- Splenic disease typically is seen on imaging as splenomegaly and less commonly as multiple focal splenic lesions. Multifocal disease can be seen in 6–33% of patients. Most splenic lesions are small, with a mean diameter of 1.0 cm [68].

Radiography

Ultrasound

- Nonspecific with diffuse increased parenchymal homogeneity or heterogeneity with innumerable hypoechoic nodules relative to the background spleen.
- There have also been reports of slightly hyperechoic nodules [68].

CT Scan

- The most common finding of sarcoidosis with splenic involvement is splenomegaly.
- In cases of nodular sarcoidosis, there may be diffuse parenchymal heterogeneity or multinodular pattern in the spleen with scattered nodules of low attenuation with a mean diameter of approximately 1.0 cm on precontrast images.
- On CECT, nodular splenic lesions are hypodense relative to the adjacent normal spleen [68].

MRI

- On contrast-enhanced MRI, sarcoidosis-related nodular splenic lesions are typically hypointense on T1- and T2-weighted imaging and are relatively hypoenhancing on postcontrast T1-weighted images [67].
- The lesions are most conspicuous on T2-weighted fat-suppressed or early phase contrast-enhanced images [49]. Sarcoidosis lesion is enhanced in a minimal and delayed pattern [69].

Hematologic Neoplasms

Clinical

- NHL is the most common primary malignancy.
- The spleen is often secondarily involved by hematologic malignancies that arise elsewhere in the body.
- Patients may present with asymptomatic splenomegaly or hypersplenism (neutropenia, thrombocytopenia, hemolytic anemia, or pancytopenia).
- In general, lymphomas occupy and expand the white pulp compartment, while leukemias infiltrate and expand the red pulp compartment.

Radiography

Imaging shows different patterns, including an enlarged spleen without a discrete mass, multifocal disease with

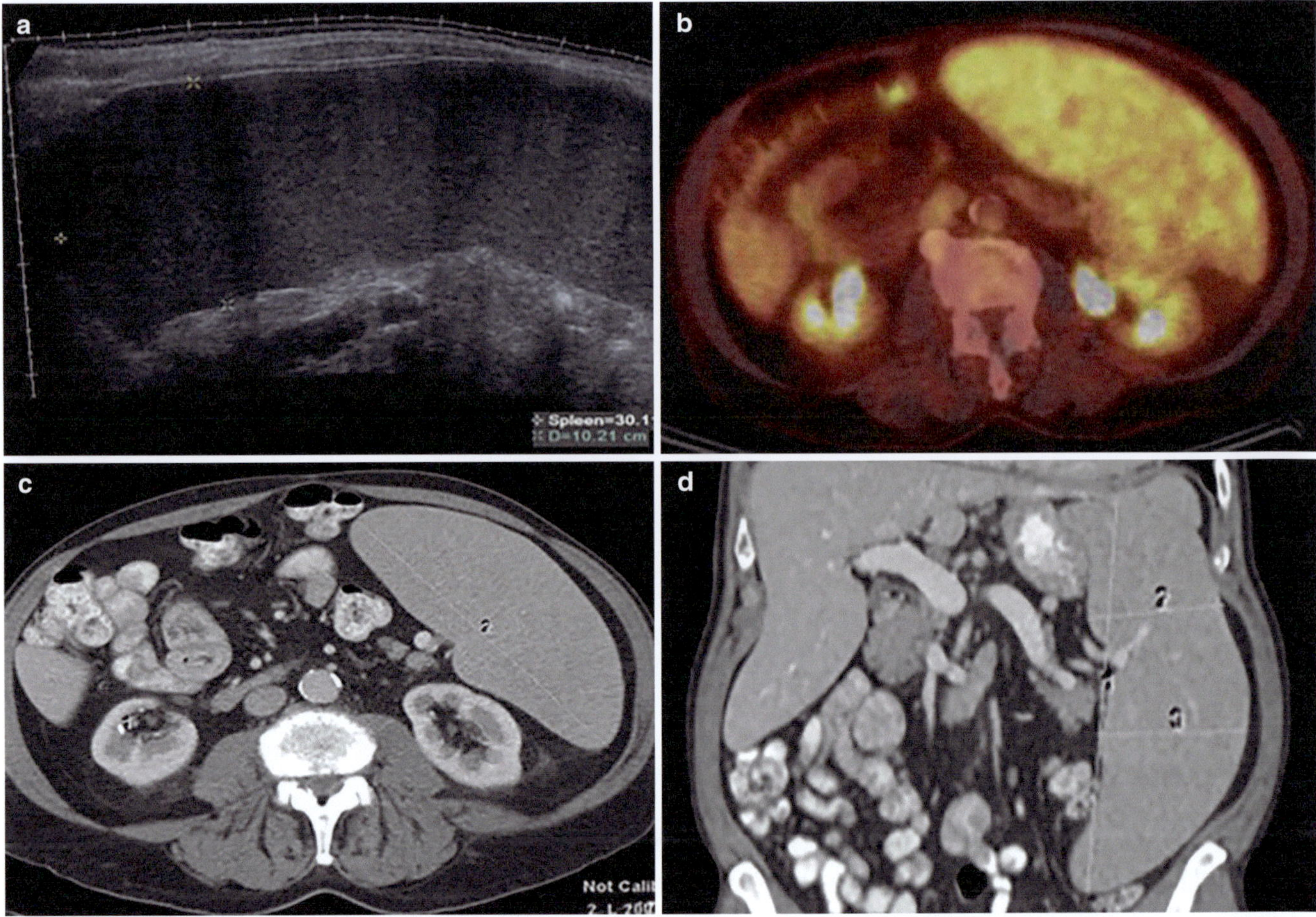

Fig. 4.16 Radiography of lymphoma of the spleen. (**a**) Longitudinal gray scale US image demonstrates markedly enlarged spleen measuring 30.1 × 10.2 × 25.2 cm in a 65-year-old man with marginal zone lymphoma. (**b**) F-18 FDG PET-CT demonstrates massive splenomegaly associated with a mild degree of diffuse increased uptake compared to the liver suspicious for active lymphomatous involvement. Axial (**c**) and coronal (**d**) CECT demonstrates massive splenomegaly associated with a homogeneous enhancement

several discrete lesions, and a solitary dominant mass or innumerable tiny nodules [70].

Ultrasound

- On gray scale US, splenic lymphoma is usually diffuse or focal hypoechoic lesions that may have a target morphology or heterogeneous pattern; this is typical of the recurrent lesions after therapy (Fig. 4.16a) [71].
- The spleen may appear heterogeneous or diffusely hypoechoic without sonographic evidence of discrete lesions.
- Diffuse miliary or micronodular infiltration is a characteristic of low-grade malignant lymphomas [72].
- Macronodular lesions are usually found in high-grade malignant lymphomas [73].
- On contrast-enhanced US arterial phase, lymphomatous splenic lesions demonstrate iso-enhancement in up to 46% of cases, moderate hypoenhancement in 50–53% of cases, and hyperenhancement online in 12.5% of cases relative to the surrounding parenchyma [74]. There is marked hypoenhancement after 1 minute in 100% of cases due to rapid washout [75].

CT Scan

- Several imaging patterns seen with splenic lymphoma on CECT (Fig. 4.16c, d).
- Normal or diffusely hypodense with poor enhancing on arterial phase imaging.
- A solitary dominant mass in some cases may be the dominant feature or multifocal disease with a severe discrete lesion measuring up to 1.0 cm in size, typically seen with AIDS-related lymphoma.
- A miliary pattern of disease with subcentimeter splenic nodules measuring up to 5 mm is another imaging pattern seen.
- Although uncommon, lesions may demonstrate cystic degeneration or necrosis.
- Lesions associated with calcification are almost never seen before treatment.
- In cases without biopsy-proven lymphoma with suspected splenic involvement, splenomegaly alone is not

diagnostic criteria for lymphomatous involvement. Lymphadenopathy at the splenic hilum is observed with non-Hodgkin lymphoma.

MRI

- Splenic lesions usually have a low-to-intermediate signal on T1-weighted images and a mild-to-moderate high signal intensity on T2-weighted images [76].
- Lesions are hypoenhancing to normal splenic parenchyma on contrast-enhanced T1-weighted images and are best visualized on delayed or venous phases.

The following hematologic entities are specific to or commonly arise in the spleen and are discussed separately below.

Splenic Marginal Zone Lymphoma

Splenic marginal zone lymphoma (SMZL) is a B-cell neoplasm composed of small lymphocytes that surround and replace the splenic white pulp germinal centers, merge with the marginal zone of larger cells, and infiltrate the red pulp.

Clinical

- Patients present with splenomegaly, anemia, and weight loss.
- Most patients are over 50 years old.
- The lymphoma involves the spleen, splenic hilar lymph nodes, bone marrow, and often peripheral blood.
- Peripheral lymph nodes are not typically involved.

Cytology of FNA and Touch Preparation

- Small- to medium-sized lymphocytes with regular to mildly irregular nuclei, slightly open chromatin, scattered small nucleoli, and a moderate amount of pale cytoplasm.

Histology of Core

- Miliary expansion of the white pulp composed of cells, as described earlier.

Comments

- **Differential Diagnosis**
  - Hairy cell leukemia.
  - Other splenic B-cell lymphomas (splenic diffuse red pulp small B-cell lymphoma and hairy cell leukemia variant).
- **Ancillary Studies**
  - Immunophenotype: CD19+, CD20+, CD5–, CD10–, CD 23–, CYCLIN D1–, CD11c–, and CD43–.
  - Loss of chromosome 7q31-32 has been described in up to 40% of SMZLs [77].

Hairy Cell Leukemia

Hairy cell leukemia is an indolent neoplasm of small to intermediate sized mature B cells with oval nuclei, abundant cytoplasm, and hairy projections; it involves the peripheral blood, bone marrow, and spleen.

Clinical

- Diffusely and markedly enlarged spleen.
- Rare neoplasm (2% of lymphoid leukemias) with median age of diagnosis at 50 years and a striking male predominance (male:female = 5:1).
- Patients present with splenomegaly, nonspecific symptoms (weakness, fatigue), and cytopenias.

Cytology of FNA and Touch Preparation

- Monotonous population of small mononuclear cells with characteristic coffee bean-shaped nuclei and scant cytoplasm with fine cytoplasmic projections.

Histology of Core

- Red pulp shows dilated sinusoids resembling blood lakes, lined by neoplastic hairy cells.

Comments

- **Differential Diagnosis**
  - Other splenic B-cell lymphomas (splenic diffuse red pulp small B-cell lymphoma and hairy cell leukemia variant)
  - Splenic marginal zone lymphoma
  - Chronic lymphocytic leukemia
  - Prolymphocytic leukemia
- **Ancillary Studies**
  - Characteristic immunocytochemistry is tartrate-resistant acid phosphatase positivity.
  - Immunophenotype: CD19+, CD20+, CD5−, CD10−, CD22bright +, CD11cbright +, CD103+, CD25+, CD123+, and annexin A1+.
  - The *BRAF* V600E mutation is present in virtually all patients with hairy cell leukemia [78, 79].

Hepatosplenic T-Cell Lymphoma

Hepatosplenic T-cell lymphoma (HSTCL) is an extranodal and systemic neoplasm derived from cytotoxic T cells usually of the gamma delta T-cell receptor type, with a predilection for the spleen and liver.

Clinical

- Affects young males who present with hepatosplenomegaly, fever, and weight loss.
- Poor prognosis.

- Can occur in young patients with Crohn disease treated with tumor necrosis factor (TNF) blockers and anti-TNF monoclonal antibodies [80].

Cytology of FNA and Touch Preparation

- Medium-sized cells with oval or folded nuclei, moderately hyperchromatic chromatin, inconspicuous nucleoli, and a pale rim of cytoplasm.

Histology of Core

- Uniformly enlarged spleen without distinct follicle formation.
- Infiltrates the cords and sinuses of red pulp with atrophy of white pulp.

Comments

- **Differential Diagnosis**
  - Splenic marginal zone lymphoma
  - T-cell large granular lymphocyte leukemia
  - Aggressive NK leukemia/lymphoma
  - Other gamma/delta T-cell lymphomas
- **Ancillary Studies**
  - The neoplastic cells express CD2, surface CD3, CD7, CD16, TIA1 with variable CD56 expression, and are negative for CD4, CD5, CD8, perforin, and granzyme B.
  - Most cases of HSTCL express the gamma/delta T-cell receptor, but rare cases express the alpha/beta T-cell receptor (TCR beta-positive).

Mastocytosis

Mastocytosis is a myeloproliferative disorder characterized by a clonal, neoplastic proliferation of mast cells that accumulates in one or more organs.

Clinical

- Heterogeneous disease ranging from skin lesions that may spontaneously regress to highly aggressive neoplasms associated with multiorgan failure and short survival.
- Two subtypes: (1) cutaneous mastocytosis with predominantly skin involvement without evidence of systemic mastocytosis, and (2) systemic mastocytosis.
- The spleen is frequently involved, while lymph node involvement is rare in systemic mastocytosis.

Cytology FNA and Touch Preparation

- Mast cells are better appreciated in Wright-Giemsa stains.
- Medium-sized cells with round, ovoid, or spindle-shaped nuclei, clumped chromatin, inconspicuous or absent nucleoli, and abundant cytoplasm with dense metachromatic granules.

Histology of Core

- Grossly, the spleen demonstrates scattered, fibrotic ill-defined granuloma-like nodules.
- Multifocal clusters, cohesive aggregates, or infiltrates of round, ovoid, or spindle-shaped mast cells.

Ancillary Studies

- Key to diagnosis is the identification of mast cells with expression of tryptase and CD117.
- Neoplastic mast cells have aberrant expression of CD25 and CD2.
- Presence of activating point mutation of *KIT* [81, 82].
- In cases with eosinophilia, studies for *PDGFR or FGFR1* rearrangement are recommended to reassign these cases to myeloid and lymphoid neoplasms with eosinophilia and abnormalities of *PDGFR* or *FGFR1*.

Vascular Neoplasms

Hemangioma

Clinical

- Most common primary neoplasm of the spleen.
- Patients are usually asymptomatic; occasionally they may present with abdominal pain or mass lesion.

Gross

- Often of the cavernous variety.
- Usually less than 2 cm but can be large and multiple, involving the entire spleen (angiomatosis).

Cytology of FNA and Touch Preparation

- Endothelial cells, spindle fibroblasts, and polymorphous lymphocytes that are nonspecific for hemangioma.

Histology of Core

- Interconnected vascular channels of varying size lined by flattened endothelial cells.

Comments

- **Differential Diagnosis**
  - Angiosarcoma and hemangioendothelioma

- **Ancillary Studies**
  - Endothelial cells positive for CD31, CD34, ERG, and Fli-1.

Littoral Cell Angioma

Clinical

- Rare neoplasm that occurs only in the spleen.
- Patients present with splenomegaly.

Gross

- Single or multiple spongy, purplish-black, well-circumscribed nodules.

Cytology of FNA and Touch Preparation

- Vascular fragments in a background of blood and lymphocytes (Fig. 4.17a, b).

Histology of Core

- Irregular vascular spaces lined by cuboidal to hobnail-shaped cells with large vesicular nuclei (Fig. 4.17c).
- Papillary projections protruding into the vascular spaces.
- No significant cellular atypia.

Comments

- **Differential Diagnosis**
  - Hemangioma
- **Ancillary Studies**
  - Shows features of both endothelial (Factor VIII, CD31 [Fig. 4.17d]) and histiocytic (CD68 [Fig. 4.17e], lysozyme) differentiation, and are negative for CD34 and CD8 [83].
  - In contrast, the normal endothelium of the venous sinuses of the spleen red pulp only expresses endothelial antigens and CD8 (Fig. 4.17f).

Angiosarcoma

Clinical

- Most common in elderly people.
- Splenomegaly; may present with rupture.

Gross

- Solitary nodule or diffuse involvement of splenic parenchyma.
- Foci of hemorrhage and necrosis are prominent.

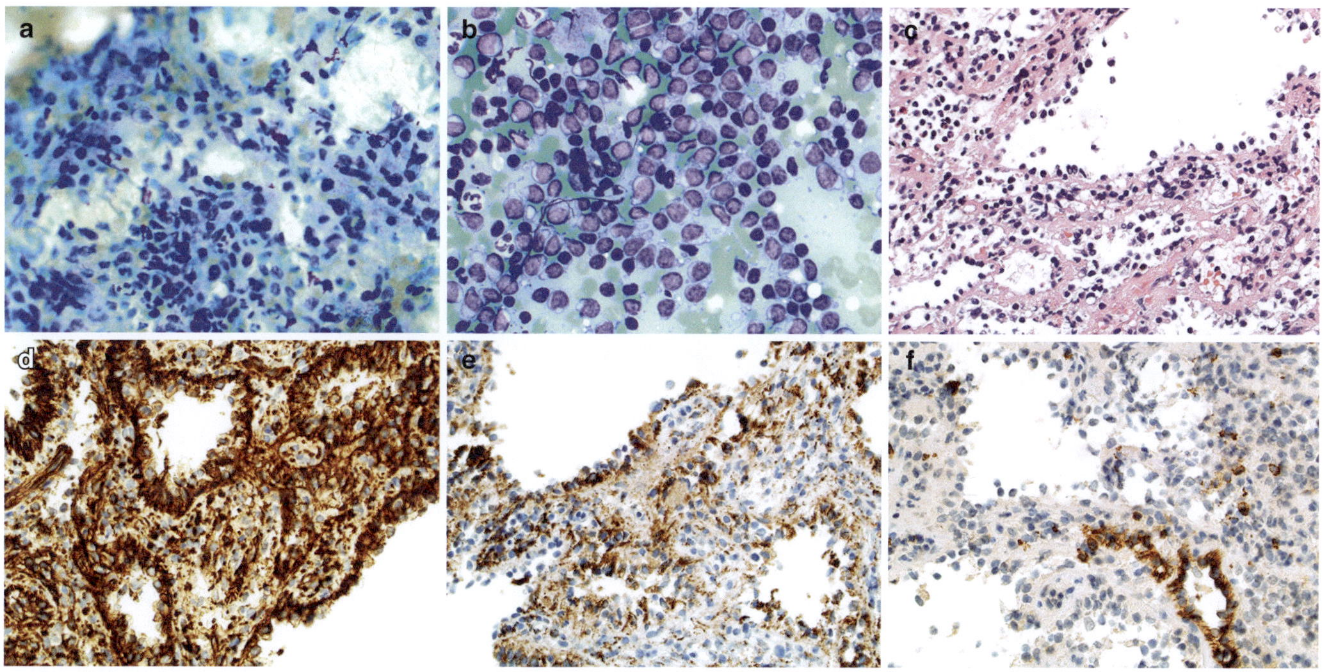

Fig. 4.17 Littoral cell angioma. (**a**, **b**) Cytomorphology of FNA of the spleen lesion; Diff-Quik stain, 600×. (**c**) Histology of needle core, hematoxylin and eosin stain, 600×. (**d–f**) Immunostains for CD31 (**d**), CD68 (**e**), and CD8 (**f**), 600×

Cytology of FNA and Touch Preparation

- Pleomorphic spindle-shaped or epithelioid cells with hyperchromatic nuclei arranged singly, in clusters, or in a syncytial pattern.
- Some cells with intracytoplasmic lumina containing red blood cells or debris.
- Occasional intracytoplasmic hyaline globules may be identified.

Core Biopsy

- Anastomosing vascular channels lined with pleomorphic endothelial cells.

Comments

- **Differential Diagnosis**
  - Hemangioma
  - Kaposi sarcoma: immunohistochemically positive for HHV8
- **Ancillary Studies**
  - Immunohistochemically positive for CD31, CD34, factor VIII, Erg, and Fli-1.

Bacillary Angiomatosis

Clinical

- Benign vascular proliferative lesion caused by the bacterium *Bartonella henselae*.
- Most commonly affects the skin, lymph nodes, liver, and spleen of immunosuppressed patients such as individuals with AIDS or organ transplant patients.
- Almost all affected patients have had recent exposure to a cat scratch or bite.

Cytology of FNA and Touch Preparation

- Small aggregates of oval, round, and spindled cells in a hemorrhagic background.
- Rare bacilli are seen in the smears (better seen with Wright Giemsa special stain).

Histology of Core

- Multiple coalescent clusters of proliferating vessels with abundant amorphous or granular eosinophilic materials.

Comments

- **Differential Diagnosis**
  - Kaposi sarcoma
  - Hemangioma
  - Angiosarcoma
- **Ancillary Studies**
  - Positive *Bartonella* serology.
  - Immunohistochemical stain for *Bartonella* bacteria.
  - PCR studies on fresh or formalin-fixed tissue.

Metastatic Malignancies

General

- Uncommon because of the lack of afferent lymphatics.
- Primaries include malignant melanoma and various carcinomas late in the course of the disease.
- The FNA cytology and core histology as well as ancillary studies are the same as those described in the lymph node section.

Extramedullary Hematopoiesis

Extramedullary hematopoiesis is typically seen in patients with severe anemia (e.g., thalassemia major) or in patients with myeloproliferative neoplasms (myelofibrosis, polycythemia vera, chronic myeloid leukemia).

Cytology of FNA and Histology of Core

- Trilineage hematopoiesis (megakaryocytes, erythroid and myeloid cells) in varying stages of maturation, with scattered lymphocytes.

References

1. Steinkamp HJ, Cornehl M, Hosten N, Pegios W, Vogl T, Felix R. Cervical lymphadenopathy: ratio of long- to short-axis diameter as a predictor of malignancy. Br J Radiol. 1995;68:266–70.
2. Kwon SY, Kim TK, Kim YS, Lee KY, Lee NJ, Seol HY. CT findings in Kikuchi disease: analysis of 96 cases. Am J Neuroradiol. 2004;25:1099–102.
3. Tsujikawa T, Tsuchida T, Imamura Y, Kobayashi M, Asahi S, Shimizu K, et al. Kikuchi-Fujimoto disease: PET/CT assessment of a rare cause of cervical lymphadenopathy. Clin Nucl Med. 2011;36:661–4.
4. Khanna R, Sharma AD, Khanna S, Kumar M, Shukla RC. Usefulness of ultrasonography for the evaluation of cervical lymphadenopathy. World J Surg Oncol. 2011;9:29.
5. Choi YJ, Lee JH, Baek JH. Ultrasound elastography for evaluation of cervical lymph nodes. Ultrasonography. 2015;34:157–64.
6. Youk JH, Kim EK, Ko KH, Kim MJ. Sonographic features of axillary lymphadenopathy caused by Kikuchi disease. J Ultrasound Med. 2008;27:847–53.
7. Eisenmenger LB, Wiggins RH. Imaging of head and neck lymph nodes. Radiol Clin N Am. 2015;53:115–32.
8. Holzapfel K, Duetsch S, Fauser C, Eiber M, Rummeny EJ, Gaa J. Value of diffusion-weighted MR imaging in the differentiation between benign and malignant cervical lymph nodes. Eur J Radiol. 2009;72:381–7.
9. Si J, Huang S, Shi H, Liu Z, Hu Q, Wang G, et al. Usefulness of 3T diffusion-weighted MRI for discrimination of reactive and metastatic cervical lymph nodes in patients with oral squamous cell carcinoma: a pilot study. Dentomaxillofac Radiol. 2014;43:20130202.

10. Asano S. Granulomatous lymphadenitis. J Clin Exp Hematol. 2012;52:1–16.
11. Armitage JO, Weisenburger DD. New approach to classifying non-Hodgkin's lymphomas: clinical features of the major histologic subtypes. Non-Hodgkin's Lymphoma Classification Project. J Clin Oncol. 1998;16:2780–95.
12. Hill BT, Weil AC, Kalaycio M, Cook JR. Pulmonary involvement by chronic lymphocytic leukemia/small lymphocytic lymphoma is a specific pathologic finding independent of inflammatory infiltration. Leuk Lymphoma. 2012;53:589–95.
13. Ghofrani M, Tantiwongkosi B, Smith AS, Wasdahl DA. Richter transformation of chronic lymphocytic leukemia presenting as a dural-based non-Hodgkin lymphoma mass. Am J Neuroradiol. 2007;28:318–20.
14. Mauro FR, Chauvie S, Paoloni F, Biggi A, Cimino G, Rago A, et al. Diagnostic and prognostic role of PET/CT in patients with chronic lymphocytic leukemia and progressive disease. Leukemia. 2015;29:1360–5.
15. Hallek M, Cheson BD, Catovsky D, Caligaris-Cappio F, Dighiero G, Dohner H, et al. Guidelines for the diagnosis and treatment of chronic lymphocytic leukemia: a report from the International Workshop on Chronic Lymphocytic Leukemia updating the National Cancer Institute-Working Group 1996 guidelines. Blood. 2008;111:5446–56.
16. Project BTN-HsLC. A clinical evaluation of the International Lymphoma Study Group classification of non-Hodgkin's lymphoma. The non-Hodgkin's lymphoma classification project. Blood. 1997;89:3909–18.
17. Hayashi D, Lee JC, Devenney-Cakir B, Zaim S, Ounadjela S, Solal-Celigny P, et al. Follicular non-Hodgkin's lymphoma. Clin Radiol. 2010;65:408–20.
18. Barrington SF, Mikhaeel NG, Kostakoglu L, Meignan M, Hutchings M, Mueller SP, et al. Role of imaging in the staging and response assessment of lymphoma: consensus of the International Conference on Malignant Lymphomas Imaging Working Group. J Clin Oncol. 2014;32:3048–58.
19. Rowley JD. Chromosome studies in the non-Hodgkin's lymphomas: the role of the 14;18 translocation. J Clin Oncol. 1988;6:919–25.
20. Korsmeyer SJ. Bcl-2 initiates a new category of oncogenes: regulators of cell death. Blood. 1992;80:879–86.
21. Zucca E, Bertoni F, Roggero E, Cavalli F. The gastric marginal zone B-cell lymphoma of MALT type. Blood. 2000;96:410–9.
22. Hussell T, Isaacson PG, Crabtree JE, Spencer J. The response of cells from low-grade B-cell gastric lymphomas of mucosa-associated lymphoid tissue to *Helicobacter pylori*. Lancet. 1993;342:571–4.
23. Swerdlow S, Campo E, Harris NL, Jaffe E, Pileri S, Stein S, Thiele J, Vardiman J, editors. WHO classification of tumours of haematopoietic and lymphoid tissues. 4th ed. Lyon: International Agency for Research on Cancer (IARC); 2008.
24. Dierlamm J, Baens M, Stefanova-Ouzounova M, Hinz K, Wlodarska I, Maes B, et al. Detection of t(11;18)(q21;q21) by interphase fluorescence in situ hybridization using API2 and MLT specific probes. Blood. 2000;96:2215–8.
25. Mozos A, Royo C, Hartmann E, De Jong D, Baro C, Valera A, et al. SOX11 expression is highly specific for mantle cell lymphoma and identifies the cyclin D1-negative subtype. Haematologica. 2009;94:1555–62.
26. Zukerberg LR, Yang WI, Arnold A, Harris NL. Cyclin D1 expression in non-Hodgkin's lymphomas. Detection by immunohistochemistry. Am J Clin Pathol. 1995;103:756–60.
27. Ahuja AT, Ying M. Sonographic evaluation of cervical lymph nodes. Am J Roentgenol. 2005;184:1691–9.
28. Tateishi U, Muller NL, Johkoh T, Onishi Y, Arai Y, Satake M, et al. Primary mediastinal lymphoma: characteristic features of the various histological subtypes on CT. J Comput Assist Tomogr. 2004;28:782–9.
29. Cronin CG, Swords R, Truong MT, Viswanathan C, Rohren E, Giles FJ, et al. Clinical utility of PET/CT in lymphoma. Am J Roentgenol. 2010;194:W91–103.
30. Hans CP, Weisenburger DD, Greiner TC, Gascoyne RD, Delabie J, Ott G, et al. Confirmation of the molecular classification of diffuse large B-cell lymphoma by immunohistochemistry using a tissue microarray. Blood. 2004;103:275–82.
31. Alizadeh AA, Eisen MB, Davis RE, Ma C, Lossos IS, Rosenwald A, et al. Distinct types of diffuse large B-cell lymphoma identified by gene expression profiling. Nature. 2000;403:503–11.
32. Kramer MH, Hermans J, Wijburg E, Philippo K, Geelen E, van Krieken JH, et al. Clinical relevance of BCL2, BCL6, and MYC rearrangements in diffuse large B-cell lymphoma. Blood. 1998;92:3152–62.
33. Johnson NA, Savage KJ, Ludkovski O, Ben-Neriah S, Woods R, Steidl C, et al. Lymphomas with concurrent BCL2 and MYC translocations: the critical factors associated with survival. Blood. 2009;114:2273–9.
34. Vitolo U, Gaidano G, Botto B, Volpe G, Audisio E, Bertini M, et al. Rearrangements of bcl-6, bcl-2, c-myc and 6q deletion in B-diffuse large-cell lymphoma: clinical relevance in 71 patients. Ann Oncol. 1998;9:55–61.
35. Rajkumar SV, Dimopoulos MA, Palumbo A, Blade J, Merlini G, Mateos MV, et al. International Myeloma Working Group updated criteria for the diagnosis of multiple myeloma. Lancet Oncol. 2014;15:e538–48.
36. Treon SP, Xu L, Yang G, Zhou Y, Liu X, Cao Y, et al. MYD88 L265P somatic mutation in Waldenstrom's macroglobulinemia. N Engl J Med. 2012;367:826–33.
37. Varettoni M, Arcaini L, Zibellini S, Boveri E, Rattotti S, Riboni R, et al. Prevalence and clinical significance of the MYD88 (L265P) somatic mutation in Waldenstrom's macroglobulinemia and related lymphoid neoplasms. Blood. 2013;121:2522–8.
38. Vose J, Armitage J, Weisenburger D, International TCLP. International peripheral T-cell and natural killer/T-cell lymphoma study: pathology findings and clinical outcomes. J Clin Oncol. 2008;26:4124–30.
39. Weisenburger DD, Savage KJ, Harris NL, Gascoyne RD, Jaffe ES, MacLennan KA, et al. Peripheral T-cell lymphoma, not otherwise specified: a report of 340 cases from the International Peripheral T-cell Lymphoma Project. Blood. 2011;117:3402–8.
40. Murphy EL, Hanchard B, Figueroa JP, Gibbs WN, Lofters WS, Campbell M, et al. Modelling the risk of adult T-cell leukemia/lymphoma in persons infected with human T-lymphotropic virus type I. Int J Cancer. 1989;43:250–3.
41. Weiss LM, Jaffe ES, Liu XF, Chen YY, Shibata D, Medeiros LJ. Detection and localization of Epstein-Barr viral genomes in angioimmunoblastic lymphadenopathy and angioimmunoblastic lymphadenopathy-like lymphoma. Blood. 1992;79:1789–95.
42. Anagnostopoulos I, Hummel M, Finn T, Tiemann M, Korbjuhn P, Dimmler C, et al. Heterogeneous Epstein-Barr virus infection patterns in peripheral T-cell lymphoma of angioimmunoblastic lymphadenopathy type. Blood. 1992;80:1804–12.
43. Odejide O, Weigert O, Lane AA, Toscano D, Lunning MA, Kopp N, et al. A targeted mutational landscape of angioimmunoblastic T-cell lymphoma. Blood. 2014;123:129–36.
44. Weiss LM, Strickler JG, Dorfman RF, Horning SJ, Warnke RA, Sklar J. Clonal T-cell populations in angioimmunoblastic lymphadenopathy and angioimmunoblastic lymphadenopathy-like lymphoma. Am J Pathol. 1986;122:392–7.
45. Feller AC, Griesser H, Schilling CV, Wacker HH, Dallenbach F, Bartels H, et al. Clonal gene rearrangement patterns correlate with immunophenotype and clinical parameters in patients with angioimmunoblastic lymphadenopathy. Am J Pathol. 1988;133:549–56.

46. Toma P, Granata C, Rossi A, Garaventa A. Multimodality imaging of Hodgkin disease and non-Hodgkin lymphomas in children. Radiographics. 2007;27:1335–54.
47. Bae YA, Lee KS. Cross-sectional evaluation of thoracic lymphoma. Radiol Clin N Am. 2008;46:253–64.. viii
48. Jhanwar YS, Straus DJ. The role of PET in lymphoma. J Nucl Med. 2006;47:1326–34.
49. Elsayes KM, Narra VR, Mukundan G, Lewis JS, Menias CO, Heiken JP. MR imaging of the spleen: spectrum of abnormalities. Radiographics. 2005;25:967–82.
50. Ahuja AT, Ying M, Ho SY, Antonio G, Lee YP, King AD, et al. Ultrasound of malignant cervical lymph nodes. Cancer Imaging. 2008;8:48–56.
51. Herndier BG, Sanchez HC, Chang KL, Chen YY, Weiss LM. High prevalence of Epstein-Barr virus in the Reed-Sternberg cells of HIV-associated Hodgkin's disease. Am J Pathol. 1993;142:1073–9.
52. Wang E, Hutchinson CB, Huang Q, Sebastian S, Rehder C, Kanaly A, et al. Histiocytic sarcoma arising in indolent small B-cell lymphoma: report of two cases with molecular/genetic evidence suggestive of a 'transdifferentiation' during the clonal evolution. Leuk Lymphoma. 2010;51:802–12.
53. Castro EC, Blazquez C, Boyd J, Correa H, de Chadarevian JP, Felgar RE, et al. Clinicopathologic features of histiocytic lesions following ALL, with a review of the literature. Pediatr Dev Pathol. 2010;13:225–37.
54. Arico M, Girschikofsky M, Genereau T, Klersy C, McClain K, Grois N, et al. Langerhans cell histiocytosis in adults. Report from the International Registry of the Histiocyte Society. Eur J Cancer. 2003;39:2341–8.
55. Gotz G, Fichter J. Langerhans'-cell histiocytosis in 58 adults. Eur J Med Res. 2004;9:510–4.
56. Go H, Jeon YK, Huh J, Choi SJ, Choi YD, Cha HJ, et al. Frequent detection of BRAF (V600E) mutations in histiocytic and dendritic cell neoplasms. Histopathology. 2014;65:261–72.
57. Badalian-Very G, Vergilio JA, Degar BA, MacConaill LE, Brandner B, Calicchio ML, et al. Recurrent BRAF mutations in Langerhans cell histiocytosis. Blood. 2010;116:1919–23.
58. King DM. Imaging of metastatic melanoma. Cancer Imaging. 2006;6:204–8.
59. Fishman EK, Kuhlman JE, Schuchter LM, Miller JA, Magid D. CT of malignant melanoma in the chest, abdomen, and musculoskeletal system. Radiographics. 1990;10:603–20.
60. Patnana M, Bronstein Y, Szklaruk J, Bedi DG, Hwu WJ, Gershenwald JE, et al. Multimethod imaging, staging, and spectrum of manifestations of metastatic melanoma. Clin Radiol. 2011;66:224–36.
61. Strobel K, Dummer R, Husarik DB, Perez Lago M, Hany TF, Steinert HC. High-risk melanoma: accuracy of FDG PET/CT with added CT morphologic information for detection of metastases. Radiology. 2007;244:566–74.
62. Saiag P, Bernard M, Beauchet A, Bafounta ML, Bourgault-Villada I, Chagnon S. Ultrasonography using simple diagnostic criteria vs palpation for the detection of regional lymph node metastases of melanoma. Arch Dermatol. 2005;141:183–9.
63. Civardi GVD, Berte R, Giorgio A, Filice C, Caremani M, Caturelli E, et al. Ultrasound-guided fine needle biopsy of the spleen: high clinical efficacy and low risk in a multicenter Italian Study. Am J Hematol. 2001;67:93–9.
64. Benter T, Kluhs L, Teichgraber U. Sonography of the spleen. J Ultrasound Med. 2011;30:1281–93.
65. Rabushka LS, Kawashima A, Fishman EK. Imaging of the spleen: CT with supplemental MR examination. Radiographics. 1994;14:307–32.
66. Robertson F, Leander P, Ekberg O. Radiology of the spleen. Eur Radiol. 2001;11:80–95.
67. Raber EL, Haba J, Beck P. Splenic sarcoidosis: a case report and review of the imaging findings of multiple incidental splenic lesions as the initial presentation of sarcoidosis. Can J Gastroenterol. 2011;25:477–8.
68. Warshauer DM, Lee JK. Imaging manifestations of abdominal sarcoidosis. Am J Roentgenol. 2004;182:15–28.
69. Koyama T, Ueda H, Togashi K, Umeoka S, Kataoka M, Nagai S. Radiologic manifestations of sarcoidosis in various organs. Radiographics. 2004;24:87–104.
70. Freeman JL, Jafri SZ, Roberts JL, Mezwa DG, Shirkhoda A. CT of congenital and acquired abnormalities of the spleen. Radiographics. 1993;13:597–610.
71. Caremani M, Occhini U, Caremani A, Tacconi D, Lapini L, Accorsi A, et al. Focal splenic lesions: US findings. J Ultrasound. 2013;16:65–74.
72. Urrutia M, Mergo PJ, Ros LH, Torres GM, Ros PR. Cystic masses of the spleen: radiologic-pathologic correlation. Radiographics. 1996;16:107–29.
73. Ishida H, Konno K, Ishida J, Naganuma H, Komatsuda T, Sato M, et al. Splenic lymphoma: differentiation from splenic cyst with ultrasonography. Abdom Imaging. 2001;26:529–32.
74. von Herbay A, Barreiros AP, Ignee A, Westendorff J, Gregor M, Galle PR, et al. Contrast-enhanced ultrasonography with SonoVue: differentiation between benign and malignant lesions of the spleen. J Ultrasound Med. 2009;28:421–34.
75. Gorg C. The forgotten organ: contrast enhanced sonography of the spleen. Eur J Radiol. 2007;64:189–201.
76. Thipphavong S, Duigenan S, Schindera ST, Gee MS, Philips S. Nonneoplastic, benign, and malignant splenic diseases: cross-sectional imaging findings and rare disease entities. Am J Roentgenol. 2014;203:315–22.
77. Mateo M, Mollejo M, Villuendas R, Algara P, Sanchez-Beato M, Martinez P, et al. 7q31-32 allelic loss is a frequent finding in splenic marginal zone lymphoma. Am J Pathol. 1999;154:1583–9.
78. Tiacci E, Trifonov V, Schiavoni G, Holmes A, Kern W, Martelli MP, et al. BRAF mutations in hairy-cell leukemia. N Engl J Med. 2011;364:2305–15.
79. Tiacci E, Schiavoni G, Forconi F, Santi A, Trentin L, Ambrosetti A, et al. Simple genetic diagnosis of hairy cell leukemia by sensitive detection of the BRAF-V600E mutation. Blood. 2012;119:192–5.
80. Kotlyar DS, Osterman MT, Diamond RH, Porter D, Blonski WC, Wasik M, et al. A systematic review of factors that contribute to hepatosplenic T-cell lymphoma in patients with inflammatory bowel disease. Clin Gastroenterol Hepatol. 2011;9:36–41 e1.
81. Kristensen T, Vestergaard H, Bindslev-Jensen C, Moller MB, Broesby-Olsen S, Mastocytosis Centre OUH. Sensitive KIT D816V mutation analysis of blood as a diagnostic test in mastocytosis. Am J Hematol. 2014;89:493–8.
82. Arock M, Sotlar K, Akin C, Broesby-Olsen S, Hoermann G, Escribano L, et al. KIT mutation analysis in mast cell neoplasms: recommendations of the European Competence Network on Mastocytosis. Leukemia. 2015;29:1223–32.
83. Du J, Shen Q, Yin H, Zhou X, Wu B. Littoral cell angioma of the spleen: report of three cases and literature review. Int J Clin Exp Pathol. 2015;8:8516–20.

Kidney, Adrenal Gland, and Paraganglia

5

Xiaoqi Lin, Joseph F. Peevey, Ali Habib, Ronald Mora, and Ahsun Riaz

Kidney

Fine needle aspiration (FNA) has high sensitivity (80–100%) [1–3], specificity (91.9–100%) [1, 3, 4], positive predictive value (89.9%) [3], negative predictive value (94%) [3], and efficacy (92.2%) [3] in the diagnosis of malignant neoplasms of the kidney. As such, cytologic evaluation of renal lesions provides accurate and critical information for appropriate patient management.

Normal Renal Tissue

Renal Tubular Cells

Most epithelial cells seen in FNA smears of non-neoplastic kidney are renal tubular cells.

- They present as flat honeycomb tubules with parallel sharp borders, nests, or occasional gland-like structures (Fig. 5.1a).
- Tubular cells varying in size with indistinct cell borders and with scant to moderate amount of cytoplasm which is delicate or finely granular in texture.
- Tubular cells with small and round nuclei containing finely granular and evenly distributed chromatin, small or inconspicuous nucleoli, and smooth nuclear membrane.

Glomeruli

- Consist of large clusters of capillary loops and mesangial cells that are surrounded by Bowman capsule (Fig. 5.1b).
- Appropriate identification of this normal structure is critical so as to not misinterpret them as tumor cells.

Renal Cysts

Clinical

- Very common.
- Possibly congenital or acquired, single or polycystic, non-neoplastic or neoplastic, and benign or malignant.

Cytology of FNA or Touch Preparation of Core

The adequacy rate for FNA of renal cystic disease is estimated to be 56%, and the false negative rate 6.25% [4].

- Benign cysts: yield clear or pale, yellow fluid with few small, bland, or mildly atypical epithelial lining cells in small three-dimensional clusters; macrophages are seen in most cases. Additionally, neutrophils and occasionally Liesegang rings (three-dimensional laminated ring-like acellular structures) are also observed [5–7]. Epithelial cells seen within these benign specimens demonstrate round nuclei and ill-defined cell borders.
- Malignant cysts: generally bloody or "chocolate"-like fluid and the presence of atypical epithelial cells, macrophages, and lymphocytes [7]. Fluid from cystic renal cell carcinoma (RCC) may show features similar to those of benign cysts [7].

X. Lin (✉)
Northwestern University, Feinberg School of Medicine, Northwestern Memorial Hospital, Chicago, IL, USA
e-mail: xlin@northwestern.edu

J. F. Peevey
Department of Anatomic and Clinical Pathology, OSF St. Anthony Medical Center, Rockford, IL, USA

A. Habib
Department of Radiology, Northwestern University, Chicago, IL, USA

R. Mora
Department of Radiology, Section of Vascular and Interventional Radiology, Northwestern University, Chicago, IL, USA

A. Riaz
Department of Pathology, Northwestern Medicine, Chicago, IL, USA

R. Nayar et al. (eds.), *Atlas of Cytopathology and Radiology*, https://doi.org/10.1007/978-3-030-24756-0_5

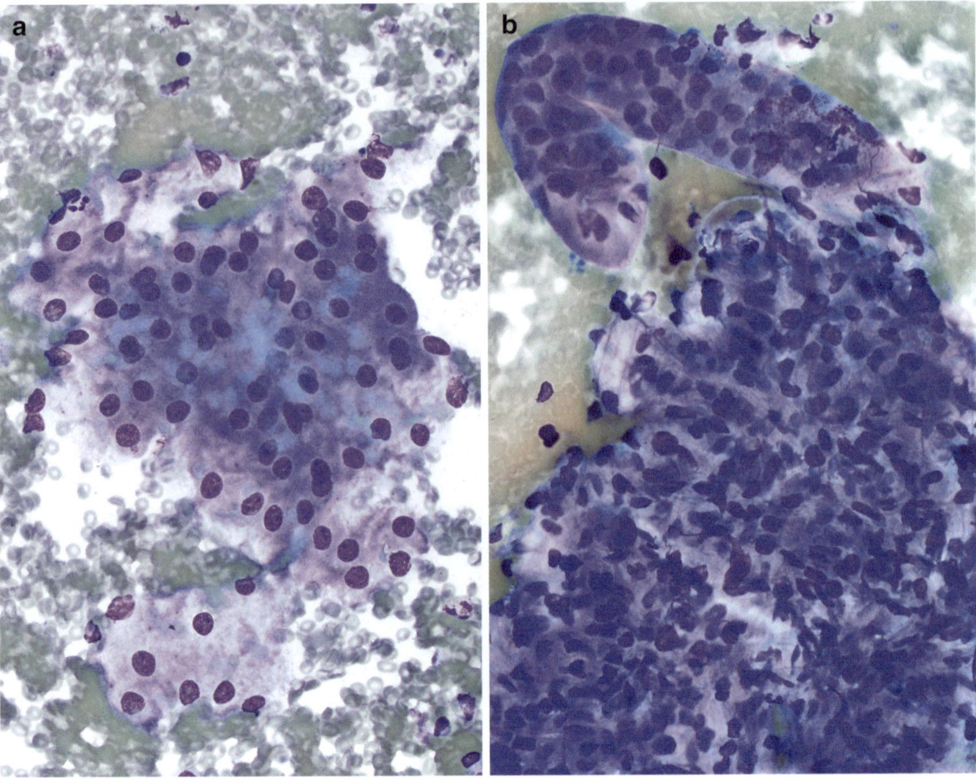

Fig. 5.1 Cytology of normal renal tissue. (**a**) Proximal renal tubule, Diff-Quik stain, 400×. (**b**) Glomerulus and proximal renal tubule, Diff-Quik stain, 400×

Comments

1. Benign epithelial cells with reactive atypia, especially with vacuolated cytoplasm; should be distinguished from RCC with cystic degeneration or cystic RCC.
2. Proximal renal tubule cells should be distinguished from oncocytoma or chromophobe type RCCs [8].
3. Chronic interstitial inflammation: Inflammatory changes can be seen in the kidneys, and the resultant distribution and nonspecific imaging characteristics may appear more nefarious in nature.
4. Renal infection: Pyelonephritis may result in wedge-shaped areas of hypoenhancement in the renal parenchyma. Renal abscesses demonstrate findings of abscesses elsewhere in the body, including a central area of fluid with an enhancing rim. On MRI, these restrict diffusion.

Benign Renal Neoplasms

Angiomyolipoma

Angiomyolipoma (AML) is a benign mesenchymal tumor composed of a variable proportion of adipose tissue, spindle and epithelioid smooth muscle cells, and abnormal thick-walled blood vessels. Angiomyolipomas are the most common benign tumors of the kidney and are more prevalent in the female population [9, 10].

Clinical

- Overall an uncommon entity, thought to represent 0.5–2% of all renal tumors. Some angiomyolipomas are associated with tuberous sclerosis [11–13].
- Male-to-female ratio is 1:4 to 1:10 in nontuberous sclerosis and 1:1 in tuberous sclerosis [11–13]. Average age is 45–55 years for patients without tuberous sclerosis and 25 to 35 for those patients with tuberous sclerosis [11–13].
- Usually asymptomatic. Patients may present with flank pain, hematuria, palpable mass, and retroperitoneal hemorrhage.

Radiology

Radiologic diagnosis of AML is complicated by the range of lipid content that an AML may contain, ranging from complete lack of fat to exhibiting macroscopic fat on cross-sectional imaging [9].

- On MRI, it is challenging to distinguish the microscopic fat of AMLs from that of clear cells on in-phase and out-of-phase T1-weighted imaging (Fig. 5.2) [14]. In addition, AMLs with lower lipid content are difficult to distinguish from papillary RCCs on T2-weighted images.
- Though AMLs are the most common benign tumor, there are abundant imaging pitfalls. Of note, if AML is >4 cm, prophylactic embolization is recommended because of the risk of rupture. Angiographically, AMLs have high vascularity and appear different from surrounding renal parenchyma.

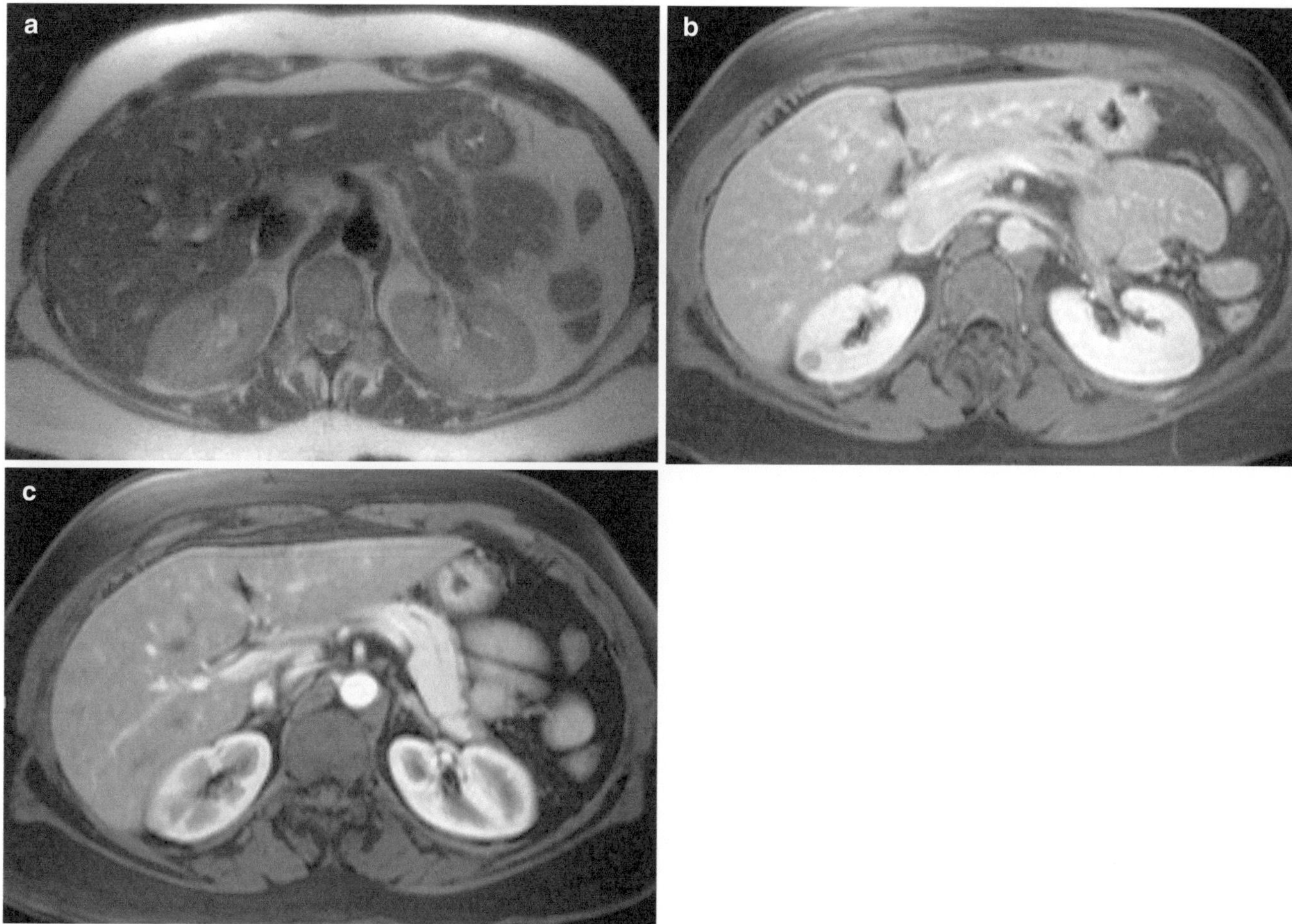

Fig. 5.2 Angiomyolipoma, radioimages. (**a**) Axial SHARP MRIs show a lesion in the right kidney that is isointense to the adjacent renal parenchyma. (**b**) Axial SHARP MRI at 17-minute delay shows a right renal lesion that is hypointense to renal parenchyma. (**c**) Axial SHARP postcontrast MRI sequence showing minimally increased ROI value consistent with enhancement

Cytology of FNA and Touch Preparation of Core

- Characteristically demonstrate a variable proportion of blood vessels and spindle and epithelioid smooth muscle spindled cells arranged in loosely cohesive or cohesive clusters as well as mature fat cells (Fig. 5.3) [15]. The nuclei of smooth muscle cells are oval to elongated with evenly distributed chromatin and no or inconspicuous nucleoli [15]. Naked nuclei are common. The cytoplasm is delicate and sometimes finely vacuolated [16]. Occasionally, smooth muscle cells and adipocytes may show atypia [15]. Mitoses and necrosis are absent [15]. Adipose tissue is not universally present [15].
- Fat necrosis can be seen, including histiocytes, multinucleated giant cells, and pleomorphic nuclei of adipocytes [17].

Comments

- Differential diagnosis includes perinephretic fat (misinterpreted as tumor adipose tissue), RCC (misinterpreted as epithelioid or atypical spindle smooth muscle cells), leiomyosarcoma (misinterpreted as atypical smooth muscle cells), and liposarcoma (misinterpreted as atypical adipocytes).
- These lesions are often sparely cellular, and positive staining of tumor cells can be very helpful in definitive diagnosis. Tumor cells are positive for melanocytic markers (HMB-45, CD63, tyrosinase, and Mart1/Melan-A), smooth muscle markers (smooth muscle actin, muscle-specific actin, desmin, and calponin), CD68, neuron-specific enolase, S-100, estrogen receptor, and progesterone receptor.

Oncocytoma

Oncocytoma is a benign renal epithelial neoplasm composed of large cells with mitochondria-rich eosinophilic cytoplasm; it is thought to arise from intercalated cells.

Clinical

- Approximately 3–7% of all renal neoplasms [18, 19].

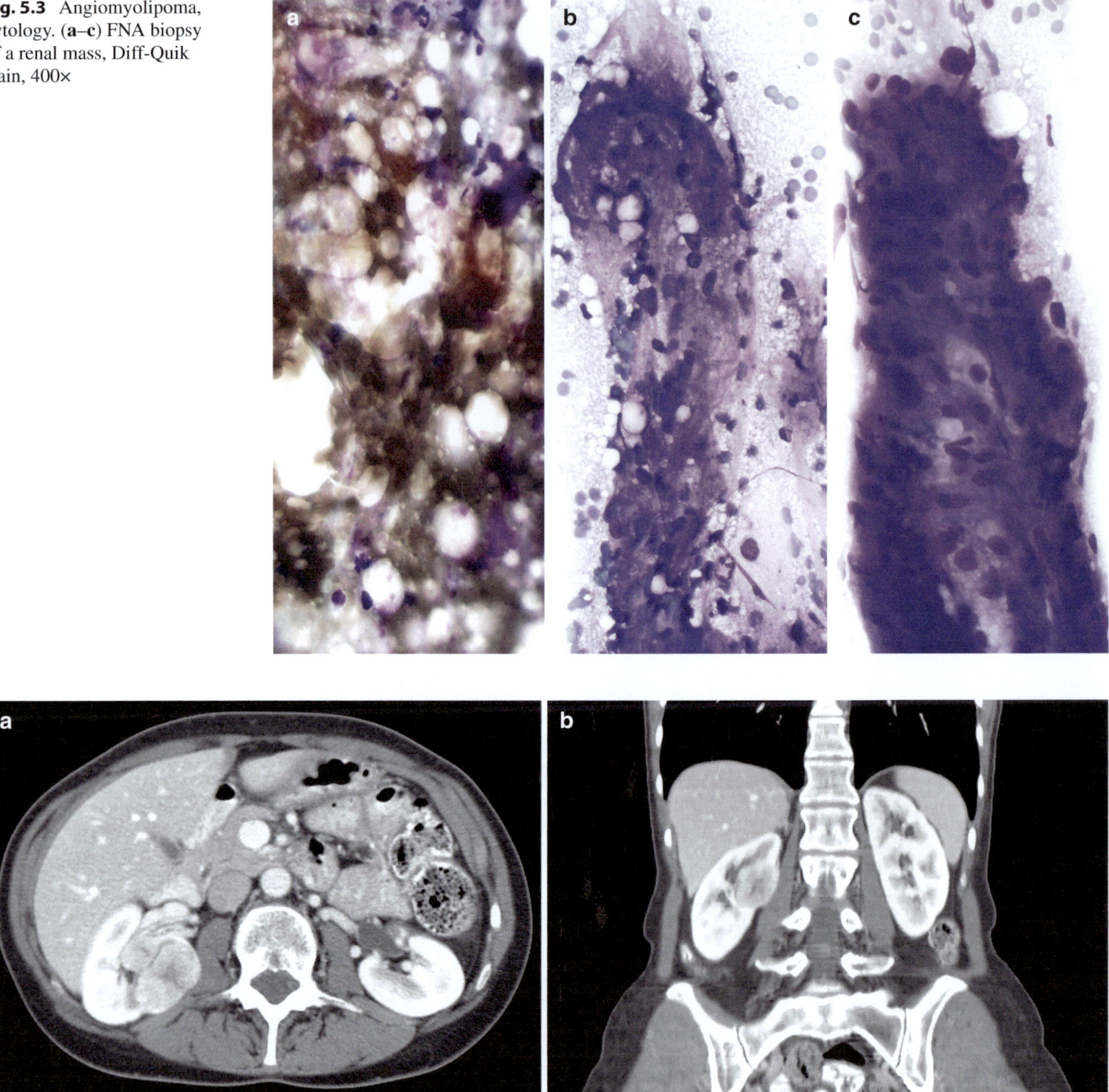

Fig. 5.3 Angiomyolipoma, cytology. (**a**–**c**) FNA biopsy of a renal mass, Diff-Quik stain, 400×

Fig. 5.4 Oncocytoma, radioimages. (**a**) CT scan shows a hyperenhancing mass in the middle pole of the right kidney which contains a central region of low density that may represent necrosis. (**b**) Coronal CT scan images show a hyperenhancing mass with a central region of necrosis

- Wide age range, with a peak in the seventh decade. Male-to-female ratio is 2:1 [20].
- Mostly asymptomatic, and a small number of patients present with hematuria, abdominal pain, and flank mass.
- Central stellate fibrous scar.
- Can be bilateral and multicentric and solid or cystic.

Radiology

- Oncocytomas have a pathologic origin similar to that of the chromophobe subtype of RCC, resulting in similar imaging features such as homogeneous features, spoke-wheel enhancement, and central stellate scar as shown in CT scan (Fig. 5.4) [21].

Cytology of FNA and Touch Preparation of Core

- Characteristically show single or small loose clusters of monotonous oncocytes (Fig. 5.5) [22].
- Oncocytes are large, polygonal or rounded with abundant and finely granular cytoplasm with well-defined cell borders [22].

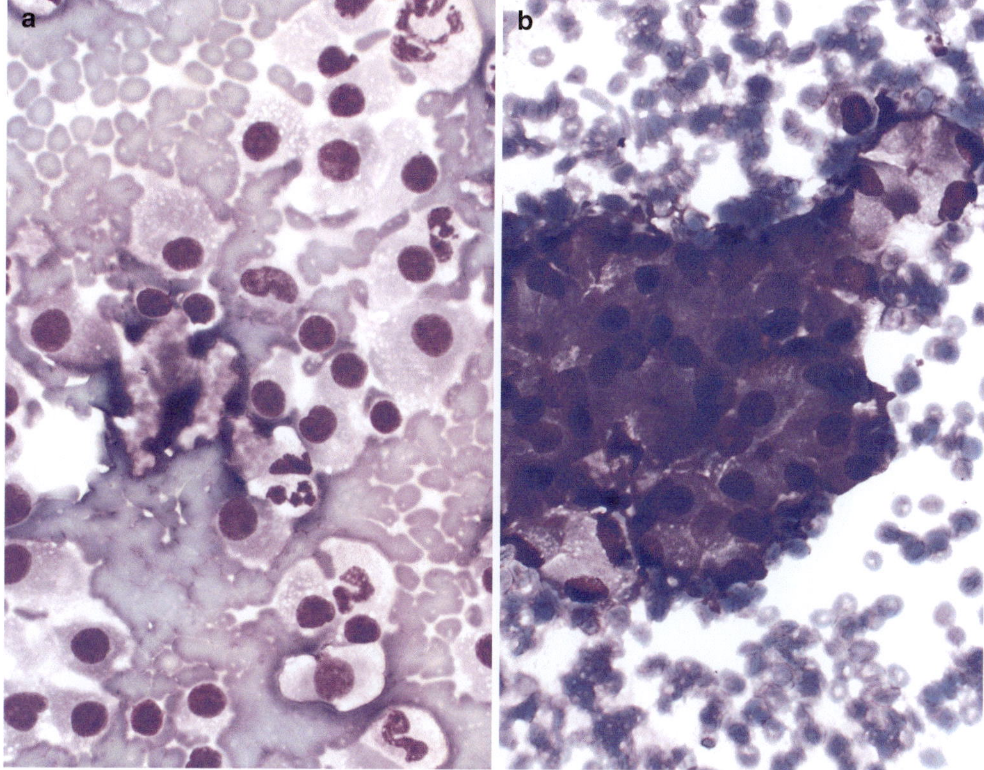

Fig. 5.5 Oncocytoma, cytology. (**a**, **b**) FNA biopsy of a renal mass, Diff-Quik stain, 600×

- The nuclei are usually small, round, regular, and centrally or eccentrically located (Fuhrman grade 2), with finely granular chromatin and no to conspicuous nucleoli [22, 23]. However, hyperchromatic or bizarre nuclei, binucleation, and nuclear enlargement can also be seen and are likely thought to represent degenerative change. Mitosis and necrosis are not usually observed.

Comments

- The differential diagnosis includes chromophobe RCC, clear cell RCC, normal renal tubular cells, and normal hepatocytes.
- The tumor cells are positive for CK7, epithelial membrane antigen (EMA), CD117, napsin A [24], E-cadherin, and S-100A1; they are less frequently positive for CD10 and alpha-methylacyl-CoA racemase (AMACR) [25]. Tumor cells are negative for the RCC antigen, vimentin [25]. There is no diffuse cytoplasmic Hale colloidal iron staining.

Malignant Renal Tumors

Renal Cell Carcinoma

RCC is a group of malignancies arising from the epithelium of the renal tubules. Based on the WHO classification (2016), it consists of familial renal cancer, clear cell RCC, multilocular cystic RCC, papillary RCC, chromophobe RCC, carcinoma of the collecting ducts of Bellini, renal medullary carcinoma, renal carcinomas associated with Xp11.2 translocations/TEF3 gene fusions, and clear cell papillary RCC [26]. Other tumors include RCC associated with neuroblastoma, mucinous tubular spindle cell carcinoma, papillary adenoma of the kidney, and unclassified RCC [27].

The clear cell subtype of RCC has worse outcomes relative to chromophobe and papillary subtypes, with a greater likelihood of metastasizing and presenting at a later stage [27–30]. The chromophobe subtype of RCC is less frequently seen than clear cell RCC and papillary RCC, with an incidence of approximately 5%. The papillary subtype of RCC is often discovered at a low grade stage and is small in size [30]. The size used to separate papillary RCC from papillary adenoma was increased from 0.5 cm to 1.0 cm in the 2016 WHO classification [27]. The five-year survival rate of papillary RCC is significantly better than that for clear cell, ranging from 82% to 92% [31, 32].

Clinical

- The ninth most common cancer in men and the fourteenth most common cancer in women [33] and >90% of all malignancies of the kidney [33].
- Male-to-female ratio is 2 to 3:1 [33, 34]. Its incidence increases steadily after 40 years of age [33].

- Clinical triad: hematuria, pain, and flank mass. Paraneoplastic endocrine syndromes can be seen [35].
- Can be solitary or cystic and single or multiple.

Radiology

- **RCC, clear cell type:** It typically exhibits heterogeneity caused by necrotic change, hemorrhage, or cystic change [32, 36]. It also exhibits features typical of most hypervascular lesions on CT (Fig. 5.6) [30].
- **RCC, chromophobe type**: The CT scan of chromophobe RCC shows a solid, homogeneous appearance with possible spoke-wheel enhancement or a stellate central scar (Fig. 5.7) [30].
- **RCC, papillary type**: The papillary subtype of RCC exhibits low signal intensity on T2-weighted MRI and is also hypervascular (Fig. 5.8).

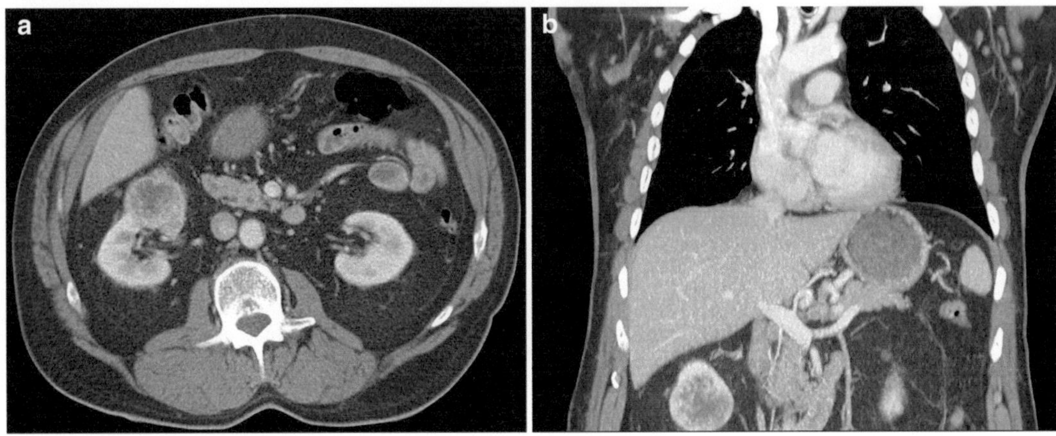

Fig. 5.6 RCC, clear cell type, radioimages. (**a**) CT scan shows an exophytic mass arising from the inferior pole of the right kidney. There is evidence of central necrosis. (**b**) CT scan on coronal view, in which the mass appears to have a central region of necrosis

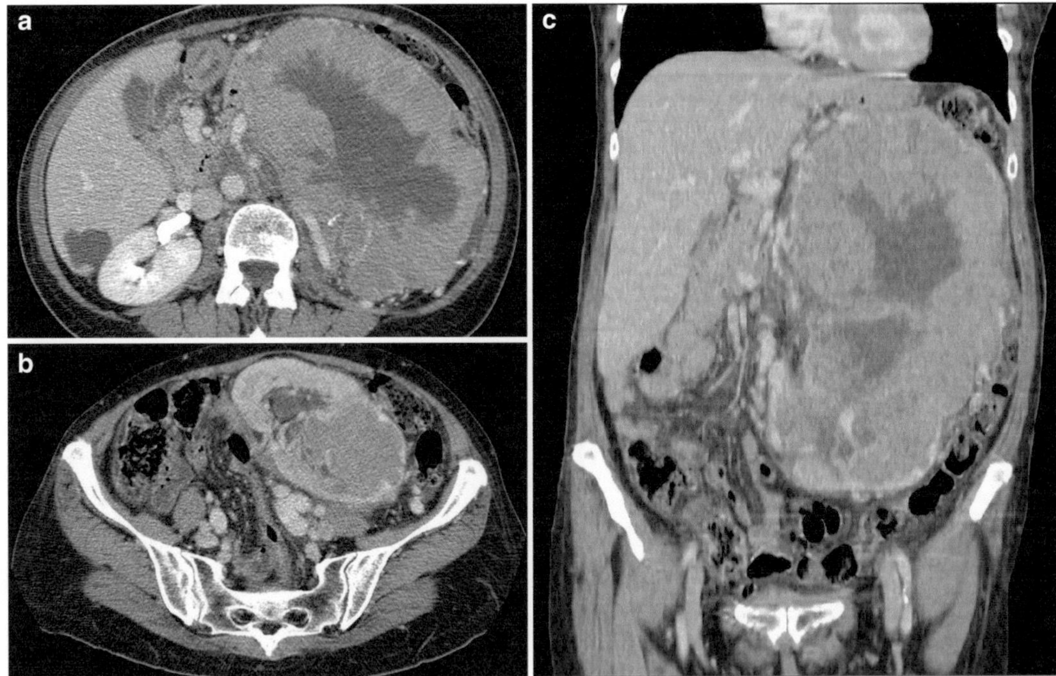

Fig. 5.7 RCC, chromophobe type, radioimages. (**a**) CT scan shows a large, heterogeneously enhancing multilobulated mass arising from the left kidney. Low density regions may represent necrosis or poorly enhancing tissue. There are coarse calcifications within the mass. (**b**) CT scan shows another view farther inferior to the large mass with associated compression and displacement of adjacent vessels. Hypoattenuating regions are again seen, possibly caused by necrosis. (**c**) CT scan shows that the true extent of the mass can be appreciated on the coronal image

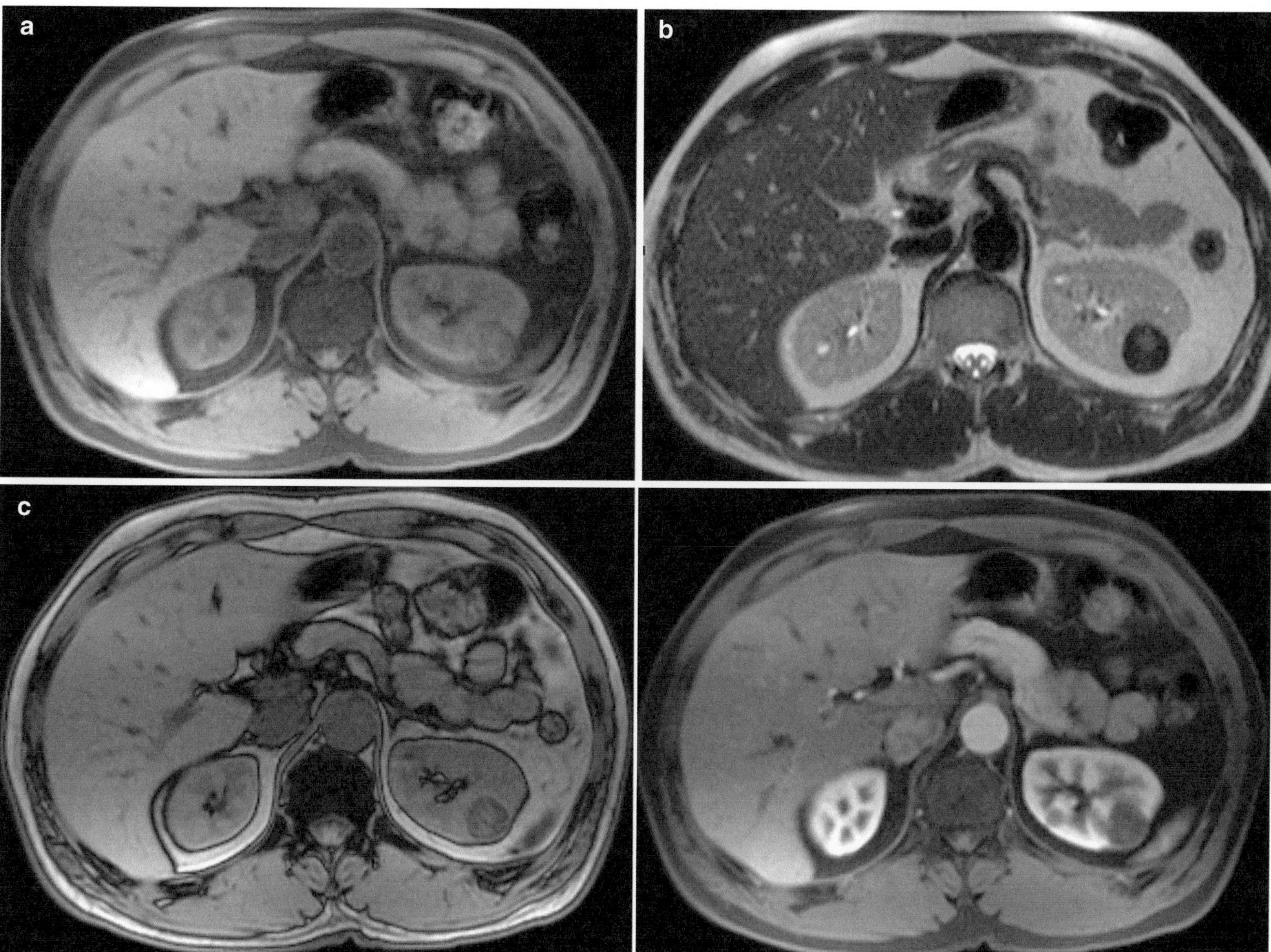

Fig. 5.8 RCC, papillary type, radioimages. (**a**) MRI (axial T1) shows a 2.5-cm lesion in the superior pole of the left kidney, which is slightly heterogeneous and showing decreased intensity on T1-weighted images. (**b**) MRI (axial HASTE) shows a hypointense lesion in the left kidney. (**c**) MRI (in-phase image) shows signal loss when compared to the out-of-phase images. (**d**) MRI (postcontrast) sequence of the lesion demonstrates mild early enhancement, which increases slowly over time

- **RCC, sarcomatoid differentiation**: The sarcomatoid differentiation can be found in any subtype of RCC. Thus, imaging features would probably be reflective of the subtype, although with aggressive features and resultant poor prognosis as shown in the CT scan (Fig. 5.9) [30].

Cytology of FNA and Touch Preparation of Core

- **RCC, clear cell type**: The most common cell type. Characteristically shows single, sheets, nests, papillary or floral-like groups, or three-dimensional clusters of clear cells with or without capillaries transversing the cells (Fig. 5.10a, b). The clear cells are large with low nuclear/cytoplasmic ratios. The cytoplasm is abundant, pale, wispy, delicate, reticulated, foamy, vacuolated, or granular. The nuclei vary from small to large, uniform to pleomorphism, bland to bizarre, smooth to irregular nuclear membrane, fine and evenly distributed chromatin to coarse and unevenly distributed chromatin, and no nucleoli to prominent nucleoli, depending on the grade of the tumor [6]. Intranuclear cytoplasmic invaginations, intracytoplasmic hyaline globules, naked nuclei, and multinucleated giant tumor cells can also be seen [6]. Necrosis, frothy background, fibrosis, hemosiderin, cholesterol, and fat may be seen in the background [6].
- **RCC, chromophobe type**: Characteristically shows clusters or single large cells with granular cytoplasm, well-defined cell borders, and a low-to-high nuclear/cytoplasmic ratio (Fig. 5.11a, b) [37]. The nuclei vary significantly in size, are often atypical, and have coarse and hyperchromatic chromatin, irregular nuclear membrane, smaller nucleoli, and peri-nuclear haloes [6]. Binucleation or multinucleation is frequently seen [6, 37].

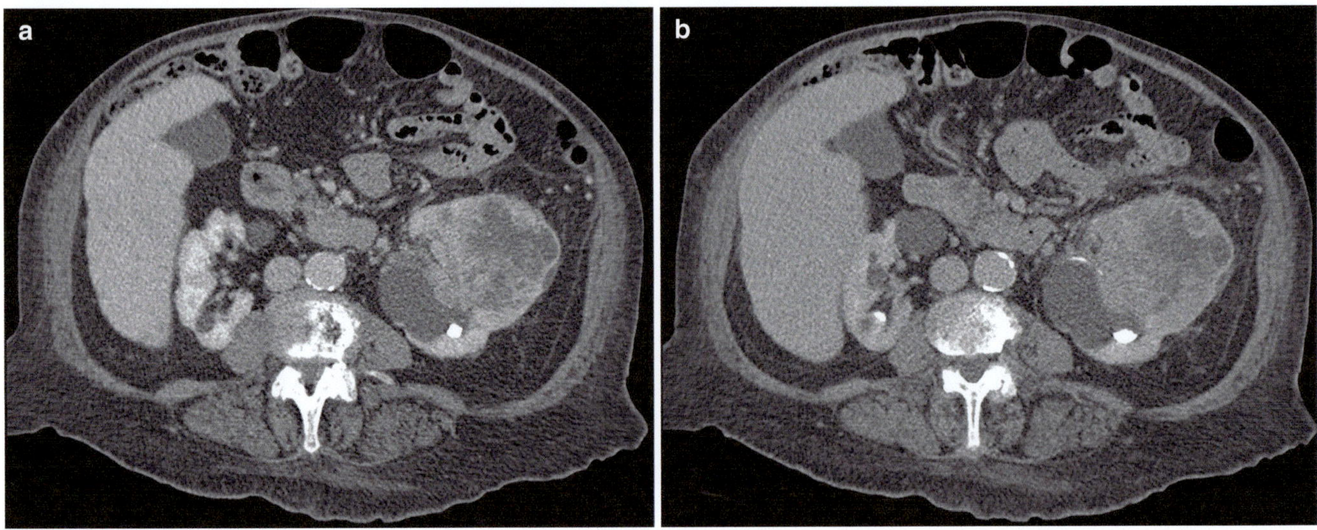

Fig. 5.9 RCC with sarcomatoid differentiation, radioimages. (**a**) CT scan shows a large, peripherally enhancing heterogeneous mass with suspected invasion of the proximal ureter as well as possible thrombosis of a renal vein branch. (**b**) CT again shows a large, heterogeneous mass obscuring the left upper pole and a portion of the renal pelvis

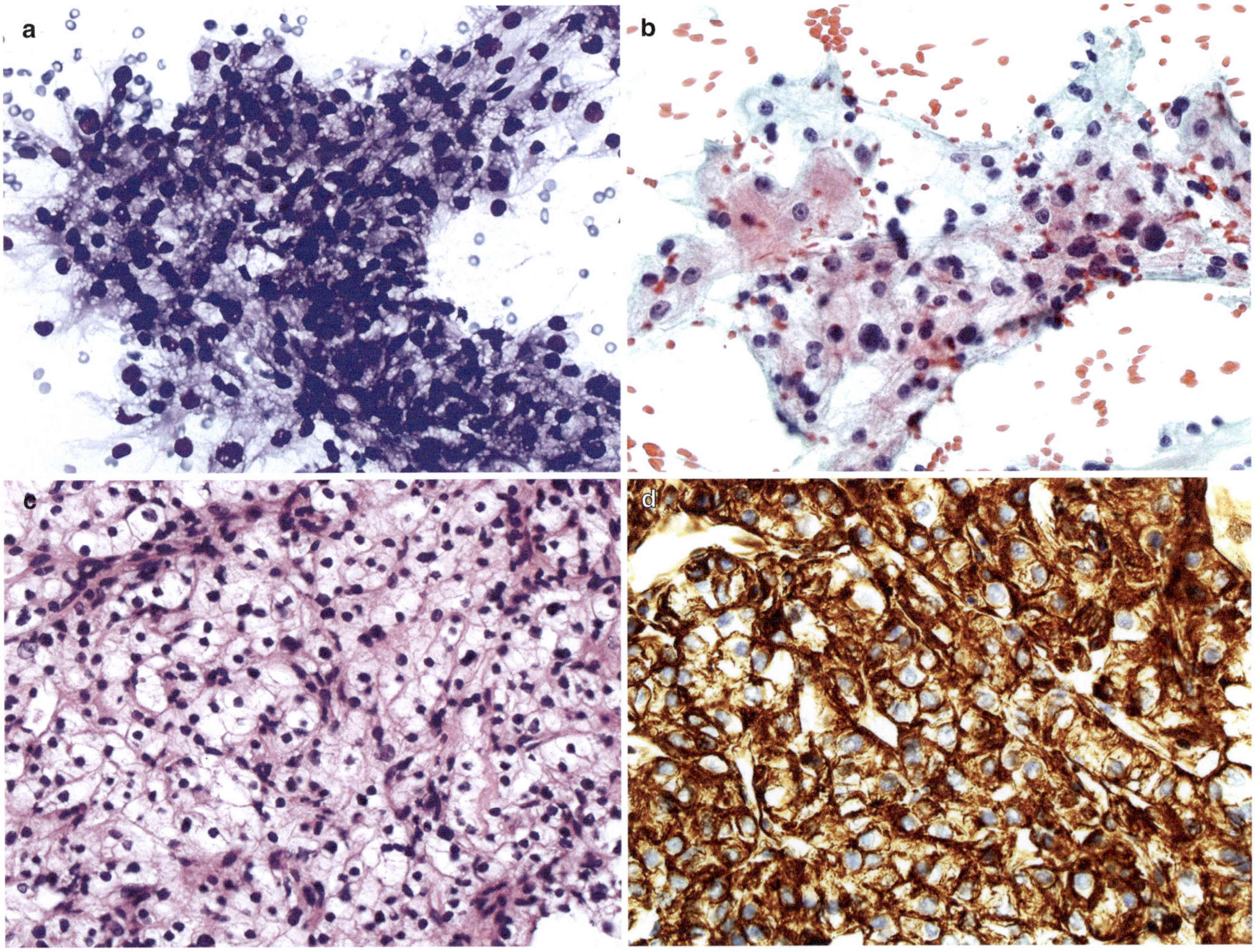

Fig. 5.10 RCC, clear cell type, cytology and histology. (**a**, **b**) Biopsy cytology of a renal mass, Diff-Quik stain (**a**) and Papanicolaou stain (**b**), 400×. (**c**) Histology of core, hematoxylin and eosin stain, 400×. (**d**) Immunostain for CA9, 400×

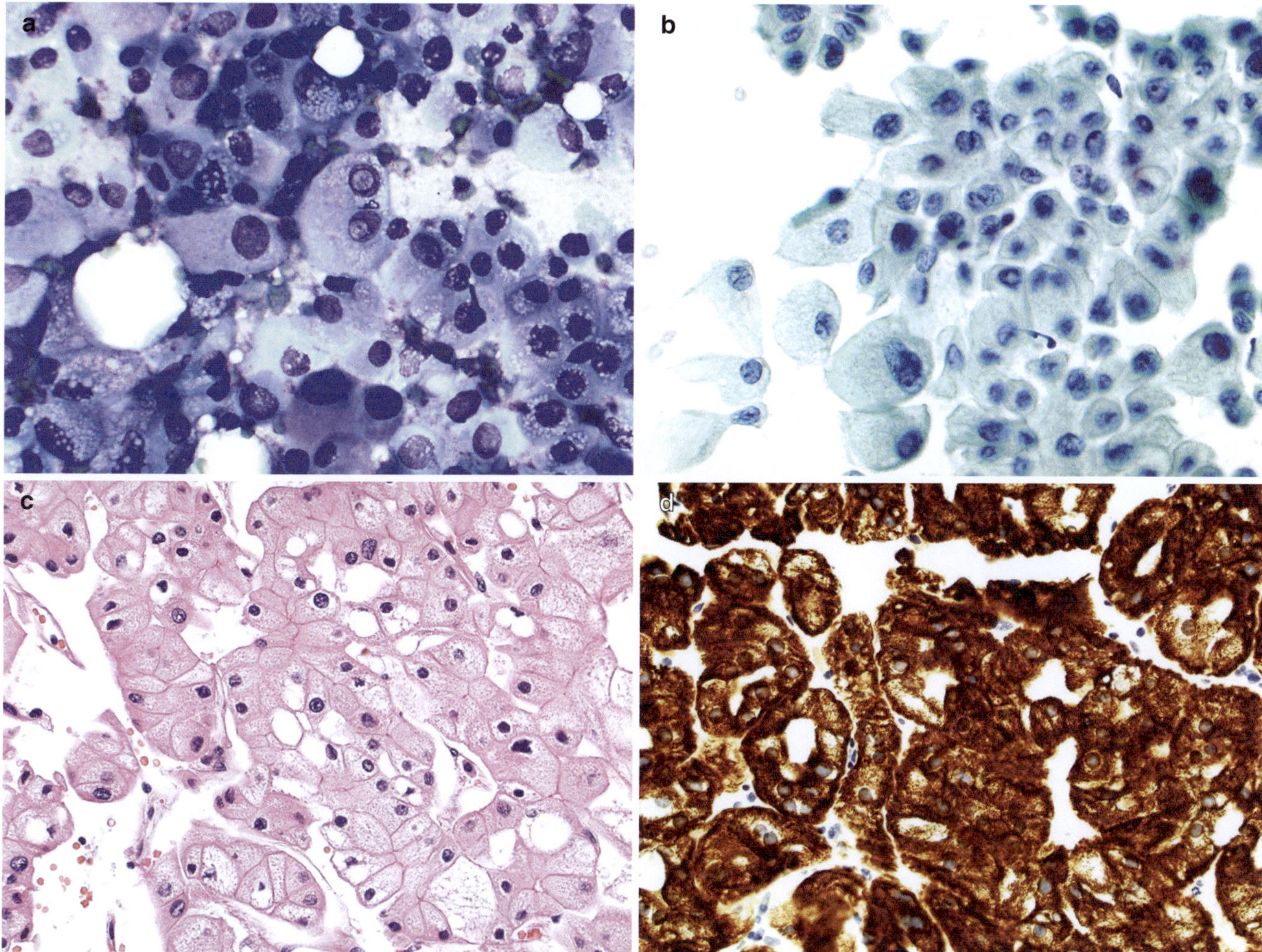

Fig. 5.11 RCC, chromophobe type, cytology and histology. (**a**, **b**) FNA biopsy of a renal mass, Diff-Quik stain (**a**) and Papanicolaou stain (**b**), 400×. (**c**) Histology of core, hematoxylin and eosin stain, 600×. (**d**) Immunostain for CK7, 600×

The cells are often referred to as "vegetable cells." Hemorrhage and necrosis are common, particularly in larger tumors.

- **RCC, papillary type**: Characteristically shows papillae composed of fibrovascular stalks surrounded by a layer of tumor cells, rounded spherules of tumor cells, single cells, and foamy or hemosiderin-laden macrophages (Fig. 5.12a). The fibrovascular stalks often contain histiocytes, with or without hemosiderin and/or lipid. The tumor cells are usually cuboidal to columnar. The nuclei are usually bland and uniform with fine chromatin, smooth to irregular nuclear membrane, small or inconspicuous nucleoli, and high nuclear/cytoplasmic ratios [6]. Pleomorphism, multinucleation, and mitotic figures are infrequent. Cytoplasm is scant and clear/pale in type 1 and abundant/eosinophilic in type 2. The tumor cells often contain hemosiderin pigment and may also contain intracytoplasmic vacuoles. Psammoma bodies, necrosis, and hemorrhage can be seen.
- **RCC, with sarcomatoid differentiation**: Characteristically shows discohesive spindle and pleomorphic cells with prominent nucleoli and delicate cytoplasm (Fig. 5.13a, b). Necrosis is frequently seen [16]. These cells show epithelial features by immunohistochemistry (IHC) and electron microscopy.
- **Collecting duct carcinoma**: Characteristically shows single or clusters of round or oval cells with tubule or papillary architectures. The nuclei are large and mildly atypical and have hyperchromatic and coarse chromatin and inconspicuous to prominent nucleoli. The cytoplasm is small to moderate in amount and finely granular with well-defined cell borders [38].

Histology of Core or Cell Block

- **RCC, clear cell type:** Sections show nests or sheets of large polygonal cells with capillary networks, foamy, clear, or granular cytoplasm, and centrally located nuclei

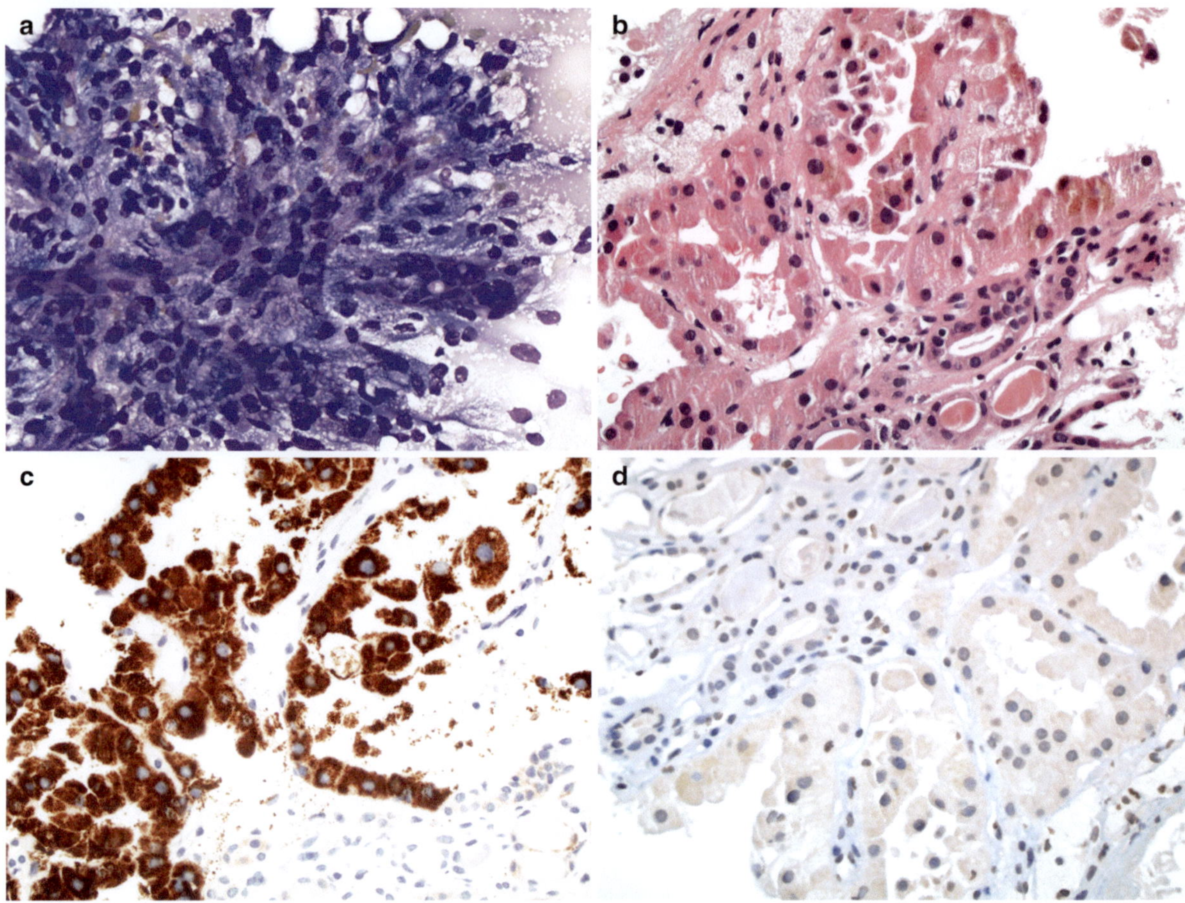

Fig. 5.12 RCC, papillary type, cytology and histology. (**a**) FNA cytology of a renal mass, Diff-Quik stain, 400×. (**b**) Histology of core, hematoxylin and eosin stain, 600×. (**c**, **d**) Immunostain for AMACR (**c**) and CA9 (**d**) 600×

Fig. 5.13 RCC, high grade, with sarcomatoid feature. (**a**, **b**) FNA biopsy of a renal mass, Diff-Quik stain, 600×

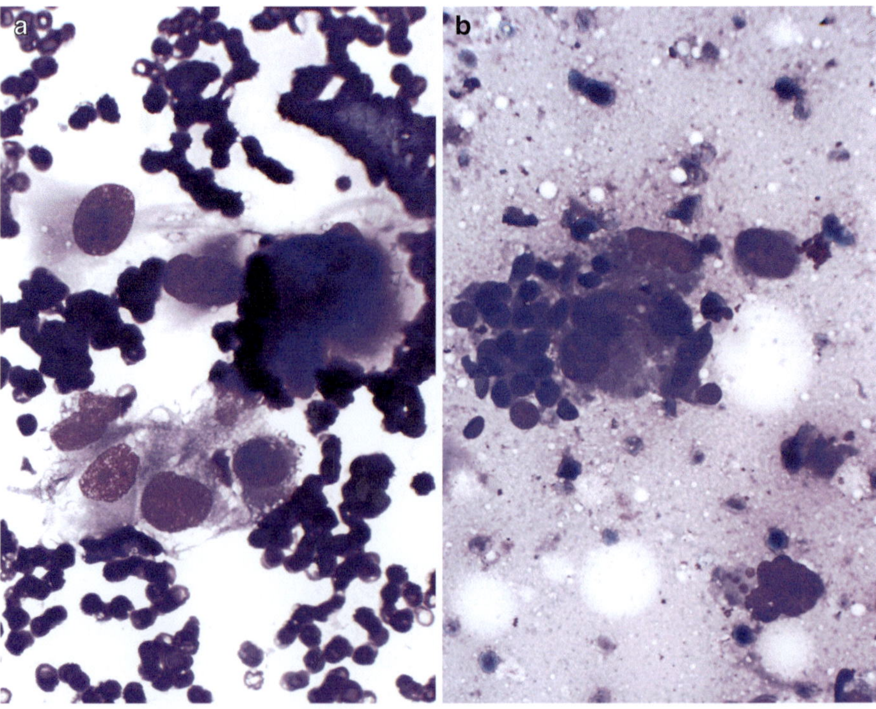

that possibly contain nucleoli, depending on grading (Fig. 5.10c).

- **RCC, chromophobe type**: Sheets of polygonal cells with abundant granular cytoplasm, well-defined cytoplasmic borders, and round or oval nuclei with perinuclear halos (Fig. 5.11c).
- **RCC, papillary type**: Papillae lined by atypical epithelial cells with nuclear atypia with or without prominent nucleoli, depending on grading of tumor; scant to abundant eosinophilic, granular, or vacuolated cytoplasm, depending on type of papillary RCC (type 1 versus type 2) (Fig. 5.12b).

Comments

- For **clear cell RCC**, the differential diagnosis includes chromophobe RCC, papillary RCC, clear cell papillary RCC histiocytes [39], degenerated tubular cells, benign adrenal cortical cells, adrenocortical neoplasms, metastatic clear cell carcinoma from other primary tumors, and angiomyolipoma. Tumor cells are positive for cytokeratins (CAM5.2, CK19, AE1), RCC antigen, CA9 (Fig. 5.10d), CD10, EMA, napsin A [24], and vimentin and less frequently or weakly and focally positive for AMACR [AU: see earlier query Already added above], CD117, and E-cadherin [25]. Tumor cells are negative for CK7 and CK20.
- For **chromophobe RCC**, the differential diagnosis includes oncocytoma/oncocytic carcinoma, clear cell RCC, and benign proximal renal tubular cells [22]. Tumor cells are positive for pan-cytokeratins, including CK7 (Fig. 5.11d), EMA, and CD117, and less frequently positive for RCC antigen, napsin A [24], E-cadherin, and CD10. The tumor cells are negative for vimentin, AMACR, and CK20 [25]. There is diffuse cytoplasmic Hale colloidal iron staining [37].
- For **papillary RCC**, the differential diagnosis includes papillary adenoma (≤1 cm), well-differentiated papillary transitional cell carcinoma, clear cell RCC [27], and carcinoma of the collecting ducts of Bellini. Tumor cells are positive for cytokeratins (CAM5.2, AE1/AE3, and CK7), RCC antigen, CD10, EMA, AMACR (Fig. 5.12c), napsin A [24], vimentin, and S-100; they are less frequently positive for CD117 and CA9 (Fig. 5.12d) [40]. The type 1 tumor cells are negative for E-cadherin, and type 2 tumor cells are less frequently positive for E-cadherin [25].
- If FNA only shows sarcomatoid features, differential diagnosis includes leiomyosarcoma, angiomyolipoma, and spindle squamous cell carcinoma or urothelial carcinoma. The tumor cells are positive for both keratins and vimentin.
- For carcinoma of the collecting ducts of Bellini, tumor cells are positive for high molecular weight cytokeratins (34βE12, CK19), vimentin, CD15, EMA, and possibly mucin. Tumor cells are negative for CD10 and CD117 [25, 41].

Urothelial Carcinoma

Clinical

- Incidence is 1.2/100,000. Accounts for about 8% of all urothelial tumors [42].
- Predominantly found in older patients (mean age 70 years) with male-to-female ratio of 2:1 [42].
- Usually multifocal [42].
- Hematuria and flank pain are the chief presenting symptoms.

Radiology

- CT imaging features of urothelial carcinoma show possible thickening of the urothelial lining or a pelvi-calyceal filling defect (Fig. 5.14).
- Occasionally, these may present as masses much like RCC; however, location in the collecting system, slight enhancement, and the absence of necrotic or cystic change increase the likelihood that the lesion is more likely to be urothelial carcinoma [43].

Cytology of FNA and Touch Preparation of Core

- Low-grade urothelial carcinoma: characteristically shows papillary aggregates of minimally atypical urothelial cells.
- High-grade urothelial carcinoma: characteristically shows single or papillary aggregates of obvious malignant urothelial cells (Fig. 5.15). The nuclei are markedly pleomorphic and have coarse, irregular chromatin and prominent nucleoli. The cytoplasm is scant to moderate, glassy to dense, and occasionally vacuolated [6].
- Micropapillary architecture might be seen in urine cytology [44] and biopsy.
- Squamous differentiation, glandular cells, clear cells, or bizarre cells may be seen.

Comments

- Differential diagnosis includes reactive urothelial cells caused by stones, inflammation, and instrumentation, metastatic carcinoma, sarcoma, high grade RCC, and papillary RCC.
- Urothelial cells are positive for CK7, p63, p40, GATA3, CK20, CK5/6, K903, and thrombomodulin. GATA3 is more sensitive than traditional markers for conventional urothelial carcinoma and micropapillary urothelial carcinoma [45]. High-grade urothelial carcinoma tends to lose expression of p63 and p40, while it retains GATA3 expression [45]. Tumor cells are negative for napsin A [24].

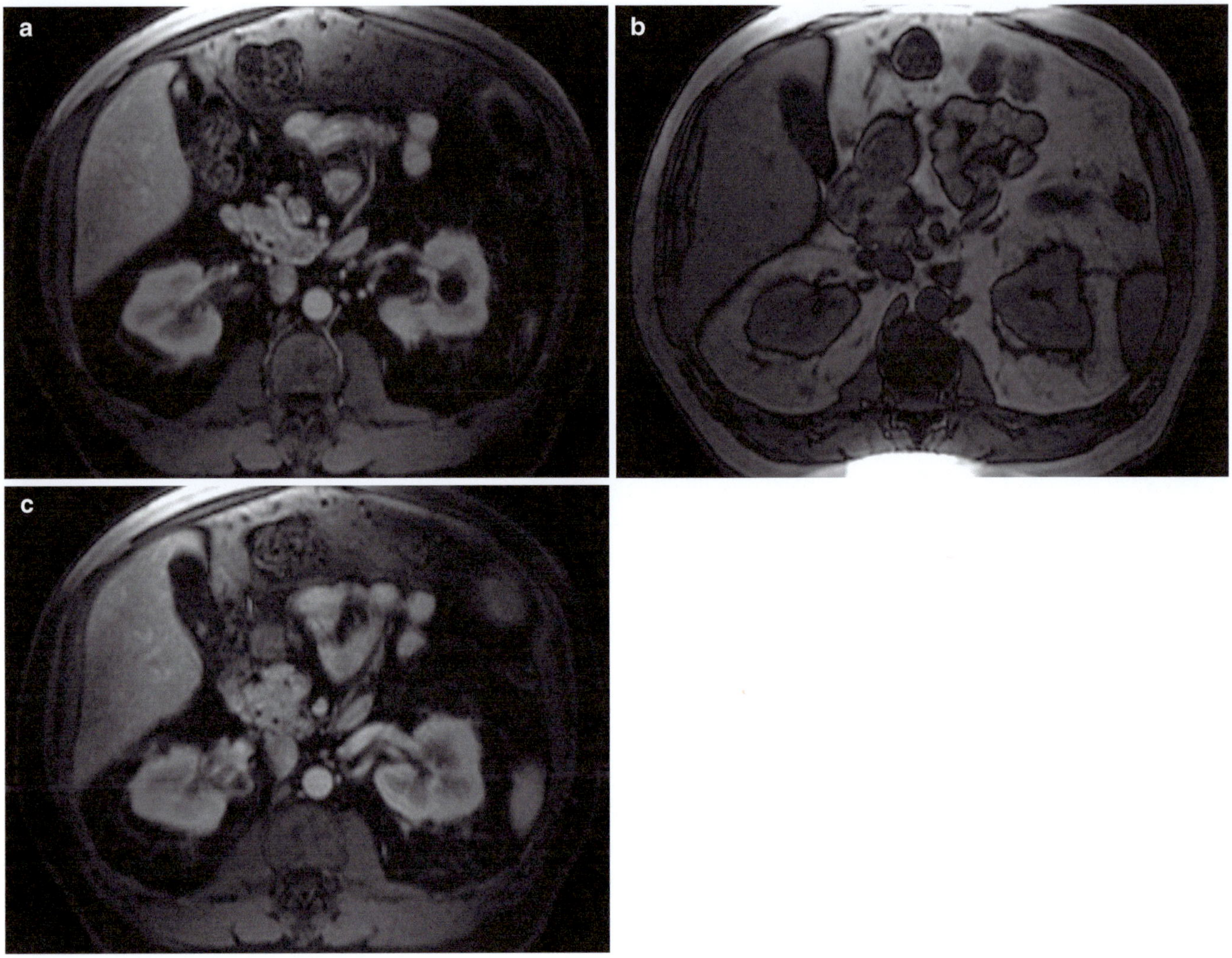

Fig. 5.14 Urothelial carcinoma, radioimages. (**a**) CT scan shows a large infiltrating mass occupying the upper half of the left kidney involving the central collecting system. Few pathologic lymph nodes are seen in the adjacent region. (**b**) Another CT scan view of the large left renal mass which enhances after contrast administration. (**c**) Early excretory phase of CT scan again shows an extensive, infiltrative mass

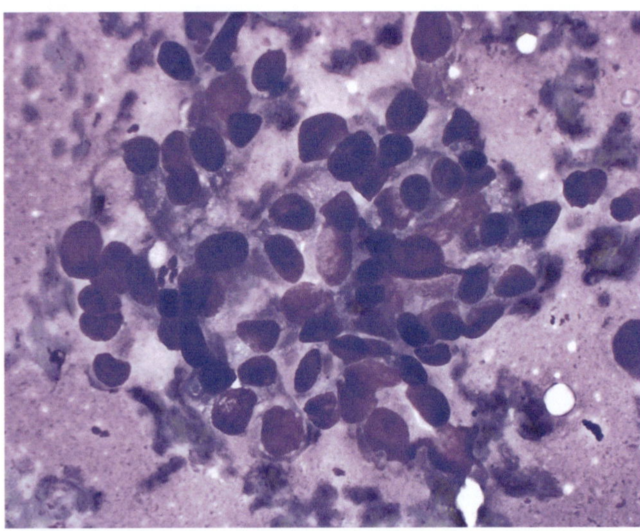

Fig. 5.15 Urothelial carcinoma, high grade. FNA biopsy of a renal mass from a patient with an enlarged retroperitoneal lymph node; Diff-Quik stain, 600×

Nephroblastoma (Wilms Tumor)

Nephroblastoma is a malignant embryonal neoplasm derived from nephrogenic blastemal cells that both replicates the histology of developing kidneys and often shows divergent patterns of differentiation [46].

Clinical

- 1/8000 children [46] and 85% of malignant renal tumors of children.
- Male-to-female ratio is 1:1 to 1:3 [46, 47]; 98% of cases are under 10 years old [46].
- Usually unilateral [46].
- Usually presents with an asymptomatic abdominal mass.

Cytology of FNA and Touch Preparation of Core

- Characteristically shows various combinations of discohesive three-dimensional sheets/groups of blastemal cells in all cases, epithelial cells in 60% of cases, stromal component in one third of cases, tubular differentiation in 26.6–85.7% of cases, and glomeruloid differentiation in 23.8–33.3% of cases [47–49]. Frequent mitoses can be seen [49].
- Blastemal cells are small- to medium-sized and round to oval. The cytoplasm is scant [48, 50]. The nuclei are round and hyperchromatic with fine chromatin, irregular nuclear membranes, and inconspicuous to distinct nucleoli [47–49]. Nuclear overlapping and molding can be seen [49]. In some cases the cells are strongly periodic acid-Schiff (PAS) -positive.
- The epithelial cells are larger than blastema cells [47, 48]. Nuclei are slightly larger than blastema nuclei, and the cytoplasm is more abundant [51]. Cohesive clusters of epithelial cells forming nests, glands, and tubules or glomeruloid bodies may be seen [47, 48].
- The stromal cells include spindle cells with a small amount of delicate cytoplasm and elongated, active nuclei (most commonly seen) set in a metachromatic, myxoid stroma [47, 48].
- Acute or chronic inflammatory cells, macrophages, and necrosis are common [50].

Comments

- The differential diagnosis includes a variety of other small blue cell tumors: embryonal rhabdomyosarcoma, Ewing sarcoma, lymphoma, desmoplastic small round cell tumor, and neuroblastoma [48].
- Tumor cells are positive for PAS, vimentin, neuron specific enolase (NSE), desmin, and cytokeratin. WT-1 is typical but not expressed in all nephroblastomas [46].

Metastasis

Clinical

- Metastases to the kidney are more common than primary renal neoplasms. Metastatic disease is the most common malignancy discovered in the kidney on autopsy [52].
- Common cancers that metastasize to the kidneys are lung, breast, colon, and malignant melanoma [53]. Several primary renal tumors (mucin-positive RCC, urothelial carcinoma, collecting duct carcinoma) can be mistaken for metastatic lesions based on cytomorphology alone. In these instances, ICH staining is very helpful.

Radiology

- Both primary and secondary lymphomas of the kidney can be seen; however, secondary lymphoma is significantly more common. If a patient has widespread lymphoma, direct extension from adjacent lymph nodes or hematogenous spread can result in renal involvement. The elevated nucleus-to-cytoplasmic ratio and the large number of cell results restricted diffusion on MRI, along with intermediate signal intensity on both T1- and T2-weighted sequences.
- On CT scan, the nephrographic phase allows for maximal spatial resolution to aid in evaluation for metastatic disease (Fig. 5.16) [54]. Renal melanoma is rare. However, when it does occur, it usually follows the features of melanoma, which are nonspecific on ultrasound and CT. However, on MRI, there is a T1 hyperintense signal and T2 hypointense signal. In addition to these findings, there is hyperenhancement.

Cytology and Histology

- Cytomorphology/histomorphology differ, depending on type of metastatic malignancy.
- Comparison with morphology of primary malignancy is important.
- A panel of immunostains can be performed to confirm the diagnosis.

IHC for napsin A has been widely used to support a diagnosis of lung adenocarcinoma with reported high sensitivity [24]; however it is also expressed in many renal neoplasms [24], therefore, care should be taken when trying to separate a renal primary from a lung primary using Napsin.

Adrenal Glands

Use of FNA biopsy for incidentally discovered adrenal masses or "incidentalomas" is controversial [55–57]. Incidental findings can be seen in approximately 0.4–4.4% of all CT studies [58, 59]. Adrenal lesions are often identified on cross-sectional imaging in symptomatic and asymptomatic patients. Because of the uncertain nature of certain adrenal imaging findings, the utility of radiologic and pathologic correlations is high in this clinical scenario. By classifying key features of different biopsy-proven pathology, imagers will find that radiologic findings can potentially streamline downstream clinical care [56]. Using FNA may make it difficult in some cases to distinguish benign from malignant adrenal cells with certainty [60]. However, reports have stated that image-guided FNA cytology is a safe and sensitive procedure and should be performed in all patients with incidentally discovered adrenal masses with high sensitivity (83.3–100%) [61, 62], specificity (96.3–100%) [61,

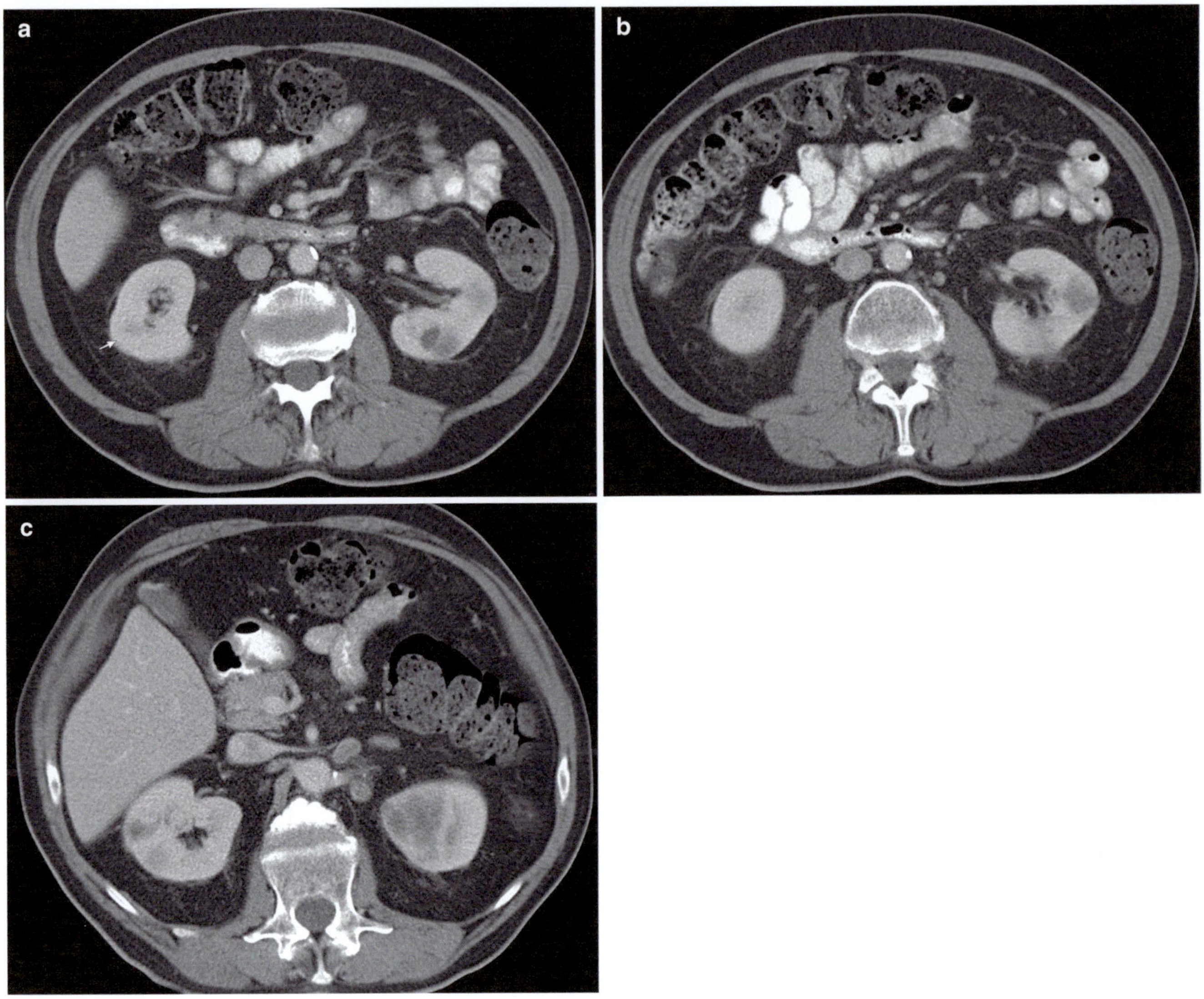

Fig. 5.16 Metastatic malignancy to the kidney, radioimages. (**a**) CT scan shows bilateral, poorly defined hypodense masses scattered throughout both kidneys. The largest is a hypodense mass in the upper pole of the left kidney. (**b**) Additional CT scan view of hypodense lesions within both kidneys. (**c**) Additional CT scan view of hypodense lesions within both kidneys

62], positive predictive value (95.8–100%) [61, 62], negative predictive value (100%) [62], and accuracy (97.6%) [62]. FNA biopsy may cause fatal hypertensive crisis or hemorrhage in pheochromocytoma, therefore biochemical testing should be performed before biopsy of adrenal masses. Complications include hypertension, hematoma of the liver, thorax, and duodenum [50], and pneumothorax [56].

Adrenal Epithelial Cells

Cytology of FNA or Touch Preparation

- Adrenal cortical cells present ias cords, small aggregates, or singly (Fig. 5.17). The cells are generally uniform and polygonal, with small to moderate, uniform and round nuclei with granular chromatin and a distinct nucleolus. Marked nuclear atypia, pleomorphism,

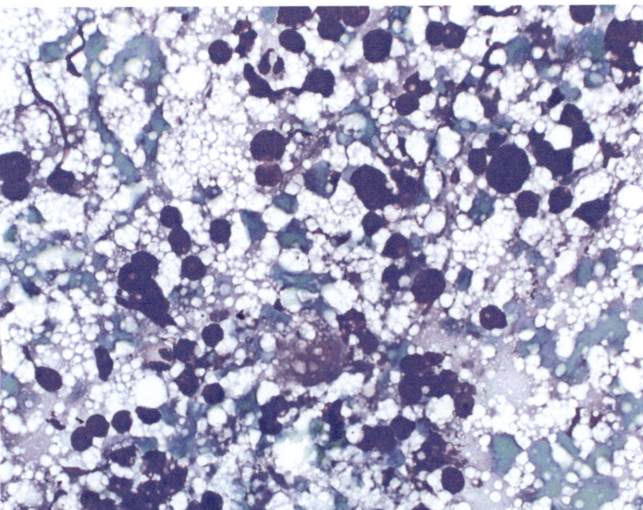

Fig. 5.17 Benign adrenal cortex cells, cytology; Diff-Quik stain, 600×

multiple large nucleoli, and binucleation may be seen. Naked nuclei are common. The cytoplasm is abundant, finely vacuolated or finely granular, and delicate with frayed cell borders.
- Adrenal medulla cells are polygonal and variable in size and shape. The nuclei have granular chromatin and a distinct nucleolus. The cytoplasm is finely granular and frequently contains lipofuscin. Intracytoplasmic hyaline globules are also commonly observed.

Inflammatory Lesions

Clinical

- When FNA is utilized to exclude a neoplasm, an inflammatory lesion may be encountered. Since it may or may not be due to infectious organisms; triage for cytologic material for microbiology studies should be be utilized.

Radiology

- It is often challenging to distinguish between inflammatory changes and neoplastic lesions in the adrenal gland.
- The overall MRI features are nonspecific, bringing adenomas, adrenal hematomas, or infection within the realm of possibility. Upon biopsy, the lesion often is found to be inflammatory change (Fig. 5.18).

Cytology of FNA and Touch Preparation of Core

- The presence of inflammatory cells (neutrophils, lymphocytes, macrophages) and benign adrenal cells (Fig. 5.19). Necrosis and/or granulomas may be seen.

Comment

- Special stains and microbiologic cultures should be performed to detect and definitively identify organisms (e.g., bacteria, mycobacteria, viruses, fungi).

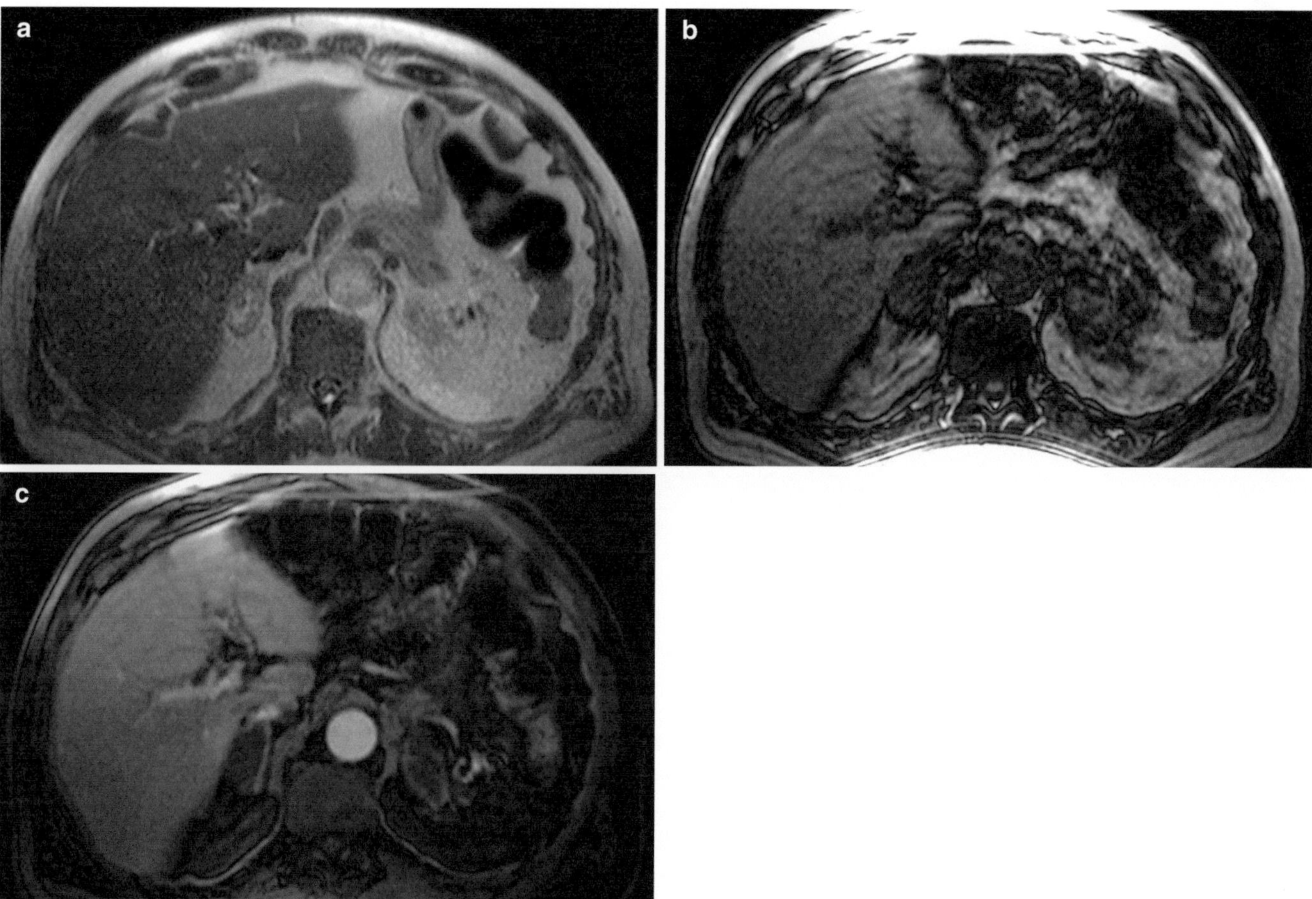

Fig. 5.18 Adrenal gland, inflammation, radioimages. (**a**) MRI (T1-weighted image) of the right adrenal nodule demonstrates heterogeneous signal intensity on precontrast images. (**b**) MRI (out of phase image) shows no definitive loss of signal on out of phase images. (**c**) MRI (postcontrast image) shows peripheral enhancement with low signal intensity

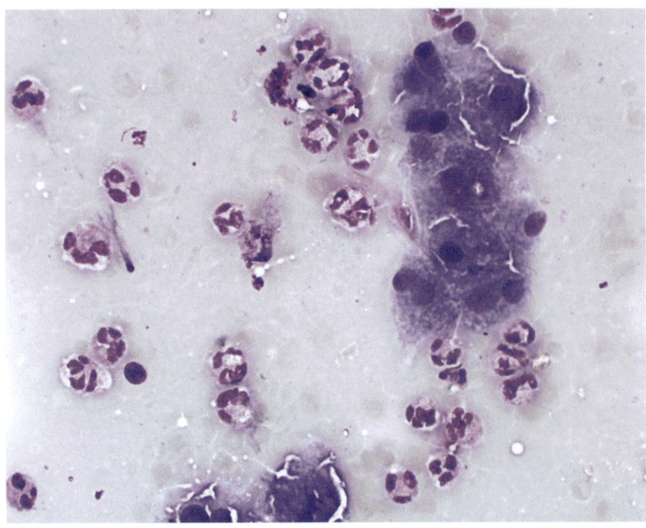

Fig. 5.19 Adrenal gland, inflammation, cytology. FNA biopsy of a lesion in the adrenal gland shows abundant neutrophils; Diff-Quik stain, 600×

Benign Adrenal Neoplasms

Adrenal Myelolipoma

Myelolipomas are benign tumors that exhibit macroscopic fat that is prominent on both CT and MRI [63]. Myelolipomas have a prevalence of 0.08–0.2% [64]. Patients are usually asymptomatic, and rarely myelolipomas may result in functional symptoms [65].

Clinical

- Uncommon benign neoplasm, 2.5% of primary adrenal tumors [66].
- In middle to late adult life without sex predilection.
- No clinical symptoms.

Radiology

- Macroscopic fat; on MRI exhibits decreased signal intensity on fat-saturated T2-weighted images and increased intensity on T1-weighted sequences (Fig. 5.20).

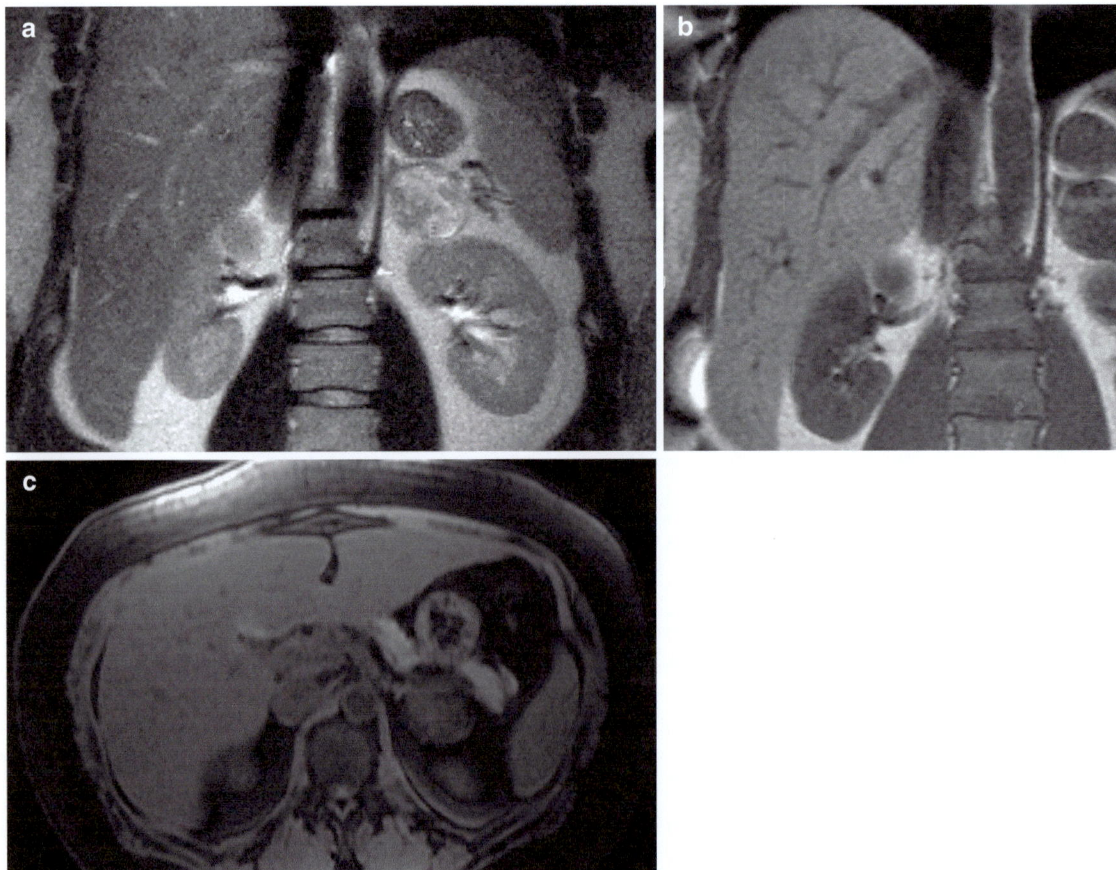

Fig. 5.20 Adrenal myelolipoma, radioimages. (**a**) MRI (T2-weighted image) shows an approximately 4-cm mass in the left adrenal gland with heterogeneous signal intensity, also shown to be mildly hyperintense on T2-weighted images. (**b**) MRI (in-phase image) is shown above, and there is heterogeneous loss of signal intensity on subsequent out-of-phase images. (**c**) MR (axial SHARP) sequence image shows increased peripheral signal intensity

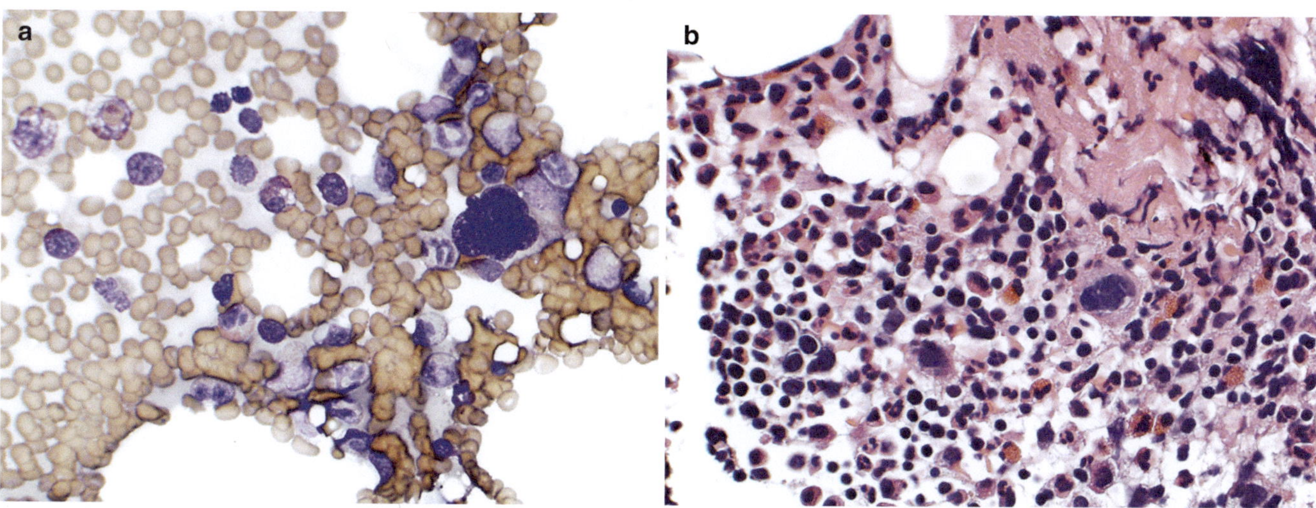

Fig. 5.21 Adrenal myelolipoma, cytology and histology. (**a**) Biopsy cytology of an adrenal lesion, Diff-Quik stain, 600×. (**b**) Histology of core, hematoxylin and eosin stain, 600×

Cytology of FNA and Touch Preparation of Core

- Characteristically bone marrow hematopoietic cells (megakaryocytes, myeloid blasts, premyelocytes, myelocytes, and erythrocytic precursors) and mature adipose tissue in variable proportions are present (Fig. 5.21a) [67].

Histology of Core

- Bone marrow trilineage hematopoiesis and adipose tissue (Fig. 5.21b).

Comments

- Special stains (chloroacetate esterase, myeloid peroxidase) or immunostains (factor VIII) can also confirm the myeloid nature of the immature cells.
- The differential diagnosis includes well-differentiated liposarcoma and hematopoietic tumors.

Adrenal Cortical Adenoma

Adrenal adenomas are the most common benign tumor of the adrenal gland with a prevalence of up to 8.9% [59].

Clinical

- Incidence on autopsy series is 1.5–7% and increases with age [68].
- No sex predilection [69].
- Eighty-five percent of adenomas are nonfunctional [68].

Radiology

The increased vascularity and elevated lipid content of adrenal adenomas results in certain key imaging characteristics on CT and MRI.

CT Scan

- Density evaluation of an adrenal lesion is highly sensitive and specific, since 70% of adrenal adenomas contain intracellular fat.
- On noncontrast imaging, <0 Hounsfield Units has a 100% specificity for adrenal adenoma and <10 Hounsfield Units has 98% specificity for adrenal adenoma. Lipid-poor adenomas are more difficult to diagnose because the CT density increases and approaches that of soft tissue. For lipid-poor lesions, the contrast washout rate can be calculated at CT.
- Adenomas typically have rapid contrast washout, whereas non adenomas tend to wash out more slowly (Fig. 5.22a, b). A 15-minute postcontrast washout image has great sensitivity (Fig. 5.22c). A >60% absolute washout and >40% relative washout are consistent with adrenal adenoma.

MRI

- The protons in fat and water differ and respond differently to sequences, with resultant weakening of signal intensity on out-of-phase sequences.
- Chemical shift imaging is an important parameter when assessing adrenal adenomas. The presence of fat within the lesion does not assure benignity, for many malignant lesions such as clear cell RCC and pheochromocytomas contain significant lipid content [70].
- Adrenal adenomas do not demonstrate restricted diffusion.

Cytomorphology of FNA and Touch Preparation of Core

- Presence of loose aggregates, fascicles, or microacini of polygonal cells (Fig. 5.23) [62, 71]. The specimen is less cellular than adrenal cortical carcinoma, and cells are smaller than carcinoma [62].

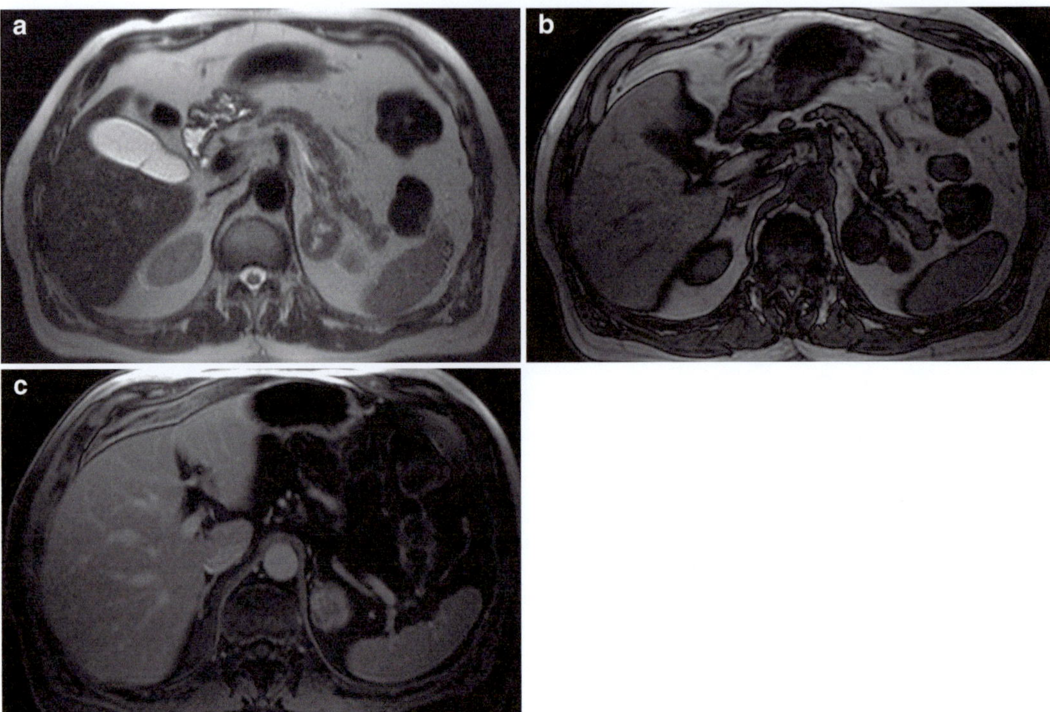

Fig. 5.22 Adrenal cortical adenoma, radioimages. (**a**) CT (T1-weighted image) precontrast images show a heterogeneous focal lesion arising from the left adrenal gland. (**b**) CT scan (out-of-phase image) shows signal dropout in the inferior portion of the lesion; however, the more cranial portion of the lesion demonstrates no significant signal dropout. (**c**) CT (postcontrast) image

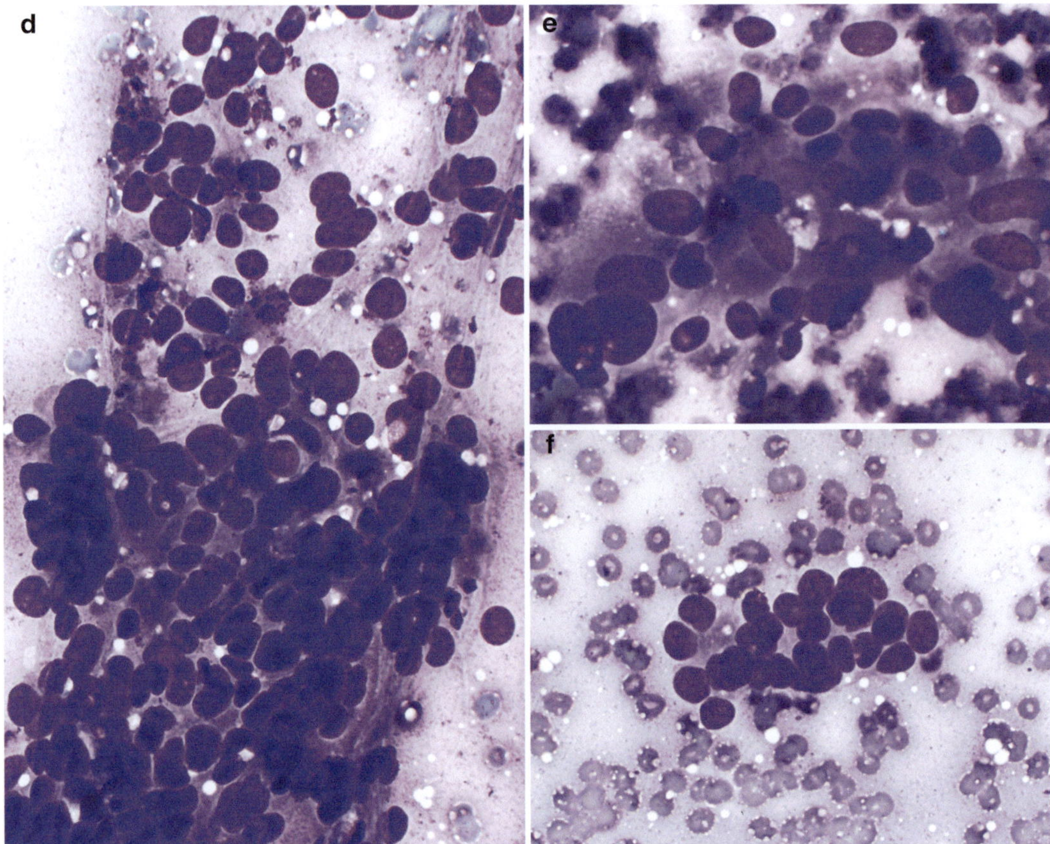

Fig. 5.23 Adrenal cortical adenoma, cytology. FNA biopsy of an adrenal lesion, Diff-Quik stain, 600×

- The nuclei are uniform and round or oval and have granular chromatin and distinct nucleoli [62, 71]. Abundant naked nuclei and intranuclear pseudoinclusions may be present [62, 71]. The cytoplasm is moderate to abundant and clear, delicate, vacuolated, or granular with indistinct cell borders [71]. Marked cytologic atypia may be present.
- A foamy background of lipid droplets is always seen [62].

Comment

1. Differential diagnosis includes non-neoplastic adrenal cortex, nodular hyperplasia, adrenal cortical carcinoma, pheochromocytoma, metastatic RCC, hepatocellular carcinoma, and small blue-cell tumor (when in the presence of aggregates of naked nuclei). It can be very difficult to distinguish cortical adenoma from adrenal cortex tissue and adenocarcinoma by FNA cytology alone. It has been reported that FNA cytology combined with clinical presentation (symptoms and endocrine function) and imaging studies (CT scan, MRI, and norcholesterol scintigraphy) may increase diagnostic accuracy to 100% [56]. However, others have stated that the cytologic features of non-neoplastic adrenal cortical tissue and adenomas are indistinguishable [72].
2. Adrenal cortical adenoma cells are positive for inhibin and melan A while negative for CK7, CK20, and chromogranin.

Primary Adrenal Malignancy

Adrenal Cortical Carcinoma

Clinical

- Frequency is 1–2 cases per 1,00,000/year with a biphasic age distribution [69, 73, 74]; comprise 3% of endocrine neoplasms and 0.02% of all malignant neoplasms [75–77].
- Mean age is 40–50 years [69]. The male-to-female ratio is 1:2.5 [69].
- Eighty percent of adrenal cortical carcinomas are functional (45% glucocorticoid, 45% glucocorticoid and androgen, and 10% androgen alone) [69]. The clinical presentation may vary; some individuals may have symptoms of hyperaldosteronism, virilization, or Cushing syndrome [73, 74, 78].
- Associated syndromes include Li-Fraumeni syndrome, Beckwith-Wiedemann syndrome, and Carney complex.

Radiology

- These masses may have calcification or regions of necrosis and hemorrhage [63].

MRI

- Heterogeneously high T2 signal and possible loss of signal on out-of-phase sequences (Fig. 5.24) [79].

Cytology of FNA and Touch Preparation of Core

- Characteristically, cellular specimen consisting of single and discohesive clusters of bland to highly pleomorphic plasmacytoid or polygonal epithelial cells (Fig. 5.25) [62, 80]. The cells are larger than those of adrenal adenoma [62].
- The nuclei may be eccentrically located and variably enlarged and contain hyperchromatic chromatin and inconspicuous to prominent nucleoli [62, 80]. Nuclear pleomorphism, bizarre-shaped nuclei, binucleation or multinucleation, spindle-shaped nuclei, and occasional naked nuclei can be seen [62, 80]. A variable number of mitoses, including atypical mitotic figures, are frequently seen [62, 80]. The cytoplasm is moderate to abundant and finely granular or vacuolated [80]. With increasing atypia, the cytoplasmic lipid content tends to decrease [62].
- Necrosis is frequently seen [62, 80]. Lipid drops and neutrophils may also be seen [80].

Comment

- The differential diagnosis includes metastatic RCC, adrenal adenoma, pheochromocytoma, neuroendocrine tumor, metastatic melanoma, and metastatic adenocarcinoma.
- ICH stains: At most focally positive for cytokeratins other than CAM5.2. Common reactive for inhibin, melan-A, and calretinin [72].

Pheochromocytoma

Clinical

- Most common tumor in adrenal medulla.
- Generally associated with clinical symptoms caused by overproduction of catecholamines, intermittent paroxysmal hypertension accompanied by sweating, palpitations, headache, diaphoresis, nervousness, nausea, vomiting, weakness, and abdominal or chest pain.

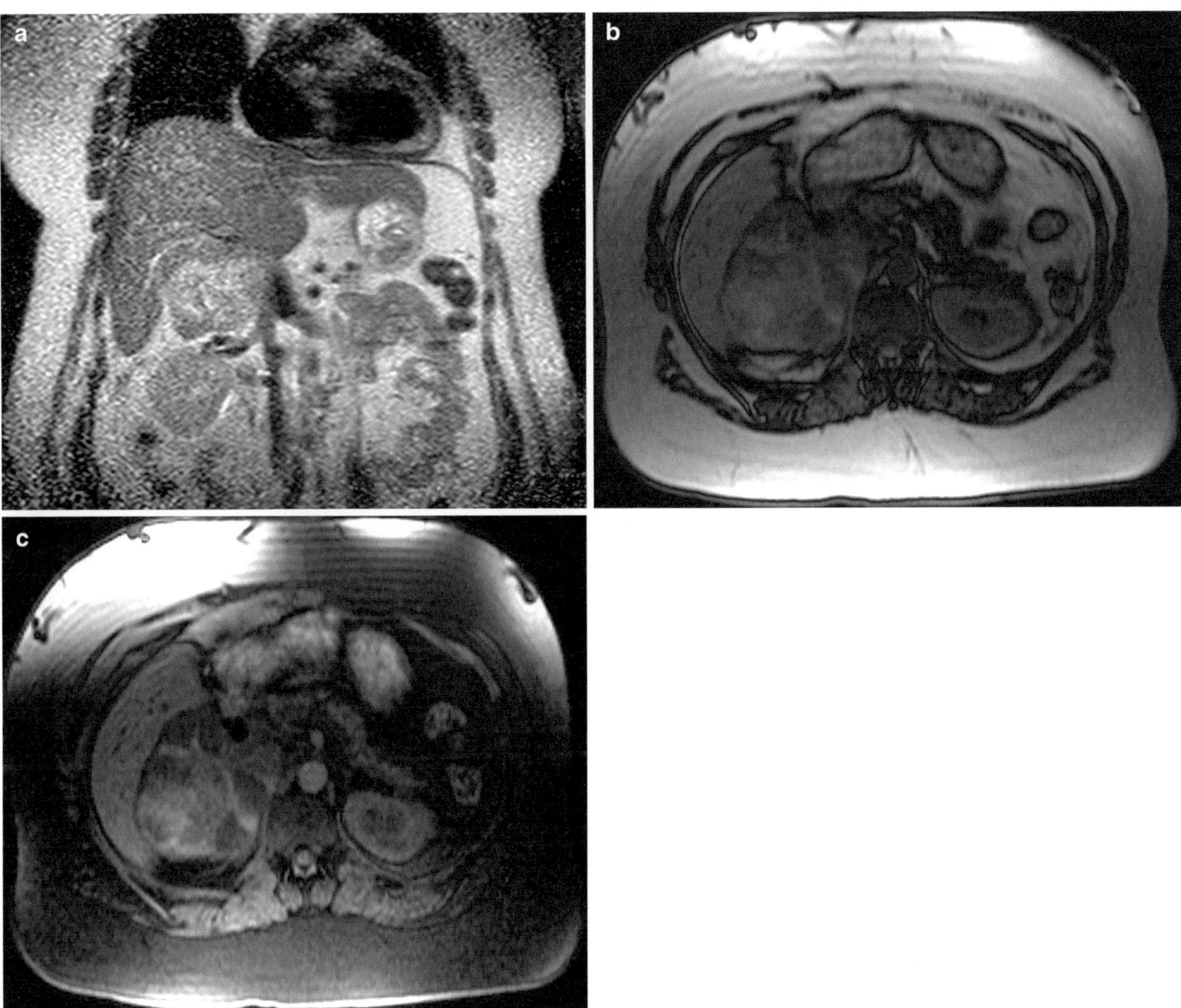

Fig. 5.24 Adrenal carcinoma, radioimage. (**a**) MRI (T1-weighted image) precontrast images show a large heterogeneous mass abutting the liver without evidence of hepatic invasion. The mass is in the expected region of the right adrenal gland. (**b**) MRI (out-of-phase image) shows heterogeneous enhancement with an overall loss of signal intensity. (**c**) MRI (postcontrast image) shows heterogeneous enhancement

Cytology of FNA and Touch Preparation of Core

- FNA findings of pheochromocytoma are similar to those of paraganglioma (*see* paraganglioma below in this chapter). Characteristically, bland to pleomorphic epithelioid or spindle cells; seen singly or in discohesive nests (zellballen) and acinar-microglandular structures or rosettes similar to those seen in paraganglioma (below) (Fig. 5.26) [81].
- The cells have single or multiple eccentrically located (plasmacytoid) round to oval nuclei with prominent nucleoli and granular chromatin [81]. Large intranuclear inclusions, binucleation or multinucleation, and naked nuclei are commonly seen [81]. The cytoplasm is abundant and is delicate, granular, or "squamoid" with ill-defined cell borders [81]. Hyaline globules and rarely melanin pigment may be seen in the cytoplasm [82].
- In cell blocks, characteristic nesting of the tumor cells (zellballen pattern) may be seen.

Comment

- Differential diagnosis: adrenal cortex neoplasm, metastatic adenocarcinoma, melanoma, and neuroendocrine neoplasms.
- Tumor cells are positive for chromogranin, synaptophysin, and NSE and negative for EMA and cytokeratins [72]. Sustentacular cells are positive for S-100.

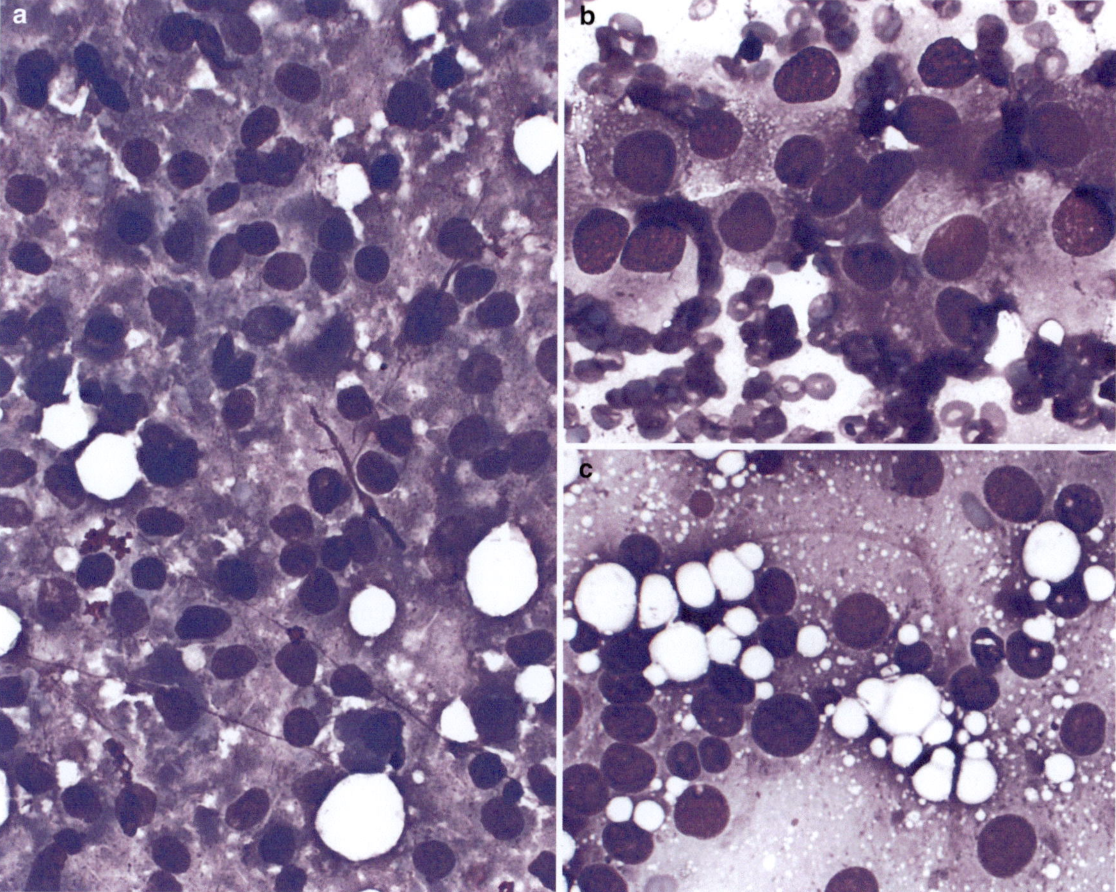

Fig. 5.25 Adrenal cortical carcinoma, cytology. FNA biopsy of a large adrenal mass; Diff-Quik stain, 600×

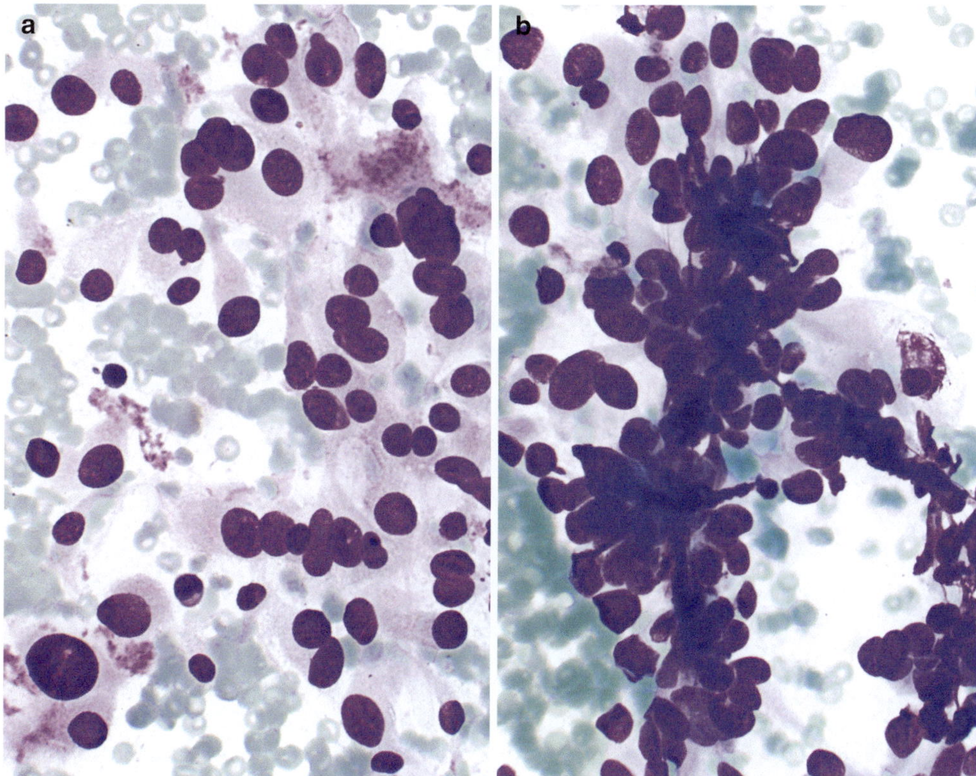

Fig. 5.26 Paraganglioma, cytology. FNA biopsy of a 3-cm retroperitoneal mass; Diff-Quik stain, 600×

- FNA biopsy should be used with caution in cases suspicious for pheochromocytoma owing to possible fatal hypertensive crisis or hemorrhage; therefore biochemical testing for pheochromocytoma should be performed before biopsy of adrenal masses.

Metastatic Malignancy

Clinical

- There is a wide range of stated prevalence of adrenal metastatic disease within adrenal incidentalomas, ranging from 2% to 30% depending on certain risk factors such as a pre-existing cancer diagnosis [63]. Metastatic malignancies are far more common than primary malignancies of the adrenal gland [83]. The adrenal is the fourth most frequent site of spread of tumors after the lungs, liver, and bone [83, 84]. Carcinomas are the most common tumor type to metastasize to the adrenal glands followed by lymphomas and melanoma [85]. Adrenal metastases are found in 27% of patients dying with carcinomas [83, 86].
- The most common primary sites are the breast, lung, kidney, stomach, pancreas, ovary, and colon [83].
- Lymphomatous involvement of the adrenal glands is an uncommon occurrence. Secondary lymphoma of the adrenal is more common than primary lymphoma, which is defined as being found only within the adrenal gland [87].

Radiology

- It is of note that the imaging features of metastatic disease are nonspecific, and that it is essential to take the patient's clinical history into consideration.
- The distribution (bilateral) and size of the lesions (>3 cm) may increase the likelihood of their being metastatic in nature [88].
- Imaging findings in lymphoma can be both discrete and diffuse. On CT evaluation, discrete lymphomatous lesions are mildly enhancing and homogeneous. Diffuse involvement of the adrenal gland may present on imaging as enlargement caused by infiltrative disease [87]. However, these classic findings are not always present, and there is significant variability in CT findings, especially in the setting of primary lymphoma [89].

Cytology of FNA and Touch Preparation of Core

- FNA and CNB are important tools to diagnose adrenal metastases.
- FNA findings vary depending on metastatic malignancies. Morphologic comparison with any known primary malignancy should be performed.

Comment

- IHC stains are very useful in differential diagnosis. Adrenal tumors are positive for melan-A and inhibin and negative for epithelial membrane antigen and keratins.

Paraganglia

Paraganglioma

Clinical

- Uncommon.
- Locations: distribution along the parasympathetic or sympathetic chains or nerves or outside the usual distribution of sympathetic and parasympathetic paraganglia, such as in the bladder, carotid body, central nervous system, gallbladder, and middle ear.
- The "ten rule": 10% are extra-adrenal, 10% are bilateral, 10% are extra-abdominal, 10% are familial (VHL, NF 1, MEN 2A/2B), 10% are pediatric, 10% are not associated with hypertension, and 10% are malignant.
- FNA should be carefully performed because of possible development of a hypertensive episode during the FNA procedure [81].

Cytology of FNA and Touch Preparation of Core

- FNA findings are similar to those of adrenal pheochromocytoma.
- Characteristic presence of single or discohesive groups of cells showing size and shape pleomorphism, forming sheets, acinar-microglandular, zellballen-type, and perivascular patterns (Fig. 5.26) [81, 90, 91].
- The cells may be round, oval, plasmacytoid, or spindled [91]. The cytoplasm is moderate to abundant and vacuolated, finely granular or "squamoid" with ill-defined cell borders [81, 90–93]. Intracytoplasmic metachromatic granules and melanin-like pigment can be seen. The nuclei are round to oval and eccentrically located with "salt and pepper" chromatin and may have prominent nucleoli [81, 90, 93]. Binucleation, multinucleation, intranuclear pseudoinclusions, nuclear grooves, and naked nuclei are commonly seen [81, 90]. Mitotic figures are more frequently seen in malignant cases [91, 92].

Comment

- Tumor cells are positive for chromagranin A, NSE, synaptophysin, and HepPar-1 (11%), while they are negative for EMA and cytokeratins. Sustentacular cells are positive for S-100.

References

1. Garcia-Solano J, Acosta-Ortega J, Perez-Guillermo M, Benedicto-Orovitg JM, Jimenez-Penick FJ. Solid renal masses in adults: image-guided fine-needle aspiration cytology and imaging techniques–"two heads better than one?". Diagn Cytopathol. 2008;36:8–12.
2. Schmidbauer J, Remzi M, Memarsadeghi M, Haitel A, Klingler HC, Katzenbeisser D, et al. Diagnostic accuracy of computed tomography-guided percutaneous biopsy of renal masses. Eur Urol. 2008;53:1003–1.
3. Zardawi IM. Renal fine needle aspiration cytology. Acta Cytol. 1999;43:184–90.
4. Andonian S, Okeke Z, Vanderbrink BA, Okeke DA, Sugrue C, Wasserman PG, et al. Aetiology of non-diagnostic renal fine-needle aspiration cytologies in a contemporary series. BJU Int. 2008;103(1):28–32.
5. Raso DS, Greene WB, Finley JL, Silverman JF. Morphology and pathogenesis of Liesegang rings in cyst aspirates: report of two cases with ancillary studies. Diagn Cytopathol. 1998;19:116–9.
6. Truong LD, Todd TD, Dhurandhar B, Ramzy I. Fine-needle aspiration of renal masses in adults: analysis of results and diagnostic problems in 108 cases. Diagn Cytopathol. 1999;20:339–49.
7. Todd TD, Dhurandhar B, Mody D, Ramzy I, Truong LD. Fine-needle aspiration of cystic lesions of the kidney. Morphologic spectrum and diagnostic problems in 41 cases. Am J Clin Pathol. 1999;111:317–28.
8. Sahni VA, Ly A, Silverman SG. Usefulness of percutaneous biopsy in diagnosing benign renal masses that mimic malignancy. Abdom Imaging. 2011;36:91–101.
9. Katabathina VS, Vikram R, Nagar AM, Tamboli P, Menias CO, Prasad SR. Mesenchymal neoplasms of the kidney in adults: imaging spectrum with radiologic-pathologic correlation. Radiographics. 2010;30:1525–40.
10. Jinzaki M, Silverman SG, Akita H, Nagashima Y, Mikami S, Oya M. Renal angiomyolipoma: a radiological classification and update on recent developments in diagnosis and management. Abdom Imaging. 2014;39:588–604.
11. Kennelly MJ, Grossman HB, Cho KJ. Outcome analysis of 42 cases of renal angiomyolipoma. J Urol. 1994;152(6 Pt 1):1988–91.
12. Steiner MS, Goldman SM, Fishman EK, Marshall FF. The natural history of renal angiomyolipoma. J Urol. 1993;150:1782–6.
13. Tong YC, Chieng PU, Tsai TC, Lin SN. Renal angiomyolipoma: report of 24 cases. Br J Urol. 1990;66:585–9.
14. Hindman N, Ngo L, Genega EM, Melamed J, Wei J, Braza JM, et al. Angiomyolipoma with minimal fat: can it be differentiated from clear cell renal cell carcinoma by using standard MR techniques? Radiology. 2012;265:468–77.
15. Crapanzano JP. Fine-needle aspiration of renal angiomyolipoma: cytological findings and diagnostic pitfalls in a series of five cases. Diagn Cytopathol. 2005;32:53–7.
16. Masoom S, Venkataraman G, Jensen J, Flanigan RC, Wojcik EM. Renal FNA-based typing of renal masses remains a useful adjunctive modality: evaluation of 31 renal masses with correlative histology. Cytopathology. 2009;20:50–5.
17. Cristallini EG, Paganelli C, Bolis GB. Role of fine-needle aspiration biopsy in the assessment of renal masses. Diagn Cytopathol. 1991;7:32–5.
18. Lieber MM. Renal oncocytoma. Urol Clin North Am. 1993;20:355–9.
19. Perez-Ordonez B, Hamed G, Campbell S, Erlandson RA, Russo P, Gaudin PB, et al. Renal oncocytoma: a clinicopathologic study of 70 cases. Am J Surg Pathol. 1997;21:871–83.
20. Hes O, Moch H, Reuter VE. Oncocytoma. In: Moch H, Humphrey PA, Ulbright TM, Reuter VE, editors. WHO classification of tumours of the urinary system and male genital organs. Lyon: International Agency for Research on Cancer; 2016. p. 43–4.
21. Wu J, Zhu Q, Zhu W, Chen W, Wang S. Comparative study of CT appearances in renal oncocytoma and chromophobe renal cell carcinoma. Acta Radiol. 2016;57:500–6.
22. Liu J, Fanning CV. Can renal oncocytomas be distinguished from renal cell carcinoma on fine-needle aspiration specimens? A study of conventional smears in conjunction with ancillary studies. Cancer. 2001;93:390–7.
23. Bishop JA, Hosler GA, Kulesza P, Erozan YS, Ali SZ. Fine-needle aspiration of renal cell carcinoma: is accurate Fuhrman grading possible on cytologic material? Diagn Cytopathol. 2011;39:168–71.
24. Zhu B, Rohan SM, Lin X. Immunoexpression of napsin A in renal neoplasms. Diagn Pathol. 2015;10:4.
25. Zhou M, Roma A, Magi-Galluzzi C. The usefulness of immunohistochemical markers in the differential diagnosis of renal neoplasms. Clin Lab Med. 2005;25:247–57.
26. Lin X. Cytomorphology of clear cell papillary renal cell carcinoma. Cancer Cytopathol. 2017;125:48–54.
27. Moch H, Humphrey PA, Ulbright TM, Reuter VE. WHO classification of tumours of the urinary system and male genital organs. Lyon: International Agency for Research on Cancer; 2016.
28. Lopez-Beltran A, Carrasco JC, Cheng L, Scarpelli M, Kirkali Z, Montironi R. 2009 update on the classification of renal epithelial tumors in adults. Int J Urol. 2009;16:432–43.
29. Hoffmann NE, Gillett MD, Cheville JC, Lohse CM, Leibovich BC, Blute ML. Differences in organ system of distant metastasis by renal cell carcinoma subtype. J Urol. 2008;179:474–7.
30. Low G, Huang G, Fu W, Moloo Z, Girgis S. Review of renal cell carcinoma and its common subtypes in radiology. World J Radiol. 2016;8:484–500.
31. Cheville JC, Lohse CM, Zincke H, Weaver AL, Blute ML. Comparisons of outcome and prognostic features among histologic subtypes of renal cell carcinoma. Am J Surg Pathol. 2003;27:612–24.
32. Gurel S, Narra V, Elsayes KM, Siegel CL, Chen ZE, Brown JJ. Subtypes of renal cell carcinoma: MRI and pathological features. Diagn Interv Radiol. 2013;19:304–11.
33. Moch H, Amin MB, Argani P, Cheville J, Delahunt B, Martignoni G, Medeiros LJ, Srigley JR, Tan PH, Tickoo SK. Renal cell tumours. In: Moch H, Humphrey PA, Ulbright TM, Reuter VE, editors. WHO classification of tumours of the urinary system and male genital organs. Lyon: International Agency for Research on Cancer; 2016. p. 12–7.
34. Parkin D, Whelan S, Ferlay J, Teppo L, Thomas D. Cancer incidence in five continents. Lyon: IARC Scientific Publications No 155. IARC Press; 2003.
35. Sufrin G, Chasan S, Golio A, Murphy GP. Paraneoplastic and serologic syndromes of renal adenocarcinoma. Semin Urol. 1989;7:158–71.
36. Prasad SR, Humphrey PA, Catena JR, Narra VR, Srigley JR, Cortez AD, et al. Common and uncommon histologic subtypes of renal cell carcinoma: imaging spectrum with pathologic correlation. Radiographics. 2006;26:1795–806; discussion, 806–10.
37. Renshaw AA, Granter SR. Fine needle aspiration of chromophobe renal cell carcinoma. Acta Cytol. 1996;40:867–72.
38. Layfield LJ. Fine-needle aspiration biopsy of renal collecting duct carcinoma. Diagn Cytopathol. 1994;11:74–8.
39. Lin X. Cytomorphology of clear cell papillary renal cell carcinoma. Cancer. 2017;125:48–54.
40. Al-Ahmadie HA, Alden D, Fine SW, Gopalan A, Touijer KA, Russo P, et al. Role of immunohistochemistry in the evaluation of needle core biopsies in adult renal cortical tumors: an ex vivo study. Am J Surg Pathol. 2011;35:949–61.
41. Adeniran AJ, Al-Ahmadie H, Iyengar P, Reuter VE, Lin O. Fine needle aspiration of renal cortical lesions in adults. Diagn Cytopathol. 2010;38:710–5.

42. Grignon DJ, Al-Ahmadie H, Algaba F, Amin MD, Comperat E, Dyrskjot L, Epstein JI, Hansel DE, Knuchel R, Lloreta J, Lopez-Beltran A, McKenney JK, Netto GJ, Paner G, Reuter VE, Shen SS, Van der Kwast T. Urothelial tumours. In: Moch H, Humphrey PA, Ulbright TM, Reuter VE, editors. WHO classification of tumours of the urinary system and male genital organs. Lyon: International Agency for Research on Cancer; 2016. p. 77–98.
43. Raza SA, Sohaib SA, Sahdev A, Bharwani N, Heenan S, Verma H, et al. Centrally infiltrating renal masses on CT: differentiating intrarenal transitional cell carcinoma from centrally located renal cell carcinoma. Am J Roentgenol. 2012;198:846–53.
44. Zhu B, Rohan SM, Lin X. Urine cytomorphology of micropapillary urothelial carcinoma. Diagn Cytopathol. 2013;41:485–91.
45. Lin X, Zhu B, Villa C, Zhong M, Kundu S, Rohan SM, et al. The utility of p63, p40, and GATA-binding protein 3 immunohistochemistry in diagnosing micropapillary urothelial carcinoma. Hum Pathol. 2014;45:1824–9.
46. Argani P, Bruder E, Dehner L, Vujanic GM. Nephroblastic and cystic tumours occurring mainly in children. In: Moch H, Humphrey PA, Ulbright TM, Reuter VE, editors. WHO classification of tumours of the urinary system and male genital organs. Lyon: IARC Press; 2004. p. 48–53.
47. Ravindra S, Kini U. Cytomorphology and morphometry of small round-cell tumors in the region of the kidney. Diagn Cytopathol. 2005;32:211–6.
48. Dey P, Radhika S, Rajwanshi A, Rao KL, Khajuria A, Nijhawan R, et al. Aspiration cytology of Wilms' tumor. Acta Cytol. 1993;37:477–82.
49. Khayyata S, Grignon DJ, Aulicino MR, Al-Abbadi MA. Metanephric adenoma vs. Wilms' tumor: a report of 2 cases with diagnosis by fine needle aspiration and cytologic comparisons. Acta Cytol. 2007;51:464–7.
50. Quijano G, Drut R. Cytologic characteristics of Wilms' tumors in fine needle aspirates. A study of ten cases. Acta Cytol. 1989;33:263–6.
51. Nayak A, Iyer VK, Agarwala S. The cytomorphologic spectrum of Wilms tumour on fine needle aspiration: a single institutional experience of 110 cases. Cytopathology. 2011;22:50–9.
52. Aras M, Dede F, Ones T, Inanir S, Erdil TY, Turoglu HT. Is the value of FDG PET/CT in evaluating renal metastasis underestimated? A case report and review of the literature. Mol Imaging Radionuc Ther. 2013;22:109–12.
53. Shimko MS, Jacobs SC, Phelan MW. Renal metastasis of malignant melanoma with unknown primary. Urology. 2007;69:384.e9–10.
54. Israel GM, Bosniak MA. Pitfalls in renal mass evaluation and how to avoid them. Radiographics. 2008;28:1325–38.
55. Quayle FJ, Spitler JA, Pierce RA, Lairmore TC, Moley JF, Brunt LM. Needle biopsy of incidentally discovered adrenal masses is rarely informative and potentially hazardous. Surgery. 2007;142:497–502; discussion, 502–4.
56. Lumachi F, Borsato S, Tregnaghi A, Marino F, Fassina A, Zucchetta P, et al. High risk of malignancy in patients with incidentally discovered adrenal masses: accuracy of adrenal imaging and image-guided fine-needle aspiration cytology. Tumori. 2007;93:269–74.
57. Nurnberg D. Ultrasound of adrenal gland tumours and indications for fine needle biopsy (uFNB). Ultraschall Med. 2005;26:458–69.
58. Bovio S, Cataldi A, Reimondo G, Sperone P, Novello S, Berruti A, et al. Prevalence of adrenal incidentaloma in a contemporary computerized tomography series. J Endocrinol Investig. 2006;29:298–302.
59. Herrera MF, Grant CS, van Heerden JA, Sheedy PF, Ilstrup DM. Incidentally discovered adrenal tumors: an institutional perspective. Surgery. 1991;110:1014–21.
60. Tikkakoski T, Taavitsainen M, Paivansalo M, Lahde S, Apaja-Sarkkinen M. Accuracy of adrenal biopsy guided by ultrasound and CT. Acta Radiol. 1991;32:371–4.
61. Lumachi F, Borsato S, Tregnaghi A, Basso SM, Marchesi P, Ciarleglio F, et al. CT-scan, MRI and image-guided FNA cytology of incidental adrenal masses. Eur J Surg Oncol. 2003;29:689–92.
62. Fassina AS, Borsato S, Fedeli U. Fine needle aspiration cytology (FNAC) of adrenal masses. Cytopathology. 2000;11:302–11.
63. Lattin GE, Sturgill ED, Tujo CA, Marko J, Sanchez-Maldonado KW, Craig WD, et al. From the radiologic pathology archives: adrenal tumors and tumor-like conditions in the adult: radiologic-pathologic correlation. Radiographics. 2014;34:805–29.
64. Olsson CA, Krane RJ, Klugo RC, Selikowitz SM. Adrenal myelolipoma. Surgery. 1973;73:665–70.
65. Kenney PJ, Wagner BJ, Rao P, Heffess CS. Myelolipoma: CT and pathologic features. Radiology. 1998;208:87–95.
66. Lam KY, Lo CY. Adrenal lipomatous tumours: a 30 year clinicopathological experience at a single institution. J Clin Pathol. 2001;54:707–12.
67. Settakorn J, Sirivanichai C, Rangdaeng S, Chaiwun B. Fine-needle aspiration cytology of adrenal myelolipoma: case report and review of the literature. Diagn Cytopathol. 1999;21:409–12.
68. Stewart PM. The adrenal cortex. In: Larsen PR, Kronenberg HM, Melmed S, Polonsky KS, editors. Williams textbook of endocrinology. 10th ed. Philadelphia: WB Saunders; 2002. p. 491–551.
69. Lloyd RV, Osamura RY, Kloppel G, Rosai J. Tumours of the adrenal cortex. In: Lloyd RV, Osamura RY, Kloppel G, Rosai J, editors. WHO classification of Tumours of endocrine organs. Lyon: International Agency for Research on Cancers; 2016. p. 161–78.
70. Elsayes KM, Mukundan G, Narra VR, Lewis JS, Shirkhoda A, Farooki A, et al. Adrenal masses: MR imaging features with pathologic correlation. Radiographics. 2004;24(Suppl 1):S73–86.
71. Stelow EB, Debol SM, Stanley MW, Mallery S, Lai R, Bardales RH. Sampling of the adrenal glands by endoscopic ultrasound-guided fine-needle aspiration. Diagn Cytopathol. 2005;33:26–30.
72. Jorda M, De MB, Nadji M. Calretinin and inhibin are useful in separating adrenocortical neoplasms from pheochromocytomas. Appl Immunohistochem Mol Morphol. 2002;10:67–70.
73. Allolio B, Fassnacht M. Clinical review: Adrenocortical carcinoma: clinical update. J Clin Endocrinol Metab. 2006;91:2027–37.
74. Wooten MD, King DK. Adrenal cortical carcinoma. Epidemiology and treatment with mitotane and a review of the literature. Cancer. 1993;72:3145–55.
75. Schteingart DE, Doherty GM, Gauger PG, Giordano TJ, Hammer GD, Korobkin M, et al. Management of patients with adrenal cancer: recommendations of an international consensus conference. Endocr Relat Cancer. 2005;12:667–80.
76. Roman S. Adrenocortical carcinoma. Curr Opin Oncol. 2006;18:36–42.
77. Ng L, Libertino JM. Adrenocortical carcinoma: diagnosis, evaluation and treatment. J Urol. 2003;169:5–11.
78. Venkatesh S, Hickey RC, Sellin RV, Fernandez JF, Samaan NA. Adrenal cortical carcinoma. Cancer. 1989;64:765–9.
79. Bharwani N, Rockall AG, Sahdev A, Gueorguiev M, Drake W, Grossman AB, et al. Adrenocortical carcinoma: the range of appearances on CT and MRI. Am J Roentgenol. 2011;196:W706–14.
80. Ren R, Guo M, Sneige N, Moran CA, Gong Y. Fine-needle aspiration of adrenal cortical carcinoma: cytologic spectrum and diagnostic challenges. Am J Clin Pathol. 2006;126:389–98.
81. Jimenez-Heffernan JA, Vicandi B, Lopez-Ferrer P, Gonzalez-Peramato P, Perez-Campos A, Viguer JM. Cytologic features of pheochromocytoma and retroperitoneal paraganglioma: a morphologic and immunohistochemical study of 13 cases. Acta Cytol. 2006;50:372–8.
82. Handa U, Khullar U, Mohan H. Pigmented pheochromocytoma: report of a case with diagnosis by fine needle aspiration. Acta Cytol. 2005;49:421–3.

83. Lloyd RV, Kawashima A, Tischler AS. Secondary tumors. In: DeLellis RA, Lloyd RV, Heitz PU, Eng C, editors. Pathology and genetics: tumors of endocrine organs. Lyon: IARC Press; 2004. p. 172–3.
84. Willis RV. The spread of tumors in the human body. 3rd ed. London: Butterworth; 1973.
85. Mayo-Smith WW, Boland GW, Noto RB, Lee MJ. State-of-the-art adrenal imaging. Radiographics. 2001;21:995–1012.
86. Abrams HL, Spiro R, Goldstein N. Metastases in carcinoma; analysis of 1000 autopsied cases. Cancer. 1950;3:74–85.
87. Leite NP, Kased N, Hanna RF, Brown MA, Pereira JM, Cunha R, et al. Cross-sectional imaging of extranodal involvement in abdominopelvic lymphoproliferative malignancies. Radiographics. 2007;27:1613–34.
88. Chong S, Lee KS, Kim HY, Kim YK, Kim BT, Chung MJ, et al. Integrated PET-CT for the characterization of adrenal gland lesions in cancer patients: diagnostic efficacy and interpretation pitfalls. Radiographics. 2006;26:1811–24; discussion, 24–6.
89. Rashidi A, Fisher SI. Primary adrenal lymphoma: a systematic review. Ann Hematol. 2013;92:1583–93.
90. Gong Y, DeFrias DV, Nayar R. Pitfalls in fine needle aspiration cytology of extraadrenal paraganglioma. A report of 2 cases. Acta Cytol. 2003;47:1082–6.
91. Varma K, Jain S, Mandal S. Cytomorphologic spectrum in paraganglioma. Acta Cytol. 2008;52:549–56.
92. Absher KJ, Witte DA, Truong LD, Ramzy I, Mody DR, Ostrowski ML. Aspiration biopsy of osseous metastasis of retroperitoneal paraganglioma. Report of a case with cytologic features and differential diagnostic considerations. Acta Cytol. 2001;45: 249–53.
93. Rana RS, Dey P, Das A. Fine needle aspiration (FNA) cytology of extra-adrenal paragangliomas. Cytopathology. 1997;8:108–13.

6 Pelvis, Peritoneum, and Omentum

Elizabeth Morency, Steven D. Huffman, and Ahsun Riaz

A variety of conditions can occur within the pelvis and the peritoneal cavity and involve omental tissue. This chapter mainly focuses on gynecologic conditions that arise in the pelvis, primarily benign and malignant ovarian or fallopian tube diseases that may then secondarily involve the peritoneal space and/or omental tissue. Benign conditions that fall under this category include endometriosis and endosalpingiosis, benign entities arising from deposits of displaced endometrial tissue, and tubal epithelium. Ovarian cysts include a spectrum of benign, unilocular simple cysts to more complex, radiologically indeterminate or pathologically borderline cysts (including serous, mucinous, and seromucinous types) to frankly malignant carcinomas. Both borderline and malignant tumors can secondarily involve the peritoneal cavity or omental tissue and represent one of the most common forms of radiologically apparent peritoneal disease. Primary peritoneal entities are rare but include primary malignant mesothelioma of the peritoneum and primary peritoneal carcinoma, both of which will be discussed. Primary peritoneal carcinoma is an interesting disease in which the presence of ovarian or tubal disease must be clinically excluded. However, there is some controversy as to its true origin. Many studies have supported the theory of the development of the disease from displaced or ectopic deposits of tubal epithelium, thus linking it to fallopian tube origin. Gynecologic malignancies are not the only entities that commonly metastasize to the peritoneal space, which is a large body cavity housing many organ systems. Other common sites of primary disease include the gastrointestinal tract, the pancreatico-biliary tract, and the genitourinary tract, among others [1–3].

Normal Findings

Benign Mesothelial Cells

- Can be seen in small clusters, in pairs, or dispersed singly.
- Dense cytoplasm seen centrally (endocytoplasm) and peripheral pale-staining (ectocytoplasm) giving a "lacy skirt" appearance.
- Paired cells with intercellular clear spaces or "windows" can be seen.
- Round nuclei with single nucleolus, occasional binucleation.

Histiocytes

- Round to ovoid nucleus, with indentation or "kidney bean" shape.
- Granular to vacuolated cytoplasm, more delicate than that of mesothelial cells.
- Can be seen clustered together but usually are scattered singly.

Inflammatory Cells

- Background lymphocytes, neutrophils, and eosinophils can be seen.
- However, usually few inflammatory cells are present unless an underlying neoplastic, infectious, or inflammatory process has occurred or the patient has received repeated diagnostic or therapeutic paracentesis causing an iatrogenic increase in inflammatory cells, particularly eosinophils.

E. Morency (✉)
Department of Pathology, Northwestern Memorial Hospital, Feinberg School of Medicine, Chicago, IL, USA
e-mail: Elizabeth.morency@northwestern.edu

S. D. Huffman
Aurora St. Luke's Medical Center of Aurora Health Care Metro, Inc., Milwaukee, WI, USA

A. Riaz
Department of Pathology, Northwestern Medicine, Chicago, IL, USA

R. Nayar et al. (eds.), *Atlas of Cytopathology and Radiology*, https://doi.org/10.1007/978-3-030-24756-0_6

Benign Conditions

Endometriosis

Clinical

- Caused by abnormal growth of endometrial tissue outside of the uterus, commonly in the area of the pelvis (surface of the pelvic organs or involving the pelvic side walls); however, it can involve extrapelvic sites [1].
- May be asymptomatic but signs and symptoms can include pelvic pain (which may worsen during menstruation), painful intercourse, painful bowel movements, or painful urination and infertility.
- A classic scenario is a subcutaneous, painful focus in/around a post-Cesarean section scar site.

Radiology

Ultrasound (US)

- On US, endometriomas are predominantly seen as complex cystic adnexal masses. They may be single or multiple and have a thin or thick wall. They demonstrate diffuse low-level internal echoes. Hyperechoic foci in the wall of an internally echogenic cyst are characteristic [4] and represent cholesterol crystals resulting from cell breakdown in chronic hemorrhage (Fig. 6.1).

Computed Tomography (CT)

- On CT, endometriomas are typically seen as a complex cystic pelvic mass. They often contain high-density fluid components. A common associated finding is hydrosalpinx (30%) [4].

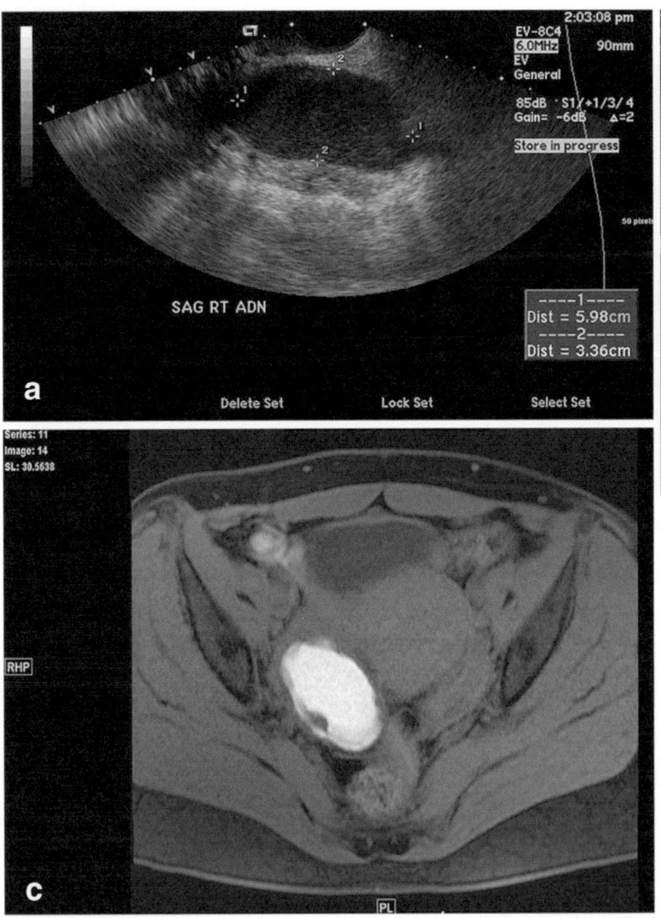

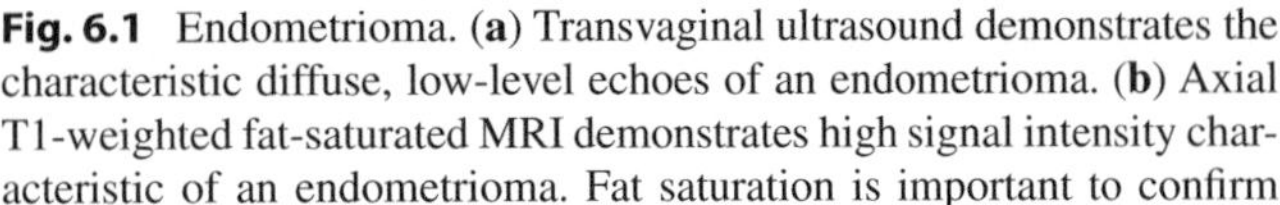
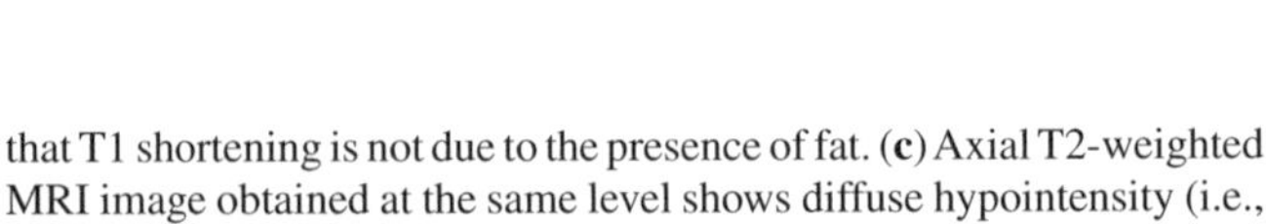

Fig. 6.1 Endometrioma. (**a**) Transvaginal ultrasound demonstrates the characteristic diffuse, low-level echoes of an endometrioma. (**b**) Axial T1-weighted fat-saturated MRI demonstrates high signal intensity characteristic of an endometrioma. Fat saturation is important to confirm that T1 shortening is not due to the presence of fat. (**c**) Axial T2-weighted MRI image obtained at the same level shows diffuse hypointensity (i.e., T2 shading) of the endometrioma

Magnetic Resonance Imaging (MRI)

- On MRI, endometriomas most often demonstrate homogeneous high intensity on T1-weighted images and low signal on T2-weighted images (T2 shading). The loss of signal on T2 is caused by the presence of methemoglobin within the cysts. The cyst wall is typically low in signal on T1 and T2, which is related either to fibrous tissue or hemosiderin. Fat-saturated T1-weighted images can improve the visualization of small implants on peritoneal surfaces (Fig. 6.1) [5].

Fine Needle Aspiration (FNA)

- Sheets and clusters of cuboidal endometrial glandular cells (Fig. 6.2).
- Clusters of spindled endometrial stromal cells.
- Hemosiderin-laden macrophages.

Core Biopsy

- Simple endometrial glands composed of bland cuboidal cells within endometrial type stroma made up of bland spindle cells within a loose matrix (Fig. 6.2c).

Endosalpingiosis

Clinical

- Usually an incidental finding, found at the time of surgery for other indications.
- Similar to endometriosis; also usually involves the pelvic region (ovarian surface, uterine serosa, peritoneal surface, and omentum), but in rare instances it can be found elsewhere.

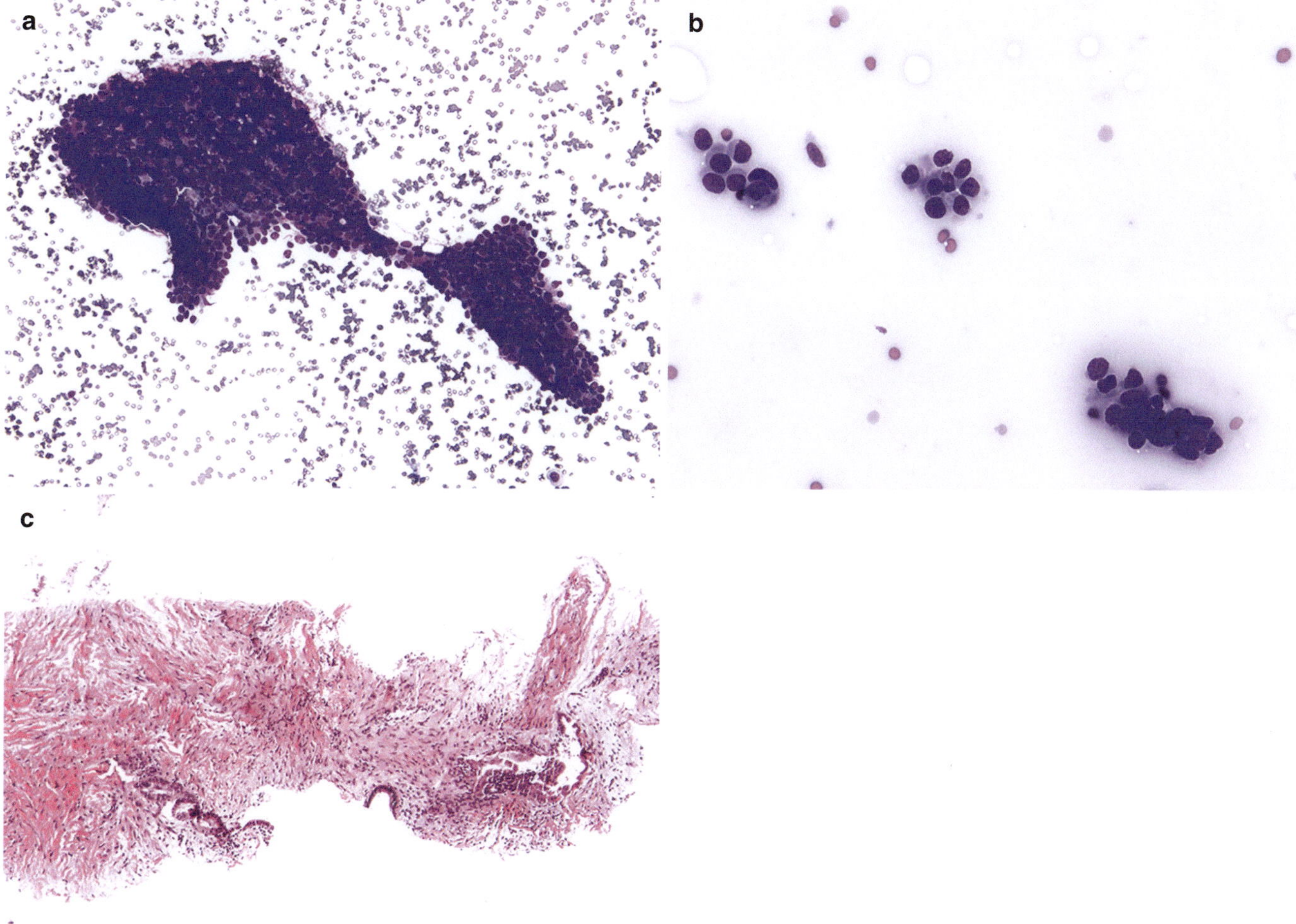

Fig. 6.2 Endometriosis. (**a**) Clusters of benign cuboidal endometrial cells as seen in this example of endometriosis involving the peritoneum in a 27-year-old patient with a history of vague abdominal pain (DiffQuik stain, 200×). (**b**) Occasionally atypia can be seen in the glandular cells, as seen in this case, and care must be taken not to misinterpret this as malignancy (DiffQuik stain, 400×). (**c**) This histological section from a core biopsy of an abdominal nodule in a 34-year-old woman shows simple endometrial glands composed of bland cuboidal cells and the subepithelial loose endometrial type stroma involving fibrous tissue (hematoxylin and eosin [H&E] stain, 100×)

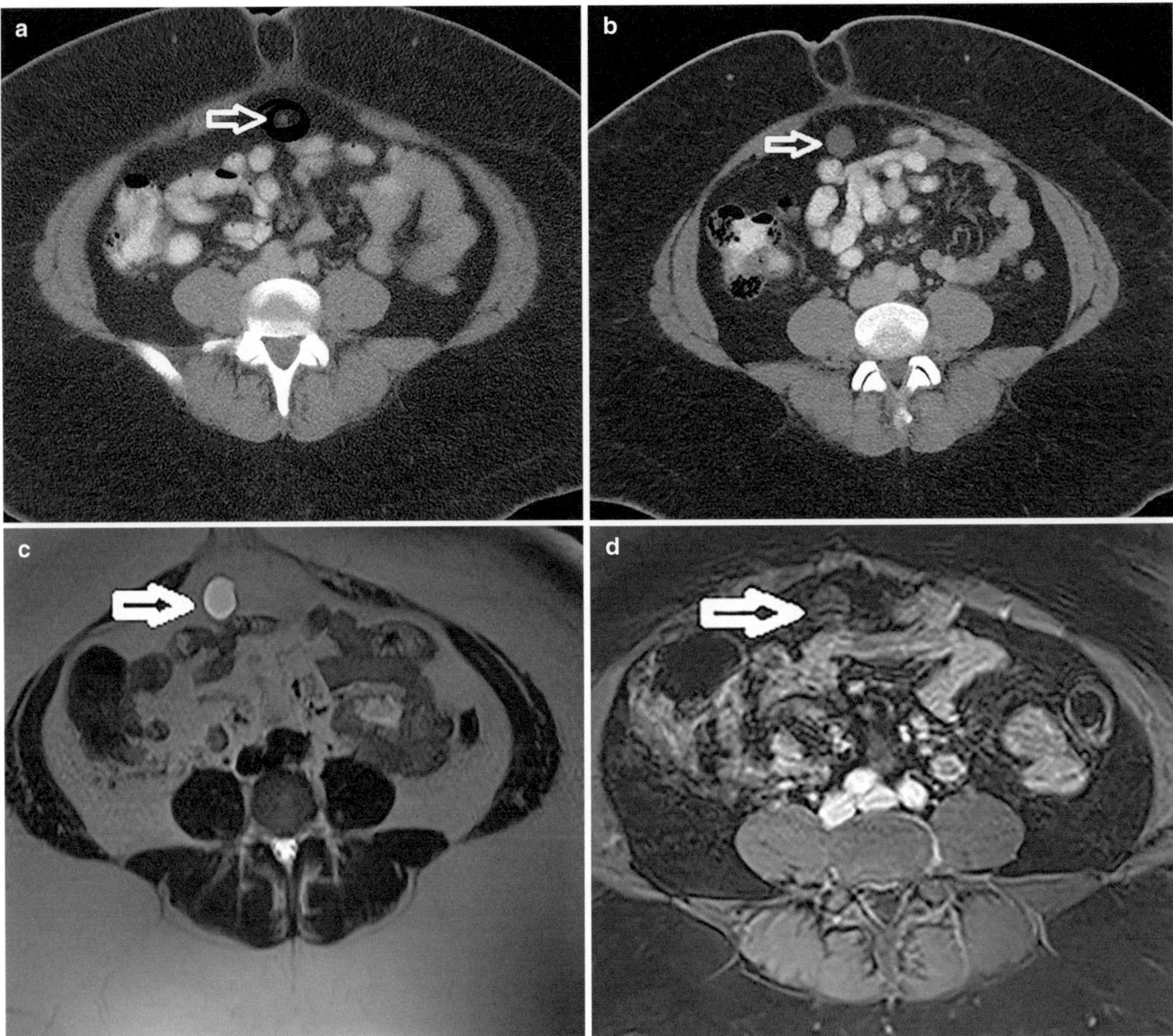

Fig. 6.3 Endosalpingiosis (*white arrow*). (**a**) CT demonstrating a very small fluid attenuating structure at baseline. (**b**) CT 2 years later demonstrates a larger rounded structure deep to the umbilicus. (**c**) T2-weighted MRI demonstrates a T2 hyperintense rounded structure. (**d**) Post-contrast T1-weighted MRI demonstrating T1 hypointense structure with minimal rim enhancement

Radiology

Ultrasound

- Cystic endosalpingiosis presents as cystic masses and is difficult to differentiate from other masses. These may be distant from the uterus (Fig. 6.3) or in proximity to the uterus in the pelvis (Fig. 6.6). Like other cystic masses, these are anechoic and may have internal septations.

Computed Tomography

- CT demonstrates masses in the abdomen and/or pelvis (Fig. 6.4), which are cystic. They may grow in size with time.

Magnetic Resonance Imaging

- The MRI findings are similar to those from CT. T1-weighted fat-suppressed postcontrast images are particularly helpful to evaluate for peripheral enhancement and no central enhancement. These are T2 hyperintense. They may have internal septations [6].

Image-Guided Biopsy

Since this method shows no definite differentiating features from other cystic peritoneal/pelvic masses, US or CT-guided biopsy might be necessary.

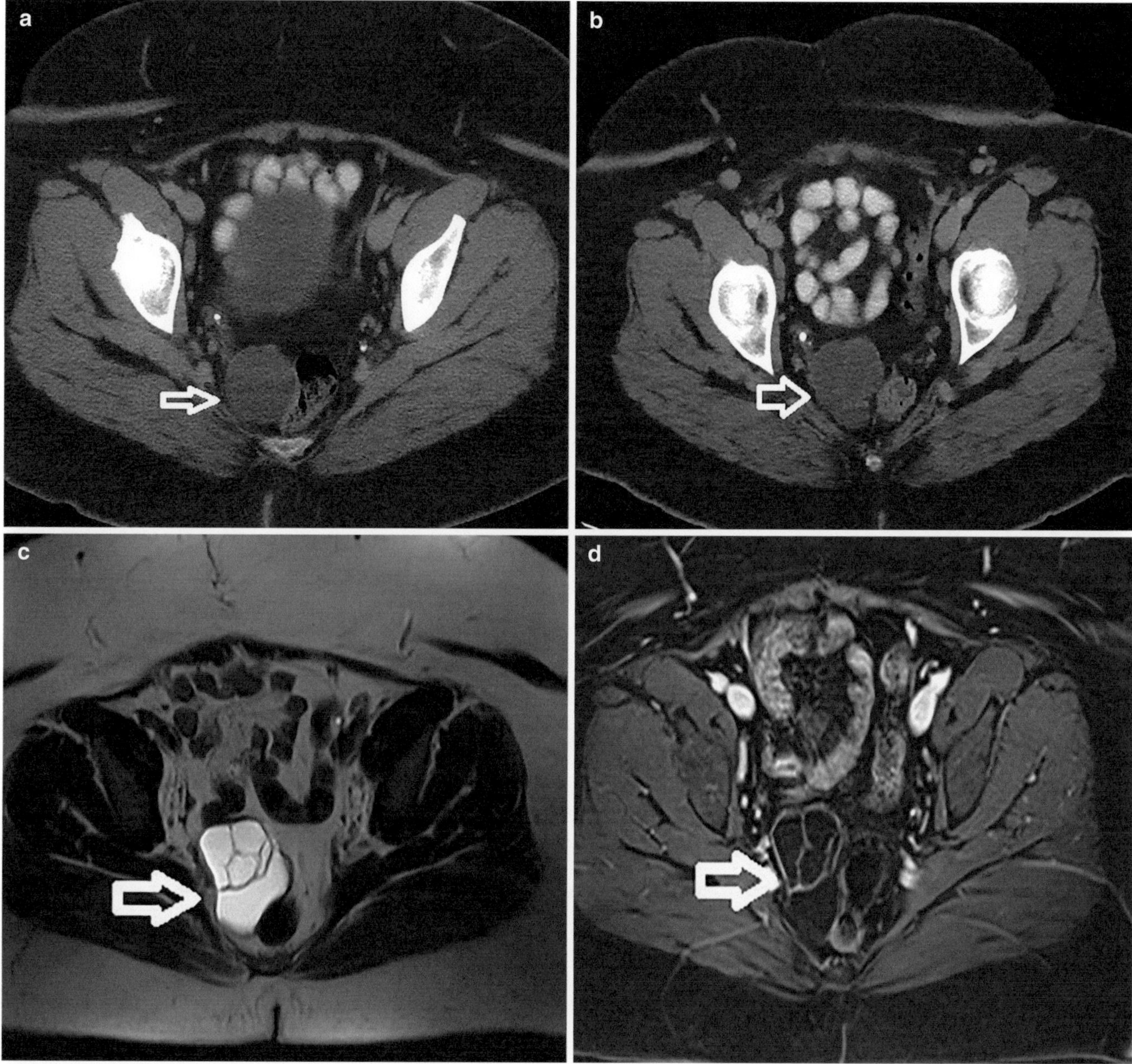

Fig. 6.4 Endosalpingiosis (*white arrow*). (**a**) CT demonstrating a small fluid attenuating structure at baseline. (**b**) CT 2 years later demonstrates a larger multilobulated structure deep in the posterior right pelvis. (**c**) T2-weighted MRI demonstrates a T2 hyperintense complex cystic structure. (**d**) Post-contrast T1-weighted MRI demonstrating T1 hypointense structure with minimal rim and internal septal enhancement

Fine Needle Aspiration

- Cuboidal, frequently ciliated, fallopian tube-like epithelial cells (Fig. 6.5).
- Psammoma bodies may be seen (Fig. 6.5) [7].

Benign Ovarian Cysts

Clinical

- Can be asymptomatic and found incidentally (e.g., during infertility work-up, pregnancy).
- Larger cysts may present with nonspecific symptoms such as dull or sharp pelvic pain, abdominal fullness, or heaviness and bloating.

Radiology

Ultrasound

- On US, cysts are thin-walled well-circumscribed lesions that are anechoic with posterior acoustic enhancement.

Computed Tomography

- On CT, cysts do not demonstrate enhancement and are water attenuated.

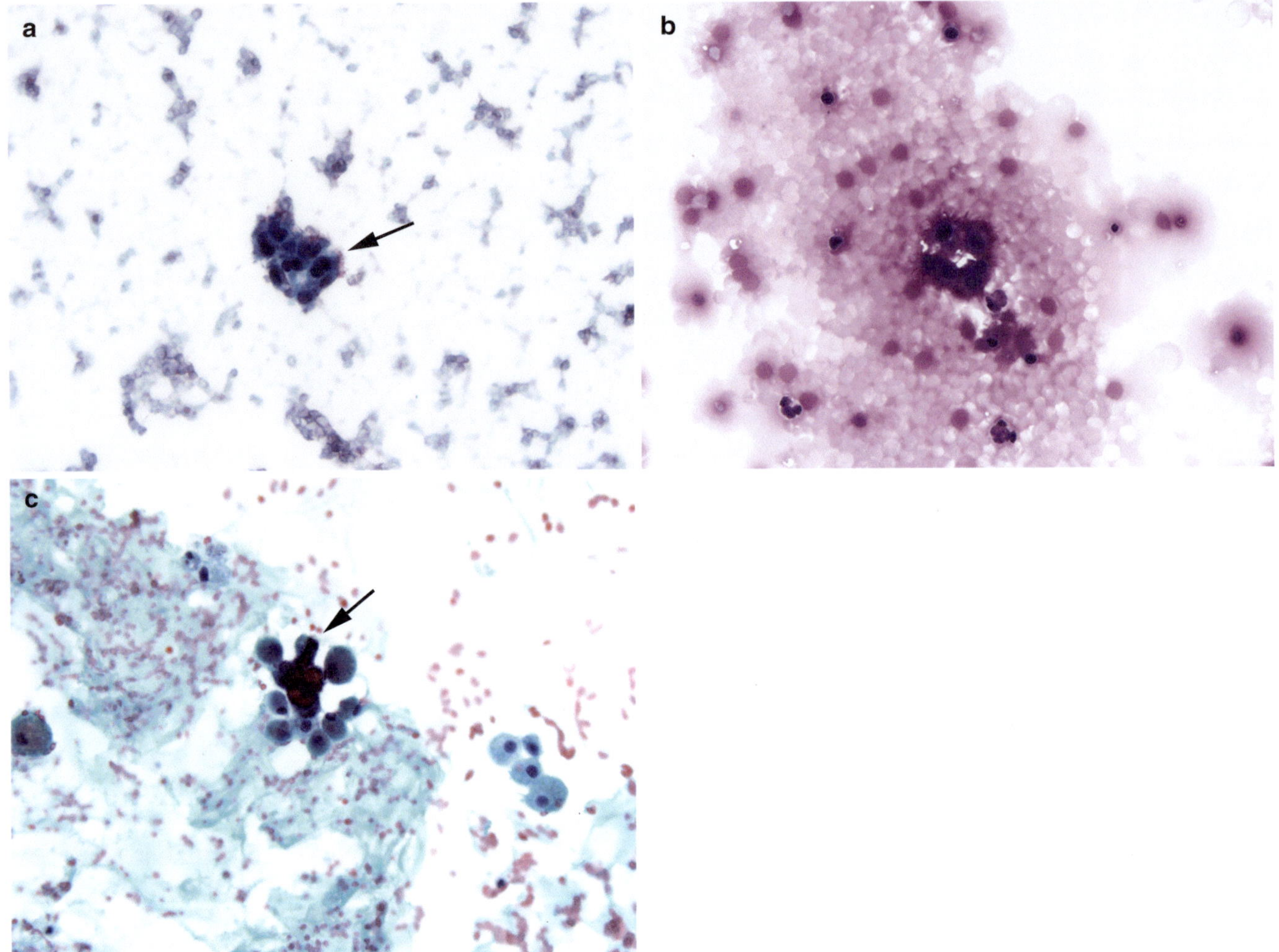

Fig. 6.5 Endosalpingiosis is similar to endometriosis but instead of the presence of ectopic endometrial tissue, it is characterized by the presence of benign glands and cysts lined by ciliated, fallopian tube-like epithelium. (**a**) Cytomorphologically, it is similar to endometriosis with clusters of bland cuboidal cells, however the presence of cilia (*arrows*) is a distinctive feature (Pap stain, 400×). (**b**) Endosalpingiosis. Another distinction from endometriosis is that endosalpingiosis is generally asymptomatic and found incidentally during surgery or imaging for other indications. In this 45-year-old woman with a history of diverticulitis, a 2.5 cm nodule was found in the mesentery. Fine needle aspiration revealed clusters of bland ciliated glandular cells, compatible with endosalpingiosis (DiffQuik stain, 400×). (**c**) In some cases, psammoma bodies, defined as calcifications with lamellated concentric bands generally found in conditions with papillary architecture, may also be found, as seen in this example (*arrow*) (Pap stain, 400×)

Magnetic Resonance Imaging

- On MRI, cysts contain simple fluid that is low signal on T1-weighted images and high signal on T2-weighted images. They contain a uniform thin, dark wall on T2. Again, there is no internal enhancement, although enhancement of the thin wall is typical [8].

Fine Needle Aspiration

- The main cytological distinction to be made is between functional and nonfunctional epithelial-lined cysts. The former includes follicular and corpus luteum cysts, while the latter encompasses endometriotic cysts, cystic surface epithelial tumors of the ovary, and mature cystic teratomas.
- Functional cysts: characterized by granulosa cells which are small, with scant indistinct cytoplasm, round to oval nuclei and coarsely granular chromatin. When degenerated, granulosa cells may mimic macrophages due to the presence of cytoplasmic microvesicles. Luteinized granulosa cells are larger and have ill-defined cell borders with abundant foamy or granular eosinophilic cytoplasm and eccentric nuclei with fine chromatin and small nucleoli. In corpus luteum cysts, luteinized cells may be seen in association with fibrin, degenerate erythrocytes], fresh blood, and hemosiderin-laden macrophages. Granulosa cells are positive for inhibin.
  - Follicular cysts are variably cellular, clusters of bland follicular cells with foamy to granular cytoplasm, small round nuclei with condensed chromatin as well

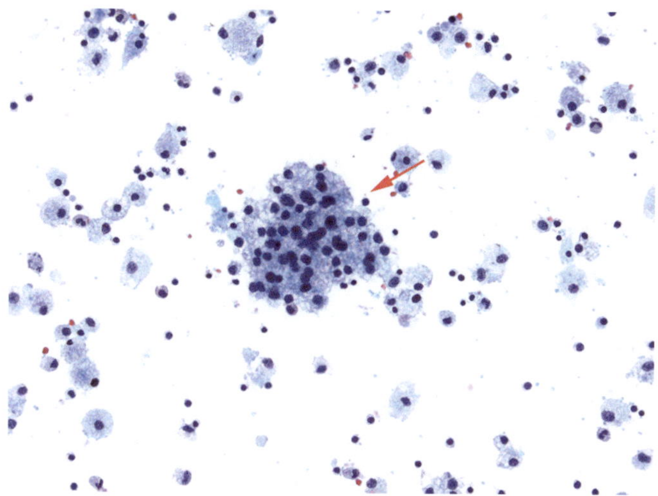

Fig. 6.6 Ovarian cysts can arise in a variety of benign and neoplastic conditions but the benign variety fall into two general categories: nonfunctional inclusion cysts, which arise from ovarian surface epithelium, and/or fallopian tube epithelium and functional cysts, including follicular and corpus luteum cysts. Cyst fluid aspirate shows a background of foamy macrophages and a cluster of follicular cells with bland round nuclei and vacuolated cytoplasm (*arrow*) characteristic of a follicular cyst (Pap stain, 200×)

as larger round nuclei with vesicular chromatin with more finely dispersed chromatin, and macrophages (Fig. 6.6) [7, 9]. They may pose a potential diagnostic pitfall due to high cellularity, cells with hyperchromatic nuclei containing conspicuous nucleoli, and the presence of mitotic figures, which may be numerous.

- Nonfunctional cysts: endometriotic cysts, cystic surface epithelial tumors of the ovary, and mature cystic teratomas They often have scant cellularity, few bland cuboidal ovarian surface/mesothelial-like cells, and macrophages.
  - Endometriotic cysts yield brownish/chocolate-colored fluid containing hemosiderin-laden macrophages with endometrial stromal and/or epithelial cells present in some cases. Often a specific interpretation beyond hemorrhagic cyst with a differential diagnosis will be rendered if all components are not seen.

Malignant Conditions

Malignant Mesothelioma

Clinical

- Strong association with previous asbestos and other occupational exposure (shipyards, military facilities, and industrial processing job sites). Occurs most commonly in the pleura and to a lesser degree in the peritoneum.
- Early in the disease it is generally asymptomatic, but with progression and late stage disease, patients can present with abdominal pain, ascites, and weight loss.

Radiology

Ultrasound/Biopsy

- Evaluating for peritoneal mesothelioma with US is difficult except in the setting of large-volume ascites. Similar to the case in omental metastases, the peritoneal fluid provides a good acoustic window to evaluate for nodularity [10]. Centrally located tumors are poorly imaged with US because of the acoustic impedance of bowel gas and mesenteric fat. Figure 6.7 demonstrates an US of the left upper quadrant with echogenic soft-tissue thickening. US is also the most commonly used method for imaging guidance to perform biopsies of these masses.

Computed Tomography

- Peritoneal mesothelioma is difficult to differentiate from omental infiltration. It has a wide range of imaging findings, from small nodules or strands of soft tissue to large masses that separate the colon or small intestine from the anterior abdominal wall. Thickening of the omentum, as seen with peritonitis, can be indistinguishable from tumor infiltration. Omental caking, similar to that seen in primary peritoneal cancer, describes diffuse infiltration of the omentum by metastatic disease (Fig. 6.7a). Ascites is often present. The masses typically enhance.

Magnetic Resonance Imaging

- The MRI findings are similar to those of CT. T1-weighted fat-suppressed postcontrast images are particularly helpful to evaluate for peritoneal enhancement.

PET-CT

- These lesions are FDG-PET avid and demonstrate increased activity [11].

Fine Needle Aspiration/Effusion Cytology

- Malignant mesothelial cells seen dispersed singly or in large clusters (greater than 12 cells) with scalloped borders (Figs. 6.8).
- Tumor cells with dense cytoplasm centrally and peripheral pale-staining cytoplasm or "lacy skirts" (Fig. 6.8).
- Enlarged irregular nuclei with prominent macronucleoli, binucleation, and multinucleation.
- Paired tumor cells with intercellular clear spaces or "windows" (Fig. 6.8).
- Tumor cells may occasionally also display cytoplasmic vacuolation (Fig. 6.8).
- Making a definitive diagnosis of mesothelioma on effusion cytology, FNA/ core biopsy has been controversial. We have published a study showing that it can be done with a high degree of accuracy when combined with clinical, radiologic, and ancillary test information [17].

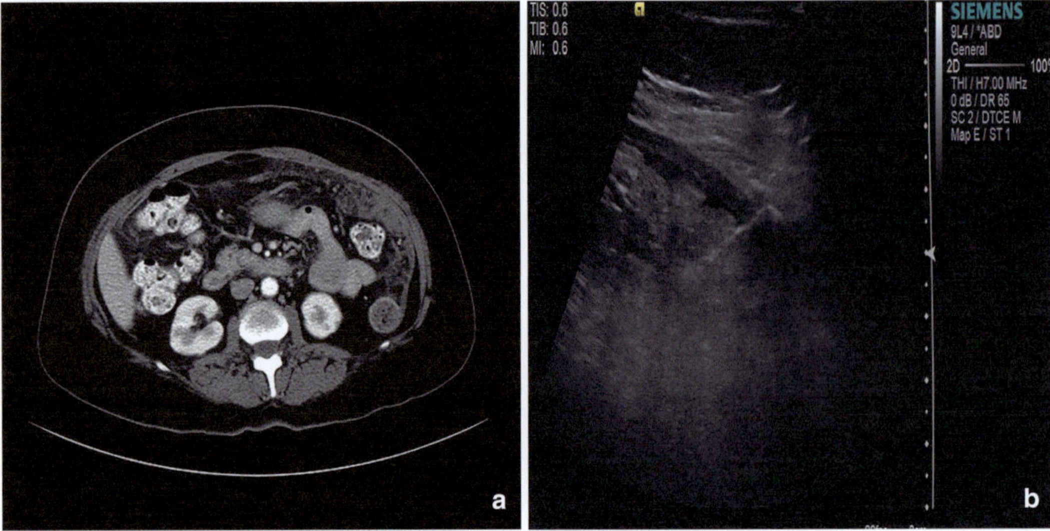

Fig. 6.7 Mesothelioma. (**a**) CT demonstrating soft tissue density and nodule thickening in the left upper quadrant. (**b**) Ultrasound demonstrating echogenic thickening of the submuscular peritoneal layer

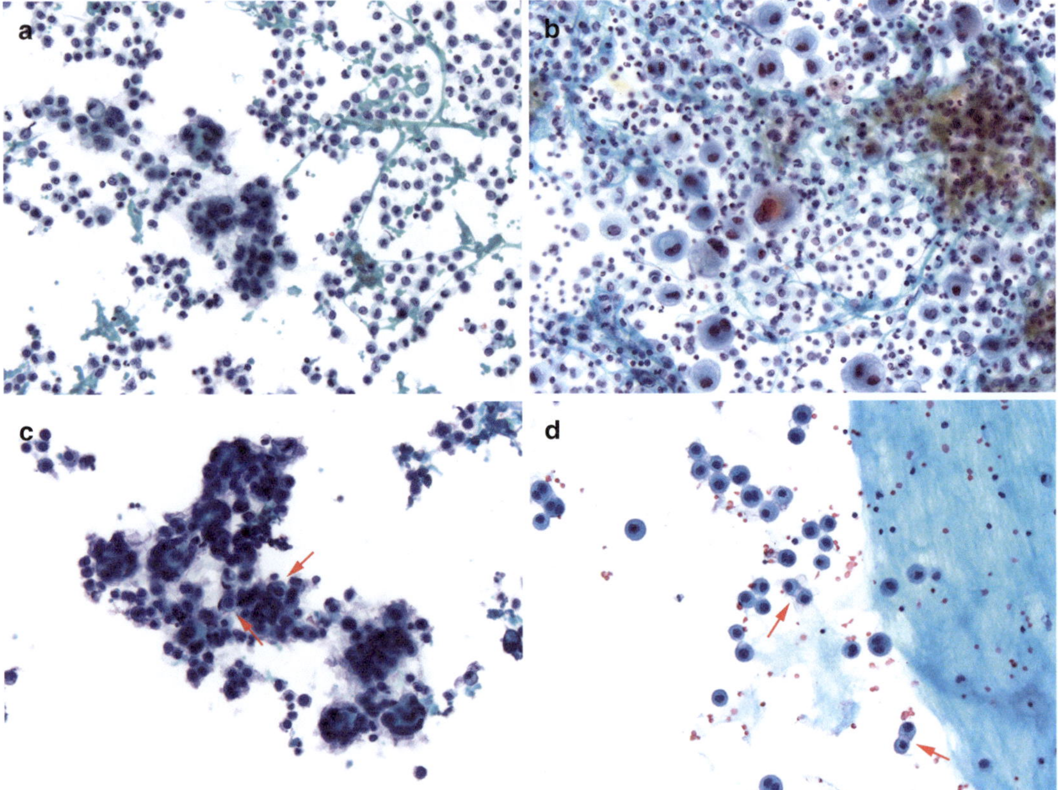

Fig. 6.8 Malignant mesothelioma is a primary serosal malignancy that is much more common in the pleural space but can occur in the peritoneal cavity as well. (**a**) It is characterized by serosal nodularity and consequent malignant effusion composed of epithelioid cells, seen singly and in large clusters with scalloped borders, with moderate to abundant dense cytoplasm and characteristic pale peripheral halo, round to ovoid centrally placed nuclei, frequent binucleation, and prominent nucleoli (Pap stain, 200×). (**b**) Pap-stained cytospin showing malignant mesothelial cells with the characteristic two-toned cytoplasm, due to long slender branching peripheral microvilli, which also explains the paler tinctorial quality of the cytoplasm around the periphery of cells and irregular nuclei with frequent binucleation. Reactive mesothelial cells can have similar morphology, so clinical and radiologic correlation is important. This peritoneal tap was from a 78-year-old woman with diffuse peritoneal studding and ascites (Pap stain, 400×). (**c**) Clusters of mesothelial cells with scalloped borders and occasional cell-in-cell pattern (*arrow*) which, although not specific to malignancy, is a sensitive marker in the appropriate clinical context (Pap stain, 200×). (**d**) Pairing of cells with intercellular spaces or "windows" is another characteristic feature of mesothelial cells and can be a helpful feature in fluid specimens when trying to distinguish between metastatic adenocarcinoma and mesothelioma. In this Papanicolaou-stained cytospin of peritoneal fluid from a 60-year-old man with mesothelioma the window between the paired mesothelial cells (*arrow*) can be appreciated (Pap stain, 200×)

Immunohistochemistry
The main differential diagnosis

- for malignant mesothelioma, especially the epithelioid type, is metastatic adenocarcinoma; therefore staining with a panel of immunostains can help differentiate the two.
- Mesothelioma: positive for calretinin, WT-1, D2–40.
- Adenocarcinoma: positive for TTF-1 (lung primary), Pax-8 (gynecologic primary), MOC-31, BerEP4, B72.3, and monoclonal CEA [12].
- A panel with two positive stains for mesothelial markers and two negative stains for adenocarcinoma has a high sensitivity and specificity for confirming the diagnosis.
- Loss of BRCA-1-associated protein (BAP1) also shows high sensitivity and specificity for malignant mesothelioma and can differentiate between reactive mesothelial cells that show retained expression [13].

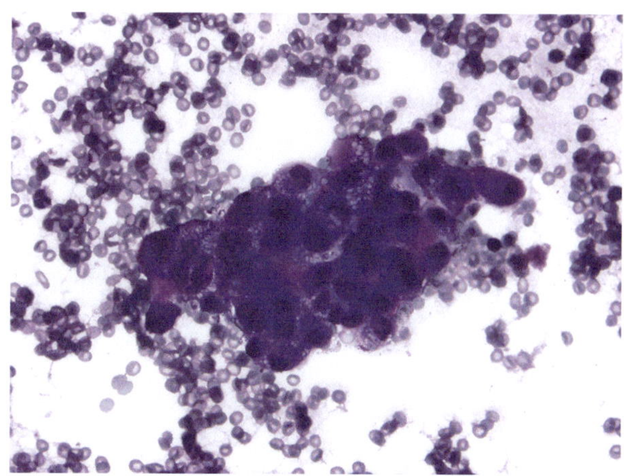

Fig. 6.9 Metastatic adenocarcinoma to the peritoneum, being much more common, is frequently in the differential diagnosis and shares some morphologic overlap with mesothelioma. This is especially due to the variability in cytomorphology of mesothelial cells. While mesothelial cells generally have denser cytoplasm than the glandular cells of adenocarcinoma, cytoplasmic vacuolization can be seen, as in this case. In these particular cases immunohistochemistry is critical in making the distinction (Diff Quik stain, 400×)

Ovarian High-Grade Serous Carcinoma

Clinical

- While primary ovarian carcinoma accounts for only about 3% of all cancers in women, it has one of the highest incidence-to-death ratios because of lack of available screening tools, the characteristic lack of early symptoms, and the consequent tendency to present at a late stage when prognosis is poor [14].
- As occurs in patients with other advanced malignancies within the peritoneal cavity, late-stage disease patients can present with nonspecific signs and symptoms such as abdominal pain, ascites, and weight loss.

Radiology

Ultrasound

- On US, ovarian cancer typically appears as a complex cystic mass. Signs of malignancy include solid components (which are the most significant predictor of malignancy) [4], irregular thick wall and septa (>3 mm), solid mural nodules and papillary projections, as well as Doppler images demonstrating blood flow within a solid component, papillary projection, or septa. Tumor extension to adjacent structures as well as ascites can also be seen with ovarian cancer.

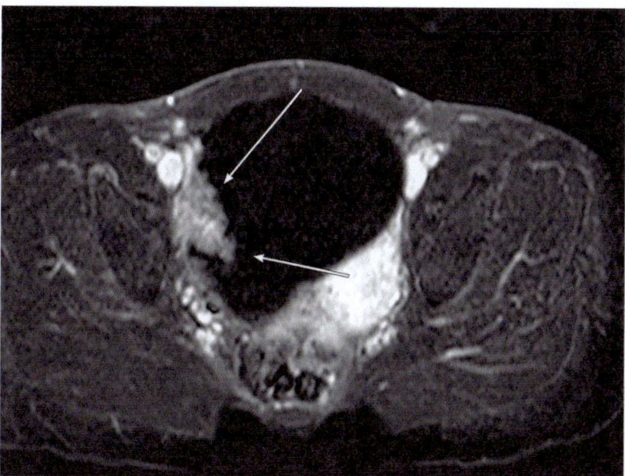

Fig. 6.10 Ovarian cancer. Axial T1-weighted fat-saturated contrast-enhanced MRI demonstrates an enhancing papillary projection in an adnexal cystic mass consistent with ovarian cancer

Computed Tomography/Magnetic Resonance Imaging

- On CT and MRI, ovarian cancer demonstrates findings similar to those on gray-scale US. In addition, enhancement of papillary projections is highly suggestive of a borderline or malignant tumor (Fig. 6.10) [8].

Fine Needle Aspiration

- Crowded three-dimensional clusters or dispersed single cells (Fig. 6.9).
- Enlarged nuclei with irregular nuclear borders, prominent nucleoli, and multinucleation.
- Tumor cells with delicate, vacuolated cytoplasm (Fig. 6.9).

Primary Peritoneal Serous Carcinoma

Clinical

- A rare primary malignancy that diffusely involves the peritoneum; it is indistinguishable clinically and cytomorphologically from primary serous ovarian carcinoma.

- Its origin has not been well characterized. However, the epithelial layer of the ovary and peritoneum share a common embryonic lineage deriving from coelomic epithelium early in life [16]. Many cases likely arise from premalignant lesions involving the fallopian tubes (serous tubal intraepithelial carcinoma).
- The clinical presentation is similar to that of ovarian serous carcinoma; however, clinically and radiologically, there is no evidence of an adnexal primary.

Radiology

Computed Tomography/Magnetic Resonance Imaging

- There is often extensive peritoneal and omental tumor and a large amount of ascites without an ovarian mass. Omental caking is usually present and may manifest as fine, nodular, soft-tissue studding or coalescent, mass-like soft tissue within the omentum [15]. Peritoneal calcifications and lymphadenopathy can also be seen. Enhancement is typical.

Fine Needle Aspiration

- Essentially cytomorphologic features identical to those seen in primary ovarian serous carcinoma.
- Crowded three-dimensional clusters or dispersed single cells.
- Enlarged nuclei with irregular nuclear borders, prominent nucleoli, and multinucleation (Fig. 6.11).
- Tumor cells with delicate, vacuolated cytoplasm.
- Psammoma bodies (Fig. 6.11).

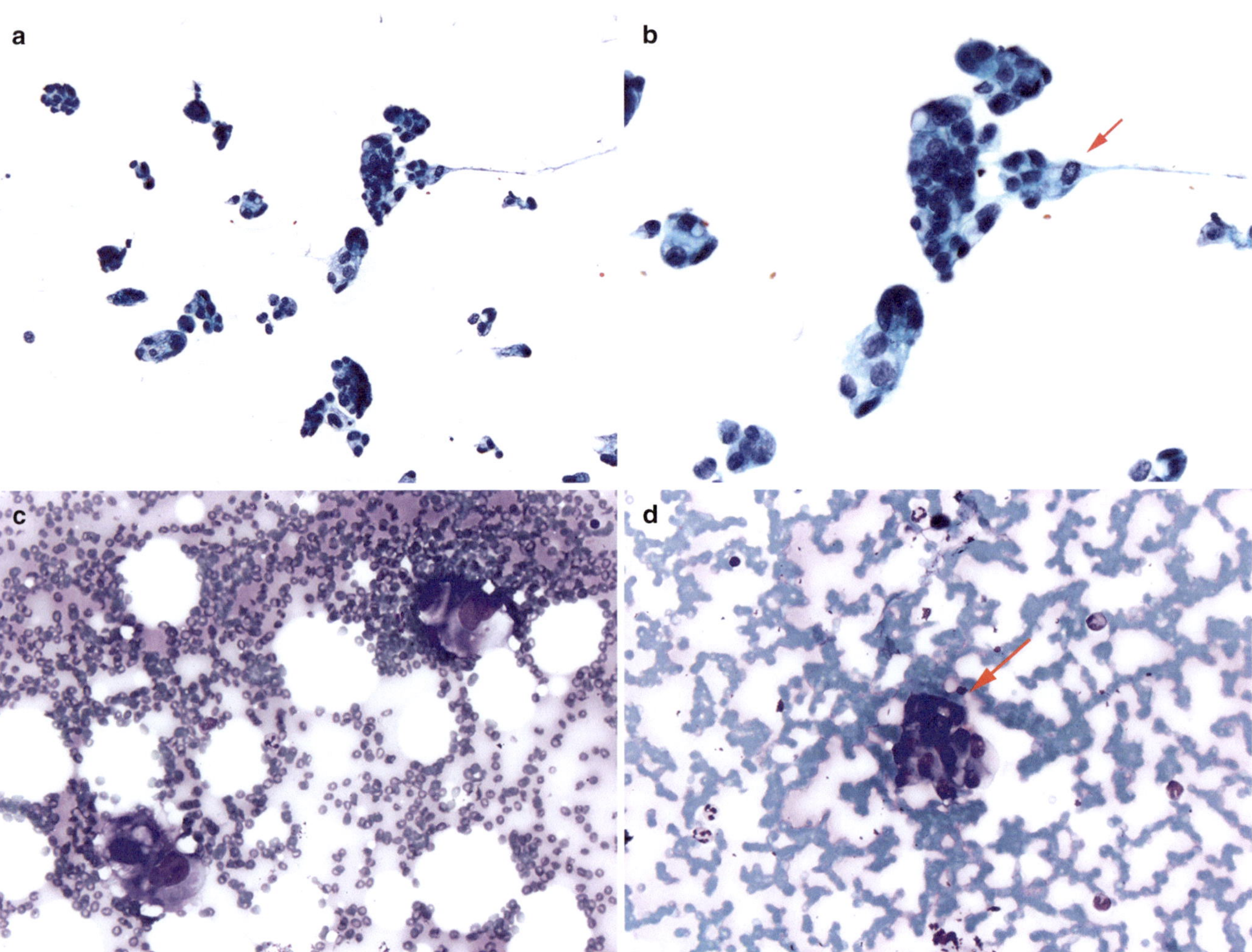

Fig. 6.11 Serous adenocarcinoma shares a similar morphology whether from ovarian, tubal, or primary peritoneal origin. (**a**) Fine needle aspirate of a peritoneal nodule in a 53-year-old woman shows crowded clusters and single tumor cells with nuclear hyperchromasia, irregular nuclear borders, occasional prominent nucleoli, and delicate vacuolated cytoplasm (Pap stain, 100×). (**b**) Medium-power Papanicolaou-stained smear shows multiple cohesive clusters of tumor cells with enlarged irregular nuclei, clumped chromatin, prominent nuclei, and cytoplasmic vacuoles. A mitotic figure is also present (*arrow*) (Pap stain, 200×). (**c**) Another high-power DiffQuik-stained image showing two small clusters of vacuolated tumor cells with markedly atypical enlarged nuclei and prominent nucleoli in a 44-year-old female patient with primary peritoneal carcinoma. There was no radiologic or clinical evidence of an adnexal primary (DiffQuik stain, 400×). (**d**) Another example of primary peritoneal carcinoma. Crowded clusters of glandular cells with anisonucleosis, or variation in nuclear size, is another feature as well as psammoma bodies (*arrow*) (DiffQuik, 400×)

Metastatic Carcinoma

Clinical

- The peritoneal cavity and omentum are frequent sites of deposits of metastatic carcinoma, and adenocarcinoma is more likely to be present in malignant effusions than squamous cell carcinoma and neuroendocrine neoplasms/small-cell carcinoma.
- Signs and symptoms may vary, depending on the site of origin. However, in the presence of peritoneal disease and the development of a malignant effusion, patients may present with the sequelae of ascites (e.g., bloating, abdominal discomfort, early satiety).

Radiology

Ultrasound

- Evaluating for omental metastasis with US is difficult except in the setting of large-volume ascites. The peritoneal fluid provides a good acoustic window to evaluate for tumor nodules as small as 2 to 3 mm. Centrally located tumors are poorly imaged with US because of the acoustic impedance of bowel gas and mesenteric fat.

Computed Tomography

- Omental infiltration has a wide range of imaging findings, from small nodules or strands of soft tissue to large masses that separate the colon or small intestine from the anterior abdominal wall. Thickening of the omentum, as seen with peritonitis, can be indistinguishable from tumor infiltration. Omental caking, similar to that seen in primary peritoneal cancer, describes diffuse infiltration of the omentum by metastatic disease (Fig. 6.12). Ascites is often present. The masses typically enhance [10].

Magnetic Resonance Imaging

- The MRI findings are similar to those seen in CT. T1-weighted fat-suppressed postcontrast images are particularly helpful to evaluate for omental enhancement. An intermediate signal intensity-enhancing soft-tissue mass in the omentum in a person with a known primary, particularly ovarian carcinoma, is highly suspicious for metastatic disease [10].

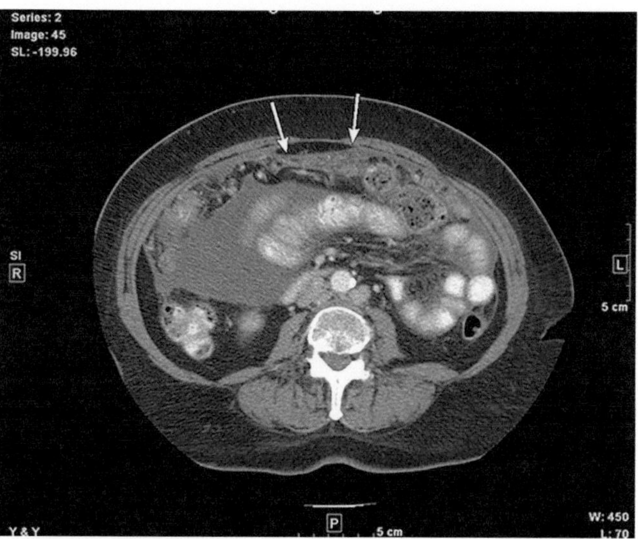

Fig. 6.12 Peritoneal carcinomatosis: contrast-enhanced computed tomography demonstrates ascites with enhancing metastases and nodular thickening involving the greater omentum

Fine Needle Aspiration/Effusion Cytology

- Adenocarcinoma
  - Large hyperchromatic, crowded three-dimensional clusters with smooth borders or dispersed single cells (Fig. 6.13).
  - Enlarged nuclei with irregular nuclear borders, prominent and multiple nucleoli, and multinucleation (Fig. 6.13).
  - Tumor cells with delicate, vacuolated cytoplasm.
  - Signet-ring cells with large cytoplasm vacuoles and eccentric nuclei pushed to one side.
- Neuroendocrine Carcinoma
  - Discohesive tumor cells in loose rosettes and dispersed singly.
  - Plasmacytoid morphology with eccentric nuclei with stippled "salt and pepper" chromatin and moderate granular cytoplasm (Fig. 6.14).

Core Biopsy

- Malignant tumor cells in glandular and papillary arrangements and crowded clusters infiltrating omental tissue with surrounding desmoplastic response, with areas of necrosis (Fig. 6.15).

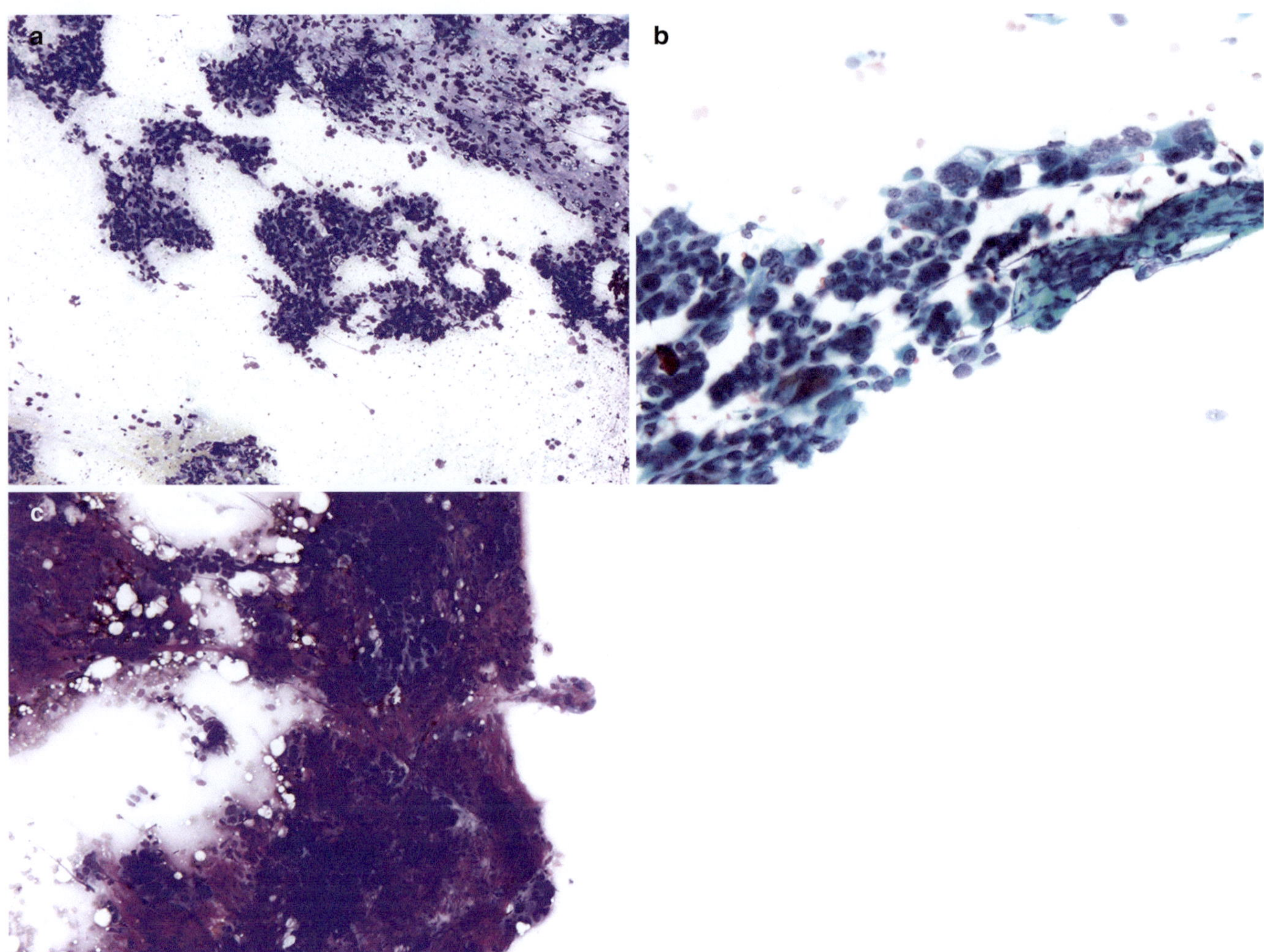

Fig. 6.13 The omentum is a sheet of fatty tissue that lies within the peritoneal cavity and extends from the greater curvature of the stomach superiorly, lies anterior to the small intestines and then reflects back on itself, splits, and encloses the transverse colon. Given the location of the greater omentum within the peritoneum it is a frequent site of metastasis for intraperitoneal primary malignancies, including ovarian, appendiceal, and intestinal primaries, among others. (**a**) This 2 cm omental metastasis is from a 65-year-old woman with a history of high-grade serous carcinoma of the ovary. Medium-power DiffQuik smear shows hypercellular specimen with crowded clusters of tumor cells with delicate cytoplasm and hyperchromatic, enlarged nuclei (DiffQuik, 200×). (**b**) Higher-power Papanicolaou-stained image displays the marked nuclear pleomorphism of this tumor including nuclear enlargement, anisonucleosis, clumped chromatin, and markedly prominent nucleoli (Pap stain, 400×). (**c**) Medium-power DiffQuik-stained image showing stromal desmoplasia or conversion of the adipose tissue, seen in the background as clear vacuoles, into dense fibrous tissue as a response to the invading tumor. The stromal fragments have a fibrillary, magenta appearance (DiffQuik stain, 200×)

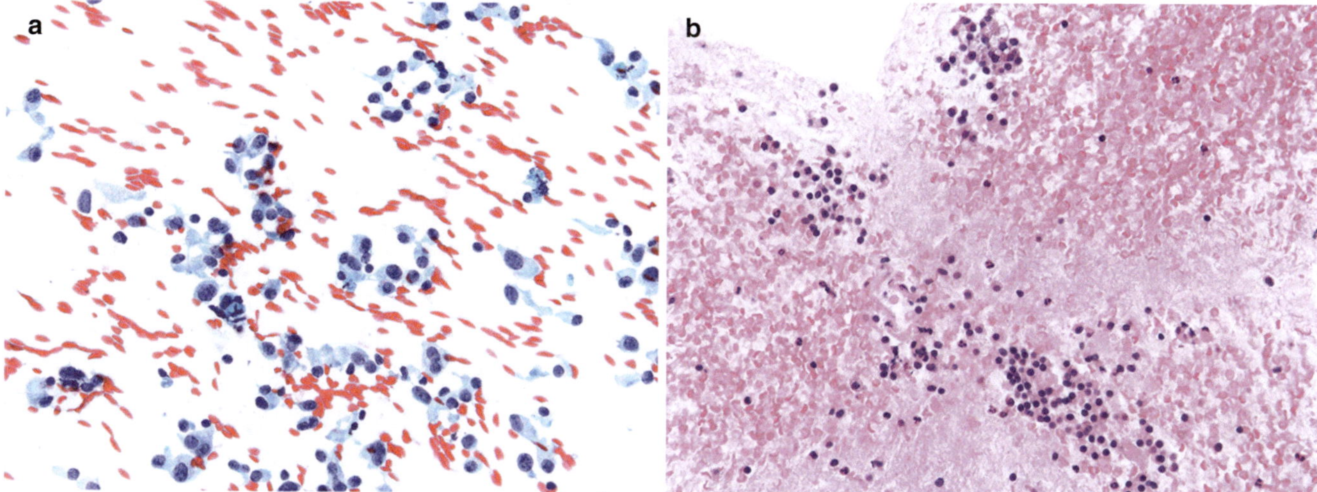

Fig. 6.14 Metastatic neuroendocrine tumors. Neuroendocrine neoplasms can arise in a number of organ systems including the lung, GI tract, and pancreas, among other sites. Given the relatively high incidence of GI tract and pancreatic primaries, metastases within the peritoneal cavity and the omentum are not unusual. (**a**) FNA from a 1.6 cm omental nodule, in a 59-year-old man with a history of a duodenal primary neuroendocrine tumor with multiple omental nodules showing sheets of discohesive plasmacytoid tumor cells with round to ovoid eccentric nuclei with irregular contours, granular "salt and pepper" chromatin, and delicate cytoplasm (Pap stain, 200×). (**b**) Cell block section from the same FNA specimen above showing similar discohesive tumor cells with plasmacytoid morphology and bland nuclear features (H&E stain, 200×)

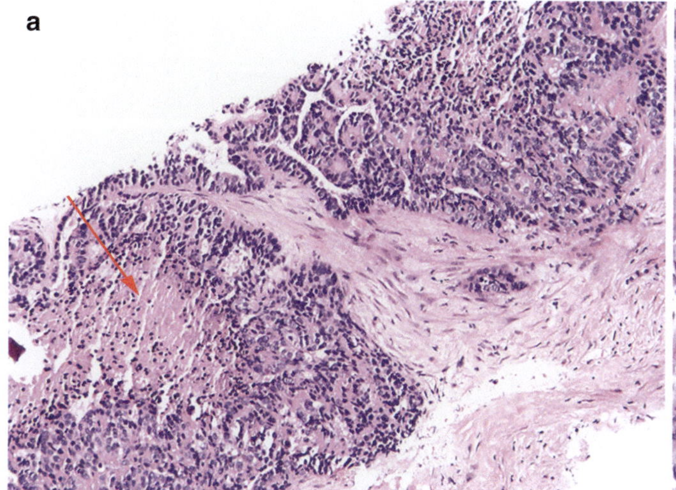

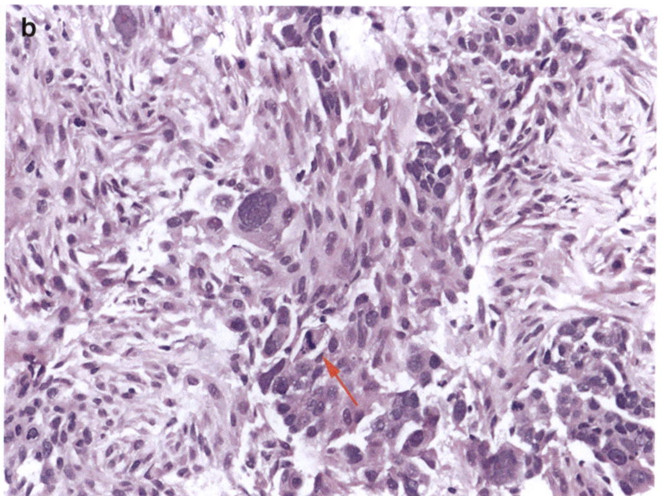

Fig. 6.15 High-grade serious carcinoma involving the omentum. (**a**) This histologic section shows malignant tumor cells in glandular and papillary arrangements infiltrating the omentum with surrounding desmoplasia, or the fibrosis that occurs in response to the invading tumor cells. Areas of necrosis can also be seen (*arrow*) indicating the high-grade nature of the tumor (H&E stain, 200×). (**b**) Higher-power image of high-grade serous carcinoma showing degree of nuclear atypia present in the tumor. There is anisonucleosis, prominent nucleoli, and a readily apparent mitotic figure (*arrow*) (H&E stain, 400×)

References

1. Cibas E. Peritoneal washings. In: Cibas E, Ducatman B, editors. Cytology: diagnostic principles and clinical correlates. 4th ed. Philadelphia: Elsevier Saunders; 2014. p. 155–69.
2. DeMay R. The art and science of cytopathology, Exfoliative cytology, vol. 1. 2nd ed. Chicago: ASCP Press; 2012. p. 268–373.
3. DeMay R. The art and science of cytopathology, Deep aspiration cytology, vol. 3. 2nd ed. Chicago: ASCP Press; 2012. p. 1146–54, 1406–36.
4. Brant WE, Helms CA. The Brant and Helms solution: fundamentals of diagnostic radiology. 3rd ed. Philadelphia: Lippincott Williams and Wilkins; 2006. p. 1584.
5. Woodward PJ, Sohaey R, Mezzetti TP Jr. Endometriosis: radiologic-pathologic correlation. Radiographics. 2001;21:193–216; questionnaire, 288–94.
6. Taneja S, Sidhu R, Khurana A, Sekhon R, Mehta A, Jena A. MRI appearance of florid cystic endosalpingiosis of the uterus: a case report. Korean J Radiol. 2010;11:476–9.

7. Ovary CE. In: Cibas E, Ducatman B, editors. Cytology: diagnostic principles and clinical correlates. 4th ed. Philadelphia: Elsevier Saunders; 2014. p. 453–70.
8. Jeong YY, Outwater EL, Kang HK. Imaging evaluation of ovarian masses. Radiographics. 2000;20:1445–70.
9. Zhou AG, Levinson KL, Rosenthal DL, VandenBussche CJ. Performance of ovarian cyst fluid fine-needle aspiration cytology. Cancer Cytopathol. 2018;126:112–21.
10. Lee JKT, Sagal SS, Stanley RJ, Heiken JP. Computed body tomography with MRI correlation. Philadelphia: Lippincott Williams and Wilkins; 2006.
11. Liu YC, Kuo YL, Yu CP, Wu HS, Yu JC, Chen CJ, et al. Primary malignant mesothelioma of the greater omentum: report of a case. Surg Today. 2004;34:780–3.
12. Davidson B. The diagnostic and molecular characteristics of malignant mesothelioma and ovarian/peritoneal serous carcinoma. Cytopathology. 2011;22:5–21.
13. Cozzi I, Oprescu FA, Rullo E, Ascoli V. Loss of BRCA1-associated protein (BAP1) expression is useful in diagnostic cytopathology of malignant mesothelioma in effusions. Diagn Cytopathol. 2018;46:9–14.
14. Li J, Fadare O, xiang L, Kong B, Zheng W. Ovarian serous carcinoma: recent concepts on its origin and carcinogenesis. J Hematol Oncol. 2012;5:1–11.
15. Levy AD, Arnáiz J, Shaw JC, Sobin LH. From the archives of the AFIP: primary peritoneal tumors: imaging features with pathologic correlation. Radiographics. 2008;28:583–607; quiz, 621–2.
16. Bhanvadia V, Parmar J, Madan Y, Sheeikh S. Primary peritoneal serous carcinoma: a rare case and palliative approach. Indian J Palliat Care. 2014;20:157–9.
17. Paintal A, Raparia K, Zakowski MF, Nayar R. The diagnosis of malignant mesothelioma in effusion cytology: a reappraisal and results of a multi-institution survey. Cancer Cytopathol. 2013;121(12):703–7.

7 Esophagus, Gastrointestinal Tract, and Pancreas

Xiaoqi Lin and Ryan Hickey

Cytologic examination of specimens from fine needle aspiration (FNA), exfoliative brushings, and needle core biopsies (NCB) are essential tests in the diagnosis of esophageal, gastrointestinal, and pancreatic lesions, staging of malignancy, and follow-up of patients. The sensitivity and specificity of cytology are increased by the concurrent use of imaging studies, immunocytochemistry, and molecular studies. The interobserver agreement among cytopathologists in the diagnosis of malignancy of the solid pancreatic lesion is variable [1].

Techniques used to obtain specimens used for cytologic examination:

- Brushing cytology is used for superficial mucosal lesions or lesions involving the mucosa of the esophagus and bile ducts [2–5]. Common bile duct and pancreatic duct brushings can be obtained during endoscopic retrograde cholangiopancreatography (ERCP) [4]. Although this less costly cancer surveillance method for gastroesophageal diseases is not used in the U.S., it is used in other countries [6, 7]. Molecular studies can increase the sensitivity and specificity of diagnosis [2].
- Also used are endoscopic ultrasound (EUS), ultrasound (US), computed tomography (CT) or magnetic resonance imaging (MRI) guided FNA or NCB for gastric/perigastric and pancreatic/peripancreatic lesions, as well for as mediastinal, perigastric, and peripancreatic lymph node staging [8]. While US- and CT-guided FNA biopsies are also alternative techniques for tissue acquisition, EUS-FNA has become the gold standard and offers greater efficacy with fewer complications.

X. Lin (✉)
Northwestern University, Feinberg School of Medicine, Northwestern Memorial Hospital, Chicago, IL, USA
e-mail: xlin@northwestern.edu

R. Hickey
Department of Radiology, Division of Vascular Interventional Radiology, New York, NY, USA

Esophagus and Gastrointestinal Tract

Barrett Esophagus and Dysplasia

Clinic

- Barrett esophagus is defined as "a change in the esophageal epithelium of any length that can be recognized at endoscopy and is confirmed to have intestinal metaplasia by biopsy" [9].
- Gastroesophageal reflux disease (GERD) is the most common type of esophagitis in the United States and may result in Barrett esophagus, dysplasia, and adenocarcinoma with an odds ratio of 7 in chronic reflux and 43.5 in longstanding and severe reflux [10–12].
- While enhanced endoscopic imaging modalities (e.g., narrow band imaging, confocal endomicroscopy) have been promising, their role is still unclear [13]. It is therefore essential to follow a methodical technique in tissue sampling (e.g., the Seattle protocol) to minimize sampling error [14].

Brushing Cytology

- Barrett esophagus: The presence of goblet cells (large cytoplasmic vacuoles compressing the nuclei to one side) embedded in cuboidal or columnar intestinal metaplastic cells arranged in small nests or acini (Fig. 7.1b) [2, 15–17]. An Alcian blue stain may be helpful to confirm the presence of goblet cells in intestinal metaplasia.
- Low grade dysplasia: The presence of small clusters or acini of columnar cells with crowded, enlarged, elongated, and hyperchromatic nuclei and increased nuclear to cytoplasm ratios (Fig. 7.1c) [16, 17].
- High grade dysplasia: The presence of two- to three-dimensional small clusters or acini of cuboidal to columnar cells with crowded, pleomorphic, enlarged, and hyperchro-

R. Nayar et al. (eds.), *Atlas of Cytopathology and Radiology*, https://doi.org/10.1007/978-3-030-24756-0_7

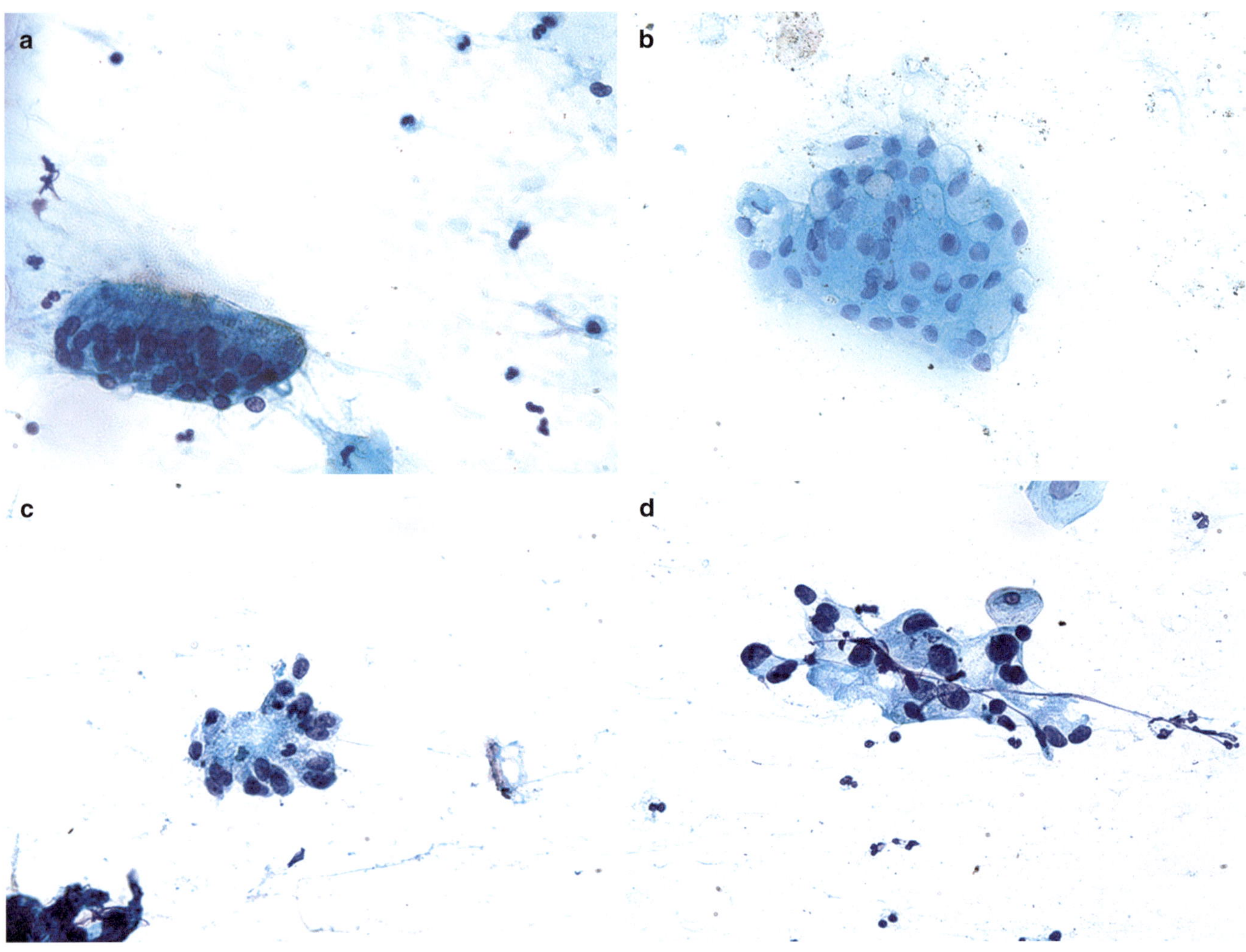

Fig. 7.1 Brushing cytology of gastroesophageal junction, Papanicolaou stain, 600×. (**a**) Benign glandular mucosa. (**b**) Barrett esophagus. (**c**) Low-grade dysplasia. (**d**) High-grade dysplasia

matic nuclei with irregular nuclear membranes and prominent nucleoli and increased nuclear-to-cytoplasm ratio (Fig. 7.1d) [16, 17]. Tumor diathesis is absent.

Histology of Core and Cell Block

- Normal junctional glandular mucosa is composed of cardiac glands (Fig. 7.2a) and/or fundic glands.
- Barrett esophagus detected by endoscopic biopsy demonstrates intestinal metaplasia defined by the presence of goblet cells (Fig. 7.2b).
- Low-grade dysplasia: Columnar cells with crowded, enlarged, elongated, pseudostratified (confined to the lower half of the glandular epithelium), and hyperchromatic nuclei with mild pleomorphism, increased nuclear-to-cytoplasmic ratio, decreased cytoplasmic mucin, and minimal architectural changes (Fig. 7.2c) [12, 16]. Endoscopic biopsy histomorphology is much more sensitive for diagnosing low-grade dysplasia than brushing cytology (sensitivity 97% versus 20%) [15]. Brushing cytology applied together with biopsy can improve the detection of dysplasia [2, 15].
- High-grade dysplasia: Marked architectural aberrations including cribriform glands, marked pleomorphism, nuclear stratification extending to the upper part of the cells and glands, decrease in or loss of mucin secretion, and frequent mitosis (Fig. 7.2d) [12, 16]. Endoscopic biopsy histomorphology and brushing cytology have similar sensitivity and specificity to diagnose high-grade dysplasia (sensitivity 90% versus 90%) and can be used together to increase the sensitivity [15].

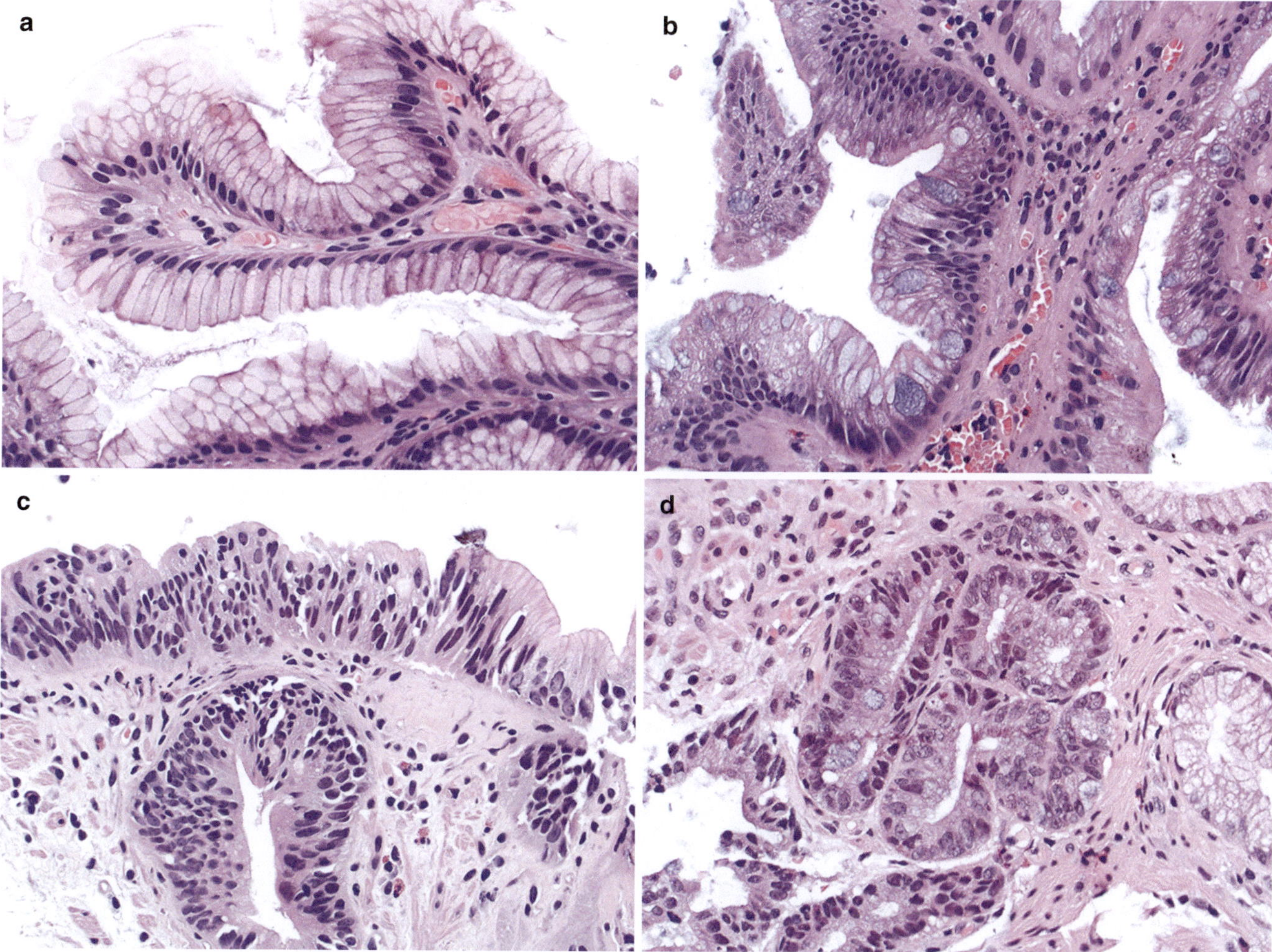

Fig. 7.2 Histology of gastrointestinal junction, hematoxylin-and-eosin (H&E) stain, 400×. (**a**) Benign glandular mucosa. (**b**) Barrett esophagus. (**c**) Low-grade dysplasia. (**d**) High-grade dysplasia

Carcinoma of the Esophagus and Gastrointestinal Tract

Adenocarcinoma

Clinical

Esophagus

- Dramatically increased in incidence in the past two to three decades; approaches or exceeds that of squamous cell esophageal cancer [12].
- One to four cases per 100,000 per year in the United States [12].
- Male-to-female ratio of 3:1–7:1.
- Retrosternal/epigastric pain or cachexia.
- Associated with Barrett esophagus in 95% of cases [12]. Other etiologies include tobacco, obesity, alcohol, and *Helicobacter pylori* [12].

Stomach

- The second most common form of esophageal cancer worldwide [18]. Increase in incidence in the past several decades worldwide but markedly decreased in incidence in the United States and England.
- Male-to-female ratio of 2:1.
- Symptoms include anemia, weight loss, and hypochlorhydria.
- Diet, bile reflux, *H. pylori* infection, excessive cell proliferation, oxidative stress, interference with antioxidant functions, and DNA damage are all causative factors [18].
- Two main histologic subtypes:
  - Intestinal type: Linked to *H. pylori*, in older patients, and located in antrum.
  - Diffuse type (signet ring cell carcinoma): Most common in younger patient; located in the body of the stomach.

Radiology for Gastric Adenocarcinoma

Radiography
- On a double-contrast barium upper GI study, gastric adenocarcinoma may present as a polypoid, ulcerated, or infiltrative lesion.
- When presenting as an ulcerated lesion, the ulcer appears intraluminal as opposed to benign; the latter appears to extend outside the limits of the gastric wall.
- Whereas benign ulcers have regular, radiating folds that reach or nearly reach the ulcer margin, malignant ulceration tends to be associated with irregular folds that are separated from the ulcer itself by a rim of malignant tissue (Fig. 7.3a) [19].

CT
- Gastric carcinoma may present as focal or generalized mural thickening or as a polypoid, enhancing lesion (Fig. 7.3b). Advanced carcinomas often demonstrate segmental or diffuse gastric mural thickening with irregular, lobulated borders and ulceration.
- Signet-ring cell cancers more often show linitis plastica changes resulting in diffuse thickening of the gastric wall and loss of the normal gastric folds [20].

Gross

- Polypoid (type I).
- Fungating (type II).
- Ulcerated (type III).
- Diffuse infiltrative (type IV).

Brushing and FNA Cytology
- Brushing cytology has sensitivity similar to that of biopsy for diagnosis of adenocarcinoma (96% versus 91%) [15].

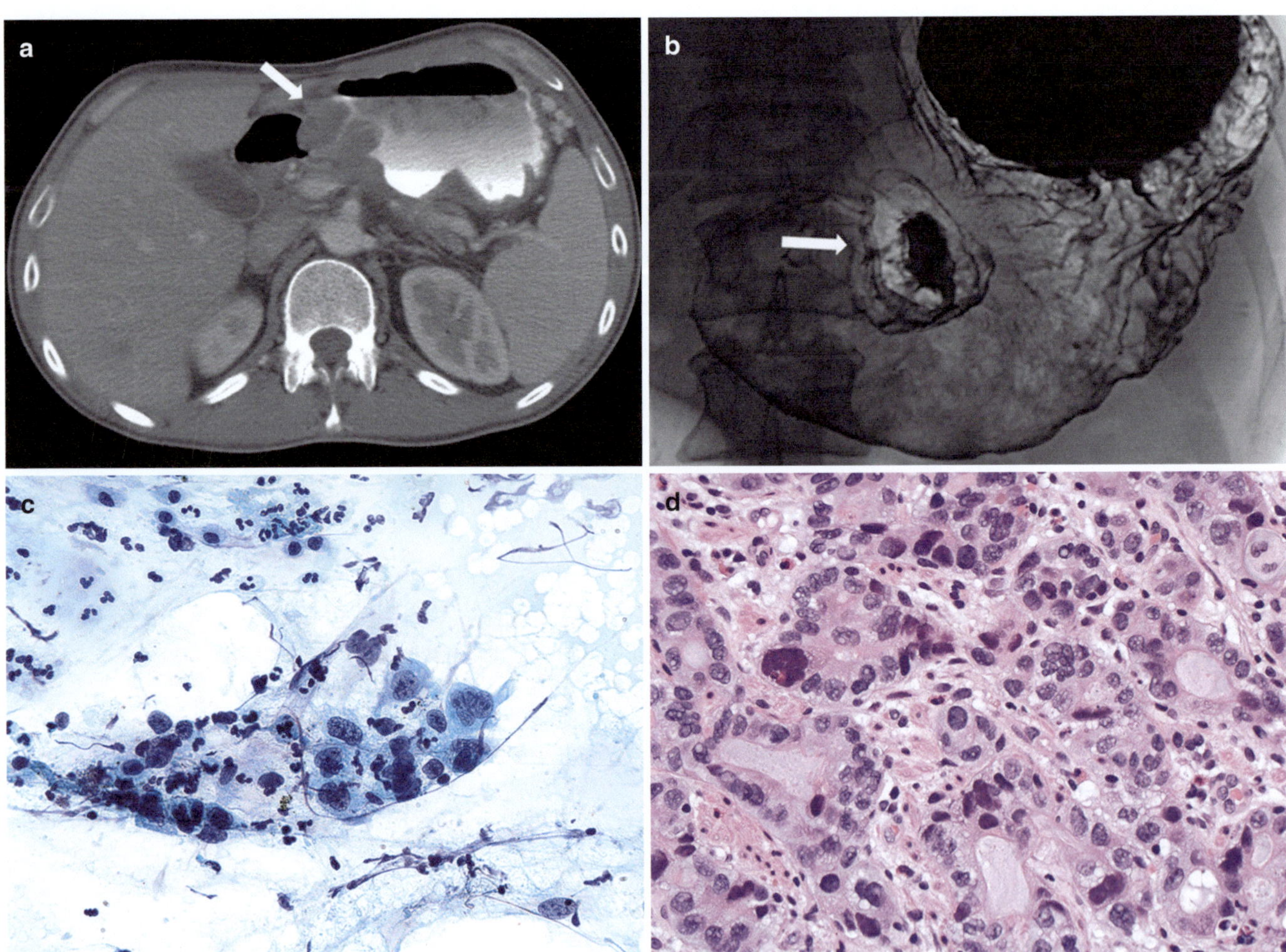

Fig. 7.3 (**a**, **b**) Radiology of gastric adenocarcinoma. (**a**) Spot image from double-contrast upper GI study demonstrating an ulcerated mass projecting into the gastric lumen. Note the thick rind of tissue "heaped up" along the circumference of the ulcer without appreciable gastric rugae (*arrow*). (**b**) Contrast-enhanced CT shows marked thickening of the antral gastric wall (*arrow*). (**c**, **d**) Pathology of adenocarcinoma. (**c**) Brushing cytology, Papanicolaou stain, 400×. (**d**) Histology, H&E stain, 400×

- EUS has become an integral component of initial esophageal and gastric cancer staging. The accuracy of EUS for T-staging is approximately 90% [21, 22].
- The presence of pleomorphic cuboidal, columnar, or polygonal cells singly or arranged in loosely cohesive and crowded three-dimensional clusters, acini, or papillae is characteristic (Fig. 7.3c) [17]. The nuclei are enlarged and hyperchromatic with abnormal chromatin and one or more prominent nucleoli [17]. The cytoplasm is delicate, granular, or vacuolar and may contain mucin.
- Signet-ring cell adenocarcinoma is characterized by the presence of single or loosely cohesive tumor cells with cytoplasmic mucin pushing hyperchromatic, dysplastic nuclei to one side.
- Single pleomorphic cells and tumor diathesis are seen.

Histology of Core and Cell Block

- Most adenocarcinomas are of the intestinal type arise from metaplastic epithelium. The tumor is composed of irregularly shaped glands that infiltrate deeper layers of the esophagus or stomach (Fig. 7.3d). Tumor cells are cuboidal to columnar with irregular nuclei containing prominent nucleoli and coarse or vesicular chromatin and eosinophilic or clear cytoplasm. Better differentiated tumors are composed of mucin-secreting columnar cells, while poorly differentiated tumors show a solid pattern of growth.
- Diffuse type: diffuse infiltration of gastric wall by single tumor cells with associated extensive fibrosis and inflammation. Intracytoplasmic mucin gives cells a characteristic signet-ring cell appearance.
- Subtypes:
  - Adenosquamous carcinoma
  - Mucinous carcinoma
  - Hepatoid carcinoma
  - Parietal gland carcinoma
  - Lymphoepithelioma-like carcinoma
  - Sarcomatoid carcinoma
  - Adenocarcinoma with rhabdoid features
  - Gastric carcinoma with osteoclast-like giant cells
- Immunoreactive to cytokeratin 7, MUC1 (intestinal type), MUC5AC (diffuse type), MUC2 (mucinous type), serotonin and somatostatin (focally positive in 80% of cases), and possibly CK20 (20%) and CDX2.

Differential Diagnosis

- High-grade dysplasia
- Metastatic carcinoma
- Reactive atypia
- Neuroendocrine neoplasm

Squamous Cell Carcinoma

Clinical

Esophagus

- Overall, the most common malignant tumor of the esophagus worldwide with great geographic diversity, <5/100,000 [23].
- Male-to-female ratio of 5:1, two to three times more common in African Americans, with median age of 65 [23].
- Risk factors:
  - Tobacco and alcohol use.
  - Food and water rich in nitrates/nitrosamines.
  - Various vitamin deficiencies.
- Localized predominantly in the middle or lower third of esophagus.
- Presents with dysphagia, weight loss, and retrosternal/epigastric pain.

Anus

- Incidence of anal carcinoma is increasing in both males and females.
- Male-to-female ratio of 3:1.
- Presents with bleeding, pain, change in bowel habits, and pruritus.
- Human papillomavirus (HPV), largely HPV 16 genotype, detected in up to 85% of anal cancers.
- Most commonly located near the pectinate line; 1% to 3% of all distal large bowel cancers.
- The majority are nonkeratinizing squamous cell carcinomas.

Brushing or FNA Cytology, Mainly for Esophageal Squamous Cell Carcinoma

- Well-differentiated squamous cell carcinoma (SCC) (keratinizing): Single or three-dimensional clusters of markedly pleomorphic cells (polygonal, bizarre, and spindle in shape) with moderate to abundant dense (keratinized) cytoplasm, slightly enlarged hyperchromatic nuclei, low nuclear to cytoplasmic ratio, and sharp cytoplasmic borders (Fig. 7.4a), in a background of necrosis.
- Moderately to poorly differentiated SCC: Loosely cohesive clusters of polygonal cells with enlarged hyperchromatic nuclei containing coarse chromatin and prominent nucleoli and scant to moderate dense cytoplasm (Fig. 7.4b) in a background of necrosis.

Anal Cytology

- Used for screening or follow-up of high-risk patients, analogous to the cervical Pap test.
- Dysplastic squamous cells, possibly bizarre in shape with prominent nucleoli, and tumor diathesis (Fig. 7.5).

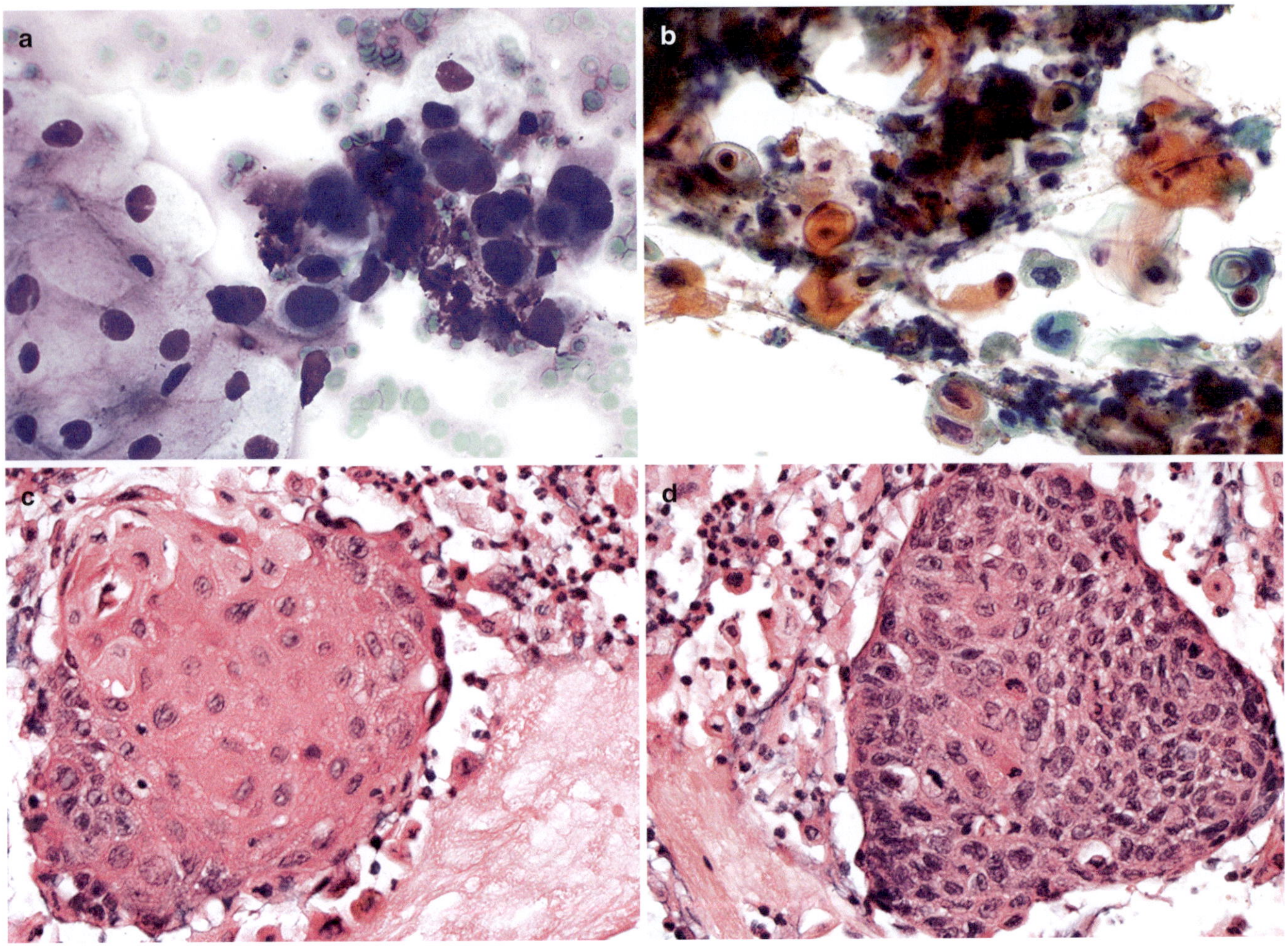

Fig. 7.4 Pathology of keratinizing squamous cell carcinoma of the esophagus. (**a**, **b**) FNA cytology, Diff-Quik stain (**a**) and Papanicolaou stain (**b**), 600×. (**c**, **d**) Cell block histology, hematoxylin and eosin stain, 400×

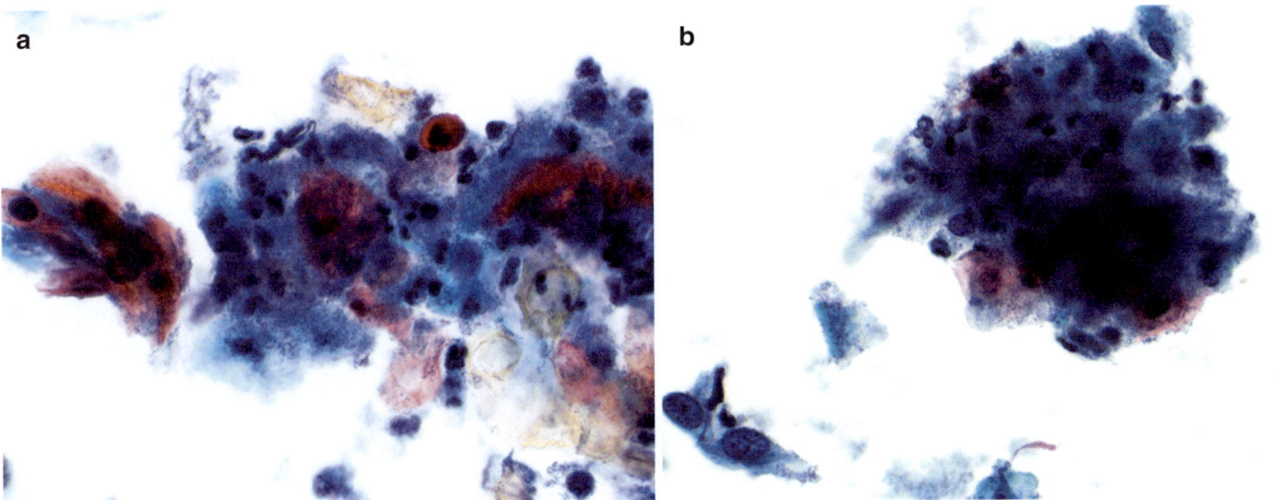

Fig. 7.5 Cytology of squamous cell carcinoma in anal Pap test, Papanicolaou-stained Thinprep slide, 600 ×

Gross

- Most commonly circumferential; often ulcerated lesions with sharply demarcated margins. Polypoid forms are less common.
- On cut surface grayish-white tumor invades the esophageal wall and in advanced cases invades surrounding structures.

Histology of Core and Cell Block

- Well-differentiated tumors show nests of polygonal epithelial cells with eosinophilic cytoplasm, intercellular bridges with keratinization, and rare basaloid cells (Fig. 7.4c).
- Moderately differentiated tumors contain a higher proportion of primitive basaloid cells arranged in irregular nests and trabeculae with focal keratinization (Fig. 7.4d).
- Poorly differentiated tumors show no evidence of keratinization and grow in solid sheets or single cells. Large bizarre pleomorphic cells may be present.
- Variants of SCC:
  - Basaloid SCC: cohesive three-dimensional clusters of cells with basaloid appearance (small, round to oval hyperchromatic nuclei and scant cytoplasm), with peripheral palisading and focal mucin secretion or focal squamous differentiation.
  - Spindle cell squamous cell carcinoma: frankly malignant mesenchymal and spindle-shaped non-keratinizing squamous cells.
  - Verrucous SCC: A type of well-differentiated SCC.
  - Lymphoepithelioma-like carcinoma.

Comments

- **Differential Diagnosis**
  - In situ neoplasia (dysplasia)
  - Pseudoepitheliomatous hyperplasia
  - Pseudodiverticulosis
  - Chemotherapy-related changes
  - Melanoma (in differential diagnosis of poorly differentiated SCC)
  - Lymphoma (in differential diagnosis of poorly differentiated SCC)
- **Immunohistochemistry**
  - Immunoreactive: cytokeratins (AE1:AE3, Cam 5.2), p63, p40, vimentin (some tumors), epidermal growth factor receptor (EGFR), cyclin D1, p16, and p53 expression.
  - Immunonegative: cytokeratin 7 (only 29% are positive), cytokeratin 20.
  - HPV tests for anal SCC and some esophageal SCC.

Adenocarcinoma of the Intestinal Tract

FNA cytology is mainly used for staging of tumors. Biopsy under endoscopy is used for diagnosis. The cytomorphology is similar to that seen in the intestinal type of gastric adenocarcinoma, often with a necrotic background.

Neuroendocrine Neoplasm

Low-Grade Neuroendocrine Neoplasm (Carcinoid)

Clinical

- Neuroendocrine neoplasm represents 2% of all tumors in the gastrointestinal tract.
- The ileum, appendix, and rectum are the most common sites.
- Presents with abdominal pain, nausea, diarrhea, weight loss, and in 10% with carcinoid syndrome (flushing, diarrhea, asthma, and tricuspid regurgitation).
- Better prognosis than gastrointestinal adenocarcinoma, gastrointestinal stromal tumor (GIST), or lymphoma.
  - Stomach:

  Three main types:
- Type I
  - Associated with autoimmune chronic atrophic gastritis and achlorhydria.
  - Located in body/ fundus and presents as small, circumscribed nodules.
- Type II
  - Associated with Zollinger-Ellison syndrome, hypertrophic, hypersecretory, and gastropathies.
  - Male-to-female ratio of 1:1.
- Type III
  - Sporadic.
  - Male-to-female ratio of 2.8:1.
  - Located in body fundus, presents as a single nodule, and is larger than 2 cm in 33% of cases.
  - Small bowel:
    - The majority occur in adults with a male-to-female ratio of 1.5:1.
    - Mostly located in the ileum and multiple in 15–35% of cases.
  - Large bowel:
    - Almost never associated with carcinoid syndrome.
  - Appendix:
    - Most common tumor of appendix.
    - Peak incidence in 3rd to 4th decades of life.

Gross

- Stomach:
  - Small, sharply outlined lesions with flat mucosa.
- Small bowel:
  - May present as small sessile polyps.

- Overlying intact mucosa.
- On cross-section, bright yellow in color.
- Large bowel:
  - May present as flat or slightly elevated lesions or as polypoid masses.
  - May be large and extend deeply through the bowel wall and spread to regional lymph nodes.
  - On cross-section, bright yellow in color.
- Appendix:
  - Firm, grayish-white well-circumscribed lesions with no capsule.

Cytology of FNA and Touch Preparation

- Cellular smears composed of small uniform cells, singly and in loosely cohesive clusters.
- Cells have high N/C ratio, delicate or granular cytoplasm, and round to slightly oval nucleus with stippled or fine granular chromatin.
- Mitosis is uncommon, and necrosis is not present.

Histology of Core and Cell Block

- Stomach
  - Macroglandular and trabecular or insular (rarely) pattern.
  - Round to polygonal cells with ill-defined cell outlines and round, monotonous-appearing nucleus with finely stippled chromatin and small nucleoli.
  - May have plasmacytoid or spindle cell features.
  - Rare mitosis, absent necrosis, and florid vascularization.
  - Three main types:
    - Type I
      - Small cells with monotonous nuclei, inconspicuous nucleoli, and fairly eosinophilic cytoplasm in microtubular-trabecular arrangement.
    - Type II
      - Grossly thickened gastric wall.
    - Type III
      - Located in body fundus, present as a single nodule, and larger than 2 cm in 33% of cases.
- Appendix:
  - Classic (insular) type: solid nests of small monotonous cells with occasional rosettes and acini.
  - Adenocarcinoid: tubular type or goblet cell type.

Comments

- **Differential Diagnosis**
  - Undifferentiated small cell carcinoma
  - Lymphoma
  - Poorly differentiated carcinoma
- **Immunohistochemistry**
  - Positive: Neuron-specific enolase (NSE), chromogranin, synaptophysin, CDX2 [24], and cytokeratins.
  - Negative: TTF-1 [24] and S-100 (except appendix).

High Grade Neuroendocrine Carcinoma

High grade neuroendocrine carcinoma includes large cell neuroendocrine carcinoma and small cell carcinoma.

Clinical

- Most common in esophagus, especially distal half.
- Male to female ratio of 2:1.
- Patient presents with weight loss and dysphagia.

Gross

- Large polypoid, fungating mass or ulcerating, stenotic lesion

Cytology of FNA and Touch Preparation

- As described in Chap. 3, Lung, Mediastinum, and Pleura.

Histology of Core and Cell Block

- As described in Chap. 3, Lung, Mediastinum, and Pleura.

Comments

- **Differential Diagnosis**
  - As described in Chap. 3, Lung, Mediastinum, and Pleura.
- **Immunohistochemistry**
  - As described in Chap. 3, Lung, Mediastinum, and Pleura.

Mesenchymal Neoplasms

Gastrointestinal Stroma Tumor (GIST)

Clinical

- Found in middle-aged and elderly individuals.
- Most common site is the stomach (more than 2/3 of cases), followed by the small intestine, mostly in the duodenum (1/3 of cases). Only 10% of cases arise in the esophagus, colon, and anorectum.
- No sex predilection except for the rare gastric epithelioid tumors arising mostly in females with Carney triad, and in the esophagus where there is a slight male predominance.
- Symptoms depend on the size and location of the tumor:
  - Mostly asymptomatic.
  - May present with abdominal pain or bleeding, nausea, vomiting, weight loss, and an abdominal mass.

Radiology

US

- GISTs often demonstrate heterogeneous echogenicity owing to areas of tumor necrosis. Because of their typically large size at the time of presentation, identification of the organ of origin is often difficult.

CT

- GISTs are usually intraluminal or exophytic and often well marginated.
- Small tumors demonstrate soft-tissue density on non–contrast images with homogeneous enhancement following contrast administration, although enhancement is typically less than that for normal liver parenchyma.
- Large tumors have variable density with heterogeneous enhancement caused by tumor necrosis, which may appear as cystic change, foci of gas, or calcifications (Fig. 7.6a) [25, 26].

Gross

- Most GISTs are well-circumscribed lesions located in submucosa or the muscularis propria.
- The overlying mucosa is either intact or ulcerated.
- The cut surface is often granular with areas of hemorrhage, necrosis, and cystic change.

Cytology of FNA and Touch Preparation

- Moderate to low cellularity.
- Single cells or small aggregate of cells with spindle or ovoid nuclei and delicate scant to moderate cytoplasm with poorly defined borders (Fig. 7.6b, c).

Histology of Core and Cell Block

Based on morphology, the majority of cases fall into one of the three categories:

- Spindle cell type (70%) (Fig. 7.6d):
  - Cells are arranged in fascicles with frequent nuclear palisading and prominent perinuclear vacuoles (fixation artifact) separated by hyalinized stroma.
  - Densely cellular spindle cells with uniform nuclei with evenly distributed chromatin and abundant eosinophilic to pale cytoplasm.
- Epithelioid type (20%) (Fig. 7.6e):
  - Most common in stomach.
  - Cells contain rim of condensed cytoplasm around the nucleus with peripheral cytoplasmic clearing.
  - Composed of sheets of epithelioid cells with round nuclei and small nucleoli.
- Mixed type (5%):
  - Consisting of both spindle and epithelioid tumor cells.

Risk for aggressive behavior is estimated based on the size, location, and mitotic count:

- Very low risk: <2 cm and <5 mitosis/50 high-power fields (HPFs).
- Low risk: 2–5 cm and <5 mitosis/50 HPFs.
- Intermediate risk: <5 cm with 6–10 mitosis/50 HPs, or 5–10 cm with <5 mitosis/50 HPFs.
- High risk: >5 cm with >5 mitosis/50 HPFs, >10 cm with any mitotic rate, or any size with >10 mitosis/50 HPFs.

Comments

- **Differential Diagnosis**
  - Smooth muscle or smooth muscle tumor (leiomyoma, leiomyosarcoma).
  - Neural tumors (schwannoma)
  - Fibromatosis.
- **Immunohistochemistry**
  - Positive: CD117 (C-kit) (Fig. 7.6f), DOG1 (Fig. 7.6g), CD 34 (70%), α-smooth muscle actin (30–40%).
  - Negative: Desmin (less than 10% stain positive), S-100 (less than 10% focally positive).

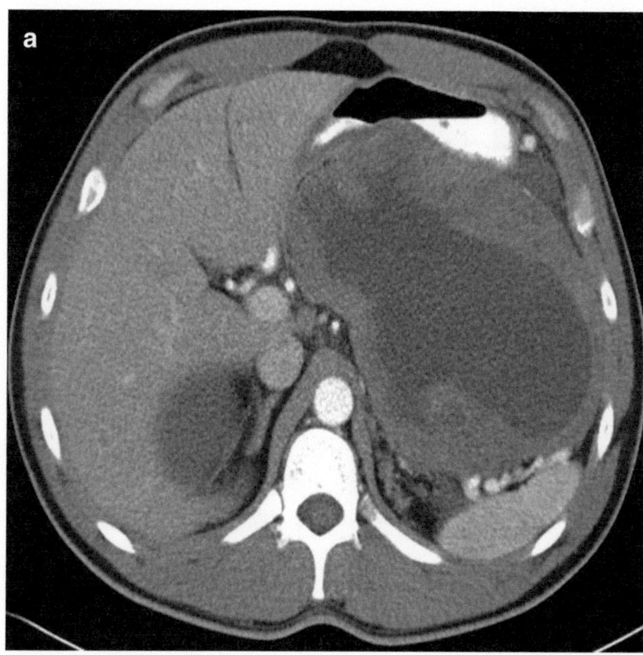

Fig. 7.6 (**a**) Contrast-enhanced CT of GIST demonstrating a large, heterogeneous mass arising from the posterior stomach. Fluid attenuation centrally indicates tumor necrosis. (**b–g**) Pathology of GIST. (**b, c**) FNA cytology, Diff-Quik stain, 600×. (**d, e**) Core and cell block histology, H&E stain, 400× and 600×, respectively. (**f, g**) Immunostains for CD117 (**f**) and Dog1 (**g**), 600 ×

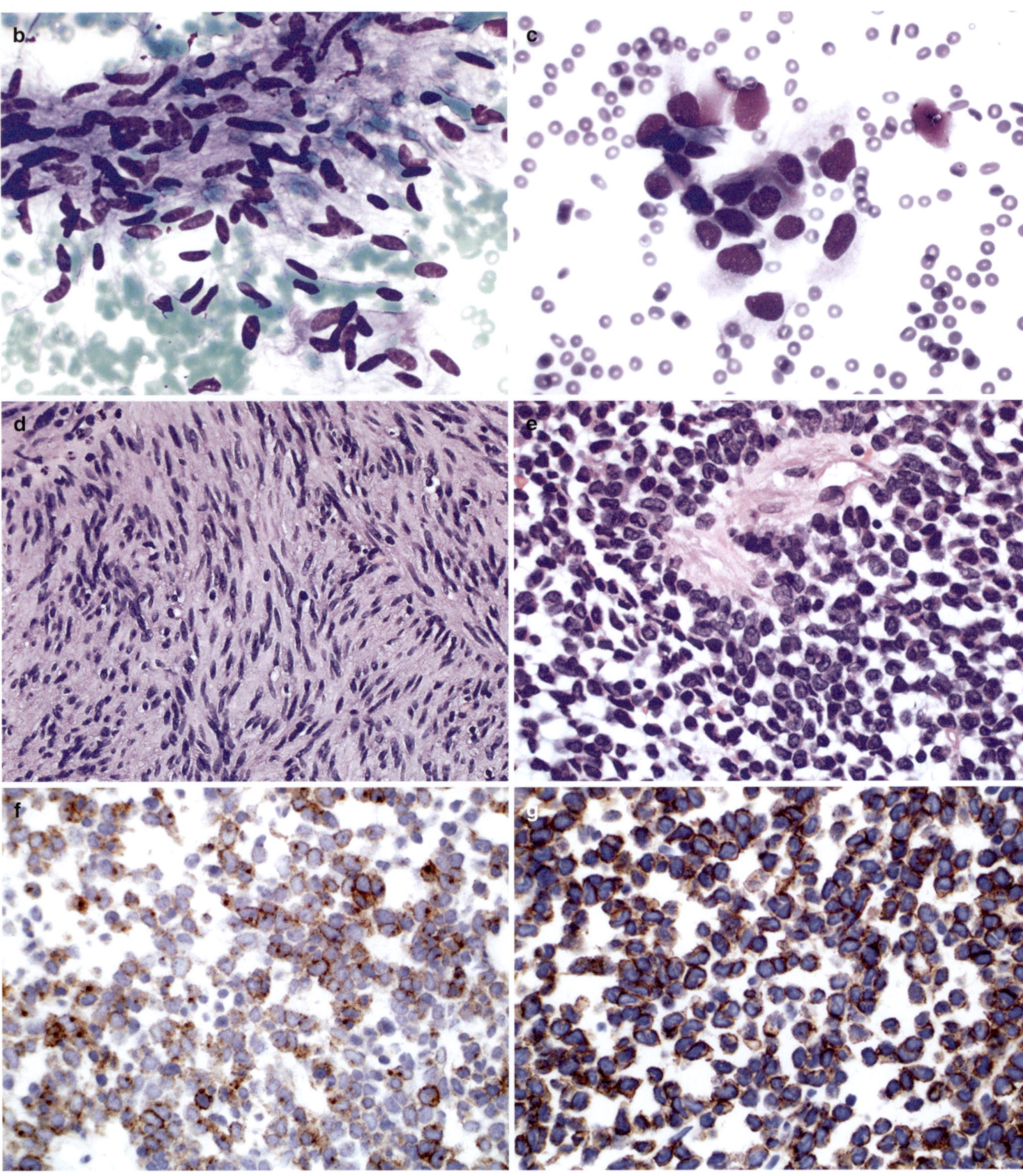

Fig. 7.6 (continued)

Leiomyoma

Clinical

- Occurs mostly at esophagus and colorectum; very rare in stomach and small bowel.
- Most common benign tumor of esophagus, especially lower esophagus.
- Males > females (2:1).
- Asymptomatic or present with dysphagia.

Gross

- Intramural sessile lesion; less commonly present as a polypoid mass.
- Up to 10 cm in diameter (usually 2–3 cm).
- Solid, gray-white on cross-section; well circumscribed.

Cytology of FNA and Touch Preparation

- Fragments of tissue composed of bland spindle-shaped cells of low or moderate cellularity.
- The cells contain cigar-shaped nuclei and eosinophilic cytoplasm with indistinct cell borders.

Histology of Core and Cell Block

- Mature-appearing smooth muscle cells arranged in fascicles and whorls.
- Absent or rare mitosis.

Comments

- **Differential Diagnosis**
  - Leiomyosarcoma.
  - GIST.
- **Immunohistochemistry**
  - Positive: α-smooth muscle actin, desmin, and caldesmon.
  - Negative: CD117 (C-kit).

Granular Cell Tumor

Clinical

- Predominantly in distal esophagus.
- Benign behavior; however, rare malignant esophageal granular cell tumors have been reported.

Gross

- 1–2 cm in diameter, firm yellow nodules or small sessile polyps.
- Mostly located in submucosa.

Cytology of FNA and Touch Preparation

- Loosely cohesive large round cells with abundant granular cytoplasm and small, uniform, eccentrically located nuclei (Fig. 7.7a, b).

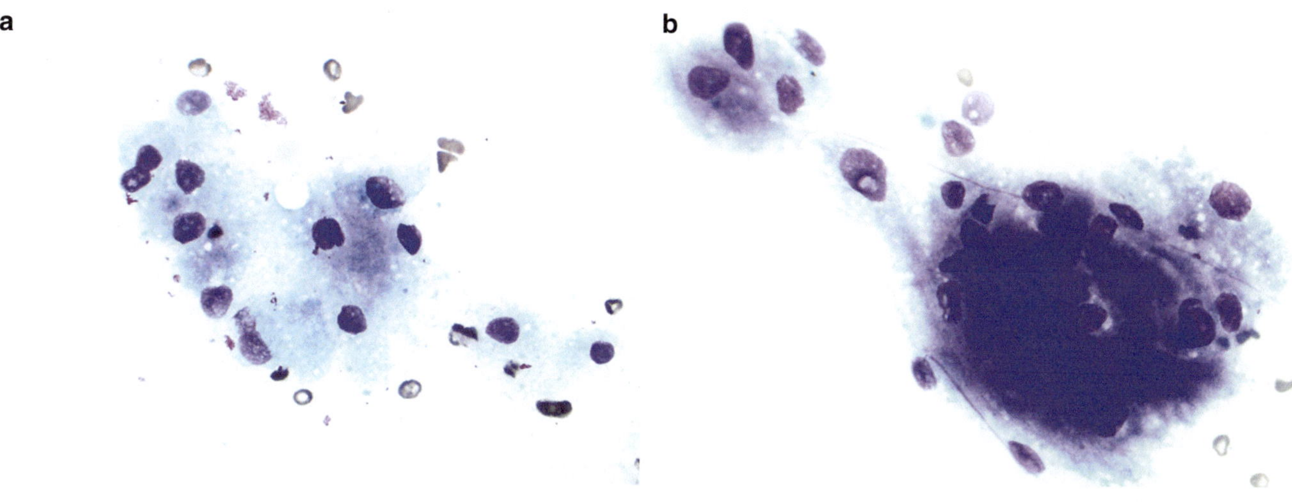

Fig. 7.7 Pathology of granular cell tumor. (**a**, **b**) Touch preparation cytology of core, Diff-Quik stain, 600×. (**c**) Histology of core, H&E stain, 600×. (**d**) Immunostain for S100, 600×

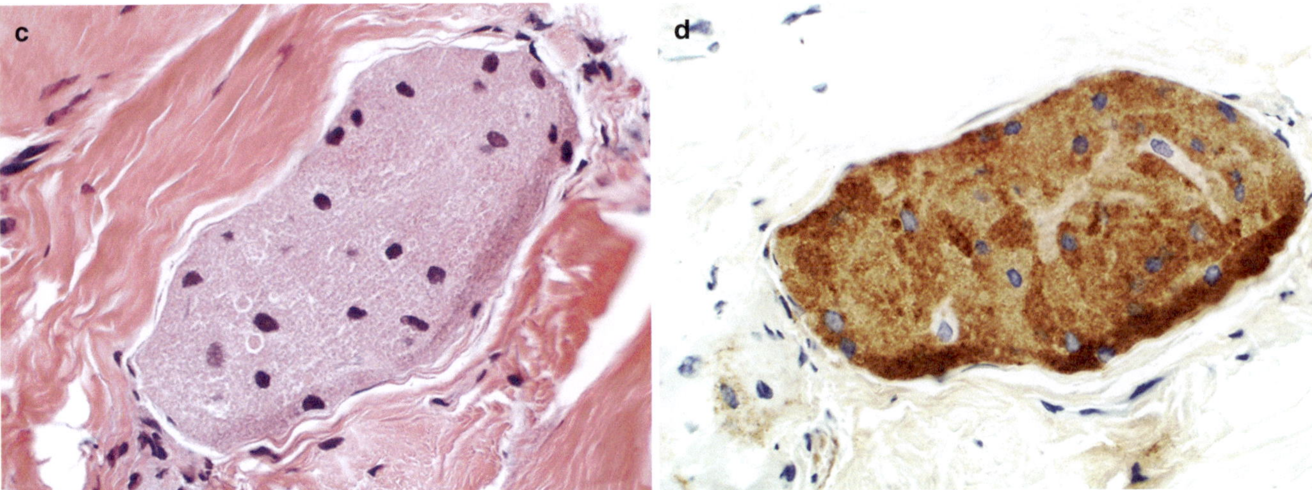

Fig. 7.7 (continued)

Histology of Core and Cell Block

- Sheets of oval to large polygonal cells with small central nucleus and abundant granular cytoplasm (Fig. 7.7c).

Immunohistochemistry

- Positive: S-100 (Fig. 7.7d).
  - Negative: Desmin, actin, CD 34, and CD117 (C-kit).

Lymphoid Tumors

Clinical

- Gastrointestinal tract lymphomas account for 4–18% of all non-Hodgkin lymphomas in Western countries, 25% of cases in the Middle East, and 10% of all gastric malignancies [27]. The stomach is most common site of primary gastrointestinal lymphoma (55–65%), followed by the small bowel and colon.
- Predisposing factors are infections (especially with *Helicobacter pylori*), celiac disease, inflammatory bowel disease, and immune deficiency syndromes [27].
- Mostly common are diffuse large B-cell lymphomas, some of which develop through progression from low grade lymphomas of mucosa associated lymphoid tissue (MALT) [27].
- Present with abdominal pain, weight loss, obstruction, or as a palpable mass.
  - Marginal zone B-cell lymphoma:
    - Women and men equally affected.
    - 88% confined to the stomach, mostly located in distal half.
    - Occur in individuals older than 50 years.
  - Diffuse large B-cell lymphoma:
    - Older adults with slight male predominance.
    - Some arise in association with marginal zone B-cell lymphoma.

Gross

- Marginal zone B-cell lymphoma:
  - Presents as erosions, shallow ulcers, mucosal granularity, thickened mucosal folds, or as diffusely infiltrative and ill-defined lesions.
  - Most are confined to the mucosa and submucosa.
- Diffuse large B-cell lymphoma:
  - Usually solitary but can be multiple.
  - Can present as large ulcerated or exophytic lesions.

Cytology of FNA and Touch Preparation

- Marginal zone B-cell lymphoma:
  - Small to medium-sized lymphocytes with slightly irregular nuclear membranes.
  - Tissue fragments (mostly present in cell block) showing infiltrate of lymphocytes and infiltration of the glands by lymphocytes (lymphoepithelial lesions).
- Diffuse large B-cell lymphoma:
  - Large lymphoid cells with irregular or lobulated nuclear membrane and thin rim of cytoplasm.

Histology of Core and Cell Block

- Marginal zone B-cell lymphoma:
  - Gastric glands may be infiltrated by lymphocytes, forming lymphoepithelial lesions.
  - Diffuse or vaguely nodular pattern.
  - Composed of monotonous to polymorphic, small to medium-sized lymphoid cells with slight nuclear membrane irregularities, possibly containing nuclear Dutcher bodies seen in one third of cases; scant to abundant cytoplasm, some showing plasmacytoid or monocytoid forms [28, 29].

- Diffuse large B-cell lymphoma:
  - Diffuse population of large atypical lymphoid cells with round, oval, irregular, or lobulated nuclei containing vesicular chromatin, one or multiple prominent nucleoli, and a moderate amount of cytoplasm.
  - Necrosis, mitoses, DNA strings, and apoptotic figures may be seen.

Comments

- **Differential Diagnosis**
  - Marginal zone B-cell lymphoma:
    - Gastritis.
    - Other low-grade lymphomas.
  - Diffuse large B-cell lymphoma:
    - Poorly differentiated carcinoma.
- **Immunohistochemistry and Flow Cytometry**
  - Marginal zone B-cell lymphoma:
    - Positive: CD20, BCL2, CD19, CD79a, PAX5, and CD43.
    - Positive for kappa or lambda light chain restriction.
    - Negative: CD5, CD10, and CD43.
  - Diffuse large B-cell lymphoma:
    - Positive: CD20, CD19, CD79a, PAX5, and CD43 (50% of cases), and possibly positive for CD10 and BCL6.
    - Possibly showing kappa or lambda light chain restriction.
  - Fluorescence in situ hybridization (FISH)
    - MALT: t11:18(q21:q21).

Pancreas

Pancreatitis

Clinical

- Progressive inflammatory disease of pancreas, caused by alcohol consumption in 70% of cases, idiopathic chronic pancreatitis (second most common type), gallstones.
- Most common in men.
- Characterized by a clinical triad: diabetes, steatorrhea, radiographic evidence of calcification.
- Elevated risk for pancreatic adenocarcinoma.

Radiology

US

- The pancreas is often poorly visualized with ultrasound because of overlying bowel gas.
- Diffuse enlargement and hypoechogenicity of the gland indicate edema, while peripancreatic fluid collections may indicate more severe disease.

CT

- Acute pancreatitis presents as focal or diffuse enlargement of the pancreas with surrounding inflammatory changes and obliteration of fat planes.
- Areas of pancreatic nonenhancement following bolus contrast administration indicate ischemia or necrosis.
- Chronic pancreatitis often shows pancreatic atrophy with main pancreatic ductal dilatation and coarse calcifications (Fig. 7.8a).

MRI

- MRI is useful to define subtle, focal, and diffuse pancreatic abnormalities with T1 fat-suppressed images. T2-weighted images help identify fluid collections and pseudocysts. Contrast-enhanced MRI also accurately depicts areas of necrosis as nonenhancement [30].

Gross

- Involves pancreas in focal, segmental, or diffuse pattern.
- Involved areas are enlarged and hard as a result of fibrosis.
- In advanced stage, the pancreas is hard and shrunken because of atrophy.

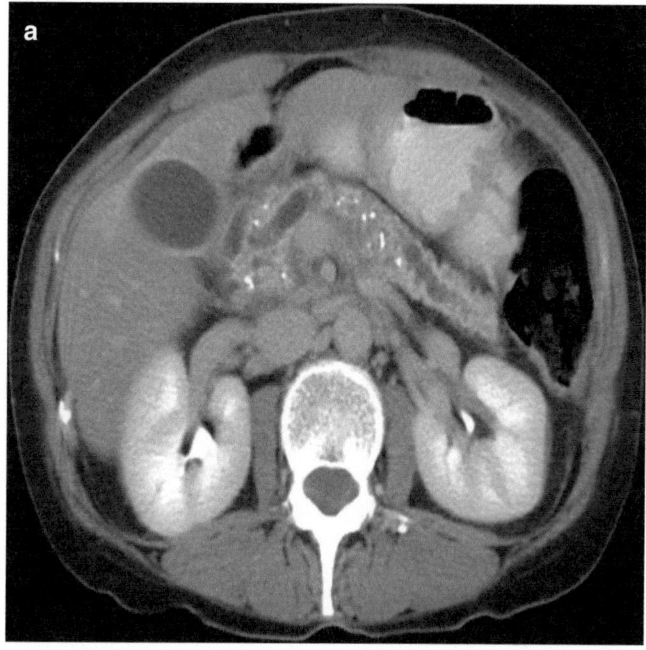

Fig. 7.8 (**a**) CT scan of chronic pancreatitis. Atrophic pancreas with marked dilatation of the main pancreatic duct and scattered coarse calcifications. (**b**, **e**) Cytology of chronic pancreatitis. EUS-FNA smear cytology, Diff-Quik stain, 400× (**b**, **d**) and 600× (**c**, **e**)

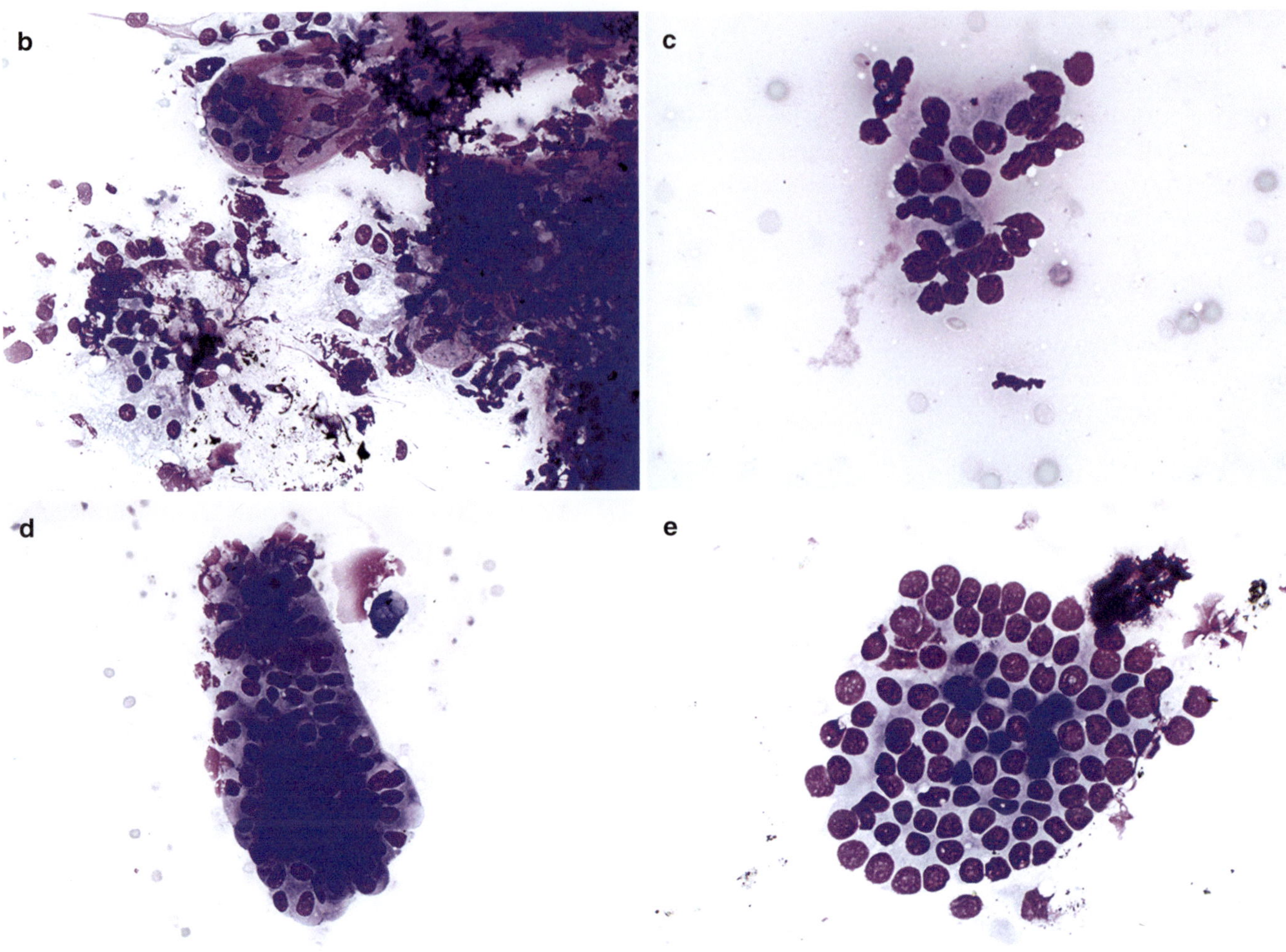

Fig. 7.8 (continued)

Cytology of FNA and Touch Preparation

- Scant to moderate cellularity consisting of lymphocytes, neutrophils, and macrophages (Fig. 7.8b).
- Ductal epithelium that may show different degrees of reactive/atypical changes and few acinar cells (Fig. 7.8d, e), and islet cells (Fig. 7.8c).
- Fragments of fibrotic tissue (Fig. 7.8b).

Histology of Core and Cell Block

- Normal lobular architecture of the acini is preserved with irregular loss of acinar tissue.
- Variable amount of chronic inflammation and fibrosis.

Differential Diagnosis

- Ductal adenocarcinoma.

Pseudocyst

Clinical

- Most common type of cystic lesion in the pancreas as result of pancreatitis.
- Presents with abdominal pain, which may resolve spontaneously, remain stable, or grow in size.
- Complications include infection, hemorrhage, rupture, or obstruction.

Radiology

CT and MRI

- Pancreatic pseudocysts may be seen as peripancreatic fluid collections with either a thin, nearly imperceptible wall or a uniformly thick, enhancing fibrous capsule.

- Pseudocyst contents should not enhance. While a history of prior pancreatitis can aid in the diagnosis, neither CT nor MRI can definitively differentiate a pseudocyst from a cystic pancreatic neoplasm [31].

Gross

- Unilocular lesion mostly located in body and tail and with rough inner surface and thick wall.
- Contents can be clear or bloody.

Cytology of FNA and Touch Preparation

- Cyst contents composed of inflammatory cells, foamy macrophages, necrotic debris, blood, calcifications, and yellow hematoidin pigment (Fig. 7.9a–f).
- Small fragments of fibrous tissue containing bland spindle cells and inflammatory cells.

Histology of Core and Cell Block

- Cyst lined by granulation tissue and inflammatory cells and lacking epithelial lining.

Comments

- **Differential Diagnosis**
  - Other types of neoplastic or non-neoplastic cysts.
  - Pancreatic abscess.
- **Ancillary Test**
  - Elevated cyst fluid amylase levels.
  - Low cyst fluid carcinoembryonic antigen (CEA).

Carcinoma

Pancreatic Ductal Adenocarcinoma

Clinical

- Accounts for 85% of all pancreatic malignant tumors and is the fourth most common cancer-related cause of death in the U.S [32].
- 10% show familiar aggregation.
- Mostly elderly patients with a M:F ratio of 1.6:1.
- Two thirds of cases located in the head of the pancreas [32].
- Multifocal in 20% of cases.

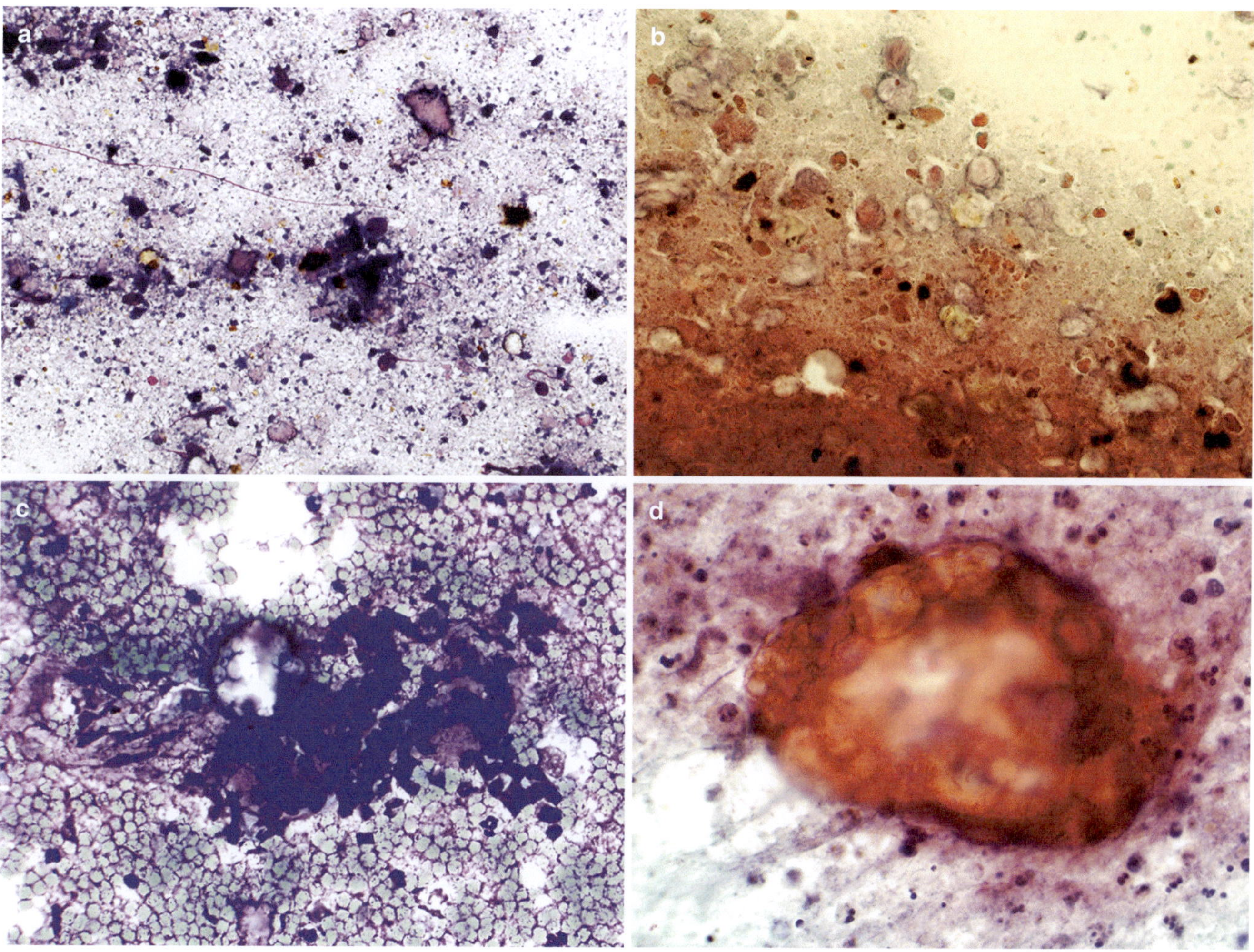

Fig. 7.9 Cytology of pseudocyst. (**a**) EUS-FNA smear cytology, Diff-Quik stain (**a**, **c**, **e**) and Papanicolaou stain (**b**, **d**, **f**), 400× (**a**, **b**) and 600× (**b**–**e**)

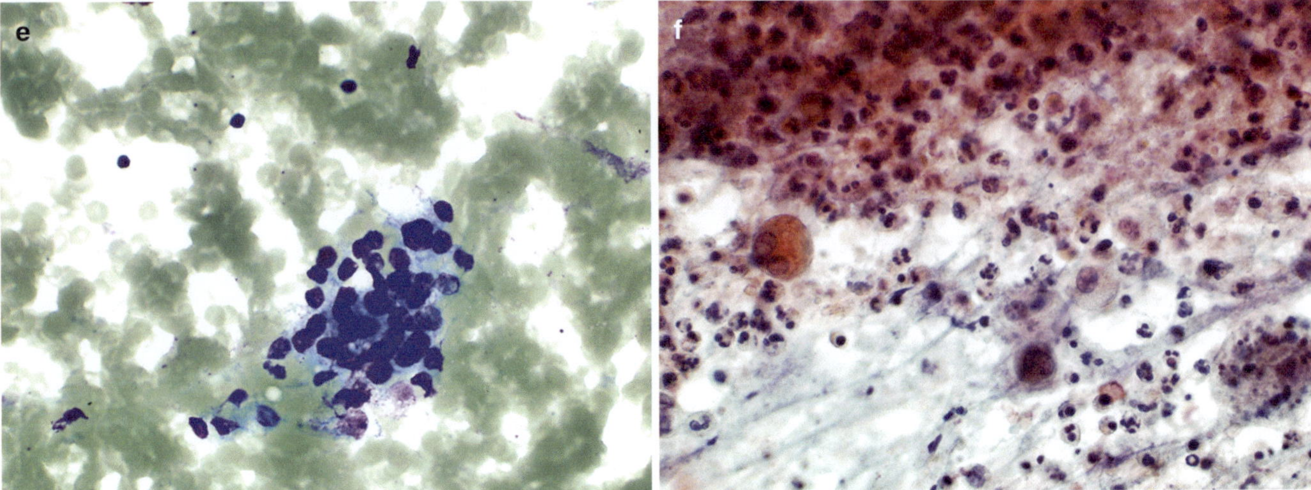

Fig. 7.9 (continued)

Radiology

CT

- Pancreatic ductal carcinoma presents as a focal, nonenhancing, or heterogeneously enhancing mass.
- Local extension into surrounding organs and vasculature at the time of initial imaging is not uncommon.
- Secondary signs of a pancreatic ductal carcinoma include both main pancreatic and biliary ductal dilatation as well as focal pancreatic atrophy.

MRI

- On fat-suppressed T1-weighted MRI, pancreatic ductal carcinoma appears hypointense relative to the normally bright pancreatic tissue.
- Tumors may be most conspicuous as areas of hypo- or nonenhancement on the arterial phase of contrast with progressive enhancement on delayed phases [33].

Gross

- Poorly delineated, firm with yellow-gray cut surface.
- Rarely undergoes cystic degeneration.

Cytology of FNA and Touch Preparation

- The needle can be guided with a variety of diagnostic imaging techniques, including endoscopic retrograde cholangiopancreatography (ERCP), percutaneous transhepatic cholangiography (PTC), ultrasound, CT and MRI. Endoscopic ultrasound-guided fine needle aspiration (EUS-FNA) has provided significant improvements in locoregional staging for pancreatic adenocarcinoma with higher sensitivity and specificity [34].
- Cellular specimen consisting of single cells, "drunken honeycomb" sheets, or loosely cohesive two- or three-dimensional glandular clusters of pleomorphic polygonal, cuboidal, or columnar cells with loss of polarity (Fig. 7.10a–d).
- The nuclei are enlarged and pleomorphic, show irregular and thickened nuclear membranes, and contain hyperchromatic, coarse, or vesicular unevenly distributed chromatin and prominent nucleoli.
- The cytoplasm is delicate, vacuolated, or squamoid, is variable in amount, and may contain mucin.
- Bizarre cells, signet-ring cells, bi- or multinucleated cells, osteoclast-like giant cells, mitoses, necrosis, and mucin can be seen.

Histology of Core and Cell Block

- Infiltrating irregular glands with pleomorphic cuboidal to columnar cells with hyperchromatic nuclei containing prominent nucleoli, irregular nuclear membranes, and scant to abundant delicate or vacuolated cytoplasm (Fig. 7.10e, f).
- Subtypes:
  - Adenosquamous carcinoma.
  - Oncocytic carcinoma.
  - Clear cell carcinoma.
  - Hepatoid carcinoma.
  - Signet-ring carcinoma.
  - Mucinous (colloid) carcinoma.
  - Giant cell carcinoma.

Comments

- **Differential Diagnosis**
  - Chronic pancreatitis.
- **Immunohistochemistry**
  - Positive: CK7 and MUC 1 (>60% of cases). Rare cases positive for CK20 and CDX2.

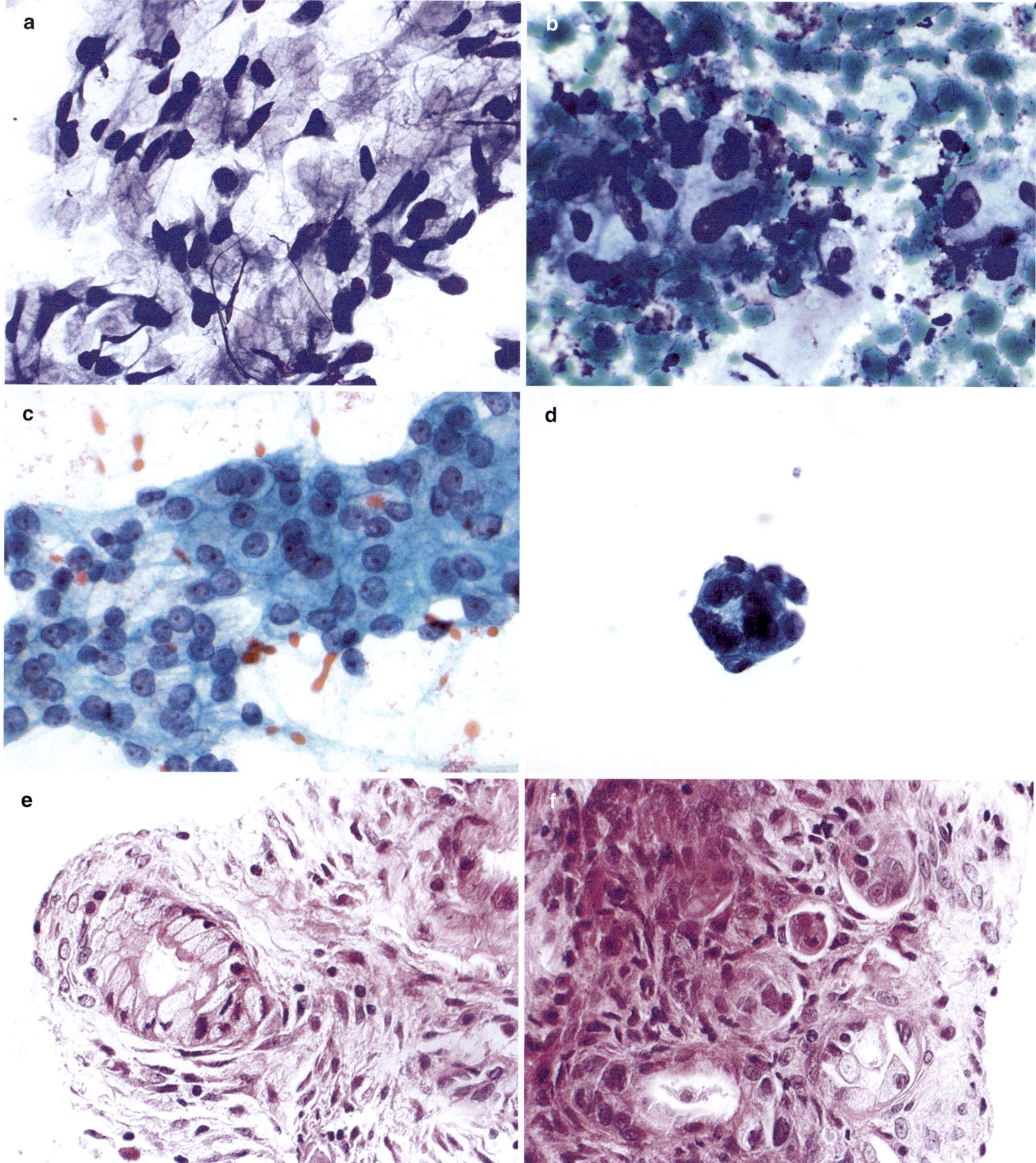

Fig. 7.10 Pathology of pancreatic ductal adenocarcinoma. (**a–d**) FNA cytomorphology, Diff-Quik stain (**a**, **b**) and Papanicolaou stain (**c**, **d**), 600×. (**e**, **f**) Histology of core, H&E stain, 600×

Acinar Cell Carcinoma

Clinical

- Accounts for 1–2% of all exocrine pancreatic neoplasms. Usually occurs in adults (mean age of 62 years old); can also occur in children.
- May arise in any portion of the pancreas [35].
- Intra-abdominal mass with or without jaundice.
- In some cases, widespread subcutaneous necrosis.

Radiology

CT

- Pancreatic acinar cell carcinomas are frequently exophytic, well-demarcated, and often have a partial or complete capsule.
- Necrosis often causes heterogeneous attenuation.
- Scattered calcifications are occasionally present and associated pancreatic ductal dilatation is rare [36].

MRI

- Acinar cell carcinomas typically demonstrate relatively low T1- and slightly higher T2- signal intensity compared to normal pancreatic tissue.
- Tumor necrosis may result in decreased T1-signal intensity and increased T2-signal intensity.
- Because they are hypovascular relative to normal pancreatic tissue, pancreatic acinar cell carcinomas do not enhance following gadolinium administration [37].

Gross

- Well-circumscribed fleshy mass; the average size is 10 cm.
- Area of hemorrhage and necrosis.

Cytology of FNA and Touch Preparation

- Moderately cellular smears consisting of polygonal cells arranged in loosely cohesive irregularly shaped clusters, trabecular formations, acini, solid sheets, small glandular clusters, or as individual cells (Fig. 7.11a, b) [38, 39].
- Cells with low nuclear cytoplasmic ratio, pleomorphic nuclei containing granular or coarsely clumped chromatin and one to two prominent nucleoli, and scant to moderate amounts of granular cytoplasm.
- Scattered, strikingly large tumor cells with giant nuclei, prominent mitoses, associated necrosis, and granular background are evident.

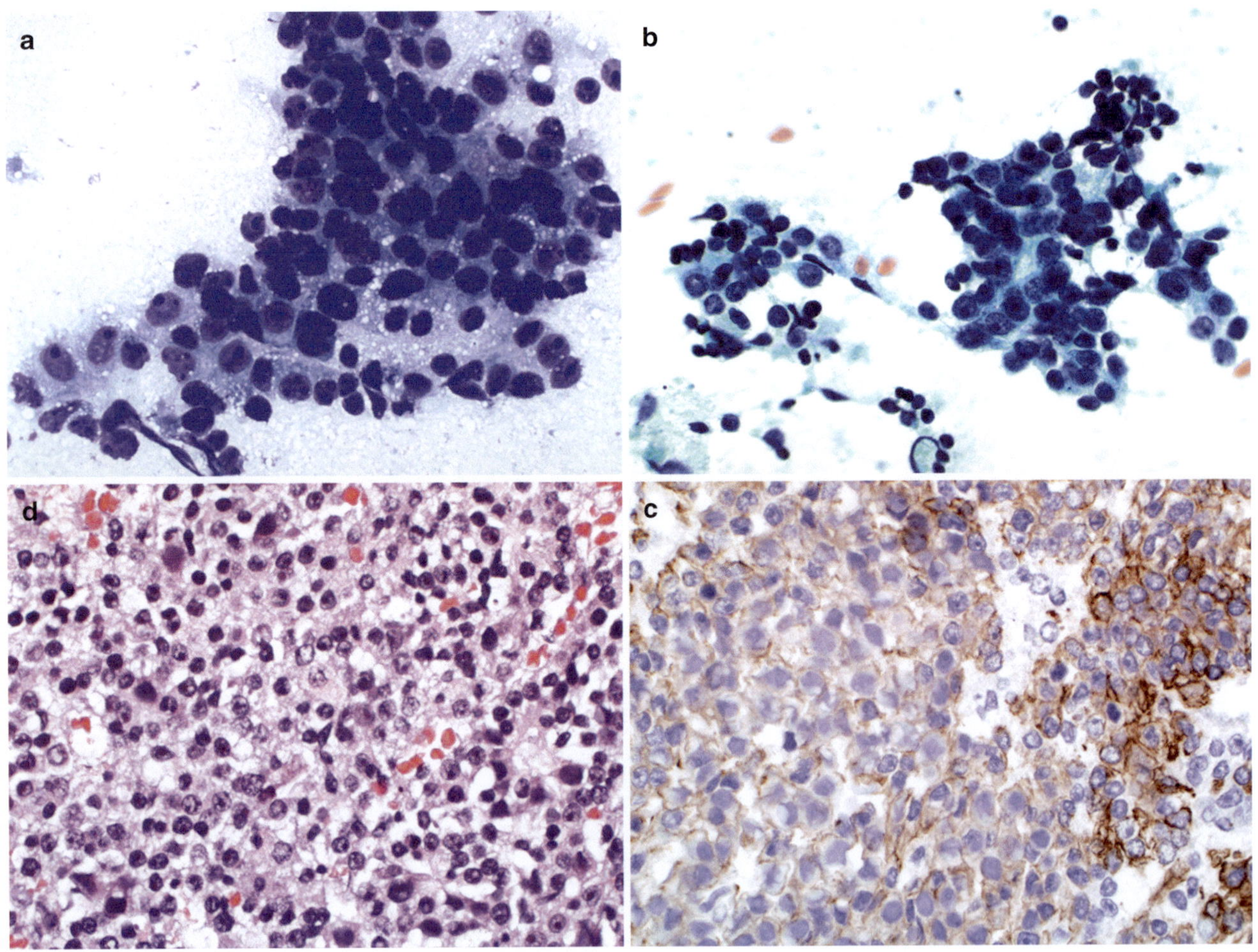

Fig. 7.11 Pathology of acinar carcinoma. (**a**, **b**) EUS-FNA cytology, Diff-Quik stain (**a**), and Papanicolaou stain (**b**), 600×. (**c**) Cell block histology, H&E stain, 600×. (**d–g**) Immunostains for AE1/AE3 (**d**), chromogranin (**e**), synaptophysin (**f**), and trypsin (**g**), 600×. Special stain for PAS-diastase, 600× (**h**)

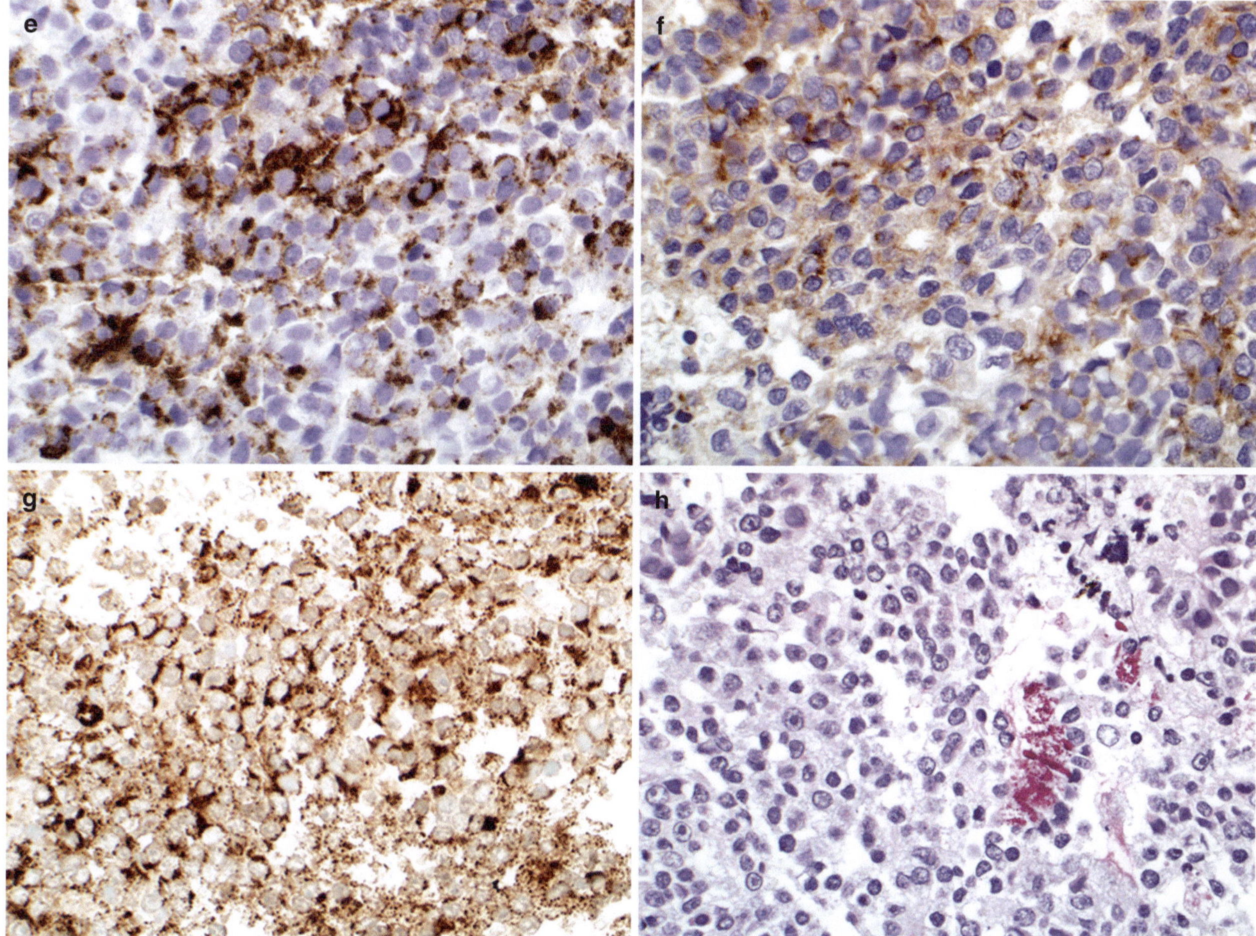

Fig. 7.11 (continued)

Histology of Core and Cell Block

- The tumor cells are arranged in solid, trabecular, or acinar arrangements with few stroma (Fig. 7.11c).
- Cellular neoplasm consisting of cuboidal cells with abundant granular cytoplasm and small round nuclei with prominent nucleoli.

Comments

- **Differential Diagnosis**
  - Well-differentiated pancreatic neuroendocrine neoplasm.
  - Solid pseudopapillary neoplasm.
  - Pancreatoblastoma.
- **Immunohistochemistry and Special Stains**
  - Positive: Trypsin (Fig. 7.11g), chymotrypsin, lipase, amylase, alpha-1-antitrypsin, alpha-1-antichymotrypsin, pan-cytokeratin (*see* Fig. 7.14d), chromogranin (1/3 of cases) (*see* Fig. 7.14e), and synaptophysin (1/3 of cases) (*see* Fig. 7.14f).
  - Negative: CK7, CK20, and CK19.
  - Positive: PAS-positive diastase-resistant cytoplasmic granules (*see* Fig. 7.14h),

Solid Pseudopapillary Neoplasm

Clinical

- Most common in the pancreatic body or tail of young women [40].
- May present as a palpable abdominal mass.
- Can rupture and present as hemoperitoneum.

Radiology

CT and MRI

- Solid pseudopapillary neoplasms often appear as large, well-circumscribed masses with a thick rim.
- CT attenuation and MRI signal intensity depend on the degree of tumor necrosis, since these tumors can range from entirely solid to mostly cystic (necrotic) in appearance [31].

Gross

- Large mass with areas of hemorrhage and necrosis.
- Surrounded by well-developed capsule in most cases.

Cytology of FNA and Touch Preparation

- Single or loosely cohesive small clusters of polygonal or plasmacytoid cells loosely attached to the capillary vessels and myxofibrous stroma (Fig. 7.12a, b) [41–43].

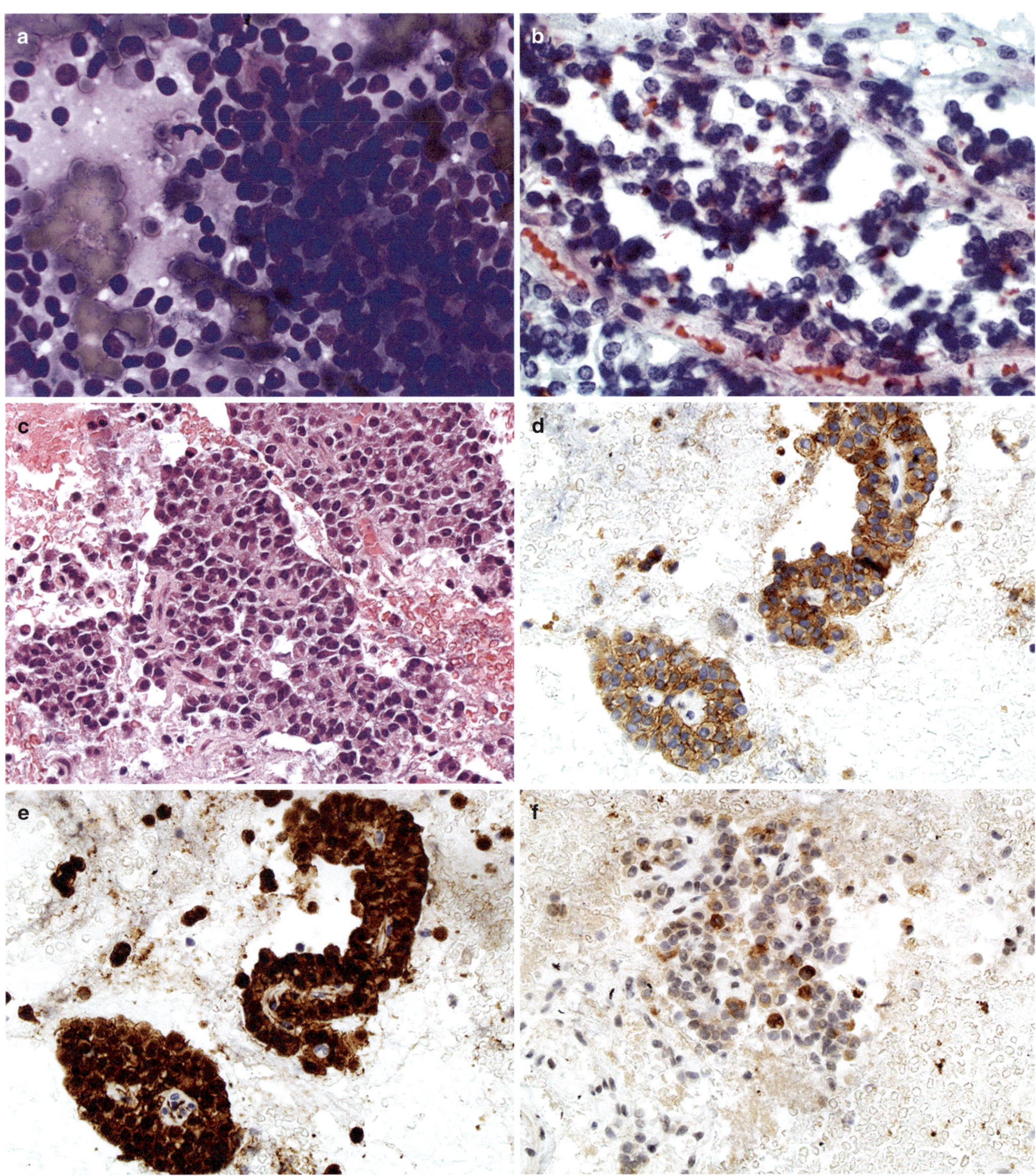

Fig. 7.12 Pathology of solid-pseudopapillary tumor. (**a**, **b**) EUS-FNA cytology, Diff-Quik stain (**a**) and Papanicolaou stain (**b**), 600×. (**c**) Cell block histology, H&E stain, 600×. (**d–f**) Immunostains for CD10 (**d**), ß-catenin (**e**), and synaptophysin (**f**), 600×

- Tumor cells are relatively uniform with scant to moderate, delicate or granular cytoplasm containing occasional small or large clear cytoplasmic vacuoles and ill-defined cytoplasmic borders.
- Round or oval nuclei containing fine, evenly distributed chromatin and small nucleoli showing smooth, regular nuclear membranes and rarely with nuclear grooves [42, 43].
- Background may be clean, hemorrhagic, or necrotic with foamy macrophages [43].

Histology of Core and Cell Block

- Composed of sheet of mostly uniform polygonal or plasmacytoid cells around capillary vessels (Fig. 7.12c).
- Cells with eosinophilic cytoplasm, often vacuolated, and round to oval nuclei with stippled chromatin and nuclear grooves.
- Some cells may contain intracytoplasmic hyaline globules.
- Mitosis and pleomorphism are uncommon.

Comments

- **Differential Diagnosis**
  - Well-differentiated pancreatic neuroendocrine tumor.
  - Acinar cell carcinoma.
- **Immunohistochemistry**
  - Positive: CD10 (*see* Fig. 7.15d), nuclear ß-catenin (*see* Fig. 7.15e), NSE, CD 56, progesterone receptor, vimentin, and α-1-antitrypsin. Also focally positive for cytokeratin, synaptophysin has variable expression (*see* Fig. 7.15f). Chromogranin is typically negative.
  - Negative: Insulin, glucagon, somatostatin, and lipase.

Neuroendocrine Tumor

Low-Grade Neuroendocrine Tumor

Clinical

- Mostly occurs in adults; few described in children.
- Typically in body and tail of pancreas.
- Can secrete hormones (functional).
- May occur as a part of MEN type I and MEN type II syndrome.

Radiology

CT

- Pancreatic neuroendocrine tumors have rich capillary networks and therefore demonstrate significant enhancement on postcontrast CT.
- Smaller tumors tend to have a homogeneous appearance, whereas larger tumors demonstrate cystic degeneration, necrosis, and calcification (Fig. 7.13a).

MRI

- On fat-suppressed T1-weighted MR images, pancreatic neuroendocrine tumors appear as well-circumscribed, hypointense lesions compared to the bright T1 signal of normal pancreatic tissue.
- On T2-weighted sequences, these tumors usually have much higher signal intensity compared to the normal pancreas, although the T2 signal can be variable (Fig. 7.13b).
- As with CT, neuroendocrine tumors demonstrate significant enhancement following gadolinium administration.

Nuclear Medicine

- Scintigraphy is useful to help diagnose a pancreatic mass as a neuroendocrine tumor provided that the tumor is well-differentiated and expresses the somatostatin receptor.
- Somatostatin-receptor scintigraphy using indium-diethylenetriaminepenta-acetic acid-octreotide 111 (^{111}In-octreotide) is the agent most commonly used and can confirm a diagnosis by demonstrating focal uptake in the region of a known pancreatic mass (Fig. 7.13c) [44].

Gross

- Pink cut surface.
- Circumscribed but does not have a well-defined capsule.

Cytology of FNA and Touch Preparation

- Hypercellular smears composed of small to medium-sized polygonal or plasmacytoid cells present singly or in loose clusters or rosettes (Fig. 7.13d, e).
- Tumor cells with round nuclei containing coarsely stippled and fine granular "salt and pepper" chromatin and inconspicuous nucleoli and minimal to moderate amounts of finely granular or delicate cytoplasm.
- Abundant naked nuclei with granular background often seen.

Histology of Core and Cell Block

- Small uniform cuboidal cells arranged in organoid growth patterns and with peripheral palisading (Fig. 7.13f).
- Tumor cells demonstrate small, round nuclei containing coarsely stippled or finely granular chromatin, smooth nuclear membranes, and acidophilic or amphophilic finely granular cytoplasm.
- Grading is based upon the mitotic count and Ki-67 index (proliferation marker).
- Perineural and vascular invasion can be seen in highly vascular stroma.

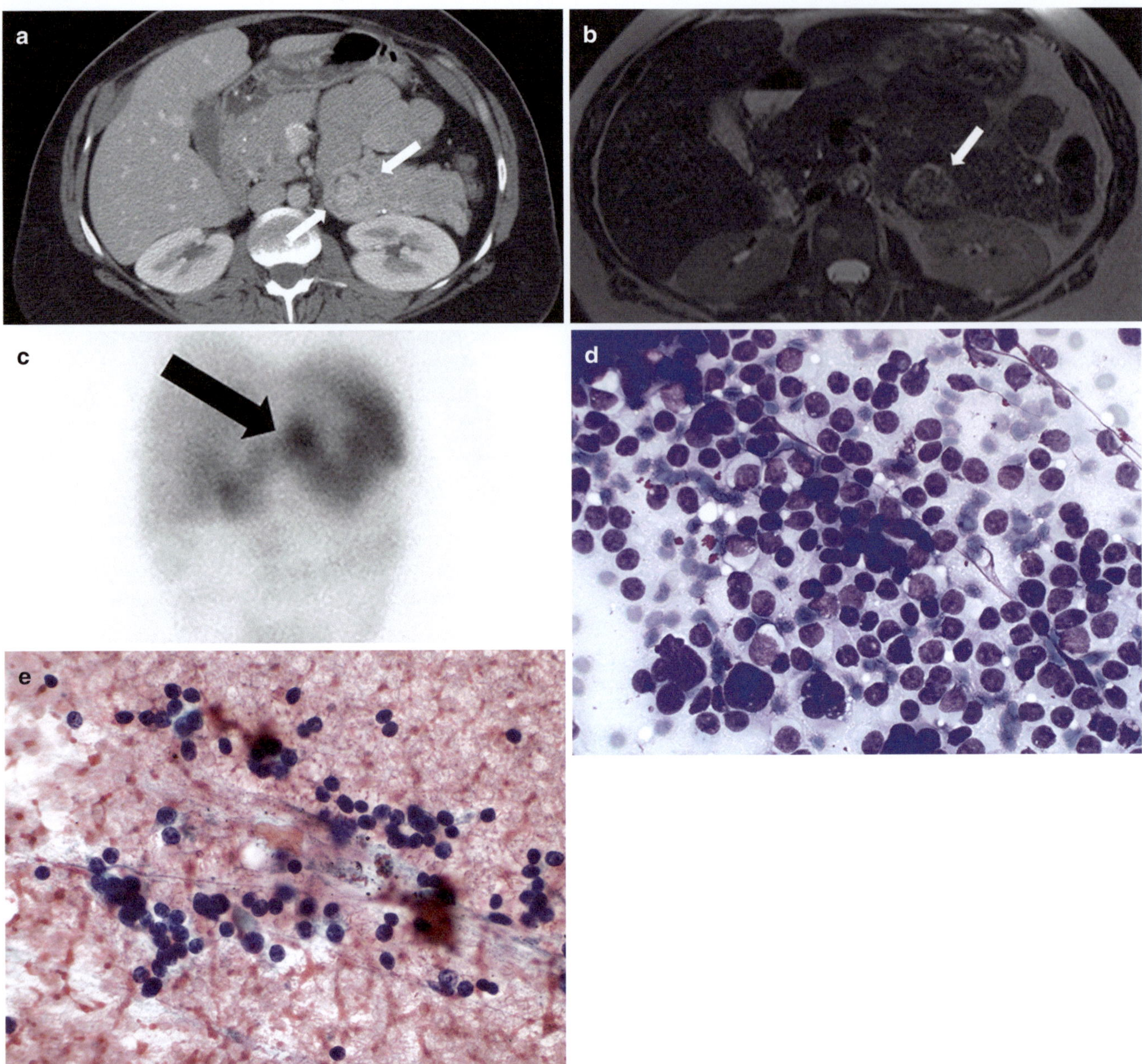

Fig. 7.13 (**a**–**c**) Pancreatic neuroendocrine tumor. (**a**) CT scan: Enhancing mass in the distal pancreas body with areas of nonenhancement consistent with tumor necrosis (*arrow*). Clinical findings and pathology were consistent with gastrinoma. (**b**) T2-weighted MRI of the same patient. The neuroendocrine tumor has a hyperintense signal compared to the normal pancreas (*arrow*). (**c**) Planar image from 111-In-octreotide study reveals uptake of the radionuclide in the region of the patient's known pancreatic mass (*arrow*). (**d**–**i**) Pathology of pancreatic low-grade neuroendocrine tumor. (**d**, **e**) EUS-FNA cytology, Diff-Quik stain (**d**), and Papanicolaou (**e**) stain, 600×. (**f**) Cell block histology, H&E stain, 600×. (**g**–**i**) Immunostains for CD56 (**g**), chromogranin (**h**), and synaptophysin (**i**), 600×

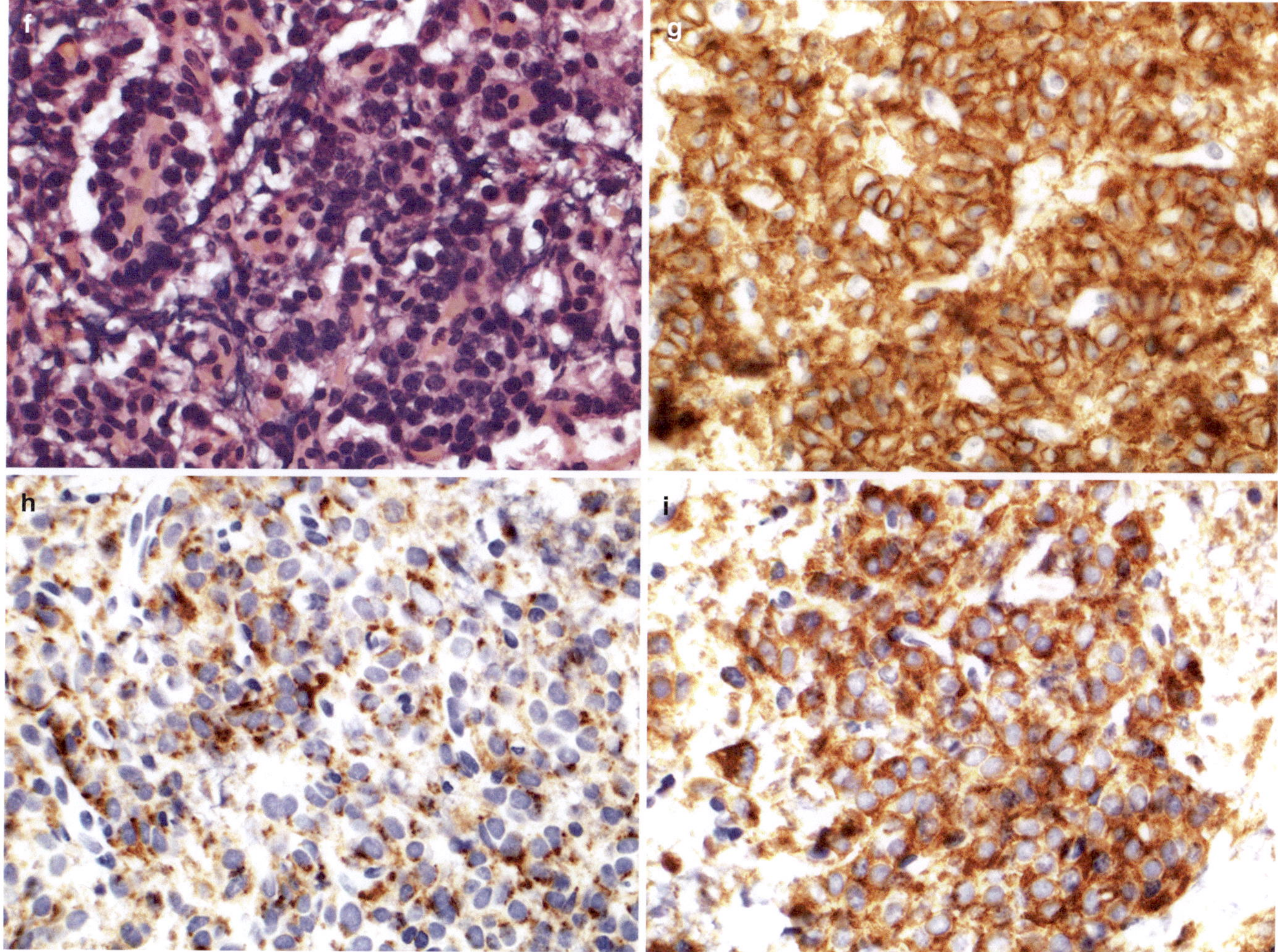

Fig. 7.13 (continued)

Comments

- **Differential Diagnosis**
  - Acinar cell carcinoma.
  - Solid-pseudopapillary neoplasm.
- **Immunohistochemistry**
  - Positive: CD56 (Fig. 7.13g), chromogranin (Fig. 7.13h), synaptophysin (Fig. 7.13i), CD57, NSE, and cytokeratin.
  - Negative: CD 10, ß-catenin, and α-1-antitrypsin.

High-Grade Neuroendocrine Carcinoma

Clinical

- Rare in pancreas.

Gross

- Solid, white to tan.
- Ill-defined borders and area of necrosis.

Cytology of FNA and Touch Preparation

- High-grade neuroendocrine carcinomas are divided into large cell neuroendocrine carcinoma and small cell carcinoma, similar to those seen in Chap. 3, Lung, Mediastinum, and Pleura.

Histology of Core and Cell Block

- Small cell type and large cell type are similar to those seen in the Chap. 3, Lung, Mediastinum, and Pleura (*see* Chap. 3).

Comments

- **Differential Diagnosis**
  - Poorly differentiated adenocarcinoma.
  - Low-grade pancreatic neuroendocrine tumor.
  - Metastasis.
- **Immunohistochemistry**
  - Positive for neuroendocrine markers: CD56, chromogranin, synaptophysin, and NSE.

Cystic Neoplasms

Serous Cystadenoma

Serous cystadenomas are also referred to as microcystic cystadenomas because of the presence of innumerable small cysts measuring less than 2 cm in size.

Clinical

- Uncommon neoplasm, occurs in elderly patients, with no sex predilection.
- Asymptomatic or present as large abdominal mass with local discomfort and abdominal pain involving the head and body/tail of pancreas.
- Generally benign; however, a malignant counterpart has been reported.
- Mostly solitary, rarely multicentric.
- Associated with von Hippel-Lindau (VHL) syndrome.
- Carcinoembryonic antigen (CEA), carbohydrate antigen (CA) 19-9, and CA 125 serum markers are almost never elevated.

Radiology

US

- Because of the multiple interfaces of the small cysts, serous cystadenomas often appear hyperechoic on US.

CT

- The tumor may demonstrate multiple small cysts of fluid density; however, it may also appear solid, depending on the size of the cysts and the relative amount of associated fibrous tissue.

MRI

- Individual cysts are often better visualized as high T2-signal intensity on MRI (Fig. 7.14a).
- While it is only present in approximately 30% of serous cystadenomas, a calcified central scar on CT or MRI is considered highly specific for the tumor (Fig. 7.14b) [31, 45, 46].

Gross

- Large multiloculated mass; average size 6 cm.
- Central scar.

Cytology of *FNA* and Touch Preparation

- Paucicellular smears consisting of loose flat nests or "honeycombed" sheets of uniform, bland cuboidal epithelial cells with small, round slightly eccentric nuclei with fine chromatin, smooth nuclear membranes, and inconspicuous nucleoli (Fig. 7.14c–e) [47, 48].
- The cytoplasm is moderate in amount and clear to finely granular or vacuolar with indistinct cell borders.
- Abundant proteinaceous material and hemosiderin-laden macrophages.
- Mitotic figures and necrosis are absent.

Histology of Core and Cell Block

- Multiple small cysts lined by glycogen-rich cuboidal cells and containing clear, watery serous fluid (Fig. 7.14f).
- Cysts usually do not communicate with the pancreatic duct system.

Comments

- **Differential Diagnosis**
  - Mucinous cystic neoplasm.
  - Lymphangioma.
  - Ductal retention cyst.
  - Well-differentiated pancreatic endocrine neoplasm.
  - Metastatic renal cell carcinoma.
- **Immunohistochemistry and Special Stains**
  - Immunoreactive: Inhibin, cytokeratin (AE1/AE3, Cam 5.2, CK7, and CK19).
  - Immunonegative: CK20, CEA (usually negative), chromogranin, and synaptophysin.
  - Positive for PAS, while negative for PAS-D.

Mucinous Cystic Neoplasm (MCN)

Mucinous cystadenomas are multilocular cystic lesions typically occurring in the body and tail of the pancreas, in which individual locules measure more than 2 cm.

Clinical

- Predominantly occur in middle-aged women [49, 50].
- If large, present with vague abdominal pain.
- Located mostly in body and tail of pancreas (90%).
- Calcification in the wall of the cyst is seen in 20% of cases.

Radiology

CT and MRI

- Hemorrhage or debris within the lobules may result in a range of CT attenuation or T1 MRI signal intensity (Fig. 7.15a, b).
- Although rare, peripheral calcifications are highly specific for mucinous cystadenoma, help distinguish the tumor from serous cystadenoma, and are highly predictive of malignancy [31, 46].

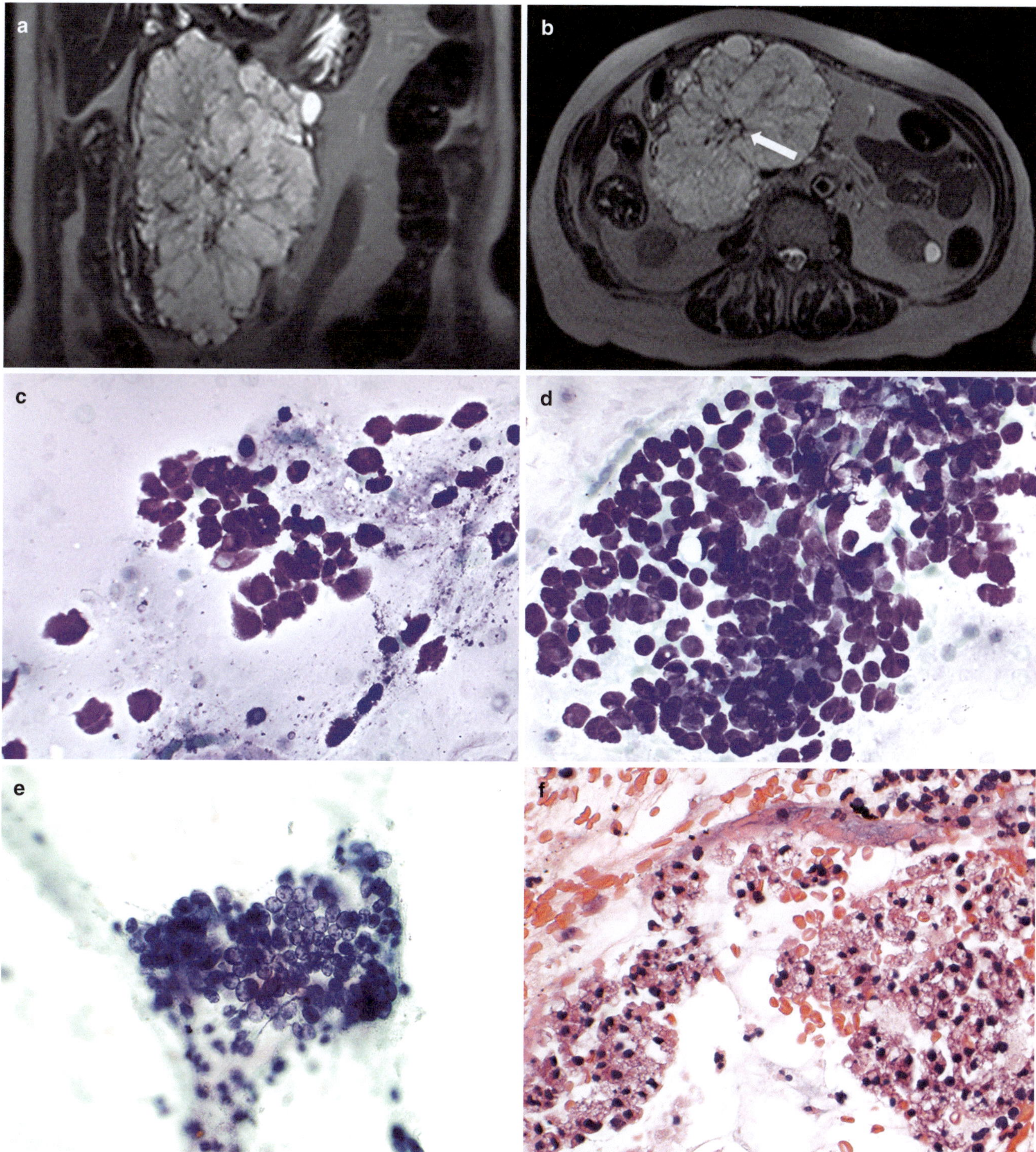

Fig. 7.14 (**a**, **b**) MRI of serous cystadenoma. (**a**) Coronal T2-weighted MR image shows large, multiloculated cystic lesion in the region of the head of the pancreas. The locules are notably <2 cm in size. Endoscopic biopsy proved this lesion to be a serous cystadenoma. (**b**) Serous cystadenoma: axial T2-weighted image in the same patient demonstrating central low attenuation in a "stellate" pattern, representing a calcified central scar (*arrow*). (**c–f**) Pathology of serous cystadenoma. (**c–e**) FNA cytology, Diff-Quik stain (**c**, **d**) and Papanicolaou stain, 600×. (**f**) Histology of cell block, H&E stain, 600×

Gross

- Solitary, large multilocular cyst with pseudocapsule.
- Rarely presents as a unilocular cyst.
- Usually does not communicate with pancreatic duct.

Cytology of FNA Nests/sheets or papillae of cohesive mucin-producing, tall columnar epithelial cells with basally located bland, round nuclei and apical mucin, loss of polarity, with or without cytologic atypia (Fig. 7.15c).

- Abundant amount of extracellular thick mucin and fibrous stroma with bland spindle cells (Fig. 7.15c).
- May be hemorrhagic or necrotic [49].

Histology of Core and Cell Block

- Cysts lined by tall, columnar mucin-producing cells, often forming papillae (Fig. 7.15d).
- The septae of the cyst contain ovarian-type stroma.
- Noninvasive MCNs are categorized as having low-grade, intermediate-grade or high-grade dysplasia [51].

Comments

- **Differential Diagnos**is
  - Intraductal papillary mucinous neoplasm.
  - Mucinous non-neoplastic cyst [52–54].
  - Serous cystic neoplasm.
  - Gastric contamination.
- **Immunohistochemistry**
  - Epithelial cells:
    - Positive: Cam5.2, CK7 (Fig. 7.15e), CK19, CA 19-9, CEA, MUC5AC, and scattered intraepithelial goblet-like cells express MUC2 [50].
    - Negative: MUC 1 (except when they become invasive), CK20 (mostly negative, positive only in rare cases), and CDX-2 (mostly negative, positive only in rare cases) (Fig. 7.15f).
  - Stromal cells:
    - Positive for ER, PR (Fig. 7.15g), and inhibin (Fig. 7.15h) [50].
- **Cyst Fluid Chemistry**
  - Elevated: CEA level above 200 ng/mL.
  - Not elevated: Amylase.

Intraductal Papillary Mucinous Neoplasm (IPMN)

Branch duct or combined main-duct and branch duct IMPNs are often difficult to distinguish from mucinous cystadenomas.

Clinical

- Most commonly located in the head of the pancreas (70%) involving the main pancreatic duct with dilation.
- Common in the elderly with a male to female ratio of 3:1.
- 35% have associated invasive carcinoma

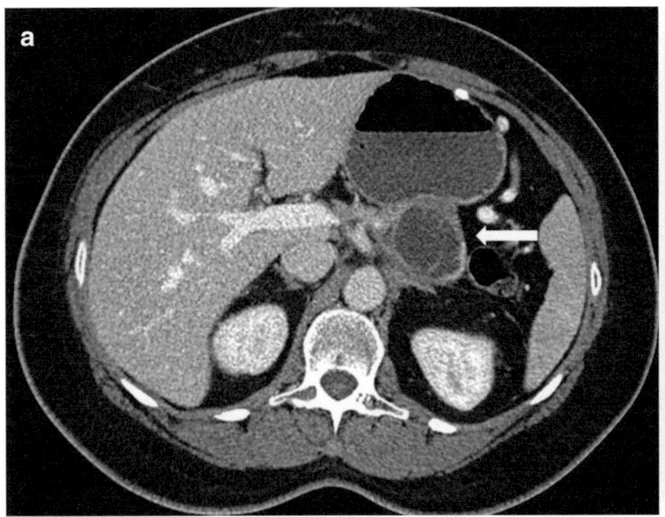

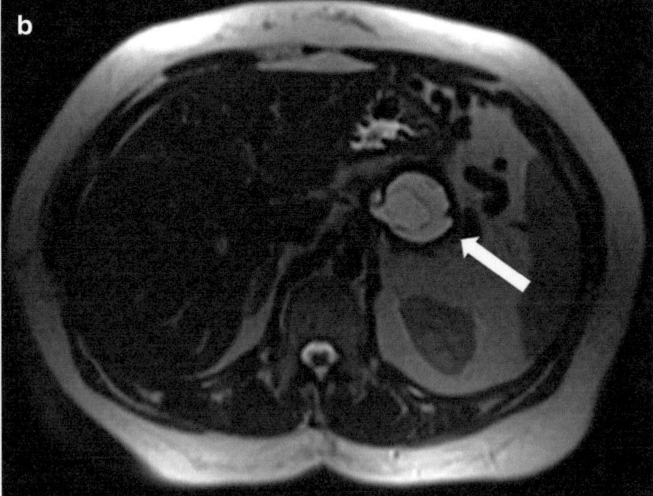

Fig. 7.15 (**a**, **b**) Mucinous cystadenoma. (**a**) Axial contrast-enhanced CT demonstrating a mucinous cystadenoma (*arrow*) at the tail of the pancreas with internal septations and fewer larger locules compared to serous cystadenoma. (**b**) T2-weighted MRI showing a mucinous cystadenoma (*arrow*) at the tail of the pancreas with clearly defined internal septations. Septations are often better visualized with MRI. (**c–h**) Pathology of mucinous cystadenoma. (**c**) EUS-FNA cytology, Diff-Quik Stain, 200×. (**d**) Histology of core, H&E stain, 400×. (**e–h**) Immunostains for CK7 (**e**), CDX2 (**f**), PR (**g**), and inhibin (**h**), 400×

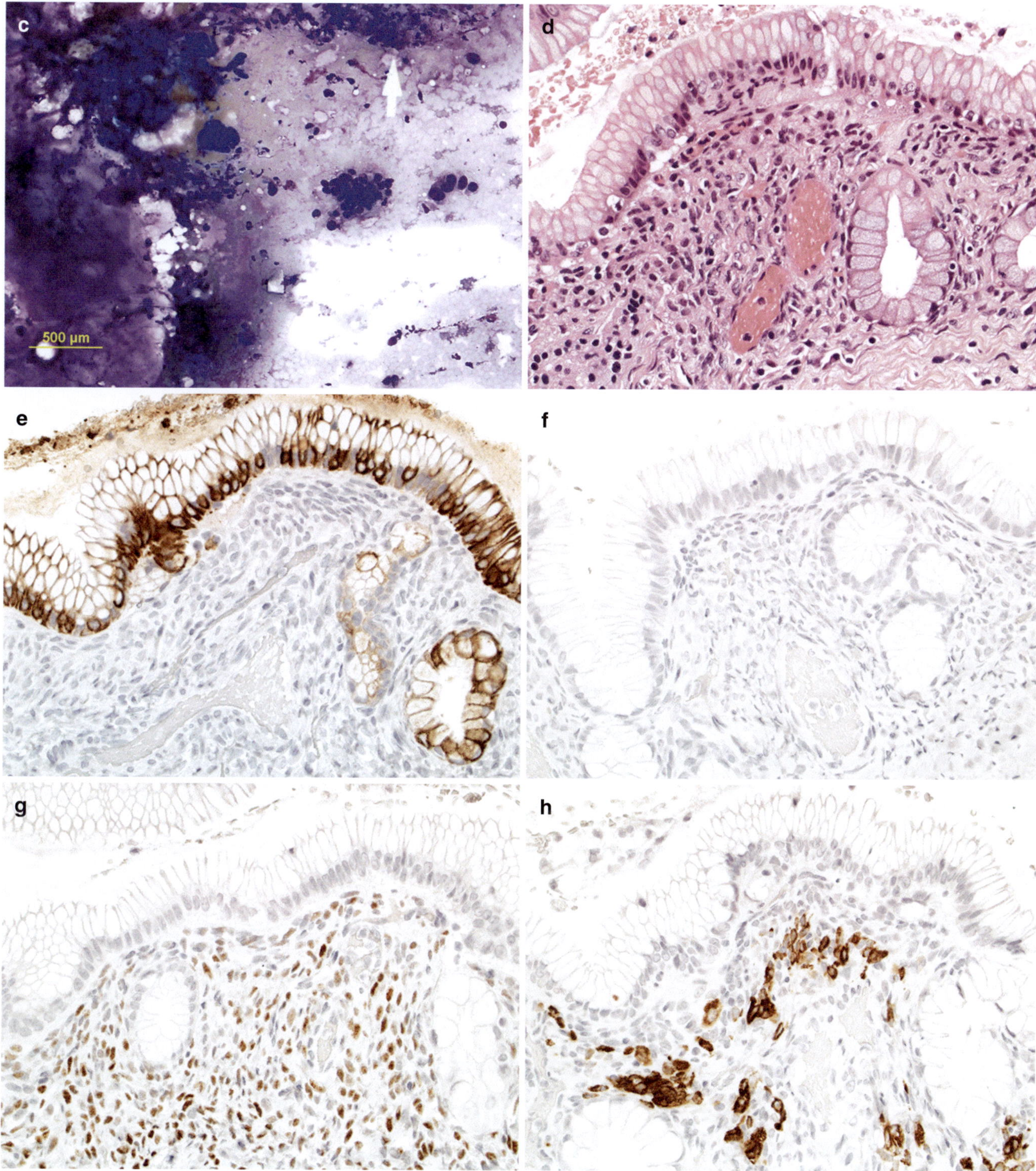

Fig. 7.15 (continued)

- Extruded mucin from the ampulla of Vater may be seen on endoscopic retrograde cholangiopancreatography (ERCP).
- Present with abdominal pain, back pain, anorexia, weight loss, and recurrent pancreatitis.

Radiology

CT and MRI:

- While thin section helical CT may be able to define the typical multilocular appearance of IMPNs as well as communication with the pancreatic ducts, MRI and MR cholangiopancreatography remain the modalities of choice for identification of these distinctive features of IMPNs [31, 46].

Gross

- Diffusely or segmentally dilated pancreatic duct or its branches.
- Papillary protrusions and thick mucin.
- Communicates with pancreatic duct or one of its branches.

Cytology of FNA and Touch Preparation

- Papillae or sheets of cuboidal to columnar, mucin-producing epithelial cells with round to ovoid, basally or eccentrically located nuclei containing fine evenly distributed granular to irregularly distributed coarse chromatin and small to prominent nucleoli (Fig. 7.16a, b) [55].
- Variable amount of extracellular mucin.
- Irregular clustering, complex papillae, and discohesiveness with single atypical cells are features of borderline and high-grade dysplasia. Micropapillary clusters and single markedly atypical cells are seen in malignant cases [55].

Histology of Core and Cell Block

- Four subtypes:
- Intestinal type: With intestinal-type papillae lined by columnar, mucin-producing epithelial cells with cigar-shaped nuclei (Fig. 7.16c).
- Gastric foveolar type: with abundant eosinophilic cytoplasm, basally oriented nuclei, and apical mucin.

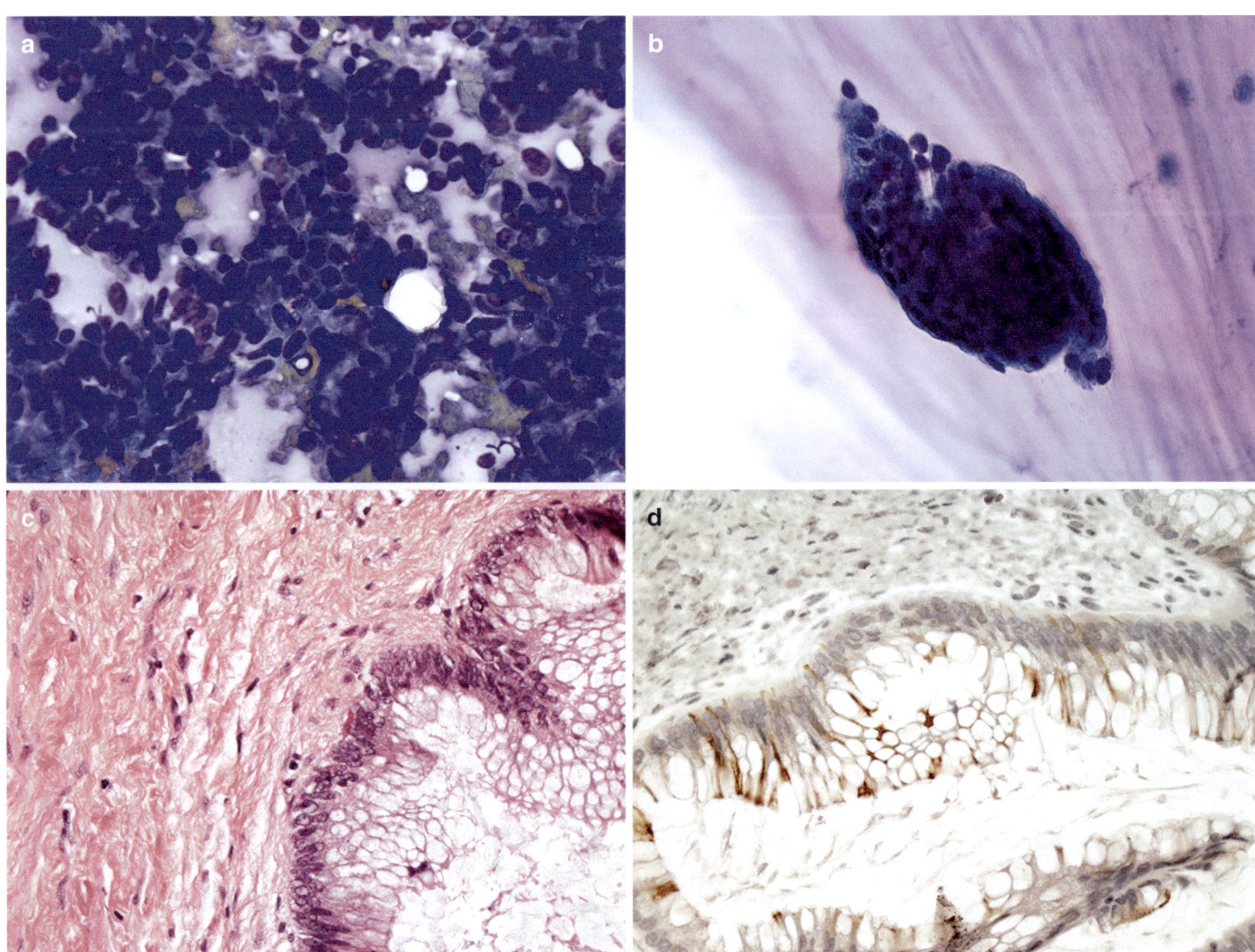

Fig. 7.16 Pathology of Intraductal papillary mucinous neoplasm. (**a**, **b**) EUS-FNA cytology, Diff-Quik stain (**a**) and Papanicolaou stain (**b**), 400×. (**c**) Core histology, H&E stain, 400×. (**d**–**h**) Immunostains for CK20 (**d**), CDX2 (**e**), MUC2 (**f**), PR (**g**), and inhibin (**h**), 400×

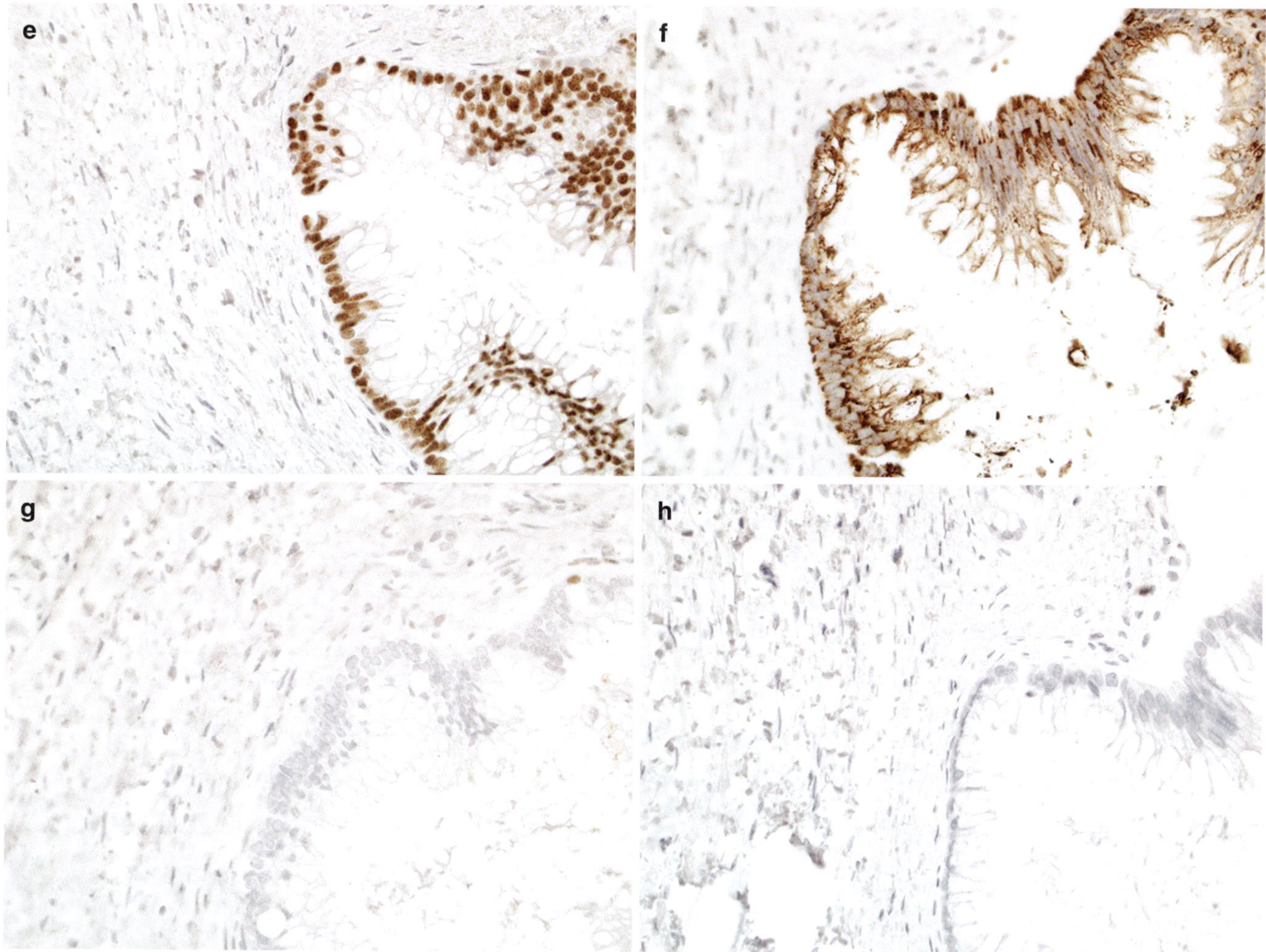

Fig. 7.16 (continued)

- Pancreaticobiliary type: With cuboidal cells lining complex papillae with bridging and cribriform architecture, with round nuclei containing prominent nucleoli.
- Oncocytic type: With moderate to abundant granular cytoplasm.
- Noninvasive IPMNs are classified on the basis of low-grade, intermediate-grade or high-grade dysplasia based at the level of nuclear atypia.

Comments

- **Differential Diagnosis**
  - Mucinous cystic neoplasm.
  - PanIN (Pancreatic intraepithelial neoplasia).
  - Serous cystic neoplasm.
  - Retention cysts.
  - Cystic pancreatic endocrine neoplasm.
  - Mucinous non-neoplastic cyst [52–54].
- **Immunohistochemistry**
  - Tumor cells positive: Cytokeratin (AE1/AE3 and Cam 5.2), CK19, CDX2 (Fig. 7.16e), MUC1, and MUC2 (Fig. 7.16f), and variably CK20 (Fig. 7.16d), CEA, and CA 19-9 [55, 56]. Increased cytoplasmic expression of caspase-3 is seen in IPMNs with invasive adenocarcinoma [57].
  - Stromal cells negative: PR (Fig. 7.16g) and inhibin (Fig. 7.16h).

Metastatic Malignancies

Radiology

CT and MRI

- Metastases to the pancreas may present as solitary (most commonly) or multiple distinct masses along the pancreas, often without the secondary findings frequently seen with primary pancreatic tumors such as pancreatic atrophy or ductal dilatation.
- Enhancement patterns reflect the characteristics of the primary malignancy, with hypovascular tumor deposits generally arising from disseminated melanoma or lung, breast, and colon cancers.

- Metastatic renal cell cancer often presents as hypervascular tumor deposits on early arterial phase imaging [58–60].

FNA Cytology and Histology of Cells Block or Cores

- The cytomorphology and histology of metastatic malignancies vary, depending on the site of origin.

Immunohistochemistry

- Immunostains for CK7, CK20, TTF1, CDX2, PAX8, PDX1, ER, and others are helpful for distinguishing metastatic malignancies from primary pancreatic tumors.

References

1. Marshall MR, Hall M, Simon V, Centeno B, Dennis K, Dhillon J, et al. Suboptimal agreement among cytopathologists in diagnosis of malignancy based on endoscopic ultrasound needle aspirates of solid pancreatic lesions: a validation study. Clin Gastroenterol Hepatol. 2018;16:1114–22.e2.
2. Lin X, Finkelstein SD, Zhu B, Ujevich BJ, Silverman JF. Loss of heterozygosities in Barrett esophagus, dysplasia, and adenocarcinoma detected by esophageal brushing cytology and gastroesophageal biopsy. Cancer Cytopathol. 2009;117:57–66.
3. Elek G, Gyokeres T, Schafer E, Burai M, Pinter F, Pap A. Early diagnosis of pancreatobiliary duct malignancies by brush cytology and biopsy. Pathol Oncol Res. 2005;11:145–55.
4. Urbano M, Rosa A, Gomes D, Camacho E, Calhau CA, Leitao M. Team approach to ERCP-directed single-brush cytology for the diagnosis of malignancy. Rev Esp Enferm Dig. 2008;100:462–5.
5. Uchida N, Kamada H, Tsutsui K, Ono M, Aritomo Y, Masaki T, et al. Utility of pancreatic duct brushing for diagnosis of pancreatic carcinoma. J Gastroenterol. 2007;42:657–62.
6. Falk GW, Chittajallu R, Goldblum JR, Biscotti CV, Geisinger KR, Petras RE, et al. Surveillance of patients with Barrett's esophagus for dysplasia and cancer with balloon cytology. Gastroenterology. 1997;112:1787–97.
7. Adams L, Roth MJ, Abnet CC, Dawsey SP, Qiao YL, Wang GQ, et al. Promoter methylation in cytology specimens as an early detection marker for esophageal squamous dysplasia and early esophageal squamous cell carcinoma. Cancer Prev Res. 2008;1:357–61.
8. Yamao K, Bhatia V, Mizuno N, Sawaki A, Shimizu Y, Irisawa A. Interventional endoscopic ultrasonography. J Gastroenterol Hepatol. 2009;24:509–19.
9. Sampliner RE. Updated guidelines for the diagnosis, surveillance, and therapy of Barrett's esophagus. Am J Gastroenterol. 2002;97:1888–95.
10. Pera M, Cameron AJ, Trastek VF, Carpenter HA, Zinsmeister AR. Increasing incidence of adenocarcinoma of the esophagus and esophagogastric junction. Gastroenterology. 1993;104:510–3.
11. Haggitt RC. Barrett's esophagus, dysplasia, and adenocarcinoma. Hum Pathol. 1994;25:982–93.
12. Odze RD, Flejou JF, Boffetta P, Hofler H, Montgomery E, Spechler SJ. Adenocarcinoma of the oesophagogastric junction. In: Bosman FT, Carneiro F, Hruban RH, Theise ND, editors. WHO classification of tumours of the digestive system. Lyon: International Agency for Research on Cancer; 2010. p. 39–44.
13. Goda K, Tajiri H, Ikegami M, Urashima M, Nakayoshi T, Kaise M. Usefulness of magnifying endoscopy with narrow band imaging for the detection of specialized intestinal metaplasia in columnar-lined esophagus and Barrett's adenocarcinoma. Gastrointest Endosc. 2007;65:36–46.
14. Wolfsen HC, Crook JE, Krishna M, Achem SR, Devault KR, Bouras EP, et al. Prospective, controlled tandem endoscopy study of narrow band imaging for dysplasia detection in Barrett's esophagus. Gastroenterology. 2008;135:24–31.
15. Saad RS, Mahood LK, Clary KM, Liu Y, Silverman JF, Raab SS. Role of cytology in the diagnosis of Barrett's esophagus and associated neoplasia. Diagn Cytopathol. 2003;29:130–5.
16. Antonioli DA, Wang HH. Morphology of Barrett's esophagus and Barrett's-associated dysplasia and adenocarcinoma. Gastroenterol Clin N Am. 1997;26:495–506.
17. Wang HH, Doria MI, Purohit-Buch S, Schnell T, Sontag S, Chejfec G. Barrett's esophagus. The cytology of dysplasia in comparison to benign and malignant lesions. Acta Cytol. 1992;36:60–4.
18. Lauwers GY, Carneiro F, Fraham DY, Curado MP, Franceschi S, Mongtgomery E, Tatematsu M, Hattori T. Gastric carcinoma. In: Bosman FT, Carneiro F, Hruban RH, Theise ND, editors. WHO classification of tumours of the digestive system. Lyon: International Agency for Research on Cancer; 2010. p. 48–58.
19. Gore RM, Levine MS, Ghahremani GG, Miller FH. Gastric cancer. Radiologic diagnosis. Radiol Clin N Am. 1997;35:311–29.
20. Ba-Ssalamah A, Prokop M, Uffmann M, Pokieser P, Teleky B, Lechner G. Dedicated multidetector CT of the stomach: spectrum of diseases. Radiographics. 2003;23:625–44.
21. Rosch T. Endosonographic staging of esophageal cancer: a review of literature results. Gastrointest Endosc Clin North Am. 1995;5:537–47.
22. Ahn HS, Lee HJ, Yoo MW, Kim SG, Im JP, Kim SH, et al. Diagnostic accuracy of T and N stages with endoscopy, stomach protocol CT, and endoscopic ultrasonography in early gastric cancer. J Surg Oncol. 2009;99:20–7.
23. Montgomery E, Field JK, Boffetta P, Daigo Y, Shimizu M, Shimoda T. Squamous cell carcinoma of the oesophagus. In: Bosman FT, Carneiro F, Hruban RH, Theise ND, editors. WHO classification of tumours of the digestive system. Lyon, France: International Agency for Research on Cancer; 2010. p. 18–24.
24. Lin X, Saad RS, Luckasevic TM, Silverman JF, Liu Y. Diagnostic value of CDX-2 and TTF-1 expressions in separating metastatic neuroendocrine neoplasms of unknown origin. Appl Immunohistochem Mol Morphol. 2007;15:407–14.
25. King DM. The radiology of gastrointestinal stromal tumours (GIST). Cancer Imaging. 2005;5:150–6.
26. Burkill GJ, Badran M, Al-Muderis O, Meirion Thomas J, Judson IR, Fisher C, et al. Malignant gastrointestinal stromal tumor: distribution, imaging features, and pattern of metastatic spread. Radiology. 2003;226:527–32.
27. Nakamura S, Muller-Hermelink HK, Delabie J, Ko YH, van Krieken JH, Jaffe ES. Lymphoma of the stomach. In: Bosman FT, Carneiro F, Hruban RH, Theise ND, editors. WHO classification of tumours of the digestive system. Lyon: International Agency for Research on Cancer; 2010. p. 69–73.
28. Arantes V, Logrono R, Faruqi S, Ahmed I, Waxman I, Bhutani MS. Endoscopic sonographically guided fine-needle aspiration yield in submucosal tumors of the gastrointestinal tract. J Ultrasound Med. 2004;23:1141–50.
29. Murphy BA, Meda BA, Buss DH, Geisinger KR. Marginal zone and mantle cell lymphomas: assessment of cytomorphology in subtyping small B-cell lymphomas. Diagn Cytopathol. 2003;28:126–30.
30. Balthazar EJ. Acute pancreatitis: assessment of severity with clinical and CT evaluation. Radiology. 2002;223:603–13.
31. Kim YH, Saini S, Sahani D, Hahn PF, Mueller PR, Auh YH. Imaging diagnosis of cystic pancreatic lesions: pseudocyst versus nonpseudocyst. Radiographics. 2005;25:671–85.
32. Hruban RH, Boffetta P, Hiraoka N, Lacobuzio-Donahue C, Kato Y, Kern SE, Klimstra DS, Kloppel G, Maitra A, Offerhaus GJA,

Pitman MB. Ductal adenocarcinoma of the pancreas. In: Bosman FT, Carneiro F, Hruban RH, Theise ND, editors. WHO classification of tumours of the digestive system. Lyon: International Agency for Research on Cancer; 2010. p. 281–91.
33. Miller FH, Rini NJ, Keppke AL. MRI of adenocarcinoma of the pancreas. Am J Roentgenol. 2006;187:W365–74.
34. Mertz HR, Sechopoulos P, Delbeke D, Leach SD. EUS, PET, and CT scanning for evaluation of pancreatic adenocarcinoma. Gastrointest Endosc. 2000;52:367–71.
35. Klimstra DS, Hruban RH, Kloppel G, Morohoshi T, Ohike N. Acinar cell neoplasms of the pancreas. In: Bosman FT, Carneiro F, Hruban RH, Theise ND, editors. WHO classification of tumours of the digestive system. Lyon: International Agency for Research on Cancer; 2010. p. 241–3.
36. Chung EM, Travis MD, Conran RM. Pancreatic tumors in children: radiologic-pathologic correlation. Radiographics. 2006;26:1211–38.
37. Mergo PJ, Helmberger TK, Buetow PC, Helmberger RC, Ros PR. Pancreatic neoplasms: MR imaging and pathologic correlation. Radiographics. 1997;17:281–301.
38. Peng HQ, Darwin P, Papadimitriou JC, Drachenberg CB. Liver metastases of pancreatic acinar cell carcinoma with marked nuclear atypia and pleomorphism diagnosed by EUS FNA cytology: a case report with emphasis on FNA cytological findings. Cytojournal. 2006;3:29.
39. Stelow EB, Bardales RH, Shami VM, Woon C, Presley A, Mallery S, et al. Cytology of pancreatic acinar cell carcinoma. Diagn Cytopathol. 2006;34:367–72.
40. Kloppel G, Hruban R, Klimstra DS, Maitra A, Morohoshi T, Notohara K, Shimizu M, Terris B. Solid-pseudopapillary neoplasm of the pancreas. In: Bosman FT, Carneiro F, Hruban RH, Theise ND, editors. WHO classification of tumours of the digestive system. Lyon: International Agency for Research on Cancer; 2010. p. 246–8.
41. Jani N, Dewitt J, Eloubeidi M, Varadarajulu S, Appalaneni V, Hoffman B, et al. Endoscopic ultrasound-guided fine-needle aspiration for diagnosis of solid pseudopapillary tumors of the pancreas: a multicenter experience. Endoscopy. 2008;40:200–3.
42. Jhala N, Siegal GP, Jhala D. Large, clear cytoplasmic vacuolation: an under-recognized cytologic clue to distinguish solid pseudopapillary neoplasms of the pancreas from pancreatic endocrine neoplasms on fine-needle aspiration. Cancer. 2008;114:249–54.
43. Bardales RH, Centeno B, Mallery JS, Lai R, Pochapin M, Guiter G, et al. Endoscopic ultrasound-guided fine-needle aspiration cytology diagnosis of solid-pseudopapillary tumor of the pancreas: a rare neoplasm of elusive origin but characteristic cytomorphologic features. Am J Clin Pathol. 2004;121:654–62.
44. Lewis RB, Lattin GE, Paal E. Pancreatic endocrine tumors: radiologic-clinicopathologic correlation. Radiographics. 2010;30:1445–64.
45. Curry CA, Eng J, Horton KM, Urban B, Siegelman S, Kuszyk BS, et al. CT of primary cystic pancreatic neoplasms: can CT be used for patient triage and treatment? Am J Roentgenol. 2000;175:99–103.
46. Sahani DV, Kadavigere R, Saokar A, Fernandez-del Castillo C, Brugge WR, Hahn PF. Cystic pancreatic lesions: a simple imaging-based classification system for guiding management. Radiographics. 2005;25:1471–84.
47. Belsley NA, Pitman MB, Lauwers GY, Brugge WR, Deshpande V. Serous cystadenoma of the pancreas: limitations and pitfalls of endoscopic ultrasound-guided fine-needle aspiration biopsy. Cancer. 2008;114:102–10.
48. Huang P, Staerkel G, Sneige N, Gong Y. Fine-needle aspiration of pancreatic serous cystadenoma: cytologic features and diagnostic pitfalls. Cancer. 2006;108:239–49.
49. Garcea G, Ong SL, Rajesh A, Neal CP, Pollard CA, Berry DP, et al. Cystic lesions of the pancreas. A diagnostic and management dilemma. Pancreatology. 2008;8:236–51.
50. Silverman JF, Zhu B, Liu Y, Lin X. Distinctive immunohistochemical profile of mucinous cystic neoplasms of pancreas, ovary and lung. Histol Histopathol. 2009;24:77–82.
51. Zamboni G, Fukushima N, Hruban RH, Kloppei G. Mucinous cystic neoplasms. In: Bosman FT, Carneiro F, Hruban RH, Theise ND, editors. WHO classification of tumours of the digestive system. Lyon: International Agency for Research on Cancer; 2010. p. 300–3.
52. Zhu B, Keswani RN, Lin X. Fine needle aspiration cytomorphology of mucinous nonneoplastic cyst of the pancreas. Pancreas. 2013;42:27–31.
53. Zhu B, Lin X. Immunoprofile of mucinous non-neoplastic cyst of the pancreas. Appl Immunohistochem Mol Morphol. 2013;21:265–70.
54. Zhu B, Finkelstein SD, Feng G, Keswani RN, Lin X. Molecular analysis of mucinous nonneoplastic cyst of the pancreas. Hum Pathol. 2016;55:159–63.
55. Salla C, Chatzipantelis P, Konstantinou P, Karoumpalis I, Sakellariou S, Pantazopoulou A, et al. Endoscopic ultrasound-guided fine-needle aspiration cytology in the diagnosis of intraductal papillary mucinous neoplasms of the pancreas. A study of 8 cases. J Oncol Pract. 2007;8:715–24.
56. Adsay NV, Merati K, Basturk O, Iacobuzio-Donahue C, Levi E, Cheng JD, et al. Pathologically and biologically distinct types of epithelium in intraductal papillary mucinous neoplasms: delineation of an "intestinal" pathway of carcinogenesis in the pancreas. Am J Surg Pathol. 2004;28:839–48.
57. Satoh K, Kaneko K, Hirota M, Toyota T, Shimosegawa T. The pattern of CPP32/caspase-3 expression reflects the biological behavior of the human pancreatic duct cell tumors. Pancreas. 2000;21:352–7.
58. Ng CS, Loyer EM, Iyer RB, David CL, DuBrow RA, Charnsangavej C. Metastases to the pancreas from renal cell carcinoma: findings on three-phase contrast-enhanced helical CT. Am J Roentgenol. 1999;172:1555–9.
59. Palmowski M, Hacke N, Satzl S, Klauss M, Wente MN, Neukamm M, et al. Metastasis to the pancreas: characterization by morphology and contrast enhancement features on CT and MRI. Pancreatology. 2008;8:199–203.
60. Scatarige JC, Horton KM, Sheth S, Fishman EK. Pancreatic parenchymal metastases: observations on helical CT. Am J Roentgenol. 2001;176:695–9.

8 Thyroid, Parathyroid, Head, and Neck

Jamie Macagba Slade, Tracey Harbert, Joseph Young, Ramona Gupta, Laura Dean, Songlin Zhang, and Ajit S. Paintal

Introduction

Palpable thyroid nodules are present in approximately 5–7% of the adult population, and of these, only a small percentage (5–10%) harbor malignancy. Ultrasound (US) imaging of the neck is typically used to characterize thyroid nodules in order to triage lesions with the highest risk of malignancy. Fine needle aspiration (FNA) is recommended for thyroid lesions with radiographically suspicious features (as outlined below). FNA biopsy of the thyroid gland is an increasingly common procedure, with approximately 300,000–500,000 biopsies performed annually in the United States [1]. The 2015 American Thyroid Association management guidelines underscore the importance of radiologic risk stratification [2].

The Bethesda System for Reporting Thyroid Cytopathology was published in 2010 and updated in 2018; it is used as a means to standardize reporting of thyroid FNA cytology. Based on these guidelines, each thyroid FNA report should begin with one of six general diagnostic categories: (1) Nondiagnostic or Unsatisfactory, (2) Benign, (3) Atypia of Undetermined Significance or Follicular Lesion of Undetermined Significance, (4) Follicular Neoplasm or Suspicious for Follicular Neoplasm, (5) Suspicious for Malignancy, or (6) Malignant. Each category has its own implied risk of malignancy and recommended clinical management.

J. M. Slade
Department of Pathology, Rush Medical College, Chicago, IL, USA

T. Harbert
Cellnetix Pathology, Olympia, WA, USA

J. Young
Department of Radiology, St. Joseph Health, St. Jude Medical Center, Fullerton, CA, USA

R. Gupta
Northwestern University Feinberg School of Medicine, Chicago, IL, USA

L. Dean
Department of Diagnostic Radiology, Cleveland Clinic, Cleveland, OH, USA

S. Zhang
Department of Pathology and Laboratory Medicine, University of Texas McGovern Medical School, Houston, TX, USA

A. S. Paintal (✉)
Northshore Medical Group, Evanston Hospital, Evanston, IL, USA

Benign Conditions

Chronic Lymphocytic Thyroiditis

Clinical

- Most common cause of hypothyroidism in areas of the world where iodine levels are sufficient.
- More frequent in middle-aged white females.
- Longstanding chronic lymphocytic thyroiditis is a risk factor for marginal zone lymphoma of the thyroid and may be associated with other autoimmune diseases. The association of chronic lymphocytic thyroiditis and papillary thyroid carcinoma is controversial [3].
- Typically associated with circulating antithyroid antibodies (e.g., antithyroglobulin, anti-TSH, and antimicrosomal).

Ultrasound

- The sonographic appearance of Hashimoto thyroiditis is well recognized. The gland is often diffusely enlarged and heterogeneous, and the parenchyma is coarsened, hypoechoic, and hypervascular [4]. The degree of hypoechogenicity may also vary with the clinical stage of Hashimoto thyroiditis, being more hypoechoic in clinically hypothyroid patients (Fig. 8.1).
- A micronodular pattern on US is highly diagnostic of Hashimoto thyroiditis with a positive predictive value of 95% [5].

R. Nayar et al. (eds.), *Atlas of Cytopathology and Radiology*, https://doi.org/10.1007/978-3-030-24756-0_8

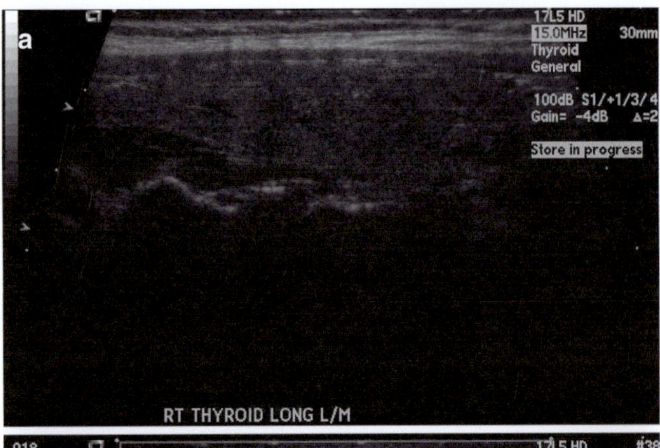

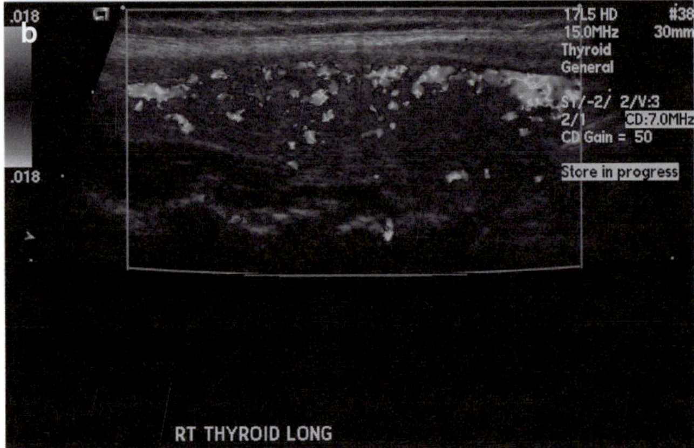

Fig. 8.1 Chronic lymphocytic thyroiditis. (**a**) The right thyroid lobe is enlarged, diffusely heterogeneous, and hypoechoic. There is a micronodular pattern throughout the right lobe. (**b**) Color Doppler imaging demonstrates diffuse hypervascularity

- Discrete nodules may, however, also occur within diffusely altered parenchyma or within sonographically normal parenchyma. The sonographic features and vascularity of nodular Hashimoto thyroiditis are extremely variable. There is overlap, with the findings typically associated with benign nodules as well as malignant nodules. Therefore, biopsy of these nodules is still necessary because there are no sonographic features that can reliably diagnose these lesions as thyroiditis and differentiate them from other lesions [6, 7].

Gross

- Firm and diffusely enlarged thyroid.
- Pale tan-yellow and nodular.

FNA

- Usually hypercellular with a mixture of Hurthle cells, abundant polymorphous population of lymphoid cells, tingible body macrophages, and histiocytic aggregates (Fig. 8.2a, b) [8].
- Variable numbers of plasma cells, lymphoid tangles, lymphoglandular bodies, germinal center fragments, skeletal muscle infiltrated by lymphoid cells, epithelioid histiocytes; rarely, granulomas may be seen in the background.
- Colloid is often scant.

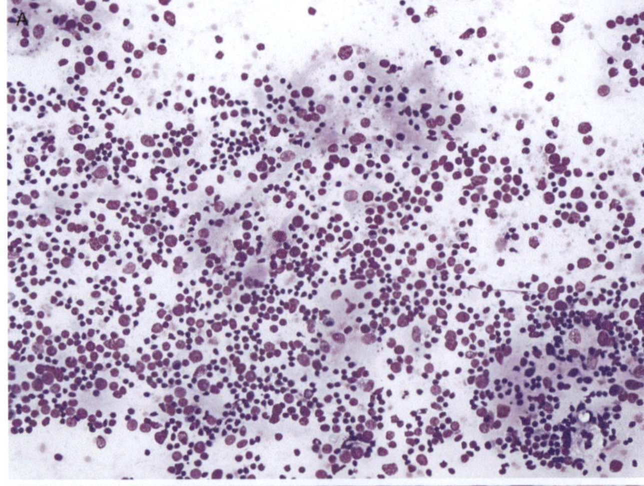

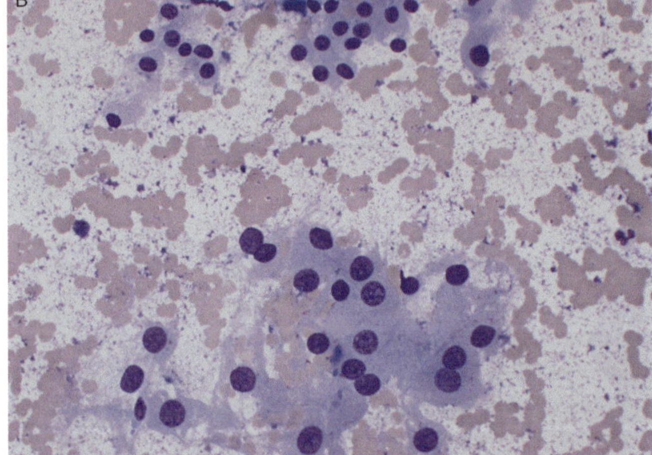

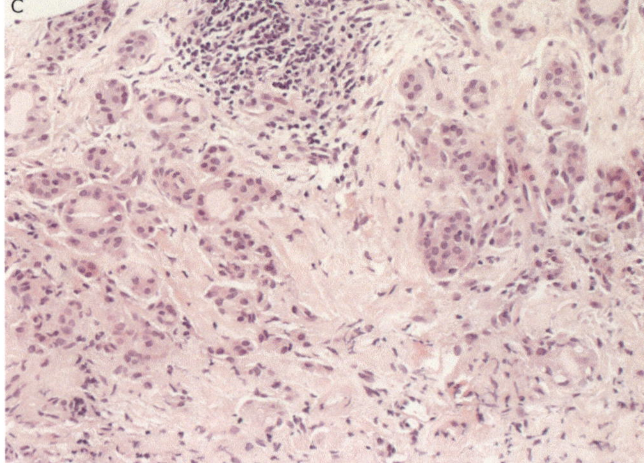

Fig. 8.2 Chronic lymphocytic thyroiditis. (**a**) A Diff-Quik (DQ) stained aspirate slide demonstrates a polymorphous population of lymphoid cells with admixed histiocytes. (**b**) The follicular cells demonstrate Hürthle cell change with abundant granular cytoplasm and enlarged, round nuclei with prominent nucleoli. (**c**) A core biopsy demonstrates interstitial fibrosis, lymphoid aggregates, Hürthle cell change, and numerous small follicles (microfollicles)

Core Biopsy

- Needle core biopsy shows small follicles with focal lymphoid infiltrate in a background of fibrosis. The follicular cells often have Hurthle cell change with abundant eosinophilic granular cytoplasm and prominent nucleoli (Fig. 8.2c).

Comment

- A microfollicular pattern is often seen in aspirates from cases in that colloid is often sparse and three-dimensional cellular clusters as well as microfollicles are frequently seen. If a lymphoid component is present in the aspirate, architectural atypia should be disregarded unless it is extremely striking.
- Similarly, in cases of chronic lymphocytic thyroiditis, nuclear enlargement, elongation, and pallor may be seen. Unless the nuclear features of papillary thyroid carcinoma are incontrovertible, this cytologic atypia should be ignored. Of note: intranuclear pseudoinclusions, if strictly defined, are not seen in cases of chronic lymphocytic thyroiditis.

Graves Disease

Clinical

- Autoimmune thyroid disease found most commonly in young women.
- Clinically presents with ophthalmopathy (exophthalmos) and dermopathy (pretibial edema).
- Increased T_3 and T_4, decreased TSH, and IgG antibodies to TSH receptor.

Ultrasound

- In Graves disease there is mild to moderate diffuse, symmetric enlargement of the thyroid gland, including the isthmus (Fig. 8.3).
- On US, there is a hypoechoic, heterogeneous, "spotty" parenchymal echo pattern [6].
- There is a marked increase in parenchymal vascularity on color Doppler, which is sometimes referred to as "thyroid inferno" [9].
- The hypervascularity tends to decrease in response to treatment [10].

Nuclear Medicine

- Technetium-99 m pertechnetate or iodine-123 scans show homogeneously increased uptake with high target to background levels. There is increased radioactive iodine uptake (normal is 8–25%), with an uptake exceeding 50–80%; this confirms the diagnosis of Graves disease.

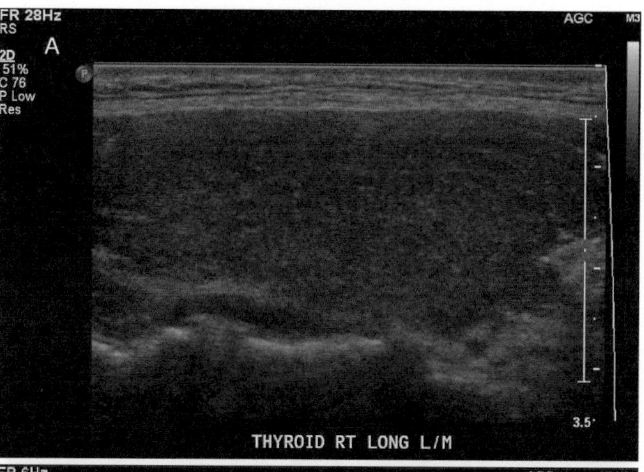

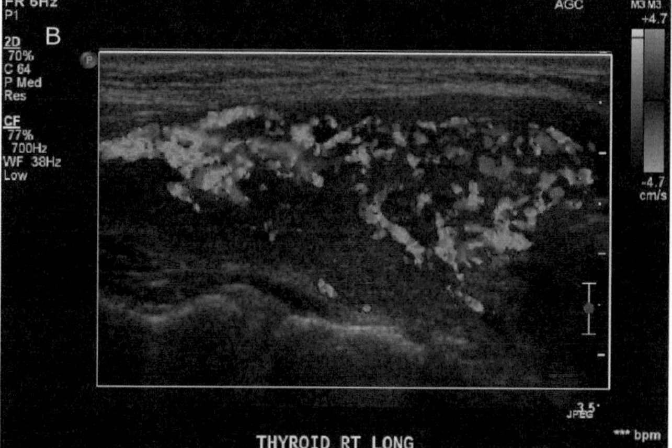

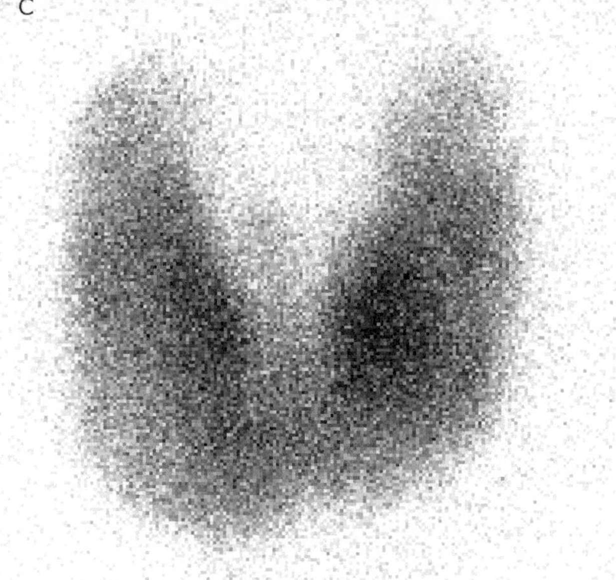

Fig. 8.3 Graves disease. (**a**) The right thyroid lobe is enlarged, heterogeneous, and hypoechoic. (**b**) Color Doppler demonstrates marked parenchymal hypervascularity or "thyroid inferno." (**c**) A 24-hour I-123 uptake scan demonstrates a markedly elevated uptake of 74% in a diffusely enlarged thyroid gland. There is diffusely prominent uptake in both lobes

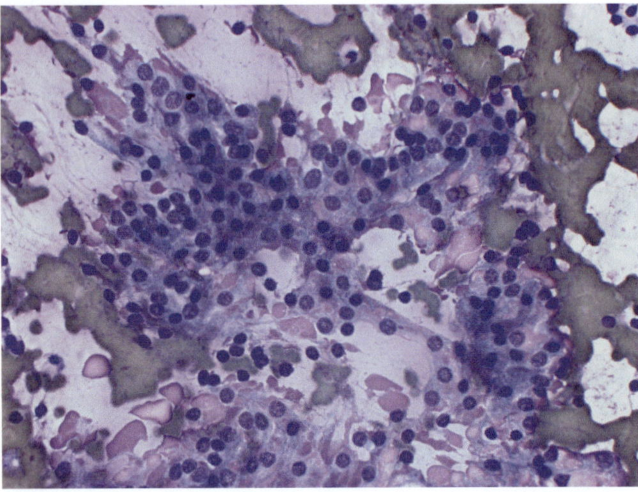

Fig. 8.4 Graves disease. The follicular cells in this aspirate slide are enlarged with large round nuclei. Marginal vacuoles containing colloid can be seen at the periphery of the cells, and magenta colloid is present in the background

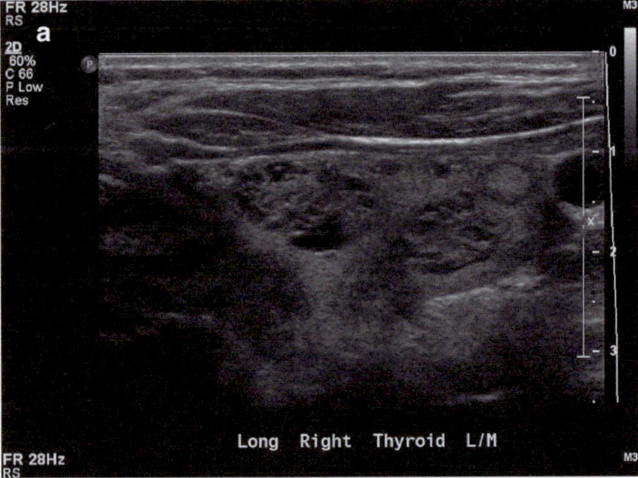

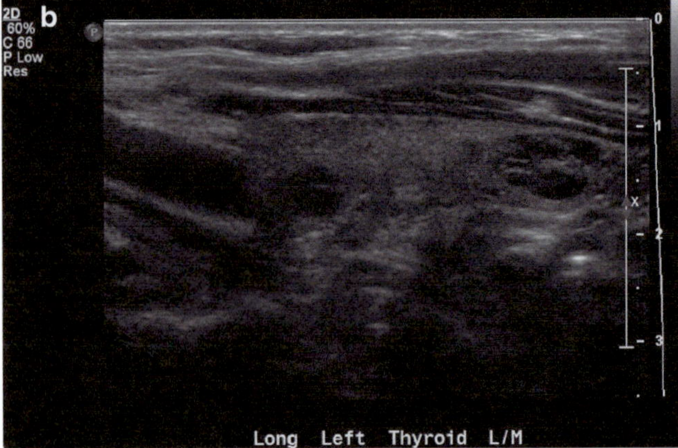

Fig. 8.5 Hyperplasia/multinodular goiter. (**a**) There is enlargement of the right thyroid lobe with several well-defined solid and mixed solid and cystic nodules of varying echogenicity. (**b**) There is enlargement of the left thyroid lobe with several well-defined solid and mixed solid and cystic nodules of varying echogenicity

Gross

- Diffusely, symmetrically enlarged thyroid with a beefy red cut surface.

FNA

- Marked cellularity
- Flame cells (fire flare): follicular cells with blebs and marginal vacuoles containing colloid (Fig. 8.4).
- Lymphocytes, Hurthle cells, and giant cells may be present. Colloid is typically scant [11].
- Three-dimensional cell groups and papillary clusters can be seen but lack the nuclear features of papillary thyroid carcinoma.

Core Biopsy

- Scant colloid with hyperplastic columnar follicular cells with papillary formations and lymphocytic infiltrate. Scalloping of colloid may be seen at the luminal surface of the follicular cells.

Comment

- While the follicular cells in Graves disease are enlarged and contain large nuclei, the nuclear: cytoplasmic ratios are low in contrast to those of papillary thyroid carcinoma.
- Papillary hyperplasia may be seen in aspirates from cases of Graves disease. As such, papillary fronds in the absence of the nuclear features of papillary thyroid carcinoma should not be considered atypical or diagnostic for malignancy.

Hyperplasia/Multinodular Goiter

Clinical

- A hyperplastic multinodular goiter in some cases may reflect impaired synthesis of thyroid hormone.
- Hyperplastic nodules can be solitary or present in a background of a multinodular thyroid gland.
- If extensive, multinodular hyperplasia may present with airway obstruction, dysphagia, or dyspnea.

Radiography

- On chest radiograph, an enlarged thyroid gland may result in tracheal deviation.

Ultrasound

- There is a well-marginated, diffuse enlargement of the thyroid gland, with multiple bilateral well-defined nodules. The main role of imaging is to identify the presence of suspicious nodules to guide biopsy (Fig. 8.5) [12].

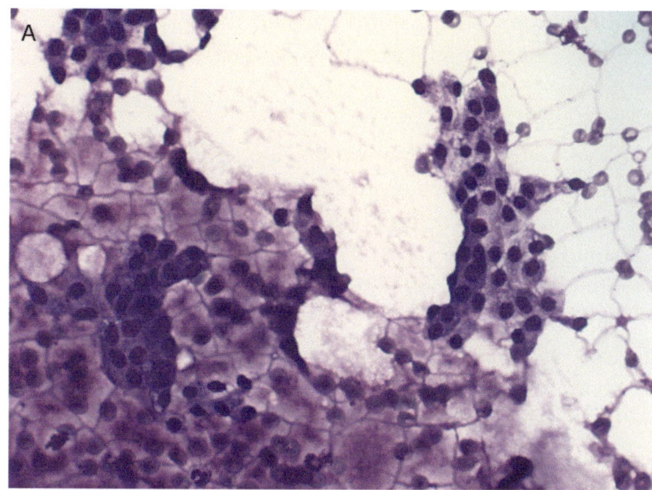

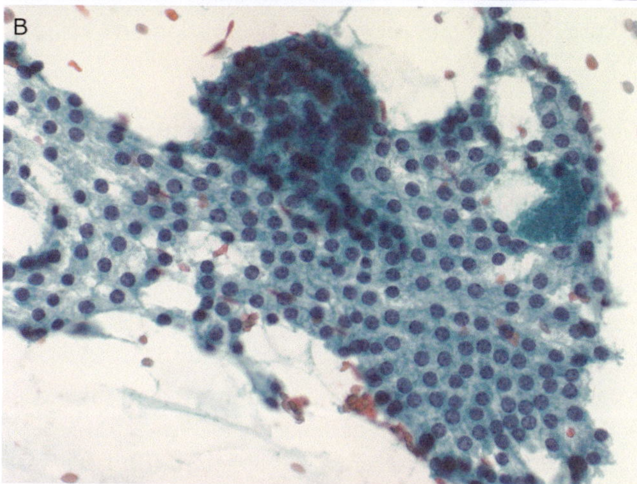

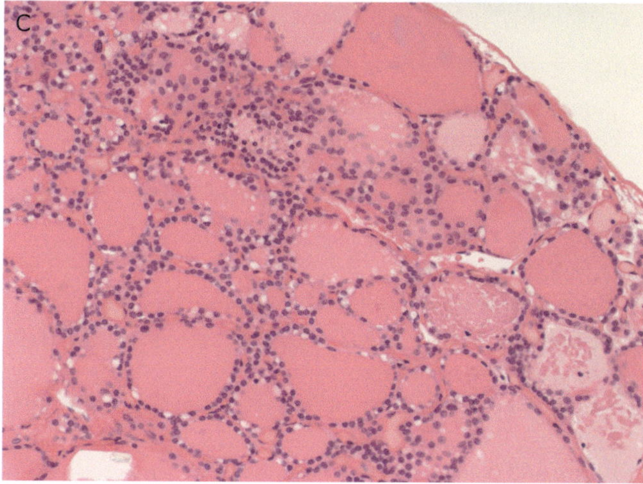

Fig. 8.6 Hyperplasia/multinodular goiter. (**a**) This DQ-stained aspirate slide contains abundant colloid in the background as well as flat sheets of thyroid follicular cells with round small nuclei. (**b**) In this Papanicolaou-stained aspirate slide, the follicular cells form a flat sheet. The granular chromatin pattern and the lack of nuclear crowding can be appreciated. (**c**) A core biopsy demonstrates numerous follicles of varying sizes

Computed Tomography (CT)/Magnetic Resonance Imaging (MRI)

- There is diffuse, heterogeneous enhancement on postcontrast imaging with multiple solid and cystic masses. CT or MRI can be used to better evaluate the mediastinal extent of the goiter and the severity of airway compression.

Gross

- Enlarged thyroid with solid and cystic nodules of various sizes; may be asymmetric.

Fine Needle Aspiration

- Benign follicular epithelial cells in a background of abundant colloid (Fig. 8.6a).
- Bland and uniform follicular epithelial cells in a flat monolayer sheet with delicate cytoplasm, round nuclei, and granular chromatin (Fig. 8.6b).
- Variable cellularity. May present with abundant colloid and rare follicular cells, or colloid may be moderate with high epithelial cellularity.
- Other cellular patterns seen include intact follicles (spherules), tissue fragments and dissociated single follicular cells, and largely cystic aspirates (colloid cysts). A minor microfollicular component may be seen.
- Hurthle cells are a variant of follicular epithelial cells with more abundant granular cytoplasm, mildly enlarged round nuclei, and prominent nucleoli.
- Involuting/degenerating nodules can show a variety of changes, some of which can cause concern radiologically or cytomorphologically. These include pigment-laden foamy macrophages and multinucleated giant cells, cyst-lining cells, mesenchymal repair, dystrophic calcifications, and usually birefringent calcium oxalate and/or cholesterol crystals and perifollicular fibrosis.

Core Biopsy

- Thyroid follicles varying in size with accumulation of colloid (Fig. 8.6c).

Comment

- A predominant microfollicular component with scant colloid, three-dimensional follicular cell clusters, and microfollicles (follicles less than 12–15 cells in circumference) may be seen in aspirates from hyperplastic thyroid nodules, thereby raising concern for the presence of a follicular neoplasm. If a significant macrofollicular component composed of abundant colloid and flat sheets of follicular cells is seen, the microfollicular component may be safely disregarded.

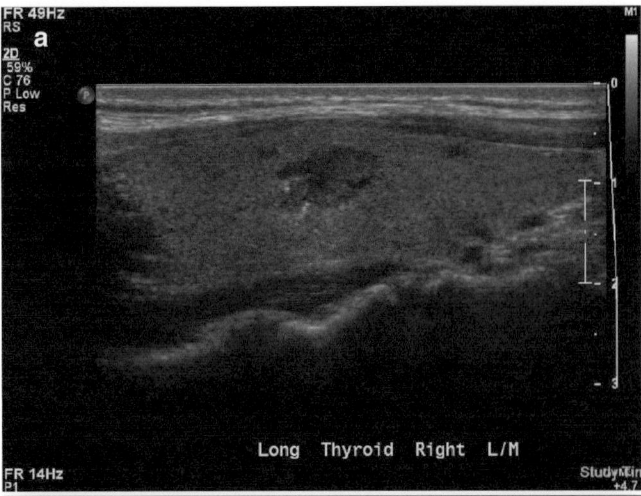

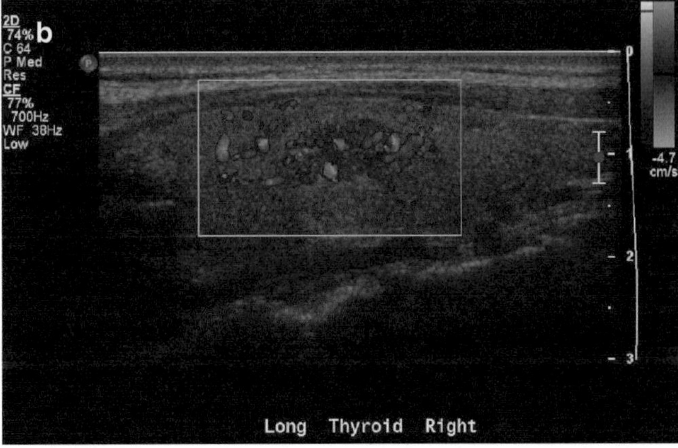

Fig. 8.7 Papillary thyroid carcinoma. (**a**) There is a well-defined hypoechoic right thyroid lobe nodule with several echogenic microcalcifications. (**b**) On color Doppler imaging, the nodule demonstrates intrinsic hypervascularity

- If using smears, we recommend that the FNA pass numbers are noted on the slides so that one can get a sense of the extent of sampling and cytologic-histologic correlation

Malignant Neoplasms: Primary

Papillary Thyroid Carcinoma (PTC)

Clinical

- The most common thyroid malignancy (85% or greater); it can be accurately diagnosed by FNA (96–100% confirmed as PTC on histologic examination).
- Usually an asymptomatic thyroid nodule; locally advanced cases may present with lymphadenopathy.
- More common in women (in Japan 9:1).
- Associated with radiation exposure, Hashimoto thyroiditis, familial adenomatous polyposis coli (FAP), Cowden syndrome, and possibly Carney complex [13].
- Overall excellent prognosis; 10-year survival rate in excess of 95%.
- Poor prognostic features include male sex, older age, gross extrathyroidal extension, and large size.

Ultrasound

- Common sonographic features are a hypoechoic texture, microcalcifications (correspond to psammomatous calcifications), well-defined margins, and intrinsic hypervascularity (Fig. 8.7) [14].
- Punctate microcalcifications are highly specific for papillary carcinoma and are seen as small echogenic foci that may or may not demonstrate posterior shadowing.
- Involved lymph nodes are usually hyperechoic to the adjacent muscle and contain microcalcifications or show cystic change [15].
- Large tumors may show signs of invasion into adjacent muscle or the esophagus, trachea, or vessels.

Computed Tomography/Magnetic Resonance Imaging

- CT or MRI may be used to stage large tumors. Although the findings are nonspecific, the primary tumor may demonstrate heterogeneous enhancement on postcontrast imaging with invasive margins, which is the key to diagnosis.

Nuclear Medicine

- Diagnostic Iodine-131 scan is performed after thyroidectomy to detect local recurrence or metastatic disease. If the scan is positive, therapeutic ablation with I-131 may be performed.

Gross

- Papillary thyroid carcinoma is grossly often a poorly circumscribed firm white scar-like lesion.
- May be well-circumscribed, diffuse, or multifocal.

Fine Needle Aspiration

- Typical aspirate is cellular with irregular sheets of follicular epithelium (Fig. 8.8a). In most cases, papillary fragments are absent or rare.
- Flat, crowded sheet of neoplastic epithelial cells with nuclear enlargement and ovoid nuclei with dense cytoplasm and conspicuous cell borders. The background frequently contains macrophages (Fig. 8.8b).
- Sheet of neoplastic cells with ovoid nuclei, fine, pale chromatin, and inconspicuous nucleoli; occasional nuclear grooves and intranuclear pseudoinclusions are typical (Fig. 8.8c) [16].
- Papillary carcinoma can have a wide variety of architectural patterns: classic papillary, follicular variant, and cystic. The most commonly seen architectural pattern is crowded monolayer sheets of cells.
- The major diagnostic features are nuclear and include:
  - Fusiform/oval nuclei with fine powdery chromatin

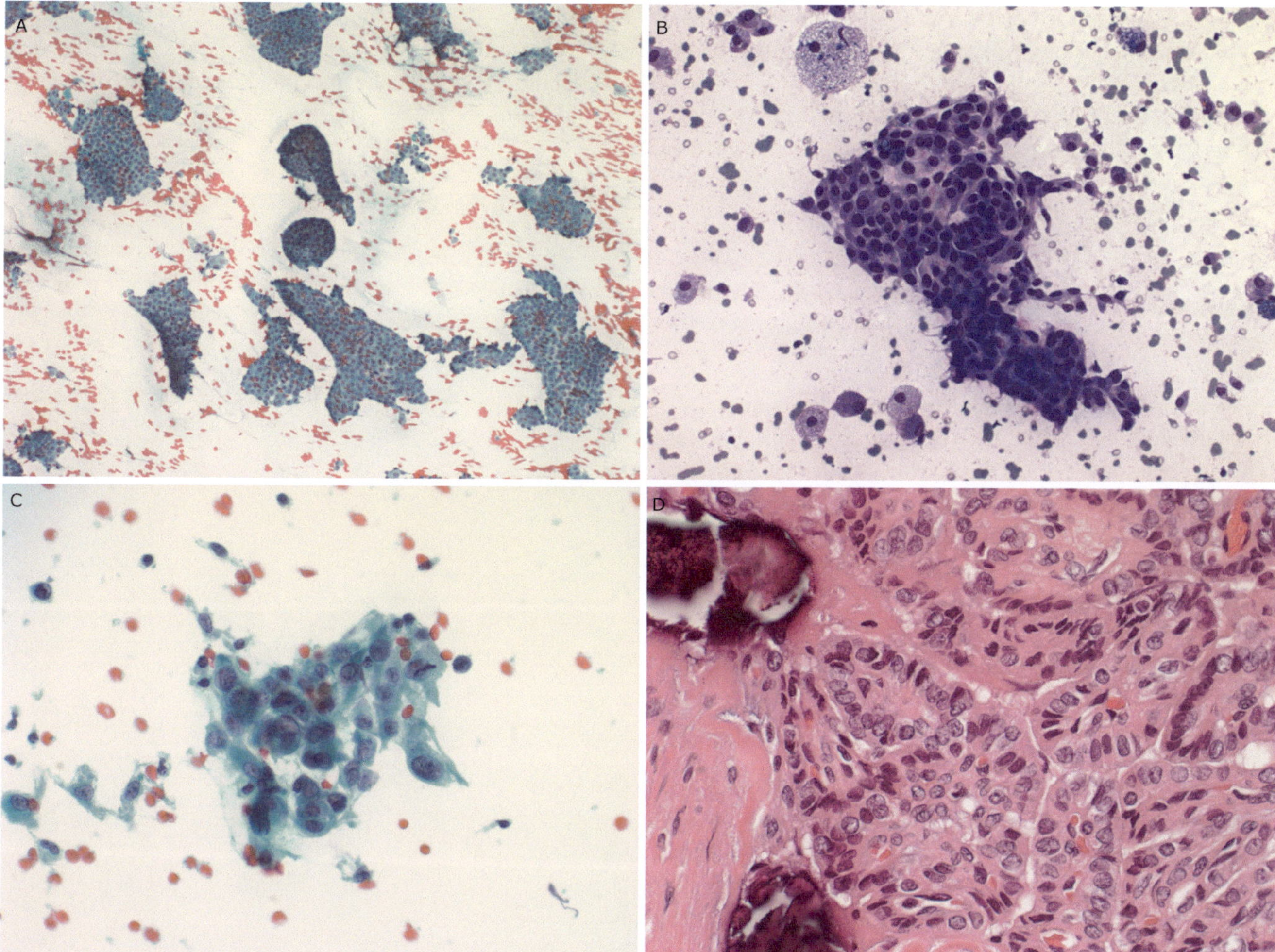

Fig. 8.8 Papillary thyroid. (**a**) Sheets of follicular cells with crowded elongated nuclei are seen in this Papanicolaou-stained aspirate slide. (**b**) Crowded sheets of follicular cells with ovoid nuclei are seen in this DQ-stained aspirate slide. Macrophages and cystic debris are seen in the background. (**c**) Scattered intranuclear pseudoinclusions can usually be identified in aspirate smears. (**d**) In this histologic section, compressed papillary fronds can be seen with crowded ovoid nuclei, nuclear pallor, and grooves. Lamellated psammomatous calcifications are visible in the background

- Intranuclear cytoplasmic pseudoinclusions
- Linear chromatin ridges (i.e., nuclear grooves)
- Single small nucleolus, often located near the nuclear membrane

• Minor diagnostic criteria include:
  - Architecture: syncytial sheets, papillary tissue fragments with fibrovascular cores, and swirl-like pattern of cell clusters [17]
  - Dense squamoid cytoplasm and septate cytoplasmic vacuoles
  - Bubble gum colloid; dense magenta colloid on modified Giemsa stain
  - Multinucleated foreign body-type giant cells
  - Psammomatous calcifications

Core Biopsy

• Papillary fronds lined by neoplastic cells with ovoid to elongated nuclei with nuclear membrane irregularities, fine chromatin with clearing, indistinct nucleoli, and occasional nuclear grooves. Psammomatous calcifications are present (Fig. 8.8d)

Comment

• The newly described entity, noninvasive follicular tumor with papillary thyroid carcinoma-like nuclei (NIFTP), is morphologically extremely similar to papillary thyroid carcinoma in cytologic preparations [18]. In resected specimens, this tumor is characterized by a follicular growth pattern, circumscription, and a lack of capsular or vascular invasion. The nuclei seen in these tumors are extremely similar to those seen in cases of papillary thyroid carcinoma. Based on currently available data, this tumor can be expected to behave in an indolent fashion when strict diagnostic criteria are used. These tumors cannot be reliably distinguished from conventional papillary thyroid carcinoma in aspirate specimens or core biopsies. This diagnosis may be considered when the nuclear features of papillary thyroid carcinoma are seen but intranuclear pseudoinclusions, true papillae, and psammoma bodies are absent [19].

- Ancillary studies such as thyroglobulin on the FNA specimen from the thyroid bed or from a lymph node to exclude metastatic disease can be useful when cytology is less than definitive.

Medullary Thyroid Carcinoma

Clinical

- Accounts for 5–10% of cases of thyroid carcinoma.
- Neuroendocrine tumor derived from either the parafollicular cells or C cells of the thyroid gland, which produce calcitonin.
- Eighty percent are sporadic; 20% are associated with MEN syndrome IIA or IIB or are familial forms of medullary thyroid carcinoma [13]. Multicentricity is seen in familial cases.
- Generally present at a higher stage than well-differentiated thyroid carcinomas. Seventy-five percent of patients with a palpable thyroid mass have metastases to the cervical lymph nodes.
- While good outcomes are seen in patients with disease confined to the thyroid (95% 10-year survival in adults), patients with regionally advanced disease have a 70% 10-year survival rate.

Ultrasound

- Medullary carcinoma is usually hypoechoic and solid, with well-defined borders (Fig. 8.9).
- Echogenic foci may be seen in 80–90% of lesions and are usually dense and coarse.
- Metastatic lymph nodes are usually hypoechoic with coarse calcifications that demonstrate posterior shadowing.
- Color Doppler imaging shows chaotic intratumoral and intranodal vascularity.
- On US, medullary carcinoma is difficult to differentiate from papillary carcinoma. The best clues for differentiation are the presence of shadowing tumoral calcification (punctuate in papillary) and hypoechoic nodes (hyperechoic in papillary) with coarse shadowing [20].

Nuclear Medicine

- Positron emission tomography (PET) scan using fludeoxyglucose (FDG) may be used when there are elevated tumor markers but no gross disease on cross-sectional imaging.
- Octreotide scintigraphy (In-111-pentreotide) or I-131-MIBG may be taken up by the tumor.

Gross

- Circumscribed nodule with a tan-yellow cut surface.
- Commonly arises in the upper and middle third of the thyroid lobe.

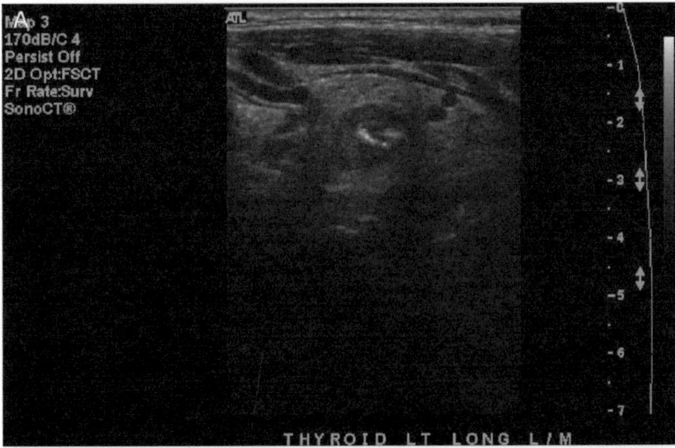

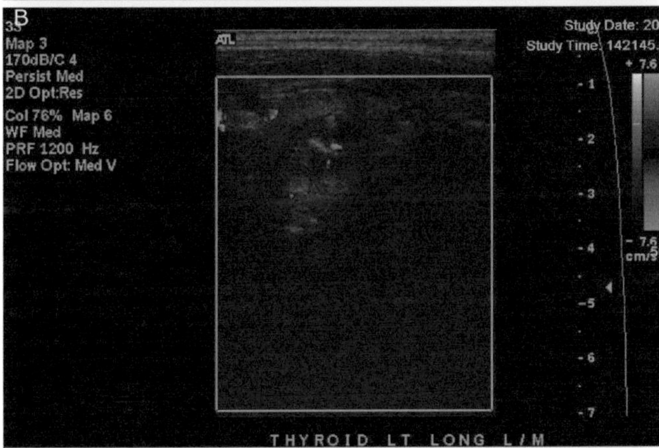

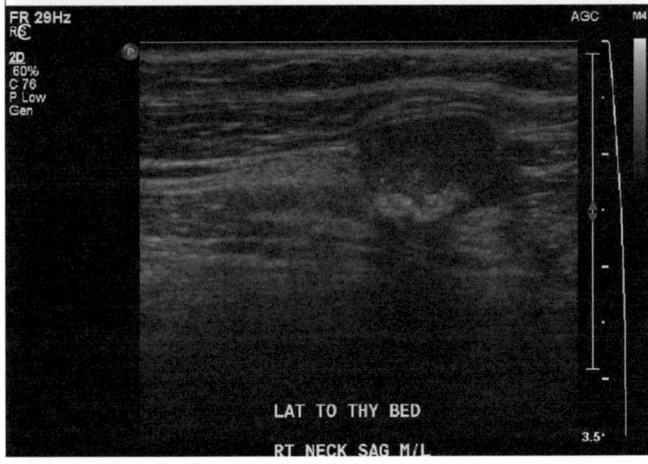

Fig. 8.9 Medullary thyroid carcinoma. (**a**) There is a well-defined hypoechoic left thyroid lobe nodule with several large coarse echogenic calcifications that demonstrate posterior acoustic shadowing. (**b**) On color Doppler imaging, there is some intratumoral vascularity. (**c**) In a different patient with metastatic medullary thyroid carcinoma, there is a hypoechoic right cervical lymph node with several coarse echogenic calcifications at the posterior aspect that demonstrate posterior acoustic shadowing

Fine Needle Aspiration

- Wide morphologic spectrum seen in aspirate smears, with cells showing variable shape and size pleomorphism [21].
- Typically hypercellular cytologic smears with single or loosely cohesive cells; however, follicular and pseudopapillary architecture can be seen (Fig. 8.10a)
- Cells may be monotonous or show marked pleomorphism; spindle, plasmacytoid, and epithelioid cells are common. Chromatin is typically finely speckled and salt and pepper in appearance (Fig. 8.10b).
- Cytoplasm often shows red metachromatic granules (Diff-Quik stain), corresponding to neuroendocrine granules (Fig. 8.10c).
- Background: amyloid material can closely mimic dense colloid but contains embedded spindled cells in many cases. The morphology of associated cells is key in recognizing this correctly.

Core Biopsy

- Neoplastic cells displaying a nested growth pattern composed of epithelioid cells with uniform, round, and monotonous nuclei and salt and pepper like chromatin. Focal area of dense, amorphous stroma (amyloid) is also seen (Fig. 8.10d).

Comment

- Medullary thyroid carcinoma may demonstrate significant morphologic overlap with Hurthle cell lesions (dense granular cytoplasm) and papillary thyroid carcinoma (intranuclear pseudo-inclusions). A microfollicular pat-

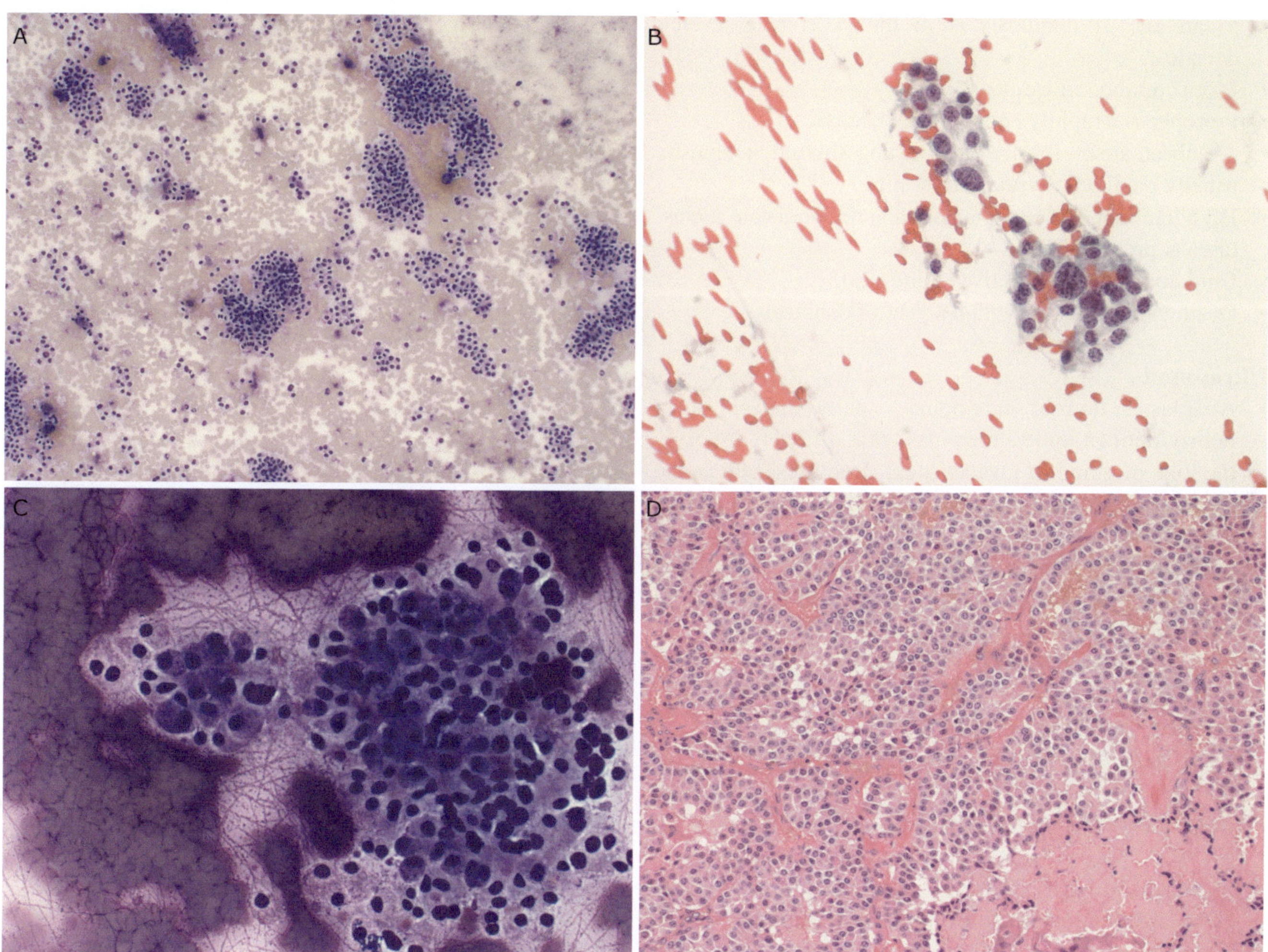

Fig. 8.10 Medullary thyroid carcinoma. (**a**) Aspirates of medullary thyroid carcinoma typically contain sheets of dyscohesive plasmacytoid cells with abundant granular cytoplasm. (**b**) A finely granular salt and pepper chromatin pattern can often be appreciated in Papanicolaou-stained aspirate slides. (**c**) The cytoplasm classically contains metachromatic (magenta) granules in DQ-stained preparations. (**d**) In histologic preparations, sheets of plasmacytoid cells with eosinophilic cytoplasm are seen. Most cases contain amorphous eosinophilic amyloid

tern can also be seen. Other differential diagnosis include plasma cell and spindle cell neoplasms. Hence medullary carcinoma has been referred to as "the melanoma of the thyroid"

- Use of immunohistochemistry on cell block material or biopsy cores to confirm the diagnosis is often reassuring, since tumor cells will be immunoreactive for chromogranin, synaptophysin, monoclonal carcinoembryonic antingen (CEA), and calcitonin.
- In the absence of suitable material for immunohistochemistry, elevated serum levels of calcitonin and CEA are strongly associated with this diagnosis and also useful to monitor recurrence.

Anaplastic Thyroid Carcinoma

Clinical

- Mean age at diagnosis is in the sixth and seventh decades.
- More common in women (3:1).
- Presents as a rapidly enlarging neck mass.
- A subset arises from a pre-existing thyroid neoplasm, usually papillary thyroid carcinoma.
- High likelihood of cervical lymph nodes or distant metastases at presentation.
- Cold nodule on radioactive iodine scan.
- Death usually occurs within a year of diagnosis.

Ultrasound

- Anaplastic thyroid carcinoma usually appears as a poorly defined hypoechoic mass that diffusely involves the lobe or gland. It invades local structures such as the trachea, esophagus, and perithyroid soft tissues (Fig. 8.11).
- Often there is necrosis or dense amorphous calcification. Color Doppler imaging shows prominent, small, chaotic intranodular vessels as well as abnormal vascularity in metastatic nodes [15].

Computed Tomography

- Anaplastic thyroid carcinoma appears as a large, ill-defined, heterogeneously enhancing primary lesion with dense calcification (58%) and necrosis (74%).
- There is often infiltration of adjacent structures such as the carotid artery, internal jugular vein, larynx, trachea, esophagus, mediastinum, and regional lymph nodes.
- Cervical lymph nodes are often involved with areas of necrosis [22].
- To differentiate anaplastic thyroid carcinoma from other lesions, tumor necrosis is the most valuable parameter. Older age (>70) and low attenuation (<100 Hounsfeld units (HU)) on postcontrast imaging are also helpful indicators [23].

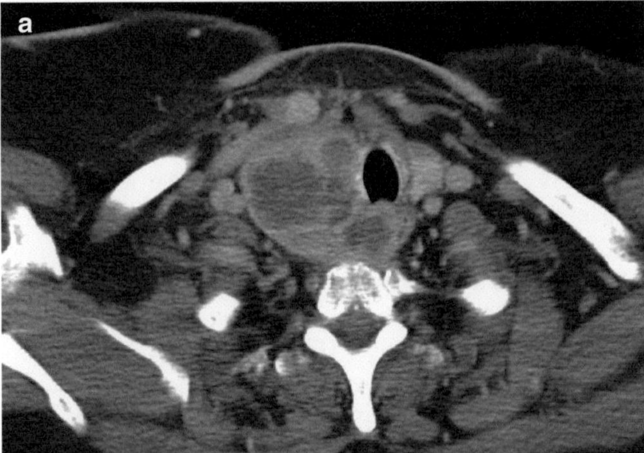

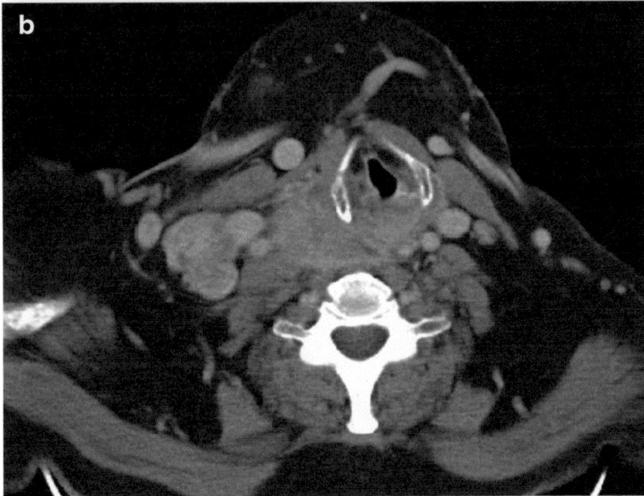

Fig. 8.11 Anaplastic thyroid carcinoma. (**a**) The right thyroid lobe is diffusely enlarged, with large areas of low attenuation representing necrosis. There is involvement of the membranous portion of the trachea. (**b**) There is a conglomeration of right cervical lymph nodes with areas of necrosis

Magnetic Resonance Imaging

- The tumor and involved lymph nodes demonstrate a diffusely hypointense T1 signal. Hemorrhage, necrosis, and calcification may result in a heterogeneous T1 signal.
- The lesion demonstrates variable T2 signal, although it is typically iso- to hyperintense.
- Postcontrast T1 imaging demonstrates moderate to marked heterogeneous enhancement [24].

Nuclear Medicine

- A technetium-99 m methylene-diphosphonate (MDP) bone scan can be used to determine bone metastases. I-131 scans are not performed in the evaluation and treatment of anaplastic carcinoma because the highly undifferentiated cells do not concentrate iodine.

Gross

- Diffusely invasive tumor often with extension to extrathyroidal structures.
- May be necrotic and hemorrhagic.

Fine Needle Aspiration

- Typically markedly cellular aspirate.
- Cells may be discohesive or in clusters with nuclear enlargement and marked pleomorphism (Fig. 8.12a). Nuclei have a coarse chromatin pattern with prominent nucleoli (Fig. 8.12b) [25, 26].
- Cell types include squamoid, giant, and spindle cell.
- Cytoplasm may be variable, with intracellular polymorphonuclear leukocytes common.
- Background may show necrotic debris and osteoclastic-like giant cells.

Core Biopsy

- Diffuse proliferation of large tumor cells with markedly pleomorphic nuclei, irregular nuclear borders, and vesicular chromatin. Mitotic figures are present (Fig. 8.12c). Tumors may morphologically or immunohistochemically resemble squamous cell carcinoma or angiosarcoma.

Comment

- Anaplastic thyroid carcinoma should show minimal morphologic or immunohistochemical evidence of thyroid differentiation. Colloid production should be absent, and the tumor cells should lack immunoreactivity for TTF1 and thyroglobulin. In most cases, weak Pax8 immunoreactivity is retained and may suggest the diagnosis.
- The main differential diagnostic consideration is usually a metastatic lesion from the lung or elsewhere, as anaplastic thyroid carcinoma does not usually show any morphologic evidence of thyroid differentiation. Correlation with the clinical and radiographic impression is extremely important. Pax8 reactivity may support the diagnosis of anaplastic thyroid carcinoma over a metastatic lesion.

Malignant Neoplasms: Metastatic Tumors to the Thyroid

General

- The most common tumors to metastasize to the thyroid gland are of the kidney, lungs, breast, hematologic malignancies, and melanoma [27].
- Secondary involvement of the thyroid gland may occur as direct extension by malignancies from contiguous organs or as a result of hematogenous/lymphatic spread from distant sites.
- Usually seen as a solitary nodule.
- Clinical history (and review of pathology slides from a prior malignancy) is one of the most important factors in the differential diagnosis of these lesions.
- Differentiation of metastatic lesions from a poorly differentiated or anaplastic thyroid carcinoma is difficult.

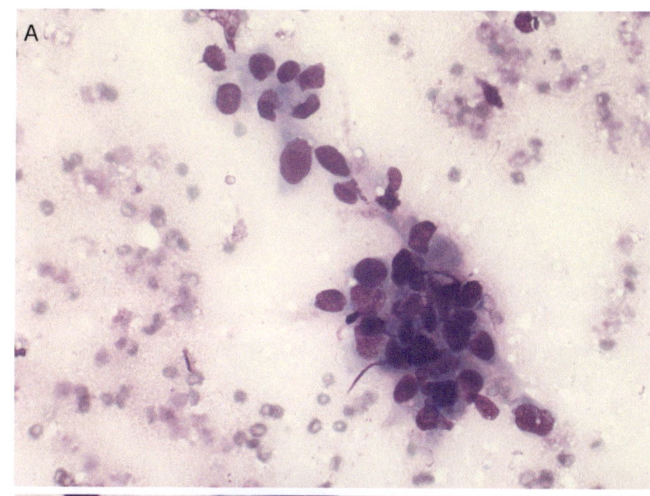

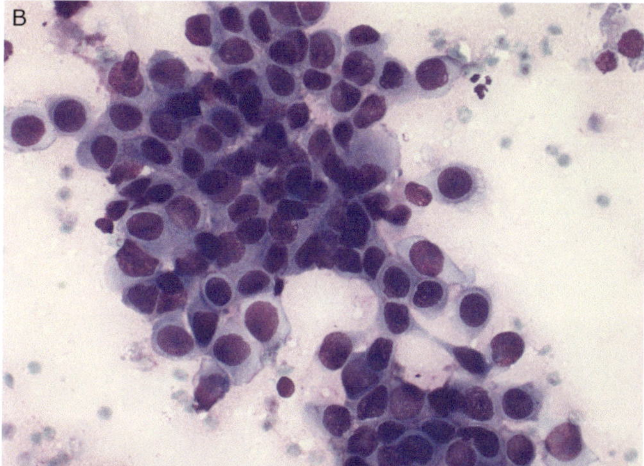

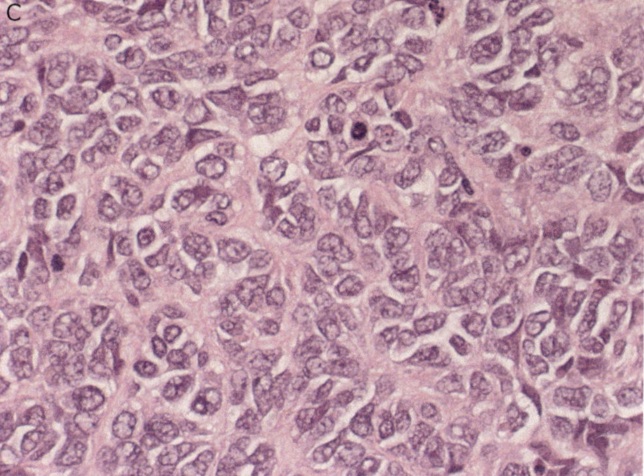

Fig. 8.12 Anaplastic thyroid carcinoma. (**a**, **b**) Irregular clusters and sheets of pleomorphic tumor cells with epithelioid and spindle cell features. No colloid production or morphologic evidence of thyroid differentiation is seen in this DQ-stained aspirate. (**c**) Sheets of pleomorphic nuclei with vesicular chromatin, irregular nuclear contours, and mitotic activity. No follicle formation is seen in this resected specimen

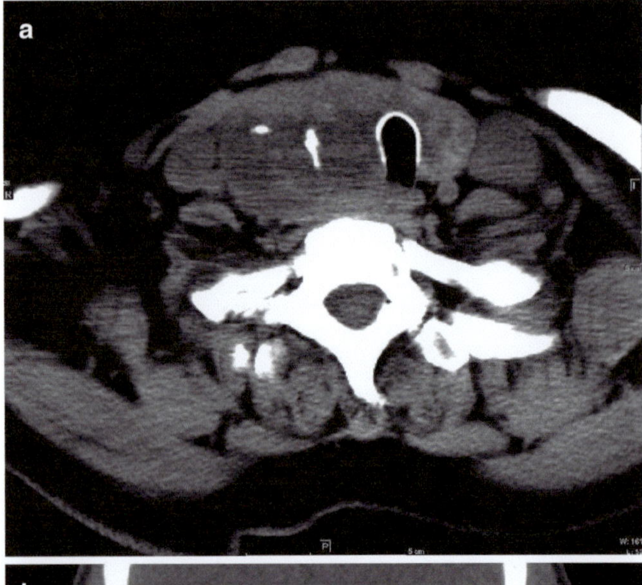

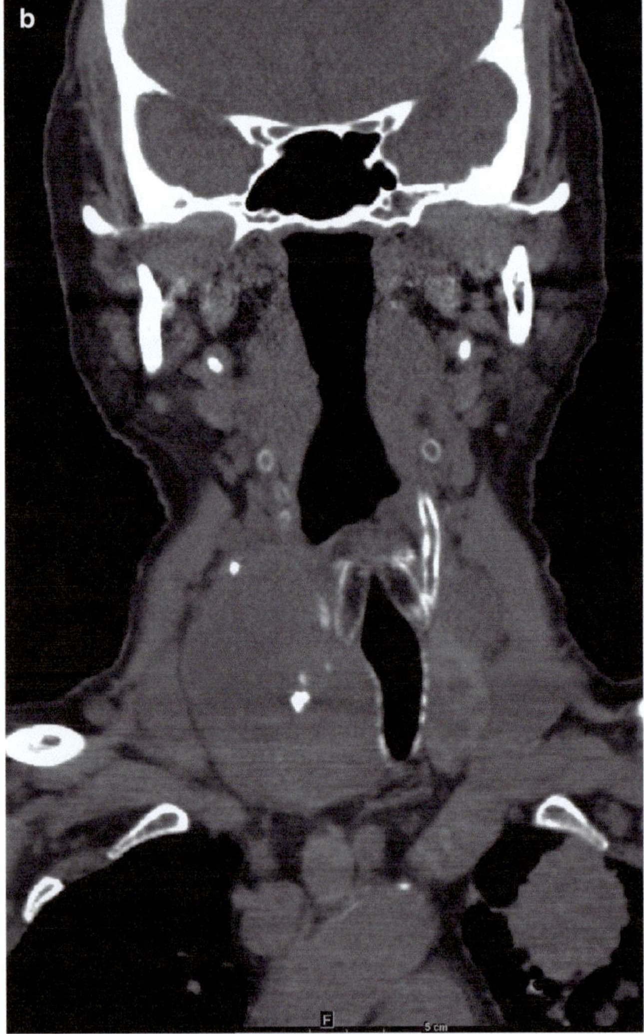

Fig. 8.13 Metastatic disease. (**a**) Axial CT image through the neck demonstrates a markedly enlarged and heterogeneous right thyroid lobe with a coarse calcification from metastatic uterine sarcoma. The enlarged right thyroid lobe causes narrowing and leftward shift of the trachea. (**b**) Coronal CT image demonstrates similar findings, with an additional exophytic left superior pole nodule

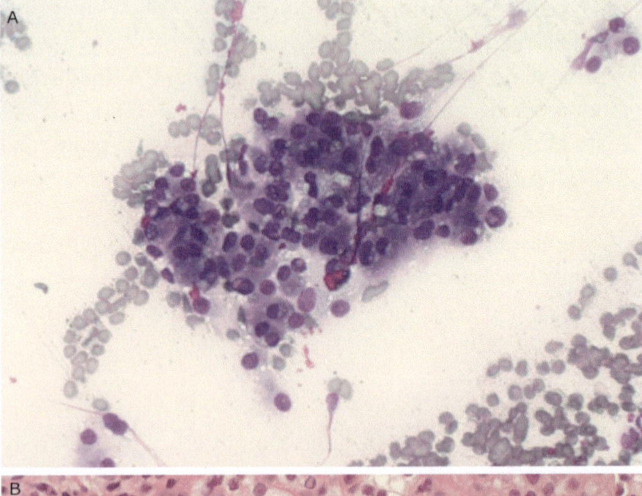

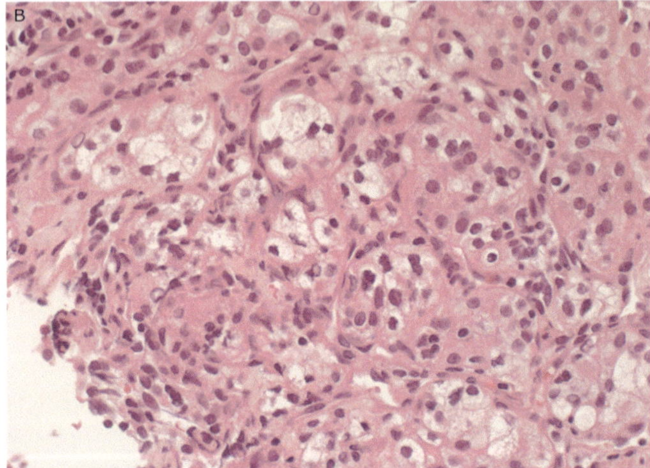

Fig. 8.14 Metastatic disease. (**a**) The tumor cells in this aspirate slide display a greater degree of pleomorphism than most forms of primary thyroid malignancy. The granular and vacuolated cytoplasm as well as the prominent nucleoli suggest a diagnosis of metastatic conventional renal cell carcinoma. (**b**) In a resected specimen, metastatic renal cell carcinoma involving the thyroid gland displays sheets of clear cytoplasm and prominent vascularity

Nuclear Medicine

- Metastases to the thyroid usually arise from breast, kidney, colon, or lung carcinoma or from melanoma primaries (Fig. 8.13). There are no distinguishing imaging features. They may be found incidentally on the FDG-PET scan.

Fine Needle Aspiration

- Varies with origin of the primary tumor.
- Metastatic renal cell carcinoma to the thyroid shows a loosely cohesive cluster of tumor cells with abundant finely vacuolated and granular cytoplasm and round eccentrically placed nuclei (Fig. 8.14a)

Core Biopsy

- Varies with the origin of the primary tumor.
- Needle core biopsy of renal cell carcinoma metastasizing to the thyroid shows infiltrating tumor cells with clear and vacuolated cytoplasm (Fig. 8.14b).

Miscellaneous Lesions

Thyroglossal Duct Cyst

General Characteristics

- The characteristic lesion is a midline cystic neck mass within the infrahyoid strap muscles.
- The majority are located at the level of the hyoid bone; however, the lesion can befound in the suprahyoid or infrahyoid neck as well [28].

Ultrasound

- The lesion appears as a well-circumscribed anechoic neck mass, usually in close proximity to the hyoid (Fig. 8.15).

Computed Tomography

- On noncontrast CT, the lesion is a benign-appearing, circumscribed fluid density mass.
- On contrast-enhanced CT, the lesion can occasionally have septations that show thin enhancement. If the cyst is superinfected, subtle enhancement of the cyst wall can be seen.

Magnetic Resonance Imaging

- On T1-weighted images, the lesion follows fluid signal intensity and is typically hypointense. If the cyst contains proteinaceous material, it can be slightly hyperintense on T1.
- On T2-weighted images, the lesion is homogeneously hyperintense. After administration of intravenous gadolinium, the characteristics are similar to those on CT, where there may be subtle enhancement of the cyst wall if there is a superinfection.

Fine Needle Aspiration

- Aspirates will often contain abundant colloid ranging in consistency from thin and watery to dense and thick [29].
- Scattered inflammatory cells, including lymphocytes and macrophages, are typical.
- An epithelial component may be seen and range from ciliated glandular cells to mature or immature squamous cells. Thyroid epithelium is not a usual finding.

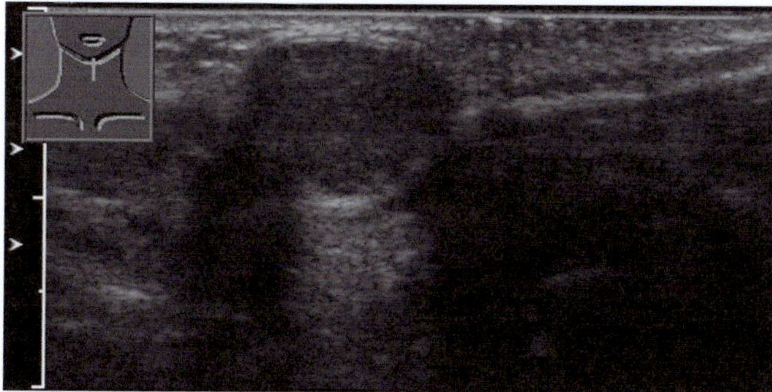

Fig. 8.15 Thyroglossal duct cyst. US image in the midline neck shows a circumscribed mass with posterior acoustic enhancement. Homogeneous echogenic reflectors within the mass are consistent with proteinaceous material, which can commonly be seen in thyroglossal duct cysts. These lesions can also be completely anechoic and have the appearance of classic cysts seen elsewhere in the body

Parathyroid Cyst

General Characteristics

- Classically, this appears as a homogeneous unilocular cyst posterior to the thyroid [30]. The lesion is seen arising from the parathyroid, most commonly the inferior parathyroid, and most commonly is on the left side.

Ultrasound

- US is the best imaging tool to differentiate the cyst from normal thyroid tissue. CT and MRI can be utilized if US findings are unclear (Fig. 8.16).
- The lesion is anechoic with posterior acoustic enhancement and no color Doppler flow.

Computed Tomography

- The appearance is that of a low density mass in the lower neck, with a thin or imperceptible wall. No enhancement is typically seen.

Magnetic Resonance Imaging

- The lesion follows fluid signal on all sequences, with a homogeneous low signal on T1 and a high signal on T2.

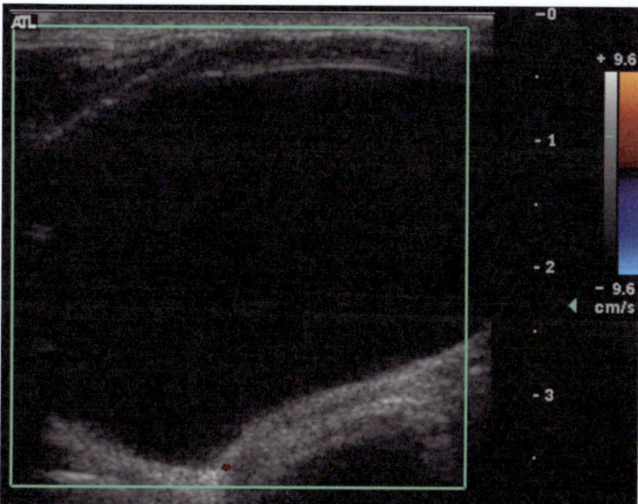

Fig. 8.16 Parathyroid cyst. Color Doppler US shows an anechoic lesion with posterior acoustic enhancement and no color flow, which is characteristic of a parathyroid cyst. This lesion is large and therefore adjacent neck structures are not visualized. However, real-time evaluation of proximity to adjacent thyroid tissue and neck vessels can help with the diagnosis

Fine Needle Aspiration

- Aspirates of parathyroid cysts are typically hypocellular or acellular and contain clear watery fluid.
- Sending the fluid for chemical analysis of PTH levels is diagnostic

Branchial Cleft Cysts

General Characteristics

- Branchial cleft cysts are rare and account for only 8% of branchial cleft remnant anomalies. Four subtypes have been described. The location is the most helpful characteristic when trying to determine which branchial cleft abnormality is present [32].
- The first branchial cleft cyst is a cystic mass located near the pinna or extending from the external auditory canal toward the mandibular angle [31, 32]. This subtype is extremely rare.
- The second branchial cleft cyst is located more inferiorly, classicly at the level of the mandibular angle and lateral to the carotid artery within the upper neck. This subtype is the most common [33].
- The third branchial cleft cyst results from failure of obliteration of the thymopharyngeal duct. The typical location is between the upper neck posterior cervical space and the anterior border of the sternocleidomastoid in the lower neck.
- The fourth branchial cleft anomaly consists of a sinus tract extending from the apex of the pyriform sinus to the left thyroid lobe. Recurrent abscesses in the superior left thyroid lobe are suggestive of this diagnosis.

Ultrasound

- The cysts are anechoic, circumscribed, simple-appearing masses most commonly in the periauricular region (first branchial cleft cyst) or at the level of the mandibular angle (second branchial cleft cyst).

Computed Tomography

- The lesion is a low-density cystic mass that is well circumscribed. There may be subtle rim enhancement. If the mass is infected, the rim enhancement may be thickened (Fig. 8.17).

Magnetic Resonance Imaging

- The lesion follows fluid signal and is low signal intensity on T1-weighted images and high signal intensity on T2-weighted images.
- There is typically no enhancement seen after administration of gadolinium, unless an infection is present.

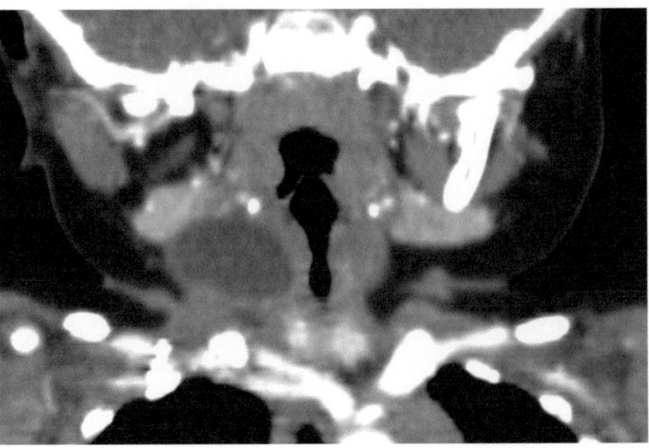

Fig. 8.17 Branchial cleft cyst, type II. Coronal low-dose contrast-enhanced CT in a child showing a circumscribed, nonenhancing low attenuation lesion in the mid-neck in the typical location of a type 2 branchial cleft cyst (level of the mandibular angle)

Fine Needle Aspiration

- Branchial cleft cysts show anucleated and nucleated squamous cells and histiocytes in a background of proteinaceous debris (Fig. 8.18).
- A prominent lymphoid component may be present in some cases.

Comment

- The most important differential diagnostic consideration is metastatic squamous cell carcinoma involving a cervical lymph node. Metastatic oropharyngeal carcinoma in particular may present as an occult primary tumor with a single enlarged, cystically degenerated lymph node, typically at level II/III. The presence of cytologic atypia or cohesive fragments of squamous cells should prompt consideration of metastatic squamous cell carcinoma, as should immunoreactivity for p16 [34]. The majority of oropharyngeal carcinomas will harbor high risk for human papillomavirus, which can be detected via RNA in situ hybridization or other methodologies [35].

Epidermal Inclusion Cyst

General Characteristics

- In the head and neck, these lesions most commonly involve the floor of the mouth [36], including the submandibular and sublingual spaces and the root of the tongue.

Ultrasound

- The lesion is a cystic, circumscribed, well-demarcated mass with fluid contents.

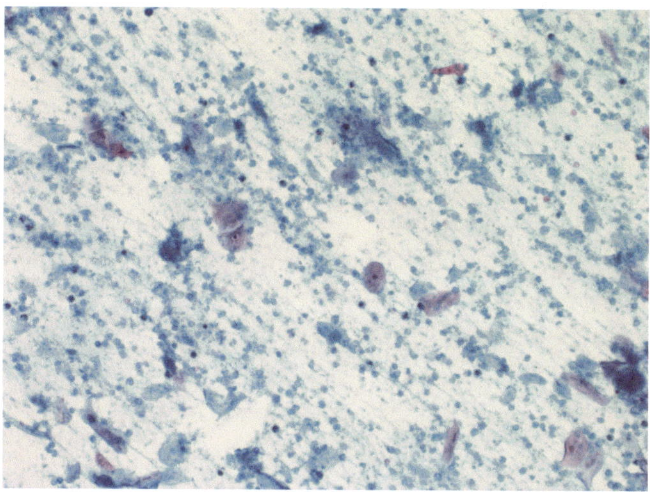

Fig. 8.18 Branchial cleft cyst: aspirates of branchial cleft cysts contain abundant granular debris and squamous cells

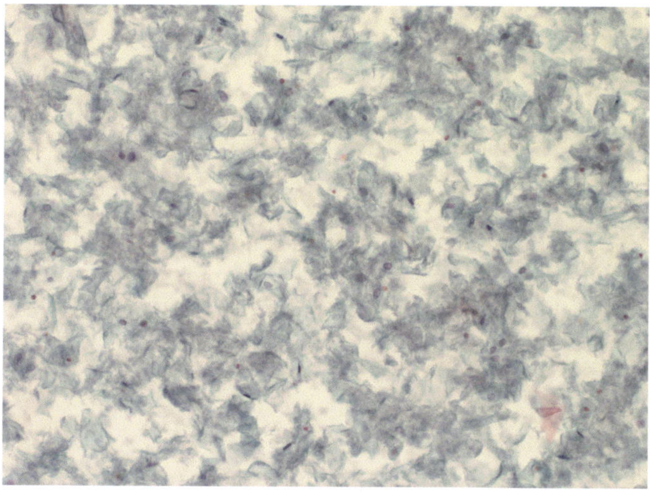

Fig. 8.19 Epidermal inclusion cyst: sheets of uniform anucleate squamous cells with a clean background

- US can be confusing with a "pseudosolid" appearance. CT and/or MRI may be needed to confirm the diagnosis.

Computed Tomography

- The lesion is a low density, unilocular, circumscribed mass that is fluid-dense with no internal complexity. Subtle rim enhancement is sometimes seen.

Magnetic Resonance Imaging

- The lesion has homogeneous fluid signal with low signal intensity on T1-weighted images and high signal intensity on T2-weighted images. The lesion may be nonenhancing or may have subtle rim enhancement.

Fine Needle Aspiration

- Epidermal inclusion cysts show numerous anucleated squamous cells (Fig. 8.19). They may get infected and contain acute inflammatory cells

Paraganglioma

General Characteristics

- These tumors are benign vascular tumors that can be seen in various locations. They are derived from primitive neural crest cells that are associated with nerve glomus bodies [37]. Eighty to ninety percent of extra-adrenal paragangliomas occur in or near the carotid body and adjacent to the jugular bulb.
- The nomenclature of paraganglioma lesions in the head and neck depends on the location, the most common being glomus jugulare (centered in jugular foramen) and carotid body paraganglioma (centered at carotid bifurcation).
- Carotid paraganglioma or carotid body tumor is the most common, often presenting as a painless neck mass.
- Glomus jugulare presents as a middle ear mass and can lead to tinnitus or hearing loss, also with possible mass effect on adjacent cranial nerves in the jugular foramen.
- Vagal paraganglioma is the least common head and neck subtype. This tumor, when large, can present as a painless neck mass with dysphagia or hoarseness in severe cases.

Computed Tomography

- On contrast-enhanced CT, the lesions are ovoid, lobulated, encapsulated masses that show avid enhancement.
- Depending on their size, they can exhibit local mass effect with displacement of adjacent fat and compression of adjacent vascular or nerve structures.

Magnetic Resonance Imaging

- The T1-weighted images demonstrate a low signal lesion with punctuate flow voids if large enough.
- The signal on T2-weighted images is intermediate to high, and there is slight hyperintensity on short T1 inversion recovery (STIR).
- After administration of intravenous gadolinium contrast medium, the lesion demonstrates homogeneous avid enhancement (Fig. 8.20).

Angiography

- Often an enlarged feeding vessel is identified with intense vascular blush of the lesion. Early draining veins are seen secondary to arteriovenous shunting.
- Because of their increased vascularity, biopsy of these lesions is contraindicated.

Nuclear Medicine

- There may be uptake of I-123 or I-131 in metastatic paraganglioma [38].
- Some lesions may show uptake of octreotide secondary to the presence of somatostatin receptors.

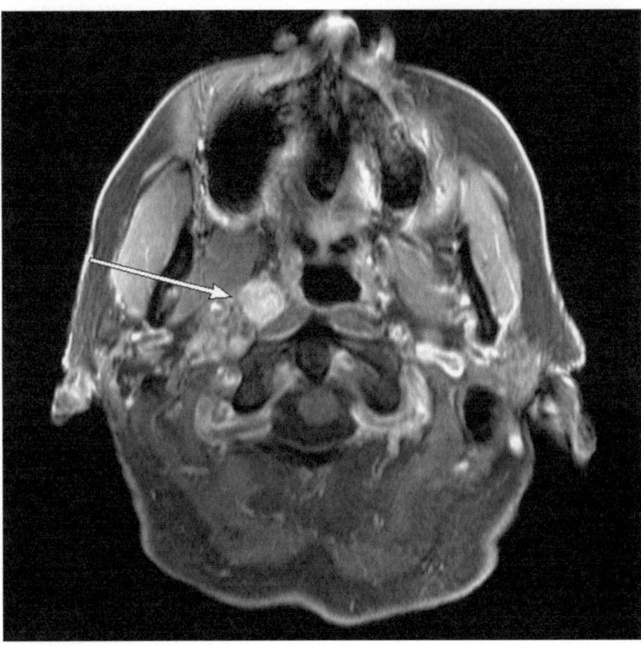

Fig. 8.20 Carotid body paraganglioma: postcontrast axial T1-MR image showing an avidly enhancing homogeneous mass in the right carotid bifurcation

Fine Needle Aspiration

- Aspirates are typically cellular and composed of spindle to polygonal tumor cells in loosely cohesive clusters or individually. A delicate capillary network is usually prominent and is intimately associated with the cellular elements [39].
- Individual tumor cells range in shape from spindle to plasmacytoid to epithelioid. The chromatin pattern is finely stippled, and cytoplasm is abundant and granular. In some cases, marked pleomorphism or intranuclear pseudo-inclusions may be seen.

Core Biopsy

- In histologic sections, paragangliomas demonstrate a sheetlike or nested growth pattern and are invested with a delicate capillary network often imparting a lobulated appearance. The borders are circumscribed and may be encapsulated.
- The nuclei are often monotonous and finely stippled. The cytoplasm is usually finely granular.

Comment

- Similar to other neuroendocrine tumors, paragangliomas of the head and neck are immunoreactive for chromogranin, CD56, and synaptophysin. S100 will label the sustentacular cells and highlight the lobular growth pattern.
- In contrast to most other neuroendocrine tumors, paragangliomas lack immunoreactivity for cytokeratins.

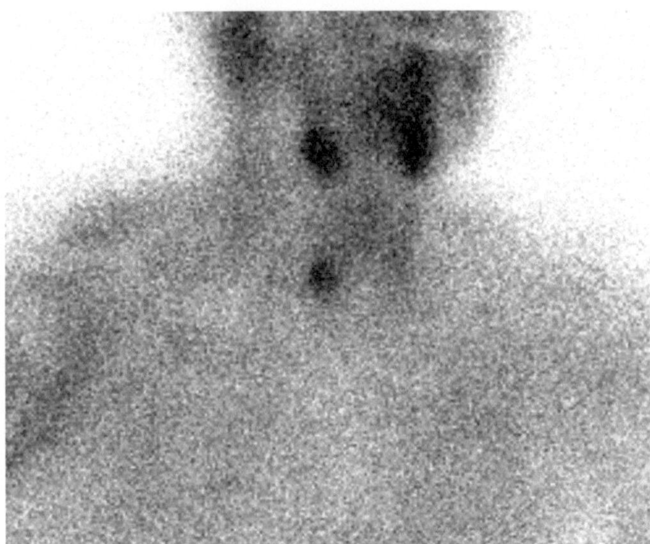

Fig. 8.21 Parathyroid adenoma. Technetium 99-m sestamibi parathyroid scan showing retention of radiotracer in a focus inferior to the right thyroid lobe

Parathyroid Adenoma

Ultrasound

- US demonstrates a homogeneous, circumscribed, hypoechoic mass adjacent to the thyroid gland [24].
- The lesion usually has increased vascularity on color Doppler imaging.

Nuclear Medicine

- Parathyroid adenomas demonstrate focal uptake and retention of radioisotope (either sestamibi or thallium), whereas there is rapid washout from normal thyroid tissue (Fig. 8.21).
- The lesions are usually 1–3 cm in size. Lesions smaller than 5 mm are not detected by nuclear medicine imaging.
- Nuclear medicine studies also allow detection of ectopic parathyroid adenomas.

Fine Needle Aspiration

- Aspirates will contain three-dimensional clusters of bland endocrine cells with nondescript cytoplasm and round nuclei with granular cytoplasm. There is a close resemblance to a follicular lesion of the thyroid. Helpful clues include the predominance of tightly cohesive three-dimensional clusters as well as naked nuclei in the background of the aspirate. Colloid is typically absent as are perivaculolar granules in the epithelial cells (Fig. 8.22a) [40].

Core Biopsy

- Normal parathyroid tissue as well as adenomas are composed of sheets of cuboidal endocrine cells, typically

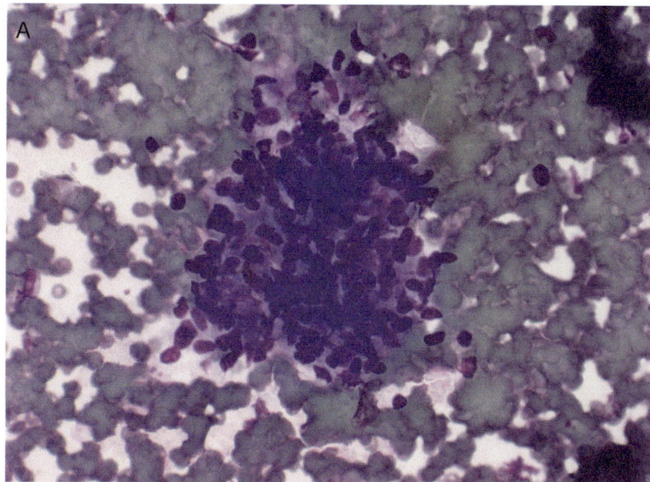

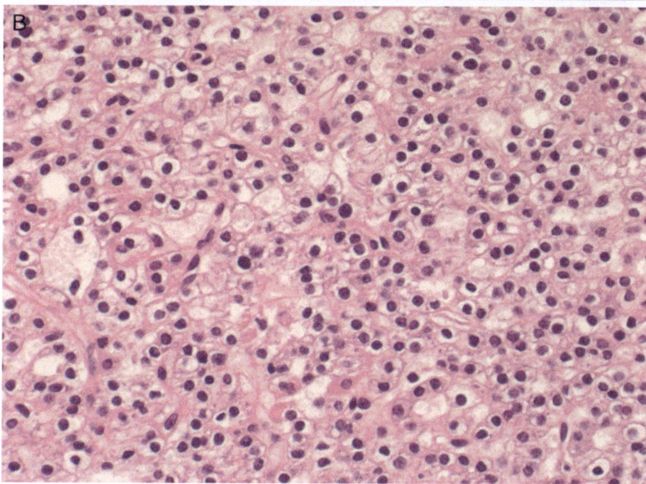

Fig. 8.22 Parathyroid adenoma. (**a**) In aspirate slides, parathyroid adenomas characteristically contain three-dimensional clusters of cuboidal cells similar to those found in thyroid follicular cells. Stripped background nuclei devoid of cytoplasm are a clue to the correct diagnosis. (**b**) In histologic sections, parathyroid lesions typically have more distinct cell boards and more hyperchromatic nuclei when compared to thyroid tissue

with well-defined cell borders and small, round hyperchromatic nuclei. A delicate vasculature is present (Fig. 8.22b).

- An admixture of clear (chief) and eosinophilic (oxyphil) cells is often seen.

References

1. Ali S, Cibas E. The Bethesda system for reporting thyroid cytopathology: definitions, criteria, and explanatory notes. 2nd ed. New York: Springer; 2018.
2. Haugen BR, Alexander EK, Bible KC, Doherty GM, Mandel SJ, Nikiforov YE, et al. 2015 American Thyroid Association Management Guidelines for Adult Patients with Thyroid Nodules and Differentiated Thyroid Cancer. Thyroid. 2016;26(1):1–133.
3. Jankovic B, Le KT, Hershman JM. Clinical review: Hashimoto's thyroiditis and papillary thyroid carcinoma: is there a correlation? J Clin Endocrinol Metab. 2013;98:474–82.
4. Simeone JF, Daniels GH, Mueller PR, Maloof F, van Sonnenberg E, Hall DA, et al. High-resolution real-time sonography of the thyroid. Radiology. 1982;145:431–5.
5. Yeh HC, Futterweit W, Gilbert P. Micronodulation: ultrasonographic sign of Hashimoto thyroiditis. J Ultrasound Med. 1996;15:813–9.
6. Langer JE, Khan A, Nisenbaum HL, Baloch ZW, Horii SC, Coleman BG, Mandel SJ. Sonographic appearance of focal thyroiditis. Am J Roentgenol. 2001;176:751–4.
7. Anderson L, Middleton WD, Teefey SA, Reading CC, Langer JE, Desser T, et al. Hashimoto thyroiditis: part 1, sonographic analysis of the nodular form of Hashimoto thyroiditis. Am J Roentgenol. 2010;195:208–15.
8. Chandanwale SS, Gore CR, Bamanikar SA, Gupta N, Gupta K. Cytomorphologic spectrum of Hashimoto's thyroiditis and its clinical correlation: a retrospective study of 52 patients. Cytojournal. 2014;11:9.
9. Ralls PW, Mayekawa DS, Lee KR, Colletti PM, Radin DR, Boswell WD, Halls JM. Color-flow Doppler sonography in Graves disease: "thyroid inferno". Am J Roentgenol. 1988;150:781–4.
10. Castagnone D, Rivolta R, Rescalli S, Castagnone D, Rivolta R, Rescalli S. Color Doppler sonography in Graves' disease: value in assessing activity of disease and predicting outcome. Am J Roentgenol. 1996;166:203–7.
11. Anderson SR, Mandel S, LiVolsi VA, Gupta PK, Baloch ZW. Can cytomorphology differentiate between benign nodules and tumors arising in Graves' disease? Diagn Cytopathol. 2004;31:64–7.
12. Harnsberger HR, Hudgins P, Wiggins R, Davidson C. Diagnostic imaging: head and neck. 1st ed. Salt Lake City, UT: Amirsys; 2004.
13. Guilmette J, Nosé V. Hereditary and familial thyroid tumours. Histopathology. 2018;72:70–81.
14. Chan BK, Desser TS, McDougall IR, Weigel RJ, Jeffrey RB Jr. Common and uncommon sonographic features of papillary thyroid carcinoma. J Ultrasound Med. 2003;22:1083–90.
15. Wong KT, Ahuja AT. Ultrasound of thyroid cancer. Cancer Imaging. 2005;5:157–66.
16. Das DK. Intranuclear cytoplasmic inclusions in fine-needle aspiration smears of papillary thyroid carcinoma: a study of its morphological forms, association with nuclear grooves, and mode of formation. Diagn Cytopathol. 2005;32:264–8.
17. Szporn AH, Yuan S, Wu M, Burstein DE. Cellular swirls in fine needle aspirates of papillary thyroid carcinoma: a new diagnostic criterion. Mod Pathol. 2006;19:1470–3.
18. Nikiforov YERR, Tallini G, Baloch ZW, Basolo F, Thompson LD, et al. Nomenclature revision for encapsulated follicular variant of papillary thyroid carcinoma: a paradigm shift to reduce overtreatment of indolent tumors. JAMA Oncol. 2016;2:1023–9.
19. Strickland KC, Howitt BE, Barletta JA, Cibas ES, Krane JF. Suggesting the cytologic diagnosis of noninvasive follicular thyroid neoplasm with papillary-like nuclear features (NIFTP): a retrospective analysis of atypical and suspicious nodules. Cancer Cytopathol. 2018;126:86–93.
20. Hoang JK, Lee WK, Lee M, Johnson D, Farrell S. US features of thyroid malignancy: pearls and pitfalls. Radiographics. 2007;27:847–60.
21. Papaparaskeva K, Nagel H, Droese M. Cytologic diagnosis of medullary carcinoma of the thyroid gland. Diagn Cytopathol. 2000;22:351–8.
22. Takashima S, Morimoto S, Ikezoe J, Takai S, Kobayashi T, Koyama H, et al. CT evaluation of anaplastic thyroid carcinoma. Am J Neuroradiol. 1990;11:361–7.
23. Lee JW, Yoon DY, Choi CS, Chang SK, Yun EJ, Seo YL, et al. Anaplastic thyroid carcinoma: computed tomographic differentiation from other thyroid masses. Acta Radiol. 2008;49:321–7.
24. Weber AL, Randolph G, Aksoy FG. The thyroid and parathyroid glands. CT and MR imaging and correlation with pathology and clinical findings. Radiol Clin North Am. 2000;38:1105–29.
25. Feng G, Laskin WB, Chou PM, Lin X. Anaplastic thyroid carcinoma with rhabdoid features. Diagn Cytopathol. 2015;43:416–20.

26. Berry B, MacFarlane J, Chan N. Osteoclastomalike anaplastic carcinoma of the thyroid. Diagnosis by fine needle aspiration cytology. Acta Cytol. 1990;34:248–50.
27. Wang H, Hoda RS, Faquin W, Rossi ED, Hotchandani N, Sun T, et al. FNA biopsy of secondary nonlymphomatous malignancies in salivary glands: a multi-institutional study of 184 cases. Cancer. 2017;125:91–103.
28. Waddell A, Saleh H, Robertson N, Khalil HS, Bridger MW. Thyroglossal duct remnants. J Laryngol Otol. 2000;114:128–9.
29. Shahin A, Burroughs FH, Kirby JP, Ali SZ. Thyroglossal duct cyst: a cytopathologic study of 26 cases. Diagn Cytopathol. 2005;33:365–9.
30. Lev S, Patel VG, Henderson VJ. Imaging of cystic lesions. Radiol Clin N Am. 2000;38:1013–27.
31. Finn DG, Buchalter IH, Sarti E, Romo T, Chodosh P. First branchial cleft cysts: clinical update. Laryngoscope. 1987;97:136–40.
32. Triglia JM, Nicollas R, Ducroz V, Koltai PJ, Garabedian EN. First branchial cleft anomalies: a study of 39 cases and a review of the literature. Arch Otolaryngol Head Neck Surg. 1998;124:291–5.
33. Sichel JY, Halperin D, Dano I, Dangoor E. Clinical update on type II first branchial cleft cysts. Laryngoscope. 1998;108:1524–7.
34. Layfield LJ, Esebua M, Schmidt RL. Cytologic separation of branchial cleft cyst from metastatic cystic squamous cell carcinoma: a multivariate analysis of nineteen cytomorphologic features. Diagn Cytopathol. 2016;44:561–7.
35. Bishop JA, Ma XJ, Wang H, Luo Y, Illei PB, Begum S, et al. Detection of transcriptionally active high-risk HPV in patients with head and neck squamous cell carcinoma as visualized by a novel E6/E7 mRNA in situ hybridization method. Am J Surg Pathol. 2012;36:1874–82.
36. Fuchshuber S, Grevers G, Issing WJ. Dermoid cyst of the floor of the mouth-- a case report. Eur Arch Otorhinolaryngol. 2002;259:60–2.
37. DeLellis RA. The neuroendocrine system and its tumors: an overview. Am J Clin Pathol. 2001;115 Suppl:S5–16.
38. Campbell L, Mouratidis B, Sullivan P. Improved detection of disseminated pheochromocytoma using post-therapy I-131 MIBG scanning. Clin Nuclear Med. 1996;21:960–3.
39. Singhi AD, Hruban RH, Fabre M, Imura J, Schulick R, Wolfgang C, Ali SZ. Peripancreatic paraganglioma: a potential diagnostic challenge in cytopathology and surgical pathology. Am J Surg Pathol. 2011;35:1498–504.
40. Domingo RP, Ogden LL, Been LC, Kennedy GC, Traweek ST. Identification of parathyroid tissue in thyroid fine-needle aspiration: a combined approach using cytology, immunohistochemical, and molecular methods. Diagn Cytopathol. 2017;45:526–32.

Salivary Glands

9

Ajit S. Paintal, Khairuddin Memon, Ahmed Gabr, Songlin Zhang, and Ahsun Riaz

Introduction

There are three pairs of major salivary glands and several hundred minor salivary glands. The parotid gland is made up of serous-type acini with the exception of a few mucinous units; the submandibular gland is mixed with a predominance of serous-type acini; and the sublingual gland is predominantly composed of mucinous-type acini. Many lesions can arise or involve the salivary glands, including non-neoplastic lesions, primary benign and malignant neoplasms, and metastatic malignancies. Fine-needle aspiration (FNA) has been accepted as an excellent although challenging method of evaluating salivary gland lesions with very good sensitivity, specificity, and accuracy. A number of reporting schemes have been utilized, with the Milan System being the latest international effort aimed at standardizing the reporting of salivary gland cytopathology in order to facilitate appropriate clinical management [1–3].

The main indication for FNA biopsy of the major salivary glands is the diagnosis of primary salivary gland neoplasia. In contrast to the masses in the thyroid gland, the majority of clinically detected masses are neoplasms. Management of most salivary gland neoplasms is based upon the broad categories of benign neoplasms, low-grade malignancies, and high-grade malignancies. Operatively, benign neoplasms and low-grade malignancies are typically treated similarly by simple resection. In the case of high-grade malignancies, a more radical resection may be indicated, and in some cases an elective neck dissection may be performed [4].

While dozens of salivary gland neoplasms with overlapping cytomorphologies have been described, fortuitously the most common benign and malignant neoplasms have relatively distinct patterns in aspiration cytology.

Normal Findings

FNA

- Aspirates of normal salivary gland parenchyma are dominated by lobules of acinar cells forming tightly cohesive spherical acini. The individual cells have indistinct cell borders, coarsely granular cytoplasm, and bland eccentric nuclei (Fig. 9.1).
- Ductal cells form flat sheets of nondescript cohesive cuboidal cells with round, evenly spaced monotonous nuclei.
- A pitfall associated with this "grapes on a stalk" pattern of normal salivary gland should be distinguished from acinic cell carcinoma (see below)

A. S. Paintal (✉)
Northshore Medical Group, Evanston Hospital, Evanston, IL, USA

K. Memon
Department of Radiology, OU Physicians, Oklahoma City, OK, USA

A. Gabr
Department of Radiology, Section of Vascular and Interventional Radiology, Northwestern University, Chicago, IL, USA

S. Zhang
Department of Pathology and Laboratory Medicine, University of Texas McGovern Medical School, Houston, TX, USA

A. Riaz
Department of Pathology, Northwestern Medicine, Chicago, IL, USA

R. Nayar et al. (eds.), *Atlas of Cytopathology and Radiology*, https://doi.org/10.1007/978-3-030-24756-0_9

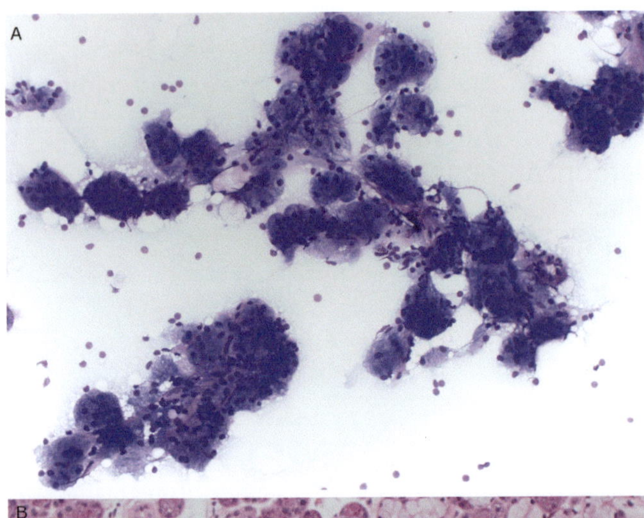

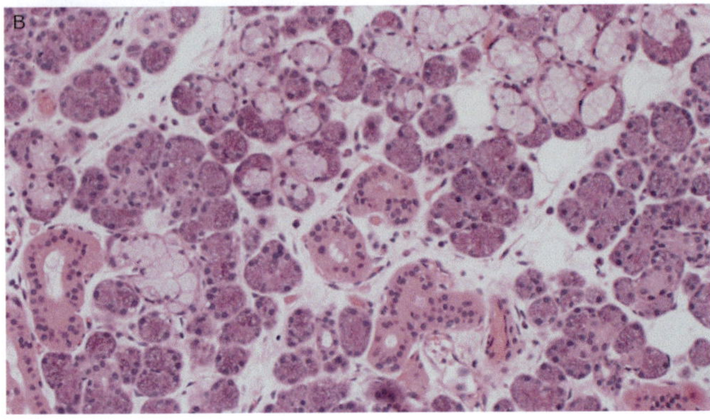

Fig. 9.1 Sialosis. (**a**) Aspirate containing acini of serous salivary gland cells forming tight grapelike clusters of cells with granular cytoplasm and bland nuclei. The acini are oriented around ductal structures composed of flattened cells with high nuclear:cytoplasmic ratios. (**b**) In histologic sections, normal salivary gland parenchyma is predominantly made up of serous cells with basophilic coarse granules and mucinous cells with clear rarified cytoplasm in various proportions. A minor ductal element is seen with well-formed lumina

Non-neoplastic Conditions

Sialosis

General Characteristics

- Diffuse non-neoplastic enlargement of the major salivary glands.
- Usually bilateral; gives a "chipmunk" facial appearance
- May occur in the settings of diabetes, alcoholism, or malnutrition.

Ultrasound (US)

- On US, sialosis appears as a diffusely enlarged gland with a normal sonographic appearance of the parenchyma, without any focal lesion.

Computed Tomography (CT)

- On CT, marked enlargement of both parotid glands may be seen with normal submandibular and sublingual glands. The attenuation coefficient of the parotid glands may be equivalent to that of fat (−55 Hounsfield units) and much lower than the normal range for parotid-gland parenchyma of −25 to 10 Hounsfield units, which is typically seen. Prominent septa of soft-tissue density may be seen within the gland parenchyma [5]. Alternatively, the size enlargement may be the only finding without change in the density of the tissue (Fig. 9.2).

Fine Needle Aspiration (FNA)

- Aspirates from patients with sialosis contain lobules of unremarkable acinar cells, fat, and sheets of ductal cells [6]. The distinction between normal salivary gland tissue and sialosis is made on the basis of clinical findings as well as the fact that the lobules of acinar tissue are significantly larger than those seen in aspirates from normal salivary glands.

Core Biopsy

- In core biopsies, sialosis resembles normal salivary gland tissue, but with larger lobules of acinar cells.

Sialolithiasis

General Characteristics

- A calcified mass (sialolith) forms within the salivary gland ductal system.
- It typically involves the submandibular gland but also may involve other major and minor salivary glands.
- May result in secondary infection.

Ultrasound

- Stones appear as strongly hyperechoic foci with distal acoustic shadowing. Small stones (<2 mm) may not shadow [7]. In cases of obstruction, the gland may appear enlarged with dilatation of the ducts proximal to the stone.

Computed Tomography

- On CT, the stones appear intensely hyperdense (Fig. 9.3), both within the duct and within the gland. In cases of obstruction, the gland may appear enlarged, hyperdense, and associated with stranding and enhancement following contrast administration. In chronic cases, fatty atrophy will be evident, with the parenchyma reduced in volume and replaced by fat.

Magnetic Resonance Imaging

- MRI is not only able to visualize larger stones but also in many instances is able to map the ductal anatomy and to assess the gland [8]. Stones appear as low-signal regions (on all sequences) outlined by high-signal saliva on T2-weighted images. In cases in which a small nonobstructive sialolith is present, the gland may appear entirely normal in appearance.

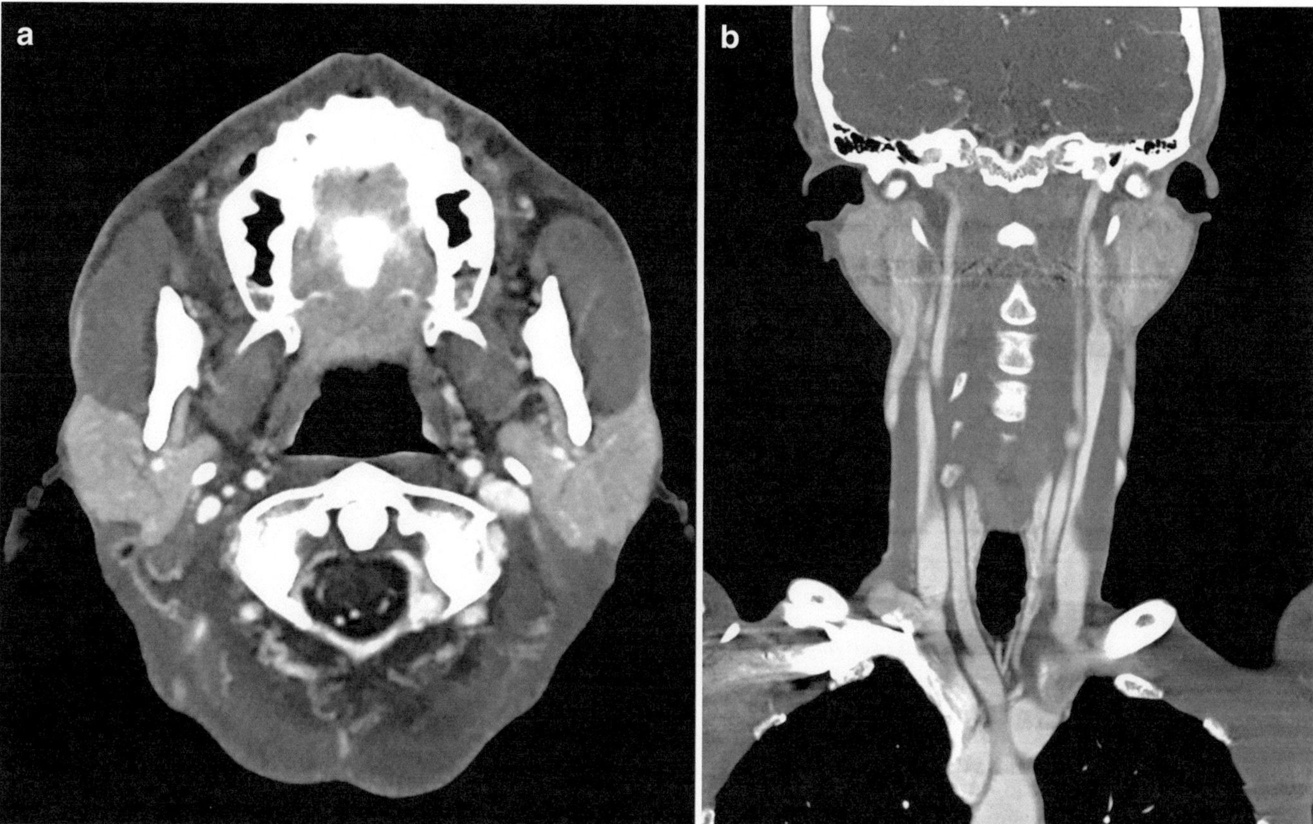

Fig. 9.2 Sialosis. Contrast-enhanced axial (**a**) and coronal (**b**) CT demonstrates moderate enlargement of the parotid glands without focal lesions; this is most compatible with sialosis

Fine Needle Aspiration

- In aspirates, stone fragments may be seen in occasional cases [9]. Other findings are relatively nonspecific and include extravasated mucin, hyperplastic epithelial fragments with mucinous metaplasia, and acute and chronic inflammation.

Core Biopsy

- Core biopsies in some cases may demonstrate ductal ectasia with chronic inflammation and stone fragments.

Sialadenitis

General Characteristics

- Inflammation of the salivary gland.
- May be acute or chronic and present with localized or systemic symptoms.
- May be infectious or noninfectious (often autoimmune) in etiology.

Ultrasound

- On US, the affected gland appears enlarged, hypoechoic, and hyperemic [10]. In chronic forms, the affected gland appears atrophic and diffusely hypoechoic with irregular margins. There may be evidence of sialectasis if there is recurrence.

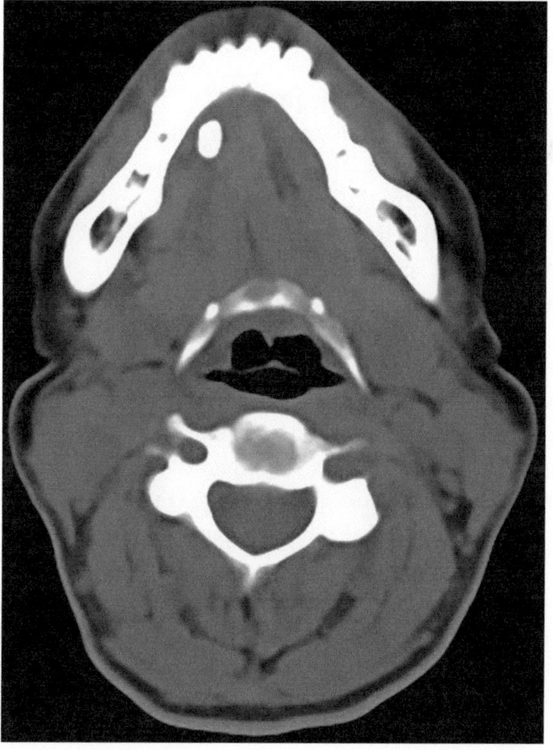

Fig. 9.3 Sialolithiasis: non-contrast CT of the salivary glands demonstrates moderate sized hyperdense stones in the right submandibular gland duct

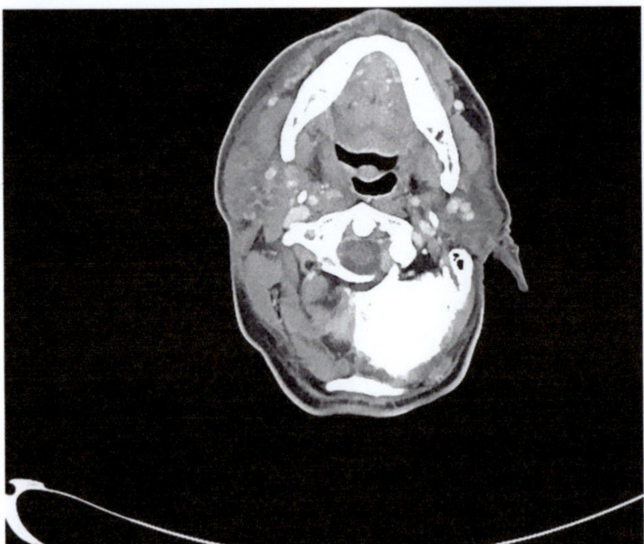

Fig. 9.4 Sialadenitis: Axial contrast-enhanced CT of the salivary gland demonstrates extensive inflammation and fat stranding in the soft tissues surrounding the right parotid gland and overlying subcutaneous tissues. No definite sialolith is visualized along the course of the right Stensen duct

Computed Tomogaphy

- On CT, the salivary gland may be enlarged with abnormal attenuation, indistinct margins, and vivid contrast enhancement with associated adjacent fat stranding (Fig. 9.4) and/or thickening of the deep cervical fasciae that are typically unilateral [10]. Enlarged intra- or extraglandular lymph nodes may also be seen but are nonspecific.

Magnetic Resonance Imaging

- The involved gland is often enlarged. The affected gland can range from well-defined to poorly defined. Signal characteristics in the majority of cases tend to be heterogeneous [10]. The gland has a low T1 signal and a high signal on T2 sequences in acute forms. The T2 signal may be low in chronic forms secondary to fibrosis.

Fine Needle Aspiration

- Aspirates from cases of chronic sialadenitis are typically hypocellular. Occasional fragments of ductal epithelium are seen with interspersed lymphoid tangles and irregular fragments of fibrotic stromal tissue (Fig. 9.5a, b) [11].
- In cases of acute sialadenitis, the aspirate is dominated by sheets of neutrophils and degenerated metachromatic material.
- Sialadenitis with crystalloid formation has a distinctive appearance, yielding cyst fluid with numerous, variably shaped amylase crystalloids in a background of histiocytes, inflammation, and reactive ductal cells.

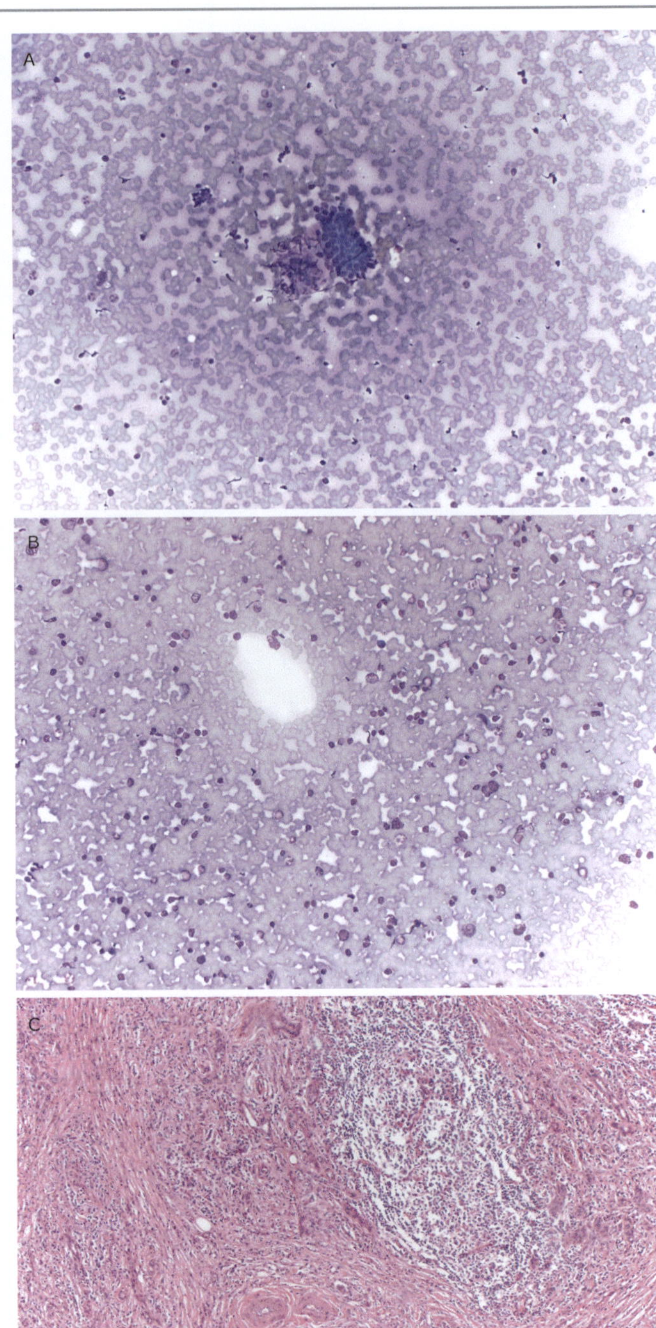

Fig. 9.5 Chronic sialadenitis: (**a**) Hypocellular aspirate containing rare clusters of nondescript basaloid ductal epithelium with high nuclear:cytoplasmic ratios. (**b**) The background of the aspirate contains numerous chronic inflammatory cells. (**c**) In histologic sections, a dense lymphoid infiltrate with germinal center formation, fibrosis, and loss of the salivary gland acinar tissue and preservation of the ductal structures is seen

Core Biopsy

- In cases of longstanding chronic sialadenitis, prominent fibrosis is seen, along with loss of the normal acinar tissue. Chronic inflammation with germinal center formation may be prominent (Fig. 9.5c).
- In cases of acute sialadenitis, the normal salivary gland structures are obscured by a neutrophilic infiltrate.

Comment

- Some cases of chronic sialadenitis are related to IgG4-mediated sclerosing disease. The findings of cellular fibrosis, a lymphoplasmacytic infiltrate, and obliterative phlebitis in a core biopsy or resected specimen may suggest this diagnosis [12]. Measurement of serum or tissue IgG4 levels may be of value in this context.

Sialocele

General Considerations

- Accumulation of saliva within tissue that typically develops as a result of an injured salivary gland.
- Often the result of trauma, either surgical or otherwise.

Ultrasound

- On US, the salivary gland cyst may appear as hypoechoic to anechoic, depending on its contents.

Computed Tomography

- On CT, sialocele will vary in its density, depending on its contents, but it would typically measure fluid attenuation (Fig. 9.6).

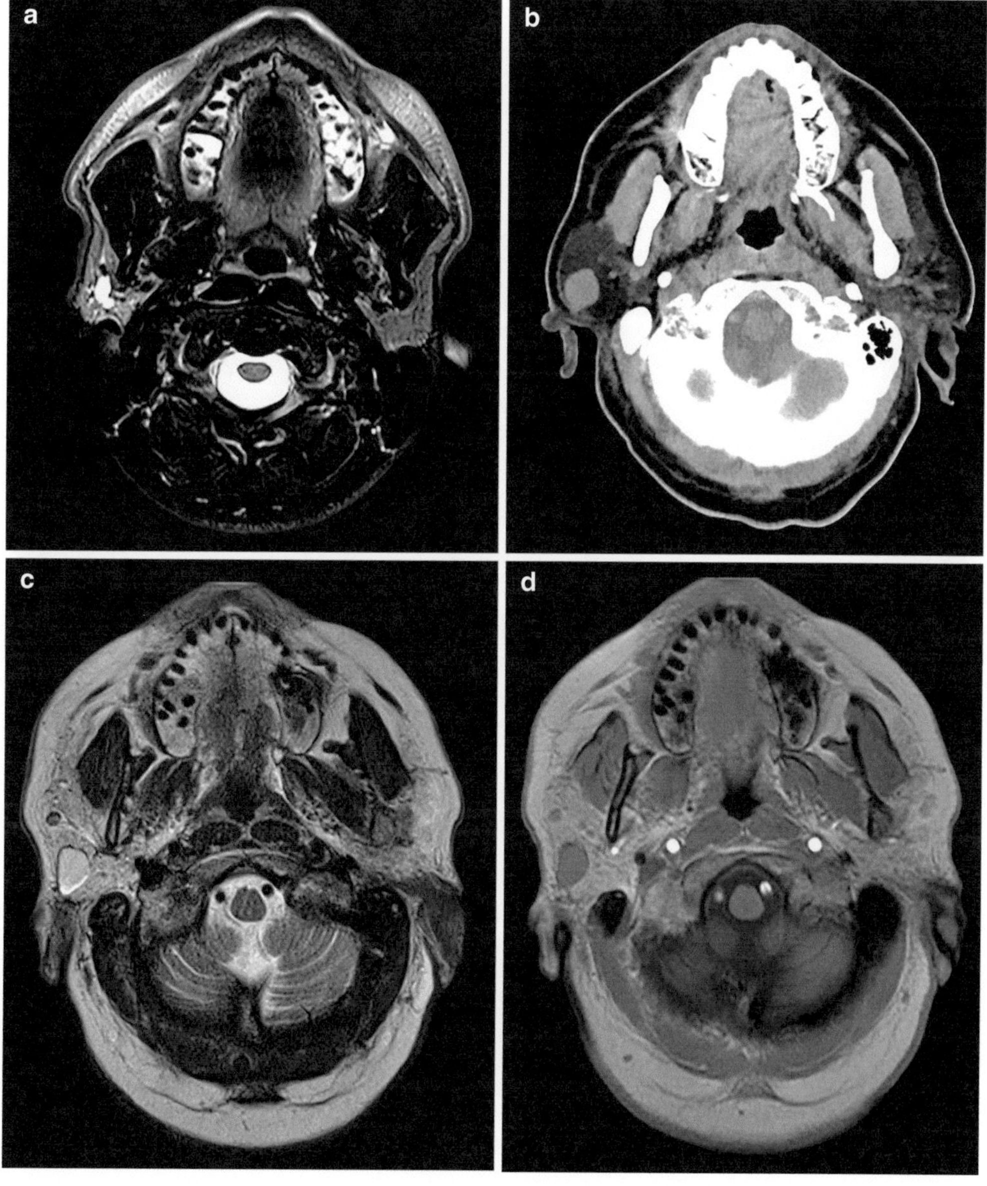

Fig. 9.6 Sialocele: (**a**) Axial T2-weighted sequence demonstrates a small sialocele and mildly dilated intraparotid ducts. (**b**) Axial noncontrast CT demonstrates a round fluid-attenuation right parotid gland lesion consistent with a cyst. On MRI the lesion appears T2 hyperintense (**c**) and T1 hypointense (**d**)

Magnetic Resonance Imaging

- T2-weighted sequence may show a sialocele to be T2 hyperintense. The cyst will be typically T1 hypointense and does not demonstrate enhancement.

Fine Needle Aspiration

- Aspirates are hypocellular and often contain mucin with occasional histiocytes (Fig. 9.7).

Comment

- The main differential diagnostic consideration is low-grade mucoepidermoid carcinoma, which may also present as a predominantly cystic salivary gland mass. Any mucinous lesion with an epithelial component should prompt strong consideration of low-grade mucoepidermoid carcinoma. Even in cases in which only mucin is present in aspirate slides, a definitive diagnosis of sialocele should not be made.

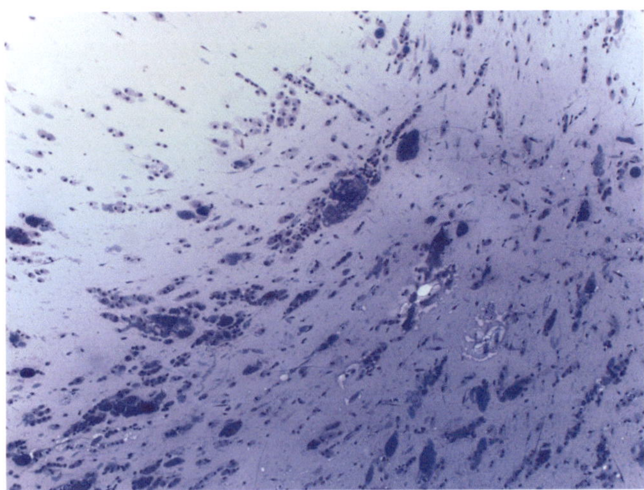

Fig. 9.7 Sialocele: aspirates are hypocellular and contain abundant mucinous material. Scattered histiocytes are seen in the background

Intraparotid Lymph Nodes

General Considerations

- Lymph nodes are commonly present within the parotid gland and may be involved by reactive hyperplasia, lymphoma, or metastatic lesions.
- A reactive intraparotid lymph node may present clinically as a parotid mass.
- Submandibular lymph nodes may be mistaken for submandibular gland masses radiographically.

Ultrasound

- The parotid gland is the only salivary gland to contain intraglandular lymph nodes. On US, they may appear as well-defined ovoid or round hypoechoic nodules with posterior sonographic enhancement and a central echogenic and central hilar vascularity on color Doppler imaging.

Computed Tomography

- On CT, lymph nodes appear as intraparotid masses, slightly hyperdense to the parenchyma. A fatty hilum may be seen. Associated lymph node enlargement may be seen in the neck (Fig. 9.8).

Magnetic Resonance Imaging

- On MRI, lymph nodes are slightly T1 hypointense and enhance on the post-gadolinium images (Fig. 9.8).

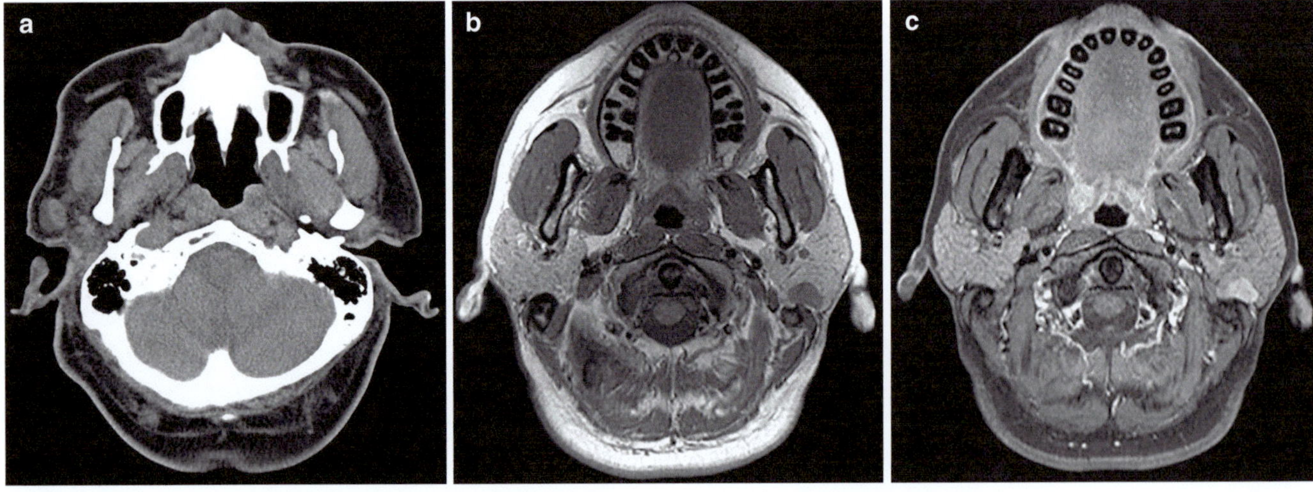

Fig. 9.8 Intraparotid lymph node. (**a**) Axial CT demonstrates an oval right parotid gland lesion consistent with a lymph node. On MRI in another patient, a left parotid lymph node appears T1 hypointense (**b**) and enhances (**c**)

Fine Needle Aspiration

- Aspirates from intraparotid lymph nodes demonstrate a polymorphous population of lymphoid cells, ranging from small lymphocytes to activated centroblasts and immunoblasts. Histiocytes, dendritic cells, and plasma cells may also be prominent (Fig. 9.9).

Core Biopsy

- Organized lymphoid tissue with germinal centers and histiocytic aggregates are typically seen in core biopsies of reactive lymph nodes.

Lymphoepithelial Lesions

General Considerations

- Often slow growing and cystic with multilocular or unilocular growth.
- May be associated with the human immunodeficiency virus (HIV) or autoimmune diseases.

Ultrasound

- On US, there may be visualization of well-circumscribed cystic spaces; these may contain multiple small septations and commonly also small mural nodules.

Computed Tomography

- The lesions may appear cystic with fluid attenuation (<20 Hounsfield units) or partly solid. These are typically multiple and bilateral (Fig. 9.10).

Magnetic Resonance Imaging

- On MRI, the lesions are typically T2 hyperintense and may demonstrate a thin rim of enhancement.

Fine Needle Aspiration

- Aspirates are characterized by a combination of granular cystic debris, polymorphous lymphocytes, and occasional angulated squamous cells (Fig. 9.11) [13].

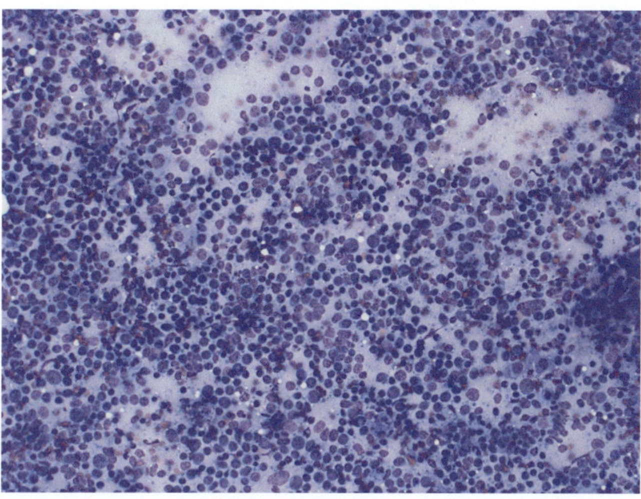

Fig. 9.9 Reactive intraparotid lymph node. Aspirates are cellular and contain polymorphous round lymphoid cells with round nuclei of varying sizes. Numerous fragments of blue cytoplasm (lymphoglandular bodies) are seen in the background

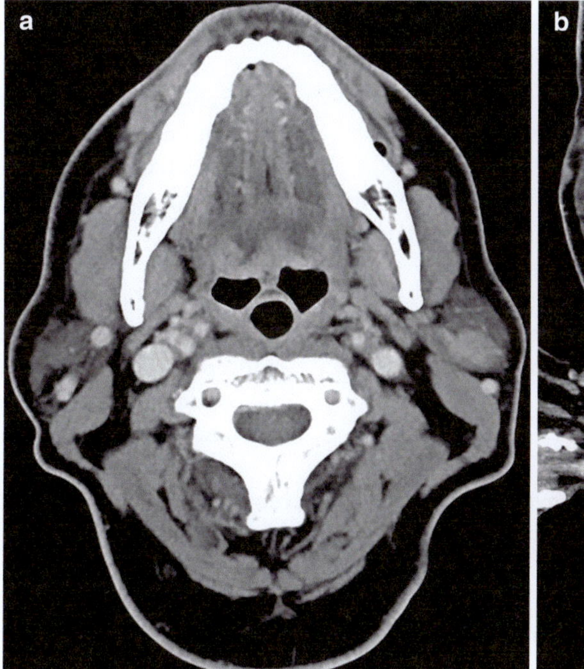

Fig. 9.10 Lymphoepithelial lesion. Contrast-enhanced axial (**a**) and coronal (**b**) CT demonstrates bilateral lobulated mixed solid and cystic lesions that appear slightly hyperdense compared to the parenchyma. In a patient with human immunodeficiency virus, these probably represent lymphoepithelial lesions

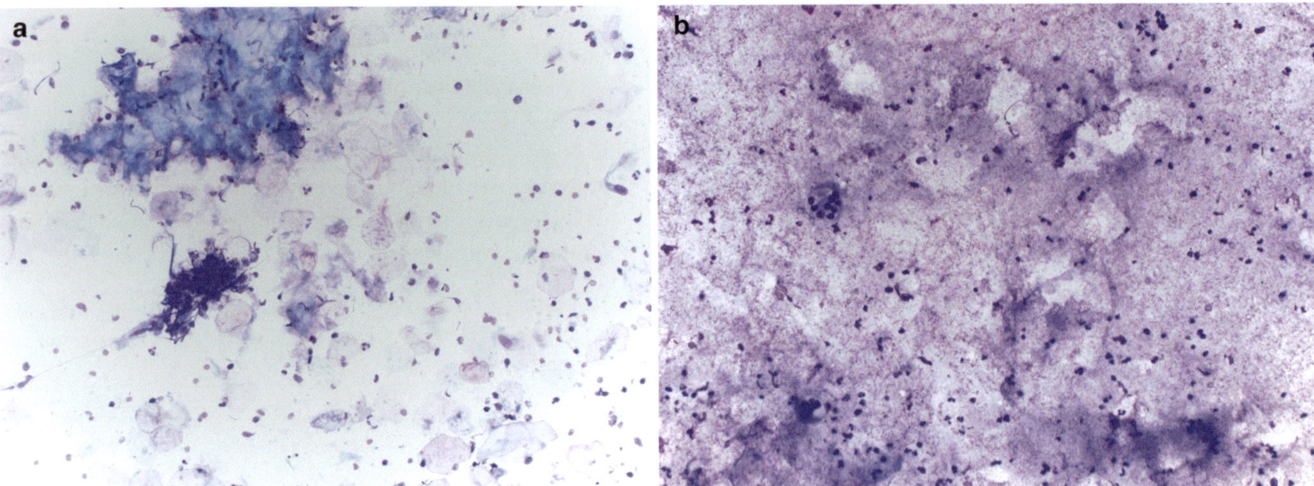

Fig. 9.11 Lymphoepithelial lesion. (**a**) Aspirates contain anucleate squamous cells, granular debris, and scattered lymphocytes and fragments of lymphoid tissue. (**b**) Granular debris, mixed inflammatory cells, and multinucleated giant cells may be seen

Core Biopsy

- In histologic sections, lymphoepithelial lesions demonstrate lymphoid stroma with cyst formation. The lymphoid stroma is typically polymorphous in nature with admixed plasma cells and macrophages.

Comment

- Other cystic salivary gland lesions with a prominent lymphoid component that may enter the differential diagnosis include acinic cell carcinoma, Warthin tumor, and lymphadenoma.

Benign Neoplasms

Pleomorphic Adenoma

General Considerations

- The most common benign salivary gland neoplasm. Occasionally carcinoma may arise in a longstanding lesion (carcinoma ex-pleomorphic adenoma).
- Instrumented lesions may metastasize (metastasizing pleomorphic adenoma). Despite the bland appearance of the metastatic lesions, a significant subset of patients die of their disease in this context.

Ultrasound

- Lesions are typically lobulated and hypoechoic ± posterior acoustic enhancement with through transmission.

Computed Tomography

- These are typically smoothly marginated or lobulated homogeneous small spherical lesions. When they are larger, they can be heterogeneous with foci of necrosis. Small calcifications are common. Enhancement is variable, depending on the size, and may be delayed [14].

Magnetic Resonance Imaging

- On MRI, the lesions are well-circumscribed and homogeneous when small. Larger tumors may be heterogeneous. They are usually of low intensity on T1, very high intensity T2-weighted images, and mostly demonstrate homogeneous enhancement (Fig. 9.12).

Fine Needle Aspiration

- Aspirates from most cases of pleomorphic adenoma are characterized by three distinct components (Fig. 9.13a–c):
  - Abundant metachromatic (magenta in Diff-Quik-stained slides) fibrillary stroma.
  - Myoepithelial cells, typically spindled, plasmacytoid, or epithelioid, present as single cells in the background or admixed intimately with stromal material.
  - Epithelial cells forming clusters, typically with glandular or squamous morphology.

Core Biopsy

- In histologic sections, pleomorphic adenomas have variable proportions of stromal material, myoepithelial cells, and epithelium. The cohesive clusters of epithelial and myoepithelial cells typically trail off and percolate into chondromyxoid stromal material (Fig. 9.13d).

Comment

- A diagnosis of pleomorphic adenoma based on cytologic findings is extremely sensitive and specific.
- Immunohistochemistry for p63 or calponin in cell block specimens or core biopsies will highlight the myoepithelial cell component. PLAG1 or HMGA2 positivity can be helpful [1].

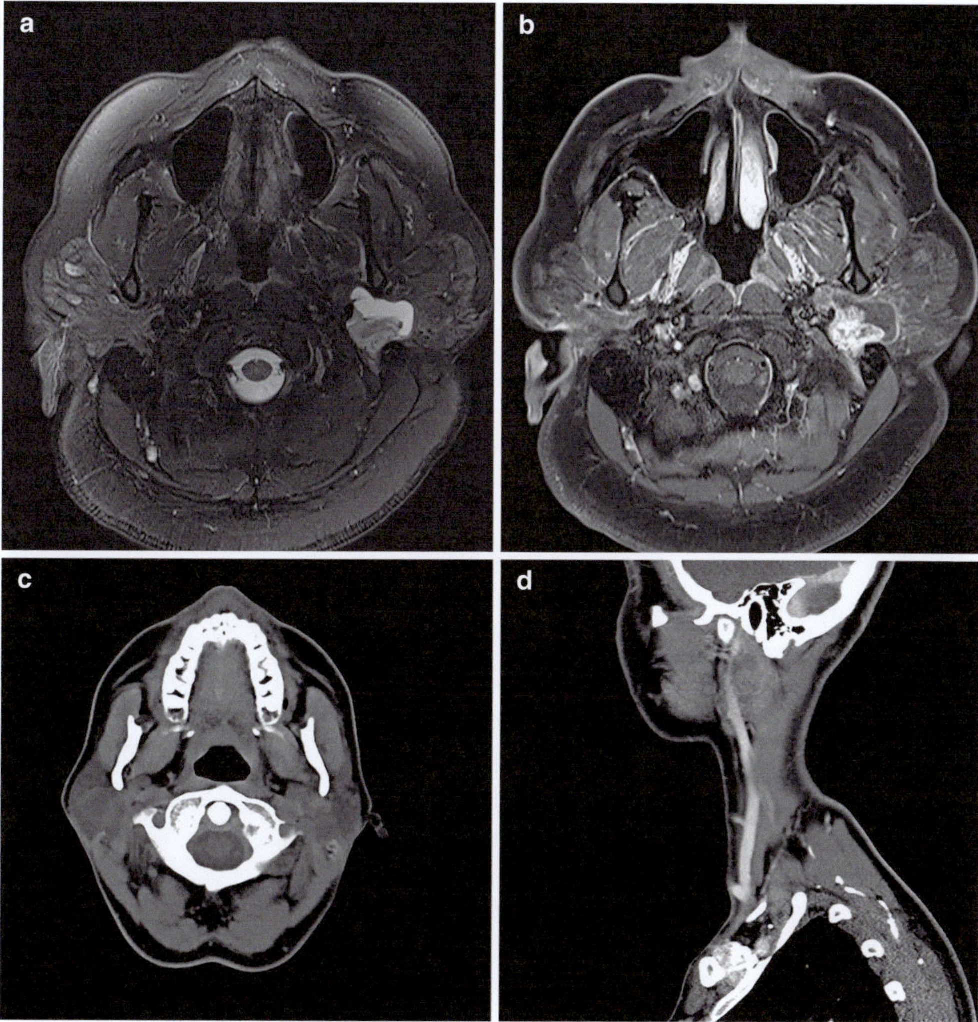

Fig. 9.12 Pleomorphic adenoma. (**a**, **b**) Pre- (**a**) and post-gadolinium MR (**b**) images demonstrate a left parotid pleomorphic adenoma that is a T2 hyperintense lesion. Axial (**c**) and sagittal (**d**) images from a contrast-enhanced CT demonstrate a heterogeneous right parotid gland pleomorphic adenoma

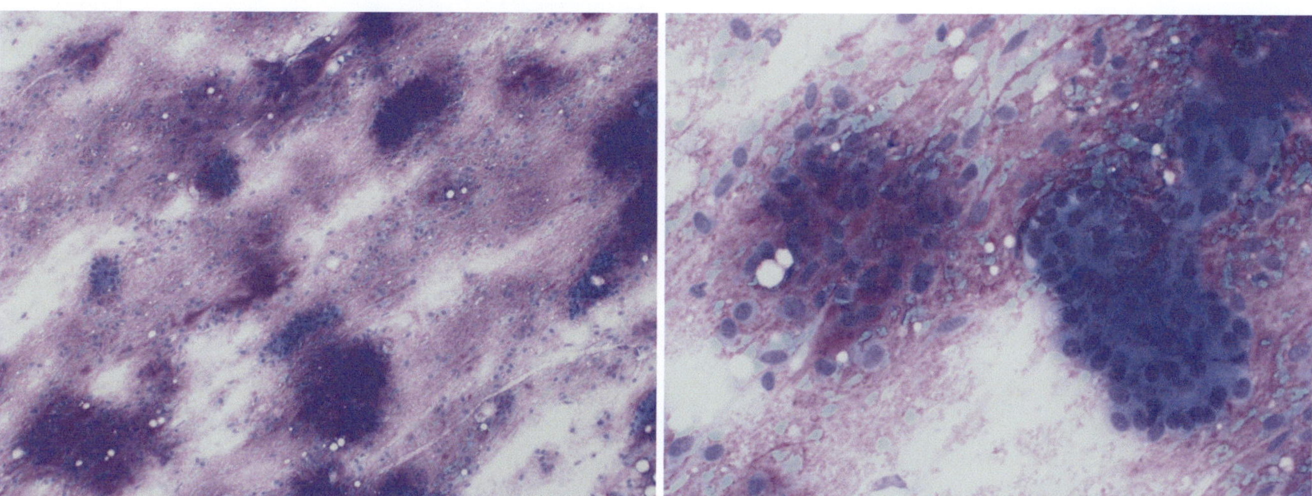

Fig. 9.13 Pleomorphic adenoma. (**a**, **b**) Diff-Quik-stained aspirates typically contain abundant metachromatic (magenta) fibrillary stroma. Clusters of epithelial cells as well as individual epithelial cells intimately admixed with stromal material are present. (**c**) In Papanicolaou-stained aspirate slides, the fibrillary nature of the stroma is more apparent. (**d**) In histologic sections, abundant chondromyxoid and hyaline stroma are seen. Clusters of epithelial cells forming glands are also seen, as are scattered myoepithelial cells trailing off into the stroma

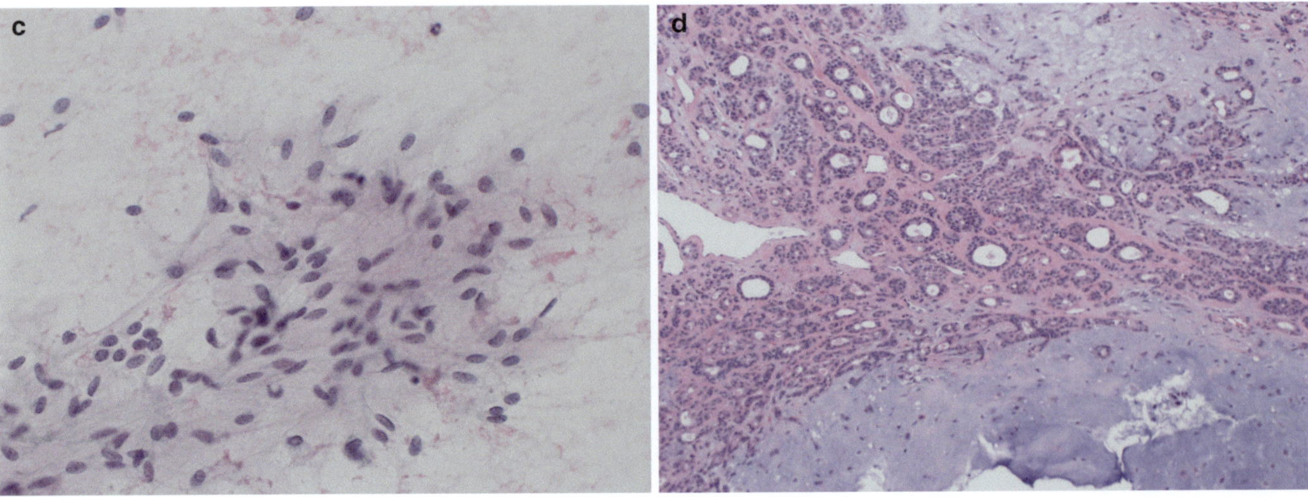

Fig. 9.13 (continued)

Warthin Tumor

General Considerations

- Warthin tumor is a common benign salivary gland neoplasm that occurs almost exclusively in the parotid gland.
- These tumors are often cystic and bilateral and frequently may be associated with smoking.

Ultrasound

- Lesions are typically oval with well-defined margins and have small anechoic areas [15]. Larger lesions are increasingly cystic.

Computed Tomography

- On CT they are well-defined heterogeneous solid cystic lesions within the superficial lobe of the parotid gland/parotid tail. No calcifications are seen. Areas of lower attenuation may reflect cystic change. Homogeneous enhancement is seen. These lesions can occur bilaterally (Fig. 9.14).

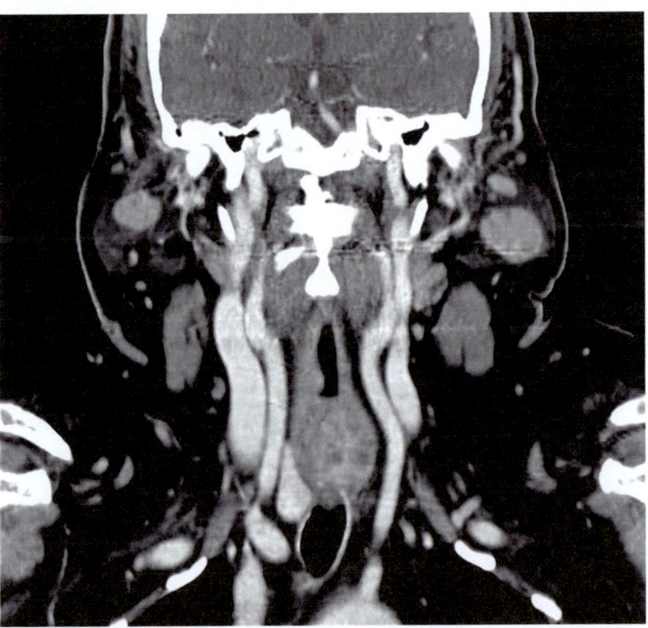

Fig. 9.14 Warthin tumor. Contrast-enhanced coronal CT demonstrates bilateral enhancing parotid masses. Because of interval increase in size, one of the lesions was removed surgically and was found to be a Warthin tumor

Magnetic Resonance Imaging

- Again, these lesions appear well defined and can be bilateral. They are low to intermediate signal on T1, heterogeneous and variable on T2, and usually show no contrast enhancement [16].

Fine Needle Aspiration

- A triphasic appearance is typical, and all three components are found in varying proportion in most cases (Fig. 9.15a–c).
  - Flat sheets of oncocytic epithelium with uniform, evenly spaced nuclei with prominent nucleoli.
  - "Grungy" granular cystic debris, markedly distinct from the mucinous cyst fluid found in mucoepidermoid carcinomas and mucoceles.
  - Lymphocytes, either crushed in small clusters, interspersed within oncocytic epithelium or individually present within cyst fluid.

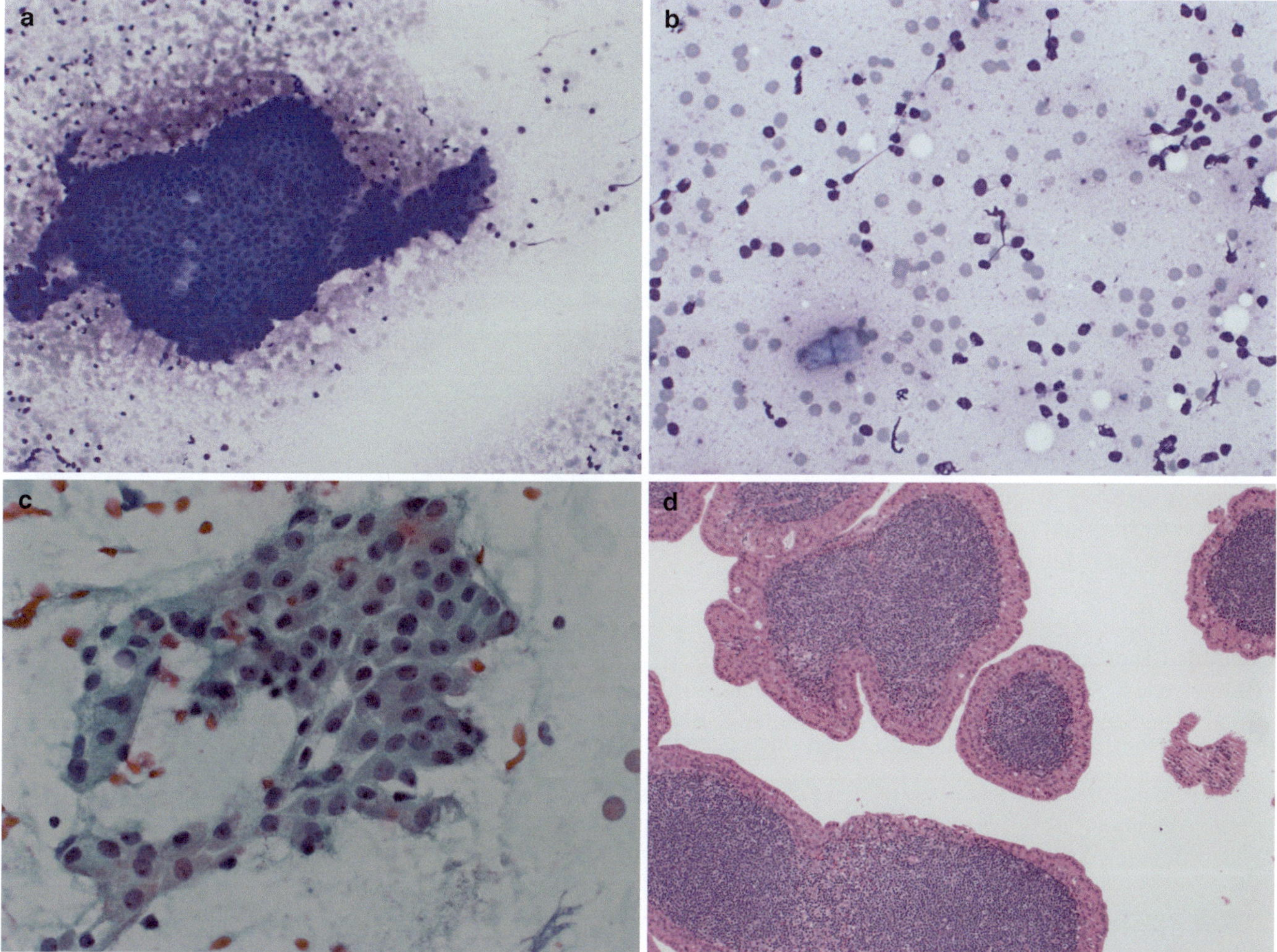

Fig. 9.15 Warthin tumor. (**a**) Flat sheets of oncocytes with small, round, evenly spaced nuclei in an aspirate smear. (**b**) The background of the aspirate contains reactive lymphocytes and granular debris. (**c**) In a Papanicolaou-stained aspirate, the granular nature of the cytoplasm as well as bland nuclei with nucleoli can be appreciated. (**d**) In histologic sections, a cystic component is often prominent. Oncocytic epithelium is typically bi-layered and closely associated with lymphoid cells. A papillary architecture may be prominent

Core Biopsy

- The oncocytic component of a Warthin tumor in histology forms bilayered ribbons and nests of epithelium intermixed with organized lymphoid tissue and cystic spaces (Fig. 9.15d).
- The three components are present in varying proportion in any given case.

Oncocytic Neoplasms

General Considerations

- Uncommon benign neoplasm composed of oncocytes (bland cells containing numerous mitochondria).

Magnetic Resonance Imaging

- Most tumors are found in the superficial parotid gland. These lesions appear hypointense relative to native parotid tissue (Fig. 9.16) [17].

Fine Needle Aspiration

- Three-dimensional clusters or trabeculae composed of bland oncocytes with abundant granular cytoplasm and uniform centrally placed nuclei (Fig. 9.17a–c).
- The flat sheet-like architecture of Warthin tumor as well as the lymphoid component and cystic debris should be absent.

Core Biopsy

- Lesions are typically well circumscribed, encapsulated, and composed of sheets of bland oncocytes with abundant eosinophilic granular cytoplasm and prominent nucleoli (Fig. 9.17d). Significant mitotic activity and necrosis should be absent.

Comment

- Oncocytoma cannot be definitively distinguished from its malignant counterpart, oncocytic carcinoma, based upon biopsy findings alone. Distinction from oncocytic carcinoma requires an assessment of necrosis, mitotic activity, atypia, and the growth pattern in a resected specimen.

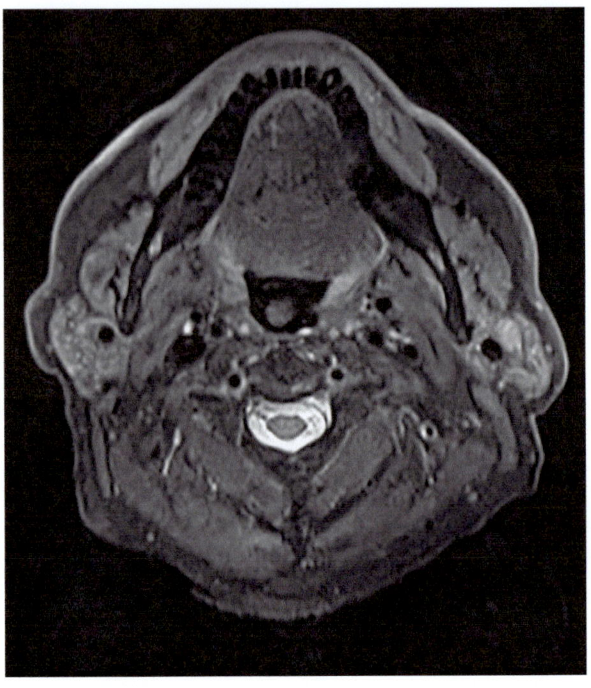

Fig. 9.16 Oncocytoma. T2 isointense to mildly hyperintense left parotid gland lesion found to be an oncocytoma at surgery

Malignant Neoplasms

Adenoid-Cystic Carcinoma

General Considerations

- Despite its bland cytology, adenoid cystic carcinoma is considered a high-grade malignancy for purposes of management. While the disease course is typically protracted, the prognosis in most cases is poor.
- While lymph node metastases are uncommon, adenoid cystic carcinoma frequently spreads along nerves and may enter the skull base. As such, complete resection is often difficult to impossible.

Computed Tomography

- Low-grade tumors tend to be well-defined in contradistinction to high-grade tumors, which appear infiltrative. Both

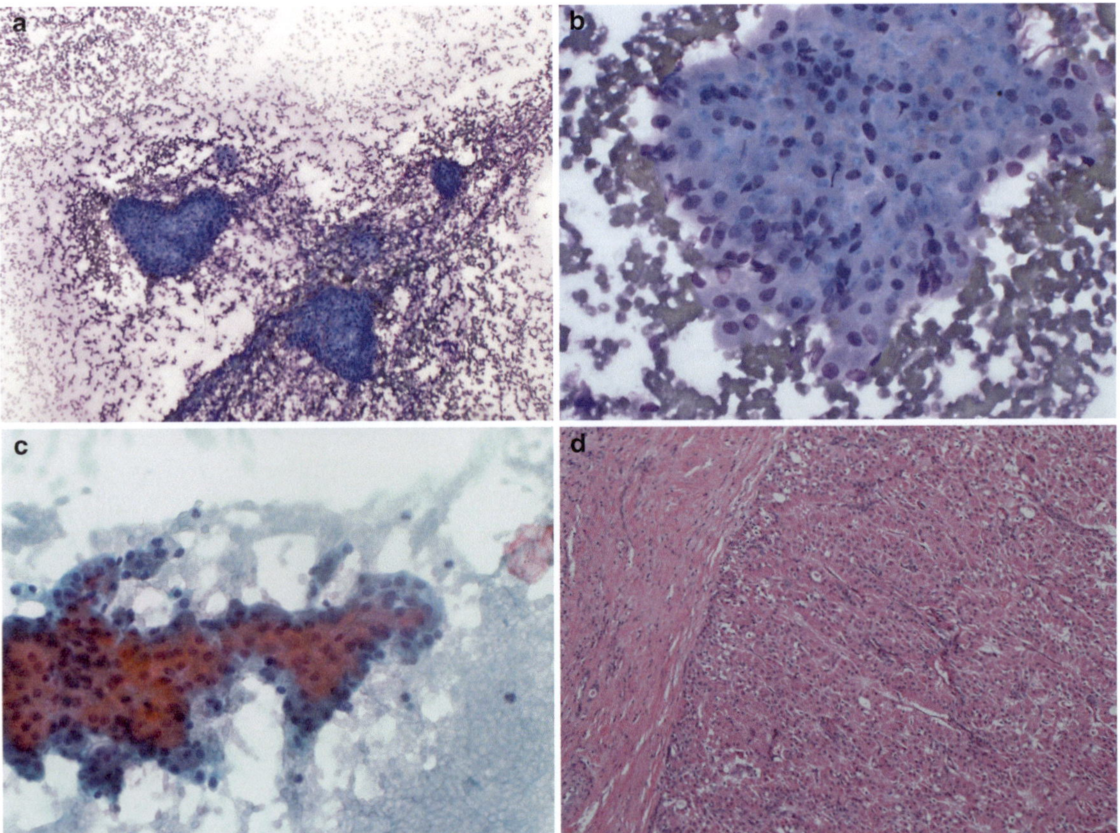

Fig. 9.17 Oncocytoma. (**a**, **b**) Irregular three-dimensional clusters of oncocytes with abundant granular cytoplasm, round nuclei, and prominent nucleoli in an aspirate specimen. (**c**) In a Papanicolaou-stained aspirate slide, the granular nature of the cytoplasm as well as the even chromatin pattern and prominent nucleoli can be seen. (**d**) In a resected specimen, a sheetlike growth pattern and uniform cells with granular eosinophilic cytoplasm are seen. The well-circumscribed nature of the lesion is consistent with a benign disease course

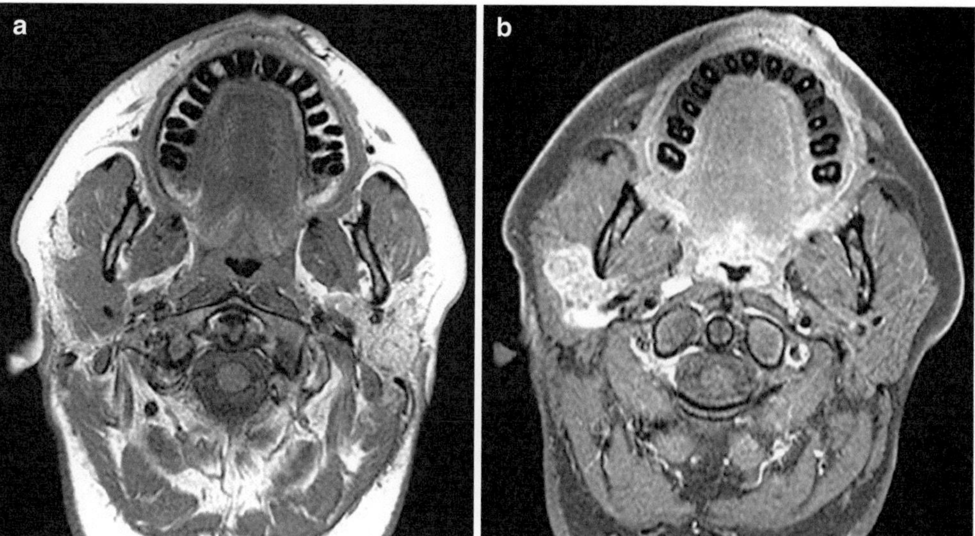

Fig. 9.18 Adenoid cystic carcinoma. T1 (**a**) and postcontrast image (**b**) demonstrate an ill-defined low T1 signal enhancing the right parotid mass, which was found to be an adenoid cystic carcinoma at surgery

subtypes are usually homogeneous. Adenoid cystic carcinomas are frequently associated with perineural spread (via cranial nerve VII) [18], better appreciated on MRI.

Magnetic Resonance Imaging

- These tumors are hypo- to isointense on T1; slightly hyperintense, with higher grades being markedly hyperintense on T2 (Fig. 9.18)

Fine Needle Aspiration

- Similar to pleomorphic adenoma, aspirates are characterized by both a cellular component and stroma (Figs. 9.19a–c) [19].
  - Uniform population of cells with bland, small, round nuclei and minimal cytoplasm. Despite the fact that this is a high-grade tumor, necrosis and pleomorphism are relatively uncommon.
  - Individual cells and groups of cells are sharply demarcated from globules of metachromatic (magenta in Diff-Quik-stained slides) stromal material. Stromal material has sharp borders and lacks the fibrillary nature of the chondromyxoid stroma seen in pleomorphic adenomas.

Core Biopsy

- The typical growth pattern seen in this tumor is cribriform; however, tumors with a tubular or solid growth pattern are not uncommon. Luminal material may be either basophilic or eosinophilic. Despite the fact that this tumor is composed of both epithelial and myoepithelial cells, most cases are strikingly monotonous in regard to their basaloid cellular composition (Fig. 9.19d).

Comment

- Adenoid cystic carcinoma may be difficult or impossible to distinguish from a variety of other benign and malignant salivary gland neoplasms in aspirated specimens and core biopsies. In the absence of numerous stromal globules, most cases are diagnosed descriptively in small biopsies.
- Similar to pleomorphic adenoma immunohistochemical stains for p63 and calponin will highlight scattered myoepithelial cells in core biopsies and cell blocks. Immunoreactivity for CD117, while characteristic, is neither sensitive nor specific [20]. In addition, most cases overexpress MYB and NOTCH, and a majority have a signature chromosomal translocation t(6;9)(q22–23;p23–24) resulting in a fusion involving the v-myb myeloblastosis viral oncogene homolog (MYB) oncogeneand the transcription factor gene NFIB [1].

Mucoepidermoid Carcinoma

General considerations

- Mucoepidermoid carcinoma is the most common salivary gland neoplasm in both adults and children.
- In contrast to most other salivary gland malignancies, mucoepidermoid carcinomas may be either high or low grade.

Computed Tomography

- Low-grade tumors appear as well-circumscribed masses, usually with cystic components. The solid components enhance, and calcification is sometimes seen. On the other hand, high-grade tumors have poorly defined margins and appear infiltrative.

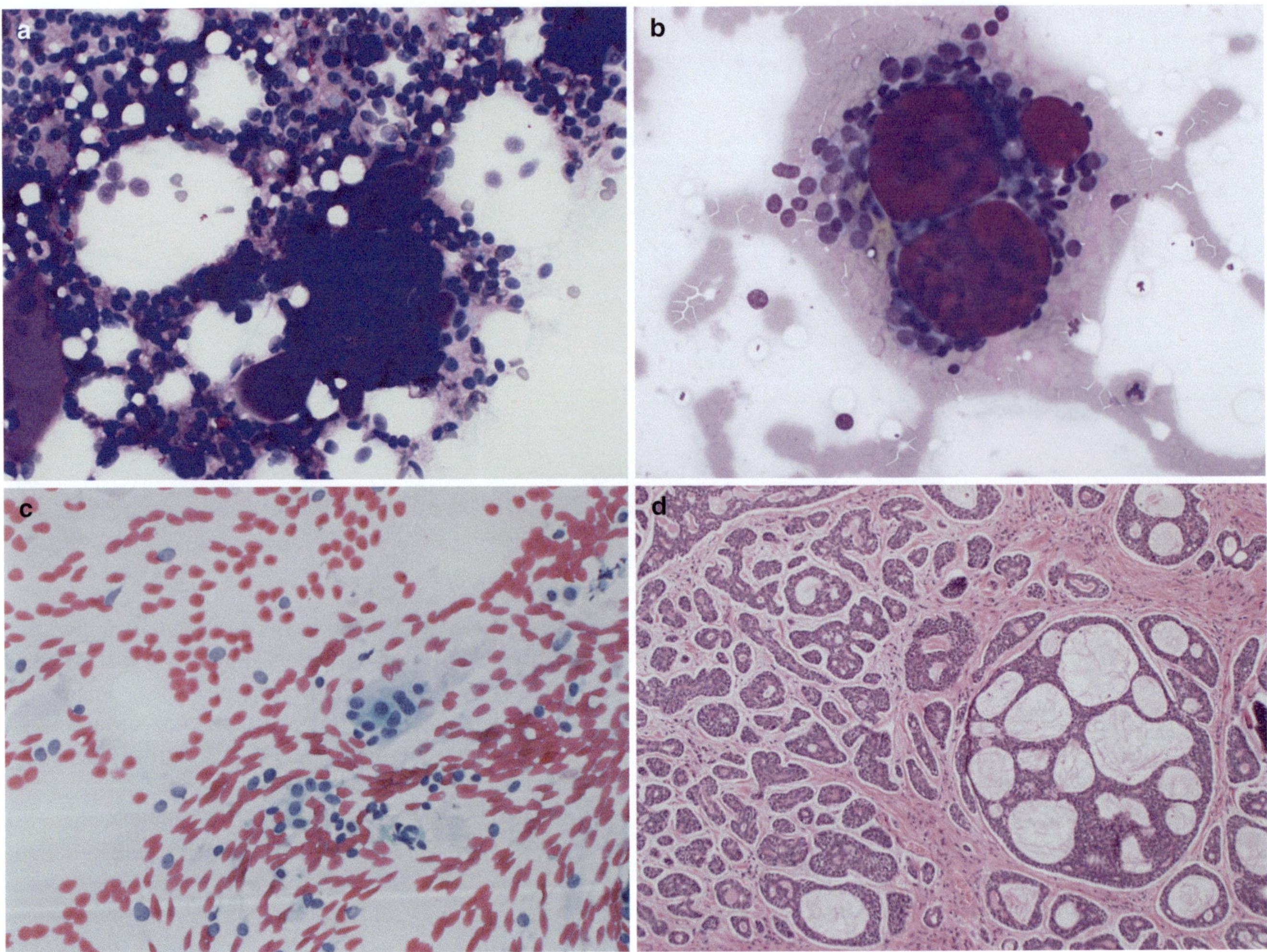

Fig. 9.19 Adenoid cystic carcinoma. (**a**, **b**) In Diff Quik-stained aspirate smears, the tumor cells are classicly basaloid with cytologic uniformity, minimal atypia, and a bland chromatin pattern. Globules of metachromatic (magenta) and even stromal material are typical. Tumor cells are not present within the stromal material. (**c**) In Papanicolaou-stained aspirate slides, bland uniform nuclei can be appreciated. (**d**) Adenoid cystic carcinoma in resected specimens may demonstrate a tubular, solid, or cribriform ("cookie-cutter") architecture with basaloid cells surrounding basement membrane material or stromal ground substance. Note the monotonous cytology

Magnetic Resonance Imaging

- Low-grade tumors are typically low to intermediate signal on T1 and T2 sequences and tend to demonstrate perineural spread (Fig. 9.20). Imaging up to the cavernous sinus and inner ear should be performed.

Fine Needle Aspiration

- Low-grade tumors are characterized by abundant mucin with clusters of squamoid cells demonstrating well-defined cell borders and angulated dense cytoplasm. Mucocytes containing rarefied cytoplasm and distended with mucin are present either in clusters or punctuating the groups of squamoid cells (Fig. 9.21a. b).
- High-grade tumors are typically composed of clusters and sheets of pleomorphic epithelial cells. Mucin is less prominent, and mucocytes are more difficult to locate. These tumors are often difficult to differentiate from other high-grade malignancies.

Core Biopsy

- Low-grade tumors are predominantly cystic and lined by an admixture of squamoid cells as well as mucin-distended goblet cells within a desmoplastic stroma (Fig. 9.21c).
- High-grade tumors often have a more solid growth pattern and a greater proportion of squamoid cells with only focal cyst formation. Goblet cells may be more difficult to find (Fig. 9.21d).

Comment

- Low-grade mucoepidermoid carcinoma is frequently underdiagnosed because cases are predominantly cystic and aspirates may contain only mucin with rare epithelial cells.
- High-grade mucoepidermoid carcinoma is difficult to distinguish from other forms of high-grade salivary gland carcinoma or metastatic squamous cell carcinoma. Of note, frank keratinization is almost never seen in cases of

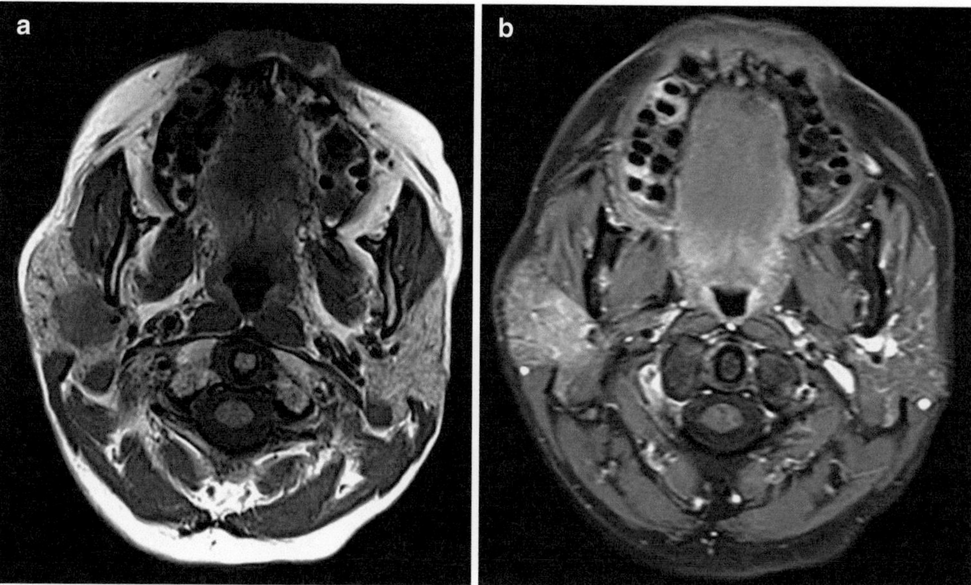

Fig. 9.20 Mucoepidermoid carcinoma: T1 hypointense (**a**) enhancing (**b**) right parotid mass found to be a mucoepidermoid carcinoma at surgery

mucoepidermoid carcinoma in contrast to cases of squamous cell carcinoma.

Acinic Cell Carcinoma

General considerations

- While intrinsically considered low-grade malignancies, occasional cases can undergo dedifferentiation (similar to other low-grade salivary gland tumors) and transform into histologically and clinically high-grade malignancies.
- Almost all cases occur in the parotid gland.

Radiology

- Imaging findings in acinic cell carcinoma are non-specific and there is an overlap with benign tumors such as Warthin tumor and pleomorphic adenoma

Fine Needle Aspiration

- Aspirate smears are typically cellular and contain haphazard clusters of cells with numerous stripped naked nuclei in the background.
- The individual tumor cells have indistinct and irregular cell borders and contain abundant coarsely granular and vacuolated cytoplasm and eccentric nuclei, which commonly display prominent nucleoli.

Core Biopsy

- Acinic cell carcinoma in core biopsies may demonstrate a sheet-like or acinar growth pattern. Occasional cases may be macrocystic. Frequently an associated lymphoid cuff may be seen and is a clue to diagnosis.
- The individual tumor cells may display lining up ("regimentation") of nuclei and the cells often have a syncytial quality with indistinct cell borders. The cytoplasm typically contains abundant coarse basophilic zymogen-rich granules.

Comment

- These tumors are typically immunoreactive for DOG1 and are highlighted with a PAS/D stain.
- The main differential diagnosis is the recently described mammary analogue secretory carcinoma (MASC). An important distinguishing feature is the absence of coarse granularity in MASC (Figs. 9.22 and 9.23).

Angiosarcoma

General Considerations

- Angiosarcomas are mesenchymal tumors of endothelial differentiation and may involve the salivary glands as either primary or metastatic lesions [21].
- While aggressive, these tumors may have a somewhat better prognosis than their soft-tissue counterparts.

Computed Tomography

- These tumors are extremely rare, and only 2% of all angiosarcomas tend to involve the salivary glands [21, 22]. They appear as large infiltrative lesions that are typically hyperenhancing. Their appearance is nonspecific, and tissue diagnosis is needed (Fig. 9.24).

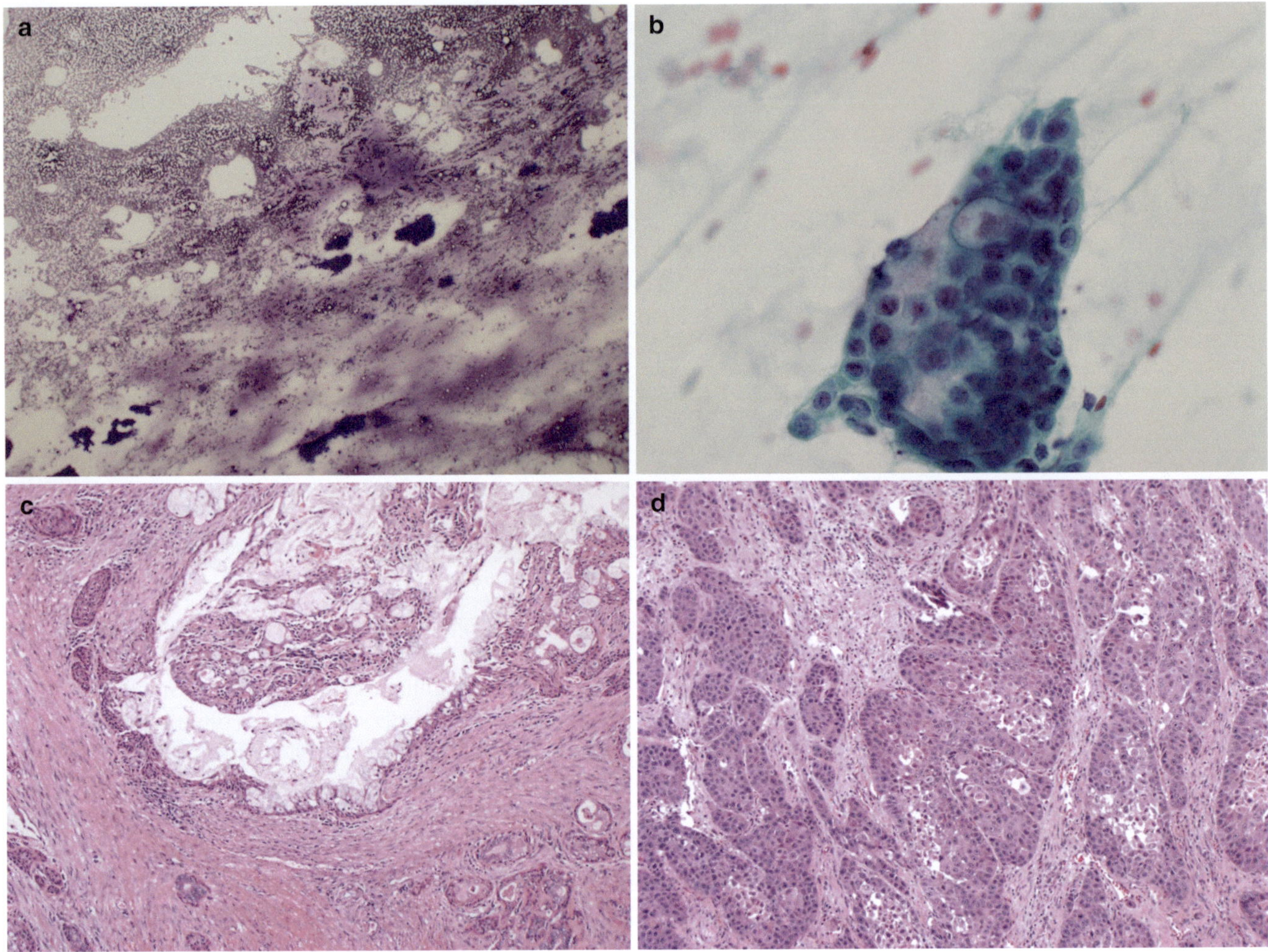

Fig. 9.21 Mucoepidermoid carcinoma. (**a**) Aspirates often contain abundant mucinous material in the background and may be hypocellular. (**b**) An admixture of squamoid cells with dense angulated cytoplasm as well as occasional mucin distended cells is seen. Intracellular mucin is pink in this Papanicolaou-stained aspirate slide. (**c**) A cystic architecture and numerous goblet cells are characteristic of low-grade mucoepidermoid carcinoma in resected specimens. (**d**) A solid growth pattern and abundance of squamoid cells are seen in resected cases of high-grade mucoepidermoid carcinoma. Mucinous goblet cells may be difficult to identify in these cases

Fine Needle Aspiration

- Aspirates are typically hemorrhagic and characterized by malignant mesenchymal cells; these can range from bland spindle cells to pleomorphic cells with vacuolated and angulated cytoplasm. The findings are nonspecific with regard to other mesenchymal tumors.

Core Biopsy

- In histology, these tumors are classicly composed of malignant endothelial cells forming anastamosing vascular channels as well as solid sheets. In some cases, intracellular lumina are present and may contain degenerating red blood cells.
- Immunhistochemical stains are positive for vascular makers.

Other more recently described salivary tumors such as secretory carcinoma, and rare tumors such as salivary duct carcinoma are beyond the scope of this discussion; the reader is referred to other resources [1].

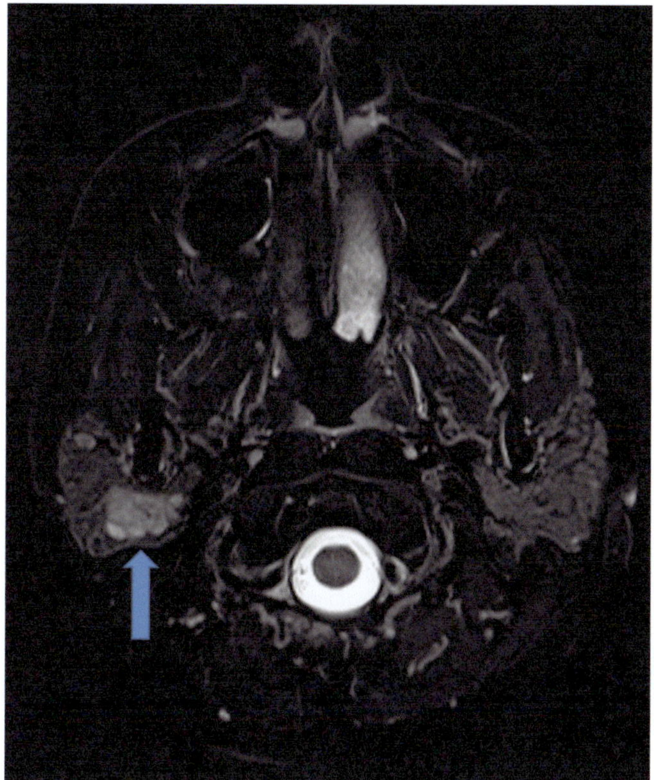

Fig. 9.22 Acinic cell carcinoma. *Arrow* indicates T2 hyperintense bosselated lesion in the right parotid gland concerning for a benign lesion such as pleomorphic adenoma or a malignant lesion such as acinic cell carcinoma. Biopsy is recommended in such cases

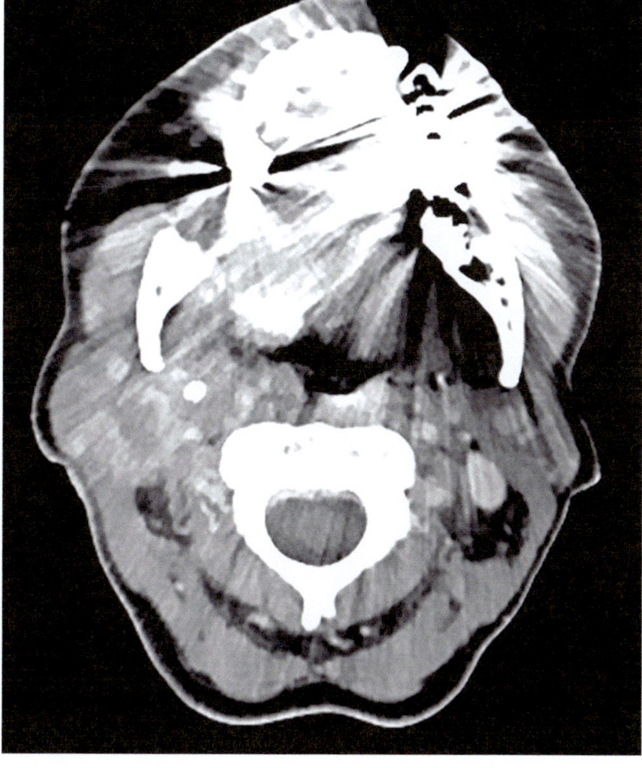

Fig. 9.24 Angiosarcoma: ill-defined enhancing mass in right parotid gland that was found to be an angiosarcoma at surgery

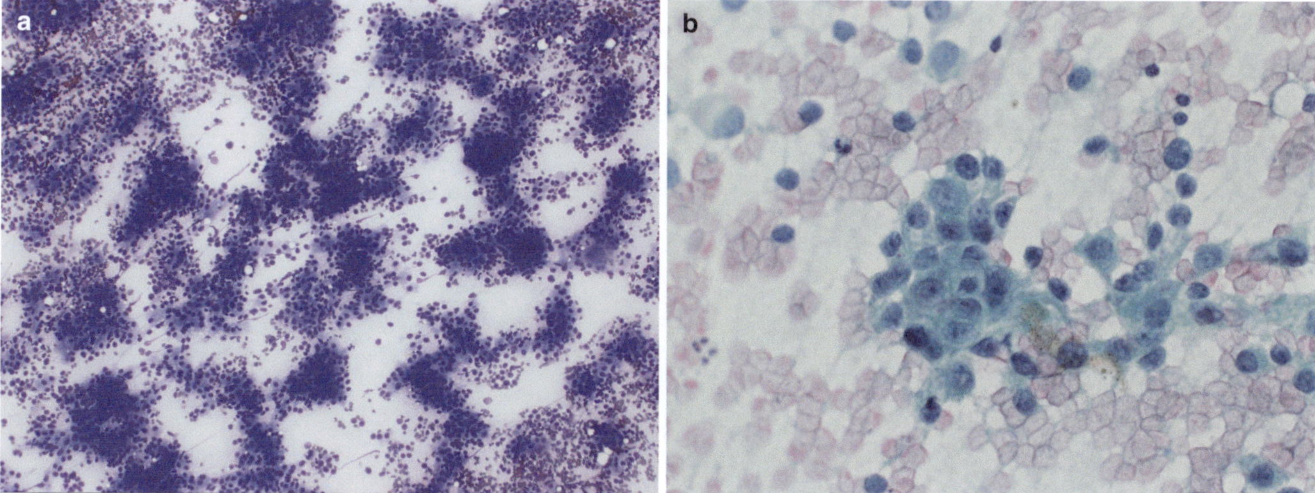

Fig. 9.23 Acinic cell carcinoma. (**a**) Aspirates demonstrate three-dimensional haphazard clusters of cells with numerous bare nuclei in the background. (**b**) At higher power, the cells demonstrate abundant coarsely granular cytoplasm, nuclear atypia, and prominent nucleoli

References

1. Faquin WC, Rossi ED, Baloch Z, Barkan GA, Foschini M, DFI K, Pusztaszeri M, Vielh P, editors. The Milan system for reporting salivary gland cytopathology. Basel: Springer; 2018.
2. Klihanienko J. Head and neck; salivary gland. In: Orell SR, Sterrett GF, Whitaker D, editors. Fine needle aspiration cytology. 4th ed. Philadelphia: Churchill Livingstone; 2005. p. 41–82.
3. Elhosseiny A. Salivary gland. In: Koss L, Melamed M, editors. Koss's diagnostic cytology and its histopathologic bases, vol. 2. 5th ed. Philadelphia: Lippincott Williams & Wilkins; 2005. p. 1229–61.
4. Seethala RR. Histologic grading and prognostic biomarkers in salivary gland carcinomas. Adv Anat Pathol. 2011;18:29–45.
5. Whyte AM, Bowyer FM. Sialosis: diagnosis by computed tomography. Br J Radiol. 1987;60:400–1.
6. Henry-Stanley MJ, Beneke J, Bardales RH, Stanley MW. Fine-needle aspiration of normal tissue from enlarged salivary glands: sialosis or missed target? Diagn Cytopathol. 1995;13:300–3.
7. Jager L, Menauer F, Holzknecht N, Scholz V, Grevers G, Reiser M. Sialolithiasis: MR sialography of the submandibular duct--an alternative to conventional sialography and US? Radiology. 2000;216:665–71.
8. Alyas F, Lewis K, Williams M, Moody AB, Wong KT, Ahuja AT, Howlett DC. Diseases of the submandibular gland as demonstrated using high resolution ultrasound. Br J Radiol. 2005;8:362–9.
9. Nasuti JF, Gupta PK, Fleisher SR, LiVolsi VA. Nontyrosine crystalloids in salivary gland lesions: report of seven cases with fine-needle aspiration cytology and follow-up surgical pathology. Diagn Cytopathol. 2000;22:167–71.
10. Yousem DM, Kraut MA, Chalian AA. Major salivary gland imaging. Radiology. 2000;216:19–29.
11. Leon ME, Santosh N, Agarwal A, Teknos TN, Ozer E, Iwenofu OH. Diagnostic challenges in the fine needle aspiration biopsy of chronic sclerosing sialadenitis (Küttner's tumor) in the context of head and neck malignancy: a series of 4 cases. Head Neck Pathol. 2016;10:389–93.
12. Geyer JT, Ferry JA, Harris NL, Stone JH, Zukerberg LR, Lauwers GY, et al. Chronic sclerosing sialadenitis (Küttner tumor) is an IgG4-associated disease. Am J Surg Pathol. 2010;34:202–10.
13. Elliott JN, Oertel YC. Lymphoepithelial cysts of the salivary glands. Histologic and cytologic features. Am J Clin Pathol. 1990;93:39–43.
14. Lev MH, Khanduja K, Morris PP, Curtin HD. Parotid pleomorphic adenomas: delayed CT enhancement. Am J Neuroradiol. 1998;19:1835–9.
15. Kim J, Kim EK, Park CS, Choi YS, Kim YH, Choi EC. Characteristic sonographic findings of Warthin's tumor in the parotid gland. J Clin Ultrasound. 2004;32:78–81.
16. Joe VQ, Westesson PL. Tumors of the parotid gland: MR imaging characteristics of various histologic types. Am J Roentgenol. 1994;163:433–8.
17. Patel ND, van Zante A, Eisele DW, Harnsberger HR, Glastonbury CM. Oncocytoma: the vanishing parotid mass. Am J Neuroradiol. 2011;32:1703–6.
18. Godge P, Sharma S, Yadav M. Adenoid cystic carcinoma of the parotid gland. Contemp Clin Dent. 2012;3:223–6.
19. Hughes JH, Volk EE, Wilbur DC. Cytopathology Resource Committee, College of American Pathologists. Pitfalls in salivary gland fine-needle aspiration cytology: lessons from the College of American Pathologists Interlaboratory Comparison Program in Nongynecologic Cytology. Arch Pathol Lab Med. 2005;129:26–31.
20. Mino M, Pilch BZ, Faquin WC. Expression of KIT (CD117) in neoplasms of the head and neck: an ancillary marker for adenoid cystic carcinoma. Mod Pathol. 2003;16:1224–31.
21. Maddox JC, Evans HL. Angiosarcoma of skin and soft tissue: a study of forty-four cases. Cancer. 1981;48:1907–21.
22. Fanburg-Smith JC, Furlong MA, Childers EL. Oral and salivary gland angiosarcoma: a clinicopathologic study of 29 cases. Mod Pathol. 2003;16:263–71.

Bone and Soft Tissue Tumors

10

Nicholas Morley and Ajit S. Paintal

Introduction

Primary tumors of bone are classified according to matrix production and differentiation. The internal tumor matrix is traditionally identified initially on plain radiographs with characteristic types of tumor matrices, including osteoid, chondroid, or fibroblastic. The osteoid matrix is characterized radiographically by "cloudlike" bone formation. The chondroid matrix is traditionally described as "rings and arcs." Fibroblastic matrix is typically radiolucent on radiographs.

Correlation between radiographic and pathologic findings is of paramount importance in the characterization of bone tumors. In what are histologically low-grade cartilaginous tumors, for example, the distinction between a benign enchondroma and grade 1 chondrosarcoma in biopsy material is almost entirely based upon the radiographic impression. Similarly, for many osteoid-producing tumors, knowledge of radiographic findings is critical for correct interpretation, since many benign as well as malignant lesions can be morphologically similar in the context of a small biopsy. In contrast to tumors at other sites, immunohistochemistry plays a very limited role in the diagnosis of matrix-producing bone tumors.

N. Morley
Department of Radiology, Marshfield Clinic, Marshfield, WI, USA

A. S. Paintal (✉)
Northshore Medical Group, Evanston Hospital, Evanston, IL, USA

Osteoid Tumor Matrix: Osteoma, Osteoid Osteoma, Osteoblastoma, and Osteosarcoma

Osteoma

Clinical

- Benign tumor composed of mature bone, typically occurring in the head and neck regions.

Plain Radiograph

- Osteomas are slow-growing, benign surface lesions [1].
- The classic appearance is an "ivory dense" cortically-based mass with sharp margins.
- The location of the lesion is helpful for diagnosis, with osteomas most commonly occurring in the frontal and ethmoidal sinuses, the calvarium, and the mandible [2].

Computed Tomography (CT)

- A homogeneously dense, usually cortically-based mass that is often incidentally detected on CT studies.

Fine Needle Aspiration (FNA)

- Since osteomas are composed entirely of dense compact bone, they do not typically yield material in aspirated specimens.

Core Biopsy

- In core biopsies and other histologic specimens, osteomas are composed entirely of dense, compact, mineralized bone [3].

Osteoid Osteoma

Clinical

- Patients with osteoid osteoma traditionally present with pain, which is worse at night and is relieved by salicylates. This presentation occurs in 30% to 50% of cases [4].

R. Nayar et al. (eds.), *Atlas of Cytopathology and Radiology*, https://doi.org/10.1007/978-3-030-24756-0_10

- Treatment options include radiofrequency (RF) ablation or surgical excision, with RF ablation showing favorable results in the appendicular skeleton and pelvis [5].

Plain Radiograph

- Osteoid osteomas are usually found in long bones, most often in the femur and tibia [6].
- Lesions are typically round, well-circumscribed, and radiolucent, but they may demonstrate a sclerotic center, which is termed the nidus.

Computed Tomography

- CT is the most valuable modality for demonstration of the nidus, particularly when osteoid osteomas occur in the posterior elements of the spine (Fig. 10.1).
- More than half of osteoid osteomas demonstrate some degree of internal matrix on CT, most frequently a central region of sclerosis. There is surrounding well-circumscribed lucency. Less frequently, the lesion may be entirely lucent or entirely sclerotic [7].
- Osteoid osteomas rarely exceed 1.5 cm in diameter, which helps to differentiate them from osteoblastomas.

Nuclear Medicine

- A radionuclide bone scan may demonstrate the double-density sign, which is related to increased vascularity.

Fine Needle Aspiration

- Findings in aspirates of osteoid osteomas are relatively nonspecific. Numerous osteoblasts and osteoclasts are typically seen.
  - Osteoblasts are characterized by abundant granular cytoplasm, eccentric nuclei, and an area of cytoplasmic clearing opposite the nucleus and adjacent to the cell membrane.

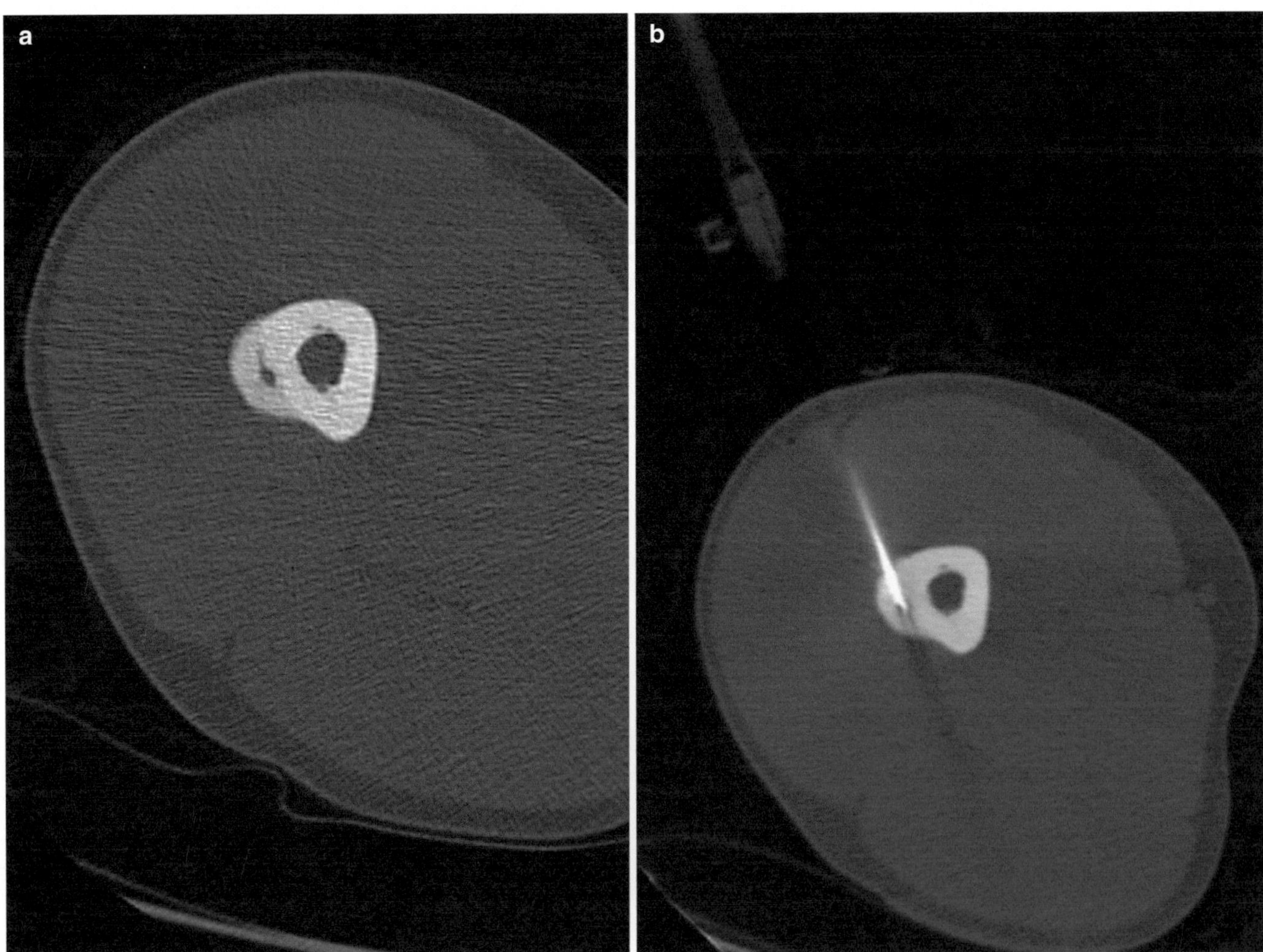

Fig. 10.1 Osteoid osteoma. (**a**) Homogeneous lucent lesion centered on the femoral cortex, representing osteoid osteoma. (**b**) Treatment was performed with CT-guided RF ablation

- Osteoclasts are multinucleated giant cells with low to intermediate nuclear:cytoplasmic ratios and round cell borders.

Core Biopsy

- Cases of osteoid osteoma are characterized in histologic sections by delicate trabeculae of woven bone with osteoblastic rimming and scattered osteoclasts. The trabeculae are separated by richly vascular stroma composed of fibroblasts and loose collagen [3].
- The centrally placed nidus is made up of thicker and more sclerotic bone.

Osteoblastoma

Clinical

- Osteoblastomas are clinicopathologically similar to osteoid osteomas, but they are larger and are accompanied by less intense pain that is not relieved by salicylates.

Plain Radiograph

- Osteoblastoma has a similar appearance to osteoid osteoma, but the lesions are generally larger than 2 cm.
- Osteoblastomas are round or oval and may contain an internal matrix [8].

Nuclear Medicine

- Osteoblastomas demonstrate methylene diphosphonate avidity.

Fine Needle Aspiration

- Findings in aspirates of osteoblastoma are relatively nonspecific. Numerous osteoblasts and osteoclasts are typically seen [9].
  - Osteoblasts are characterized by abundant granular cytoplasm, eccentric nuclei, and an area of cytoplasmic clearing opposite the nucleus and adjacent to the cell membrane.
  - Osteoclasts are multinucleated giant cells with low-to-intermediate nuclear:cytoplasmic ratios and round cell borders.

Core Biopsy

- Cases of osteoblastoma are characterized in histologic sections by delicate trabeculae of woven bone with osteoblastic rimming and scattered osteoclasts. The trabeculae are separated by richly vascular stroma composed of fibroblasts and loose collagen.
- Areas of sclerosis and chondroid matrix formation may be seen in addition to osteoblasts with bizarre nuclei.
- Correlation with radiographic findings is critical in order to exclude osteosarcoma.

Osteosarcoma

Clinical

- In contrast to chondrosarcoma, osteosarcoma tends to occur in a bimodal distribution with peaks in the second decade as well as later in life.
- Secondary osteosarcoma can occur in the context of radiation, Paget disease, and bone infarction.
- Osteosarcoma most commonly affects the long bones in the lower extremities.
- Osteosarcomas are characterized by the production of an osteoid matrix both pathologically and in radiographic studies.
- Metastatic disease is not uncommon in the setting of high-grade osteosarcoma.

Plain Radiograph

- Typically, osteosarcoma manifests as a long-bone, metaphyseal lesion with aggressive features. These include mixed areas of lysis and sclerosis, cortical destruction, periosteal new bone, and soft-tissue mass (Fig. 10.2) [10].
- While there are eight subtypes of osteosarcoma according to the World Health Organization, conventional osteosarcoma is the most common and demonstrates cloudlike bone formation in the intramedullary space [11].
- Osteosarcomas may also arise from the periosteum, in which case they are termed juxtacortical osteosarcomas.

Magnetic Resonance Imaging

- MRI is useful for demonstrating the extent of soft-tissue involvement.
- The extent of involvement of the medullary canal is also better shown on MRI.

Fine Needle Aspiration

- Aspirates of osteosarcoma may have a variety of morphologic appearances.
  - While the majority of tumors contain frankly malignant pleomorphic tumor cells in epithelioid and/or spindle cell forms, lower grade tumors may be morphologically bland.
  - In cases of osteoblastic osteosarcoma, an osteoid matrix is present in the background or interspersed between tumor cells. The osteoid matrix is hyaline or densely fibrillary and metachromatic (magenta) on the Diff-Quik stain (Fig. 10.3a) [12].
  - In cases of chondroblastic osteosarcoma, chondroid matrix (metachromatic and less dense than the osteoid matrix) will be present [13].
  - In fibroblastic osteosarcoma, matrix may be absent. In these cases and particularly in small biopsies, the radiographic impression is key to allow the distinction from chondrosarcoma and malignant fibrous histiocytoma.

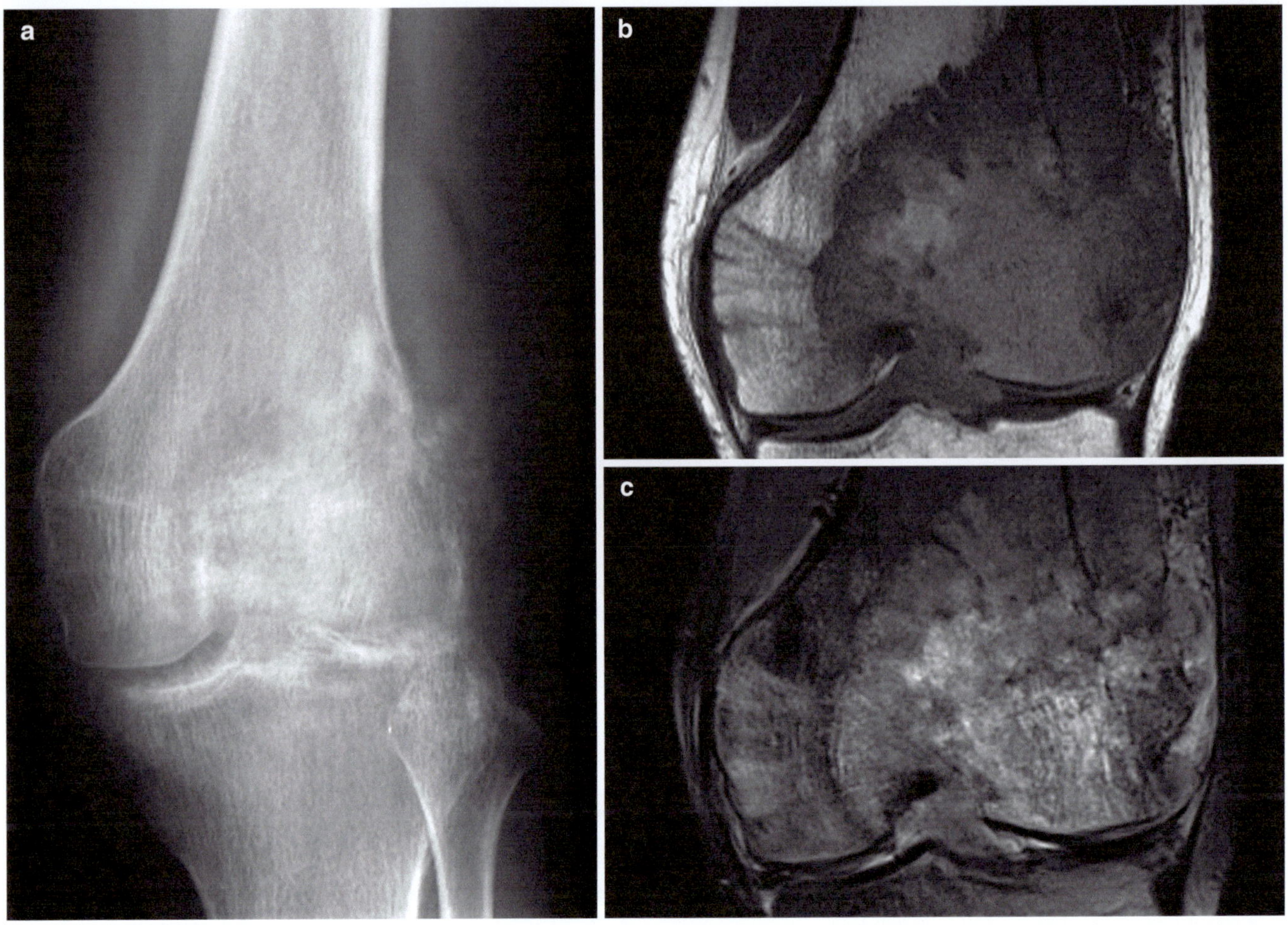

Fig. 10.2 Osteosarcoma. (**a**) Frontal radiograph of the knee demonstrating an aggressive lesion with cortical destruction, periosteal reaction, and osteoid matrix. Pathologic analysis confirmed the diagnosis of osteosarcoma. Coronal T1 (**b**) and coronal T2 (**c**) images demonstrate the extent of cortical breakthrough and soft-tissue extension to better advantage. The mass effect on adjacent structures is also better evaluated on MRI

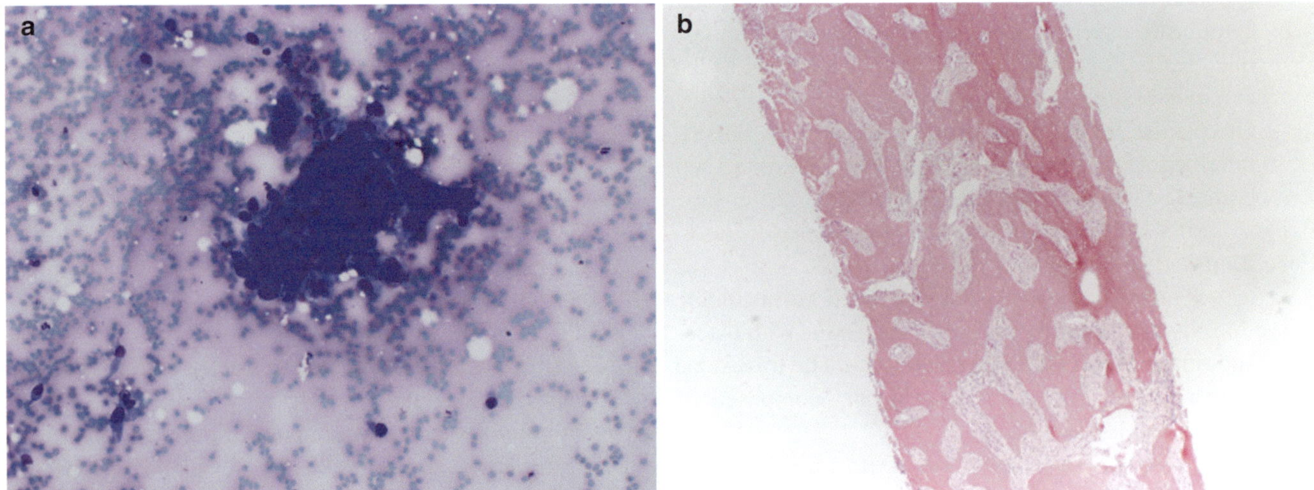

Fig. 10.3 Osteosarcoma. (**a**) Polygonal tumor cells with delicate lacy osteoid matrix are seen in this aspirate specimen. (**b**) In histologic sections, thick trabeculae of woven bone are seen in a fibroblastic background

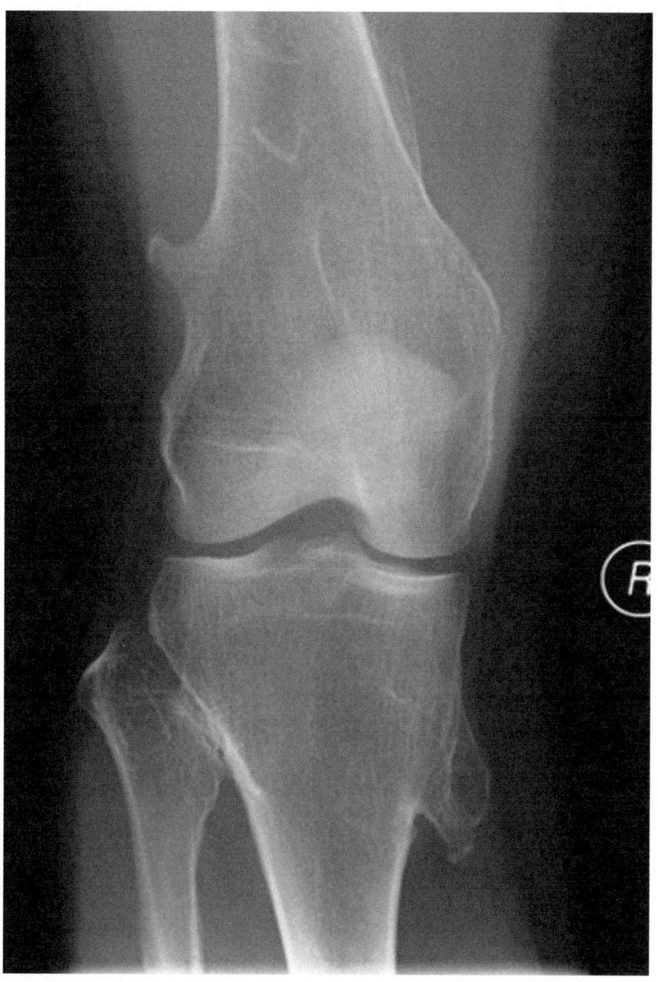

Fig. 10.4 Osteochondroma. Frontal radiograph of the knee demonstrating multiple osteochondromas as pedunculated exostotic lesions arising from the metaphyseal regions about the knee. Multiple osteochondromas have a higher risk of malignant transformation to chondrosarcoma

Core Biopsy

- The appearance of osteosarcoma in histologic sections varies greatly, depending on the grade of the tumor and the degree of differentiation. Typical high-grade osteoblastic osteosarcoma is composed of frankly malignant tumor cells intimately admixed with a lacy osteoid matrix. Lower-grade tumors may have thickened bony trabeculae and be cytologically bland (Fig. 10.3b). In these cases, correlation with radiographic findings is critical in suggesting the correct diagnosis.
- In chondroblastic osteosarcoma, a cartilaginous matrix is present and punctuated by lacunae. In cases of fibroblastic osteosarcoma, the tumor is morphologically identical to a pleomorphic undifferentiated sarcoma of soft tissue in that a matrix may be entirely lacking.

Chondroid Tumor Matrix: Osteochondroma, Enchondroma, Chondroblastoma, and Chondrosarcoma

Osteochondroma

Clinical

- Osteochondromas are the most common benign bone tumors.
- Complications of osteochondroma are typically related to mass effect, including vascular compromise, muscular or bursal irritation, or neurologic sequelae [14]. However, malignant degeneration may also occur, with transformation into chondrosarcoma.

Plain Radiograph

- The majority are located about the knee or proximal humerus.
- Osteochondromas are exophytic, typically metaphyseal lesions and may be sessile (broad-based) or pedunculated. They demonstrate continuity of the periosteum, cortex, and marrow with the underlying bone with an overlying cartilage cap (Fig. 10.4).

Magnetic Resonance Imaging

- MRI demonstrates the continuity of the osteochondroma with the underlying bone as well as the cartilaginous cap.
- Complications related to mass effect are well appreciated on MRI [15].
- Transformation to chondrosarcoma is a well-documented complication, and this risk correlates with a cartilage cap thickness greater than 2 cm. This is reproducibly measured on MRI. Cartilage cap thickness is measured from the junction of the T2 low-signal intensity mineralization with the near-fluid signal intensity cartilage to the surface of the cartilage, ignoring the undulations in the interface between them [16].

Fine Needle Aspiration

- Osteochondromas do not typically yield cellular aspirates because they are predominantly made up of mature hyaline cartilage and bone. Aspirates may contain bone marrow elements and fragments of cartilaginous or bony matrix.

Core Biopsy

- Findings in core biopsy depend on which portion of the lesion is sampled. The underlying bony stalk is made up of trabecular bone and typically contains normal bone marrow elements.
- The cartilaginous cap is composed of mature hyaline cartilage that may display some degree of myxoid degeneration. The interface between the cartilaginous cap and the bony stalk is characterized by active enchondral ossification.

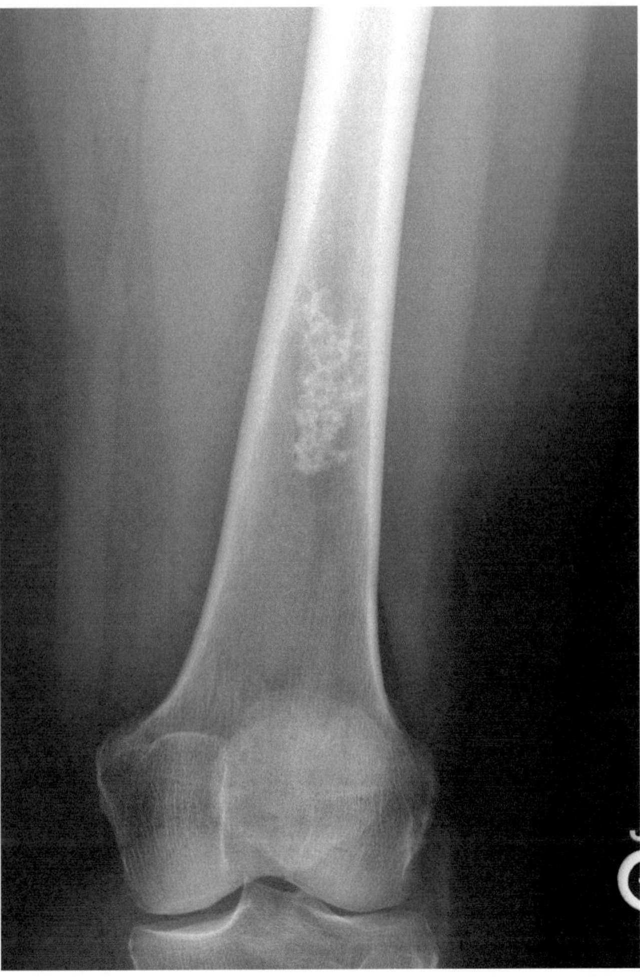

Fig. 10.5 Enchondroma. Frontal radiograph of the distal femur demonstrating the classic appearance of an enchondroma, with a lucent lesion containing a central ring-and-arc chondroid internal matrix

Enchondroma

Plain Radiograph

- Enchondromas present as well-marginated medullary lucencies. The most commonly affected locations include the hands and feet as well as the femur, humerus, and tibia.
- Lesions usually arise near an epiphysis and cause osseous expansion with endosteal scalloping and cortical thinning (Fig. 10.5).
- These benign lesions often demonstrate a typical internal chondroid matrix superimposed on a background of lucency. This may involve minimal stippling to larger areas of heterogeneous density [17].

Computed Tomography

- Enchondromas demonstrate typical lobulated margins and an internal chondroid matrix.
- Lesion size can be accurately assessed by CT.
- CT helps to separate enchondromas from chondrosarcomas by better demonstrating other aggressive features, such as cortical destruction or periosteal reaction. Enchondromas typically measure less than 5 cm in greatest dimension [7].

Fine Needle Aspiration

- Aspirates contain a metachromatic fibrillary chondroid matrix with clear round lacunae with bland round chondrocytes

Core Biopsy

- Lesions are characterized by hyaline cartilage containing bland chondrocytes in the lacunae.
- Myxoid change, increased cellularity, and cytologic atypia suggest malignancy but may be pronounced in enchondromas involving the small bones of the hands and feet [12].
- Enchondromas are almost invariably circumscribed lesions without permeation of the trabeculae.

Chondroblastoma

Clinical

- RF ablation has been described as an alternative to surgery for some cases of chondroblastoma, depending on the risk of mechanical collapse and lesion size [18].

Plain Radiograph

- Chondroblastomas demonstrate geographic bone destruction with well-defined margins [19].
- Lesions are centered at the epiphysis in tubular long bones.

Magnetic Resonance Imaging

- Chondroblastomas demonstrate low to intermediate T1 signal and T2 heterogeneity [20].
- Postcontrast images demonstrate mild tumoral enhancement.
- Adjacent soft-tissue and bone marrow edema may also be present.

Fine Needle Aspiration

- These tumors are characterized by a triphasic appearance.
  - Polygonal mononuclear cells with bland, grooved nuclei predominate. These cells are characterized by dense cytoplasm and may contain hemosiderin pigment [21].
  - Osteoclast type giant cells.
  - Fragments of a metachromatic fibrillary or amorphous chondroid matrix that may be calcified.

Core Biopsy

- Chondroblastomas typically display sheets of polygonal mononuclear cells with relatively well-defined cell borders and uniform round nuclei that may be grooved and somewhat hyperchromatic (Fig. 10.6). Scattered throughout are multinucleated osteoclast-like giant cells. Interstitial "chicken wire" calcifications and a chondroid

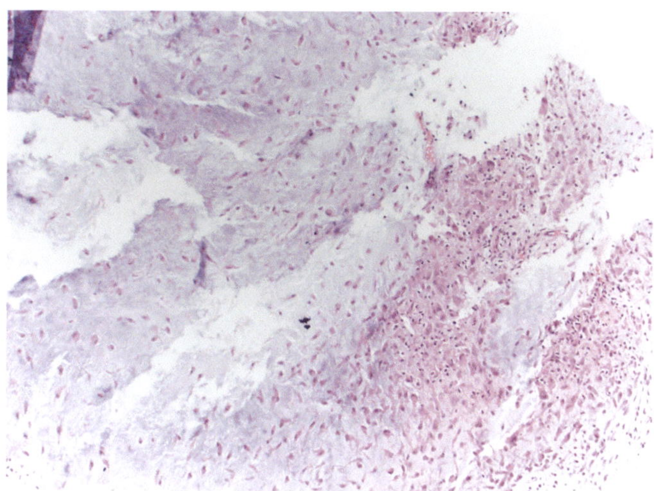

Fig. 10.6 Chondroblastoma. Histologic sections show lobules of chondroid matrix with bland spindled cells reminiscent of chondromyxoid fibroma. At the periphery are more cellular areas composed of polygonal cells with interspersed giant cells

matrix may be present and allow distinction from other giant cell rich lesions such as aneurysmal bone cyst and giant cell tumor of bone.

Chondrosarcoma

Chondrosarcoma

- Chondrosarcomas most frequently involve long bones and occur in older individuals. Although these tumors may grow large and be locally advanced, metastatic spread is less common than in other sarcomas.
- Secondary chondrosarcoma may occur in the settings of Ollier and Mafucci syndromes, synovial chondromatosis, and preexisting osteochondroma.

Plain Radiograph

- While there is occasionally overlap with features seen in enchondromas, chondrosarcomas typically demonstrate aggressive features that include cortical destruction, periosteal thickening, and endosteal scalloping (Fig. 10.7) [22].
- Lesions may include mixed lytic and sclerotic regions, with periosteal reactions ranging from thick, unilaminar, more benign-appearing periosteal reaction to a spiculated, aggressive appearance.

Magnetic Resonance Imaging

- Classicly, a chondroid matrix of a chondrosarcoma appears as alternating high T2 signal intensity lobules with heterogeneous areas of low T2 signal intensity. The low T2 signal intensity areas represent areas of calcification within the matrix.
- The extent of soft-tissue involvement is much better delineated on MRI.

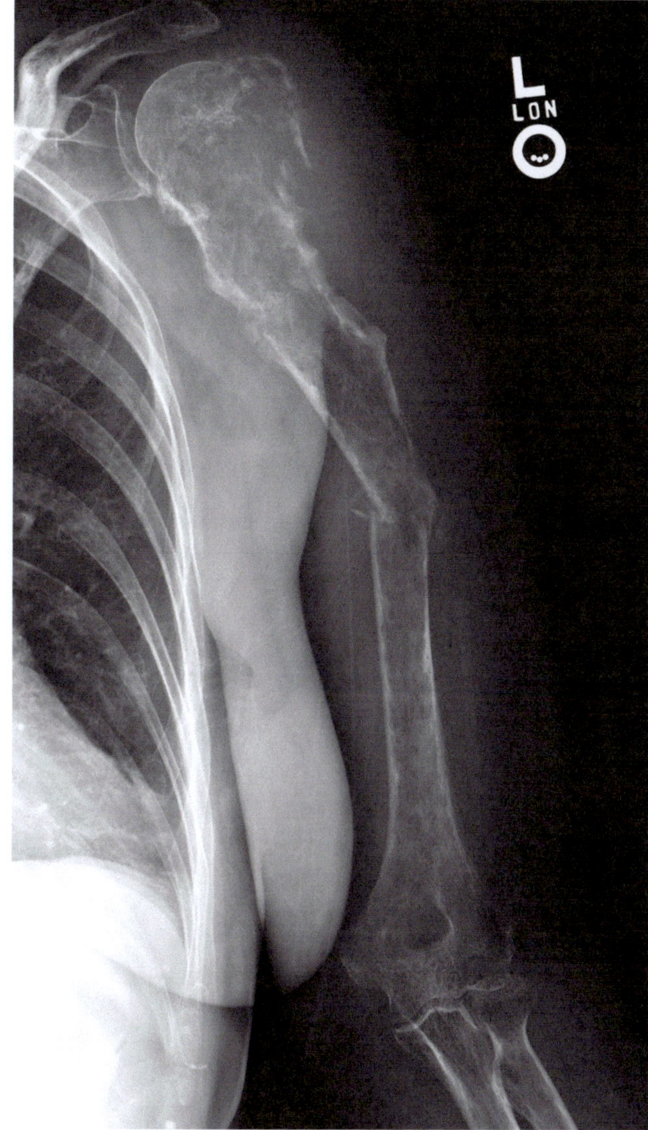

Fig. 10.7 Chondrosarcoma. Radiograph of the humerus demonstrates a chondroid matrix with diffuse cortical destruction and a lesion size much greater than 5 cm. Pathologic analysis confirmed the diagnosis of chondrosarcoma. Compare with the benign-appearing enchondroma in Fig. 10.5

- Larger lesion size correlates with a higher likelihood of malignancy.

Fine Needle Aspirates

- Aspirates are characterized by malignant chondrocytes within lacunae accompanied by an abundant chondroid matrix [23].
  - Chondrocytes are typically round cells with abundant clear to granular cytoplasm and round nuclei. They reside within rounded spaces (lacunae) within the chondroid matrix of the tumor.
  - The chondroid matrix is intensely metachromatic, with varying degrees of myxoid and fibrillary change.

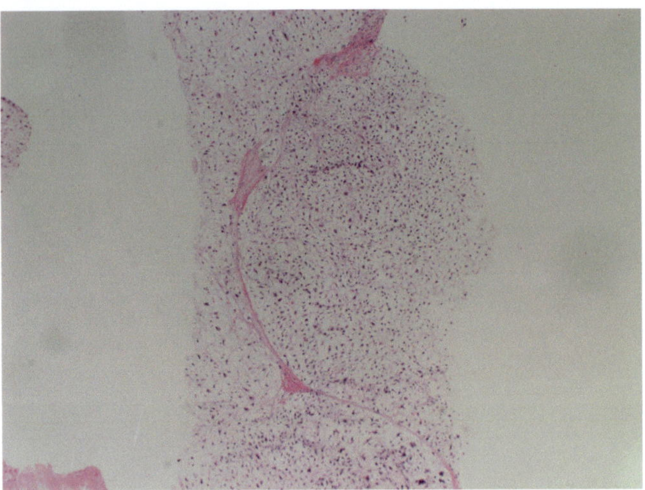

Fig. 10.8 Chondrosarcoma. Core biopsy demonstrating crowded atypical chondrocytes growing in lobules and producing a pale blue chondroid matrix

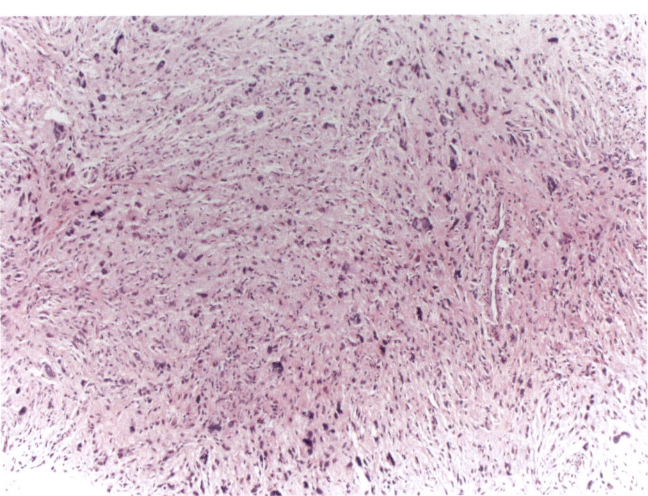

Fig. 10.9 Malignant fibrous histiocytoma. Sheets of pleomorphic highly atypical cells within a fibroblastic matrix. No evidence of differentiation along any specific lineage is seen

  - The degree of cytologic atypia impacts the overall morphologic picture. Cases of low-grade chondrosarcoma are morphologically indistinguishable from chondroma in aspirates. High-grade chondrosarcomas, in contrast, may contain little matrix and may be composed of sheets of overtly malignant cells.

Core Biopsy

- In core biopsies, the appearance of chondrosarcomas varies, based on the grade of the lesion.
  - Low-grade chondrosarcomas are predominantly made up of myxoid stromata with or without myxoid change. The overall cellularity may be low, and cytologic atypia may be minimal (normal chondrocyte nuclei should be lacking in internal nuclear detail) (Fig. 10.8).
  - In high-grade or dedifferentiated chondrosarcomas, the degree of cellularity is greater and the chondroid matrix may be absent in small biopsies. The chondrocytes are overtly malignant, and necrosis and myxoid change involving the stroma may be seen.

Fibrous Tumor Matrix: Malignant Fibrous Histiocytoma

Malignant Fibrous Histiocytoma

Clinical

- Malignant fibrous histiocytoma (MFH) of bone is a rare high-grade sarcoma lacking an overt line of differentiation that preferentially involves the long bones. It may occur as a primary lesion or secondary to radiation, bone infarction, or Paget disease of bone.

Plain Radiograph

- Lesions are osteolytic, with nonspecific aggressive features, including a wide zone of transition, permeative bone destruction, periosteal reaction, and ill-defined margins.

Magnetic Resonance Imaging

- Descriptions of the MRI appearance of MFH are limited.
- Universally, soft-tissue extension is described. MFH is T1 iso- to hyperintense to muscle, and short time inversion recovery (STIR) iso- to hypointense [24].

Fine Needle Aspiration

- Aspirates from cases of MFH show overtly malignant spindle to epithelioid cells. In typical cells, there is marked variation in both the size and shape of tumor cells. The cytoplasm is usually delicate and angulated and may contain some vacuolation. A chondroid and osteoid matrix is not seen.

Core Biopsy

- The usual cases show overtly malignant spindle cells, usually within a fibroblastic stroma. By definition, an overt line of morphologic differentiation should be absent and no osteoid or chondroid matrix should be visible either radiographically or in biopsy specimens (Fig. 10.9). Giant cells and areas of lymphohistiocytic inflammation are often seen.

Diffuse Osseous Processes: Multiple Myeloma and Metastatic Disease

While both multiple myeloma and metastatic disease may present as solitary foci, a multiplicity of abnormalities is often a characteristic finding.

Multiple Myeloma

Clinical

- Improvements in therapy for multiple myeloma, including stem cell transplant and new chemotherapeutic agents such as lenalidomide and bortezomib, have increased the median survival rate from 2.5 to 8.5 years [25].

Plain Radiograph

- Initial screening for lesions in a patient with multiple myeloma is typically performed with a skeletal survey.
- Lesions are described as "punched out," which signifies a lytic lesion without reactive sclerosis in the skull or pelvis. In the appendicular skeleton, the degree of associated sclerosis is variable [26].

Computed Tomography

- CT is rarely used in the imaging of multiple myeloma; however, occasionally CT can demonstrate small lytic osseous lesions to better advantage [27].
- CT may be valuable for determining the degree of osseous instability in a patient with multiple myeloma.

Magnetic Resonance Imaging

- Myeloma lesions are typically low signal on T1 images, with high T2 and STIR signals (Fig. 10.10) [27].
- Focal plasmacytoma may stand out as an area of T1 hypointensity against a background of normal marrow.
- There may be diffuse hypointensity of the marrow signal on T1, compatible with diffuse myelomatous involvement [28].
- Myeloma lesions often enhance after administration of gadolinium.

Fine Needle Aspiration

- Aspirates are characterized by sheets of plasma cells. Plasma cells are characterized by well-defined cytoplasmic borders, eccentric round nuclei, perinuclear clearing, and clock face chromatin. Binucleated forms may be seen.
- In a subset of cases, amorphous dense fragments of amyloid may be present.

Core Biopsy

- Similar to the findings in aspirates, core biopsies contain sheets of monotonous plasma cells containing abundant amphophilic cytoplasm. The nuclei are eccentrically placed with a clock face chromatin pattern and perinuclear clearing (Fig. 10.11).

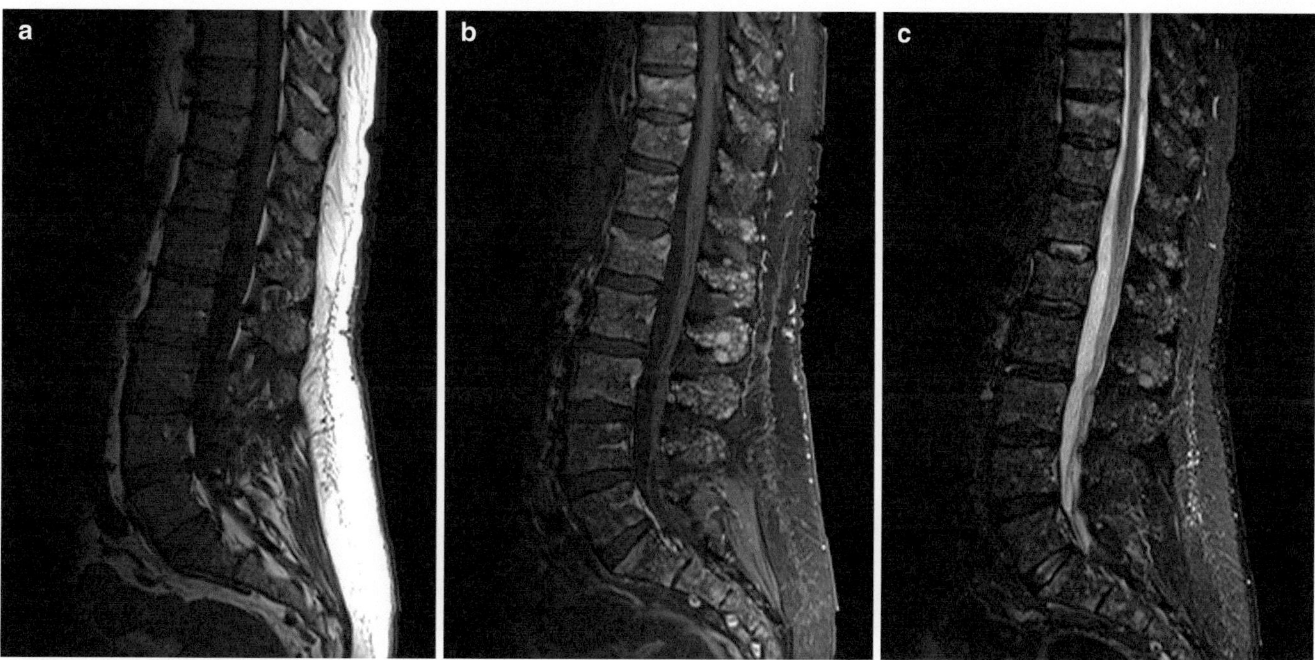

Fig. 10.10 Multiple myeloma. Sagittal lumbar spine MRI in a patient with multiple myeloma demonstrating diffuse intrinsic T1 hypointensity (**a**), heterogeneous diffuse foci of enhancement (**b**), and STIR hyperintensity (**c**)

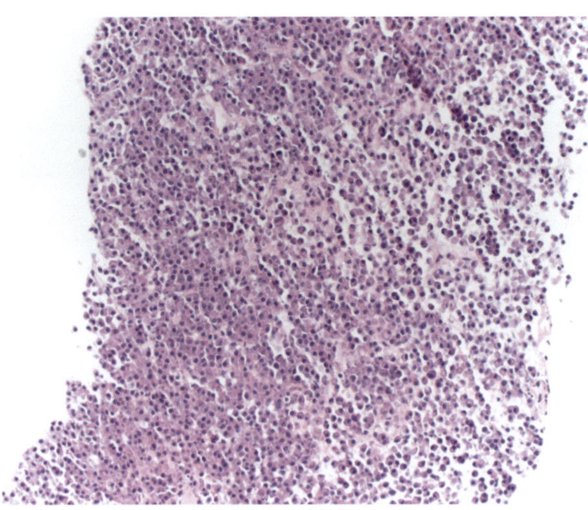

Fig. 10.11 Multiple myeloma. Core biopsy demonstrating sheets of bland dyscohesive plasma cells with eccentric bland nuclei and amphophilic cytoplasm

- Amorphous amyloid with a cracked appearance and associated giant cells may be present.
- In some cases, the plasma cells display marked nuclear pleomorphism and loss of the typical features (anaplastic myeloma). In these cases, finding occasional morphologically normal plasma cells in the background can serve as a useful clue.

Osseous Metastatic Disease

Clinical

- Metastatic carcinomas to bone greatly outnumber primary bone tumors.
- The tumors that are most likely to give rise to osseus metastases are breast carcinoma, lung adenocarcinoma, conventional renal cell carcinoma, prostatic adenocarcinoma, and follicular thyroid carcinoma.

Nuclear Medicine

- Positron emission tomography (PET)/CT is very useful in the detection of osseous metastatic disease. Lesions showing concordant fluorine 18-fluorodeoxyglucose (FDG) uptake and an underlying osseous abnormality by CT have a 98% positive predictive value for the presence of osseous metastasis [29].
- Methylene diphosphone (MDP) bone scans demonstrate MDP uptake in osseous metastatic lesions. However, limitations include differentiation from other lesions that demonstrate increased MDP uptake such as degenerative changes and photopenic metastatic lesions [30].
- Cortical lesions, rather than those that strictly involve the medullary cavity, are those that are detected by MDP bone scintigraphy [31].

Magnetic Resonance Imaging

- Metastatic disease is typically characterized by T1 hypointensity, postcontrast enhancement, and T2/STIR high signal [32].

Fine Needle Aspiration

- Findings in aspirate specimens from metastatic lesions depend on the line of differentiation and site of origin.
- In general, metastatic carcinomas tend to be more cohesive and uniform than primary bone sarcomas. The cell contours are usually rounder and palisading, and gland formation may be seen in cases of metastatic adenocarcinoma.

Core Biopsy

- The appearance of metastatic lesions in bone biopsies depends upon the site of origin of the tumor.
- In metastatic adenocarcinomas, gland formation and mucin production may be seen. Fibrosis may be extensive, and obscure malignant cells can be detected in some cases.

Other Tumors: Lipoma, Peripheral Nerve Sheath Tumors, Chordoma, and Synovial Sarcoma

Lipoma and Liposarcoma

Clinical

- Lipomas and their malignant counterpart, liposarcomas, are the most common soft-tissue tumors in adults.
- Liposarcomas are a heterogeneous group of tumors that vary greatly with regard to common sites of origin, genetics, and morphology.
- Lipomas may occur in the soft tissues or within the bone as intraosseous lipoma.
- While soft-tissue liposarcoma has been described, osseous liposarcoma is a rare and poorly defined vanishing entity.

Plain Radiography

- Intraosseous lipoma is usually a calcaneal well-defined lucent lesion on radiography. Findings are often nonspecific, which can relate to the degree of internal necrosis.

Computed Tomography

- Lipomas are characterized by their homogeneous low attenuation on CT compatible with a fat-containing lesion. Intraosseous lipomas may demonstrate areas of necrosis, with corresponding higher attenuation on CT (Fig. 10.12) [33].
- Liposarcomas also contain fat; however, the degree of homogeneity and interspersed soft-tissue density septa depends on the degree of differentiation of the tumor [34].

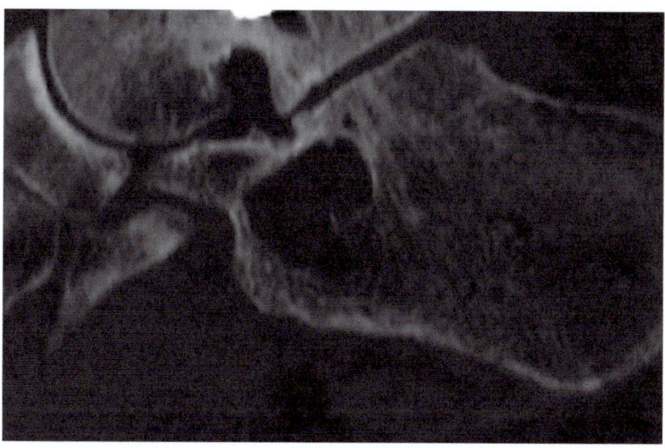

Fig. 10.12 Intraosseous lipoma. Sagittal reformatted CT image demonstrating a fat attenuation lesion in the calcaneus. This is a characteristic location for intraosseous lipoma

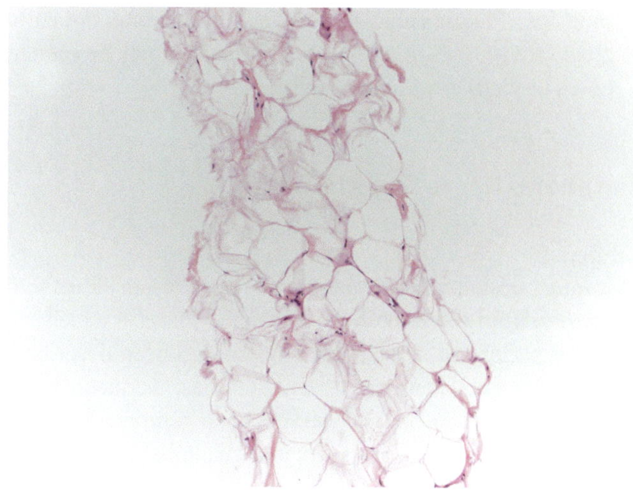

Fig. 10.13 Lipoma. Core biopsy showing sheets of uniform adipocytes with small indistinct nuclei

Magnetic Resonance Imaging

- Thick enhancing septa are characteristic of liposarcoma and demonstrate an association with malignancy rather than with benign lipoma [35].

Fine Needle Aspiration

- Aspirates of lipomas typically contain irregular clusters of adipocytes with large optically clear vacuoles and peripherally placed inconspicuous nuclei. Morphologically, lipomas are indistinguishable from normal fat in aspirates.
- Aspirates of well-differentiated liposarcomas are almost indistinguishable from those of lipoma. Occasional adipocytic cells may display hyperchromatic enlarged nuclei [36].
- Cases of myxoid liposarcoma are characterized by an admixture of adipose tissue and small round blue cells, some of which may contain microvacuoles. Delicate vascularity may be prominent. Cytologic atypia is minimal in most cases. Granular metachromatic myxoid matrix material is often present in the background.
- Dedifferentiated and pleomorphic liposarcomas are high-grade malignant mesenchymal neoplasms. In aspirates, they are probably indistinguishable from malignant fibrous histiocytomas, since adipocytic differentiation is usually minimal [37].

Core Biopsy

- In histologic material, lipomas are composed of sheets of adipocytes without increased vascularity or nuclear atypia (Fig. 10.13). In small biopsies, lipomas cannot be reliably distinguished from normal adipose tissue.
- Well-differentiated liposarcomas resemble lipomas in most cases and are difficult to diagnose definitively in small biopsies. Helpful morphologic features include fibrous septa, multivacuolated lipoblasts, and most importantly, atypical stromal cells containing hyperchromatic enlarged nuclei (Fig. 10.14). In ambiguous cases, performing FISH (fluorescence in situ hybridization) to detect *MDM2* amplification (invariably present in cases of well-differentiated liposarcoma) is diagnostic.

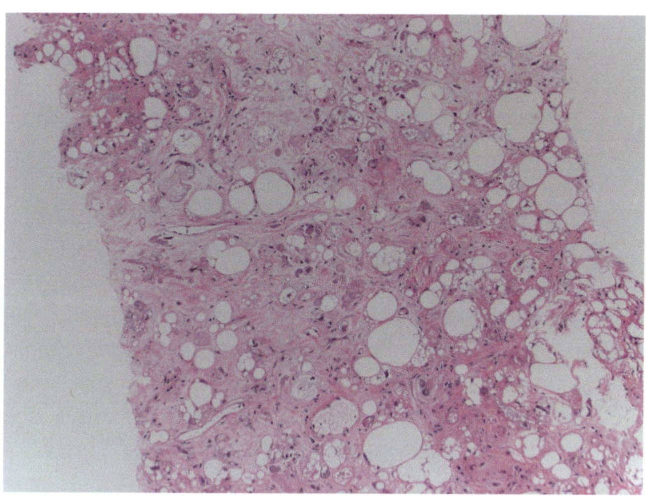

Fig. 10.14 Well-differentiated liposarcoma. Core biopsy specimen demonstrating lobules of adipocytes of varying sizes within a delicate fibrous stroma. Numerous multivacuolated lipoblasts with large indented nuclei are present, as are large atypical stromal cells with hyperchromatic nuclei

- Myxoid liposarcoma is typically made up of sheets of adipocytes and a myxoid matrix with a prominent plexiform ("chicken wire") vascular pattern. In aggressive cases, a component of bland small round blue cells (round cells) is present.
- Dedifferentiated liposarcoma and pleomorphic liposarcoma resemble malignant fibrous histiocytoma in small

biopsies. Pleomorphic tumor cells containing optically clear fat vacuoles (pleomorphic lipoblasts) may be seen in cases of pleomorphic liposarcoma.

Peripheral Nerve Sheath Tumors

Clinical

- Tumors arising from the peripheral nerve sheath either tend to grow from nerves or in the paraspinal space. A wide variety of peripheral nerve sheath tumors has been described, including schwannomas, neurofibromas, perineuriomas, and malignant peripheral nerve sheath tumors. Only the last-named tumor behaves in a malignant fashion.

Magnetic Resonance Imaging

- Peripheral nerve sheath tumors (PNSTs) are located along major nerve distributions.
- Lesions typically demonstrate a fusiform shape.
- The "split fat" sign, which is seen in PNST, is a peripheral rim of fat visualized on T1 images. A "target" appearance of peripheral T2 hyperintensity is also characteristic of nerve origin lesions [38].
- Malignant peripheral nerve sheath tumors (MPNSTs) also result in atrophy in the distribution of the affected nerve.

Fine Needle Aspiration

- Aspirates of neurofibromas and schwannomas contain fragments of metachromatic fibrous stroma and bland spindle cells as well as buckled nuclei. Single cells with a similar morphology may also be present in the background of the aspirate. Aspirates of schwannomas may also contain histiocytes and cellular fragments with palisading of spindle cell nuclei [39].
- In most cases, malignant peripheral nerve sheath tumors present with monotonous spindle cells with elevated nuclear:cytoplasmic ratios, irregular hyperchromatic nuclei, and scant delicate cytoplasm. Some cases exhibiting a greater degree of atypia are indistinguishable from cases of MFH [40].

Core Biopsy

- In histologic sections, neurofibromas are relatively circumscribed but unencapsulated tumors composed of bland spindle cells, collagenous stroma, and myxoid change. Mast cells may be present. Mitotic activity should be absent.
- Schwannomas consist of an encapsulated uniform population of bland spindle cells with areas of hypercellularity and hypocellularity. Nuclear palisading is typical and is regarded as a classic morphologic finding, as are hyalinized vessels. Areas of fibrosis and foamy histiocytes are common degenerative changes seen in these tumors.
- Malignant peripheral nerve sheath tumors (MPNSTs) are usually made up of short perpendicular intersecting fascicles of monotonous spindle cells with elevated nuclear:cytoplasmic ratios and hyperchromatic irregular nuclei (Figs. 10.15 and 10.16). Mitotic activity may be brisk, and necrosis can be extensive.

Chordoma

Clinical

- Chordoma is a rare tumor that arises from vestiges of the notochord along the neuraxis. This tumor usually arises from the clivus or coccyx.

Magnetic Resonance Imaging

- The majority of chordomas have both intraosseous and extraosseous portions. This is a major point of differentiation between chordomas, which have a poor prognosis, and the less aggressive benign notochordal cell tumors, which tend to remain compartmentalized within their tissue of origin (Fig. 10.17) [41].
- Chordomas are midline structures and are commonly centered on the clivus, with extraosseous extension.
- High T2 signal and lobulated contours are characteristic findings [42].

Fine Needle Aspiration

- Typical chordomas have an extremely characteristic appearance in aspirate specimens.
  - Abundant fibrillary metachromatic stroma are typically seen, intimately admixed with groups of cells as well as individual cells (Fig. 10.18a) [43].
  - Round epithelioid tumor cells are abundant from nests and cords, and they contain "bubbly" cytoplasm with multiple well-defined vacuoles ("physaliphorous cells").

Core Biopsy

- While they are not always observed in core biopsies, chordomas are invariably lobulated tumors. Abundant loose myxoid stroma is present, within which the round tumor cells form cords and nests. Individual tumor cells contain abundant clear vacuolated cytoplasm (Fig. 10.18b).

Synovial Sarcoma

Clinical

- Most synovial sarcomas occur in extra-articular locations in younger individuals in the second or third decades of life. Despite its name, this tumor typically does not involve or resemble synovium. Monophasic synovial sarcoma is the most common subtype of this soft-tissue tumor [44].

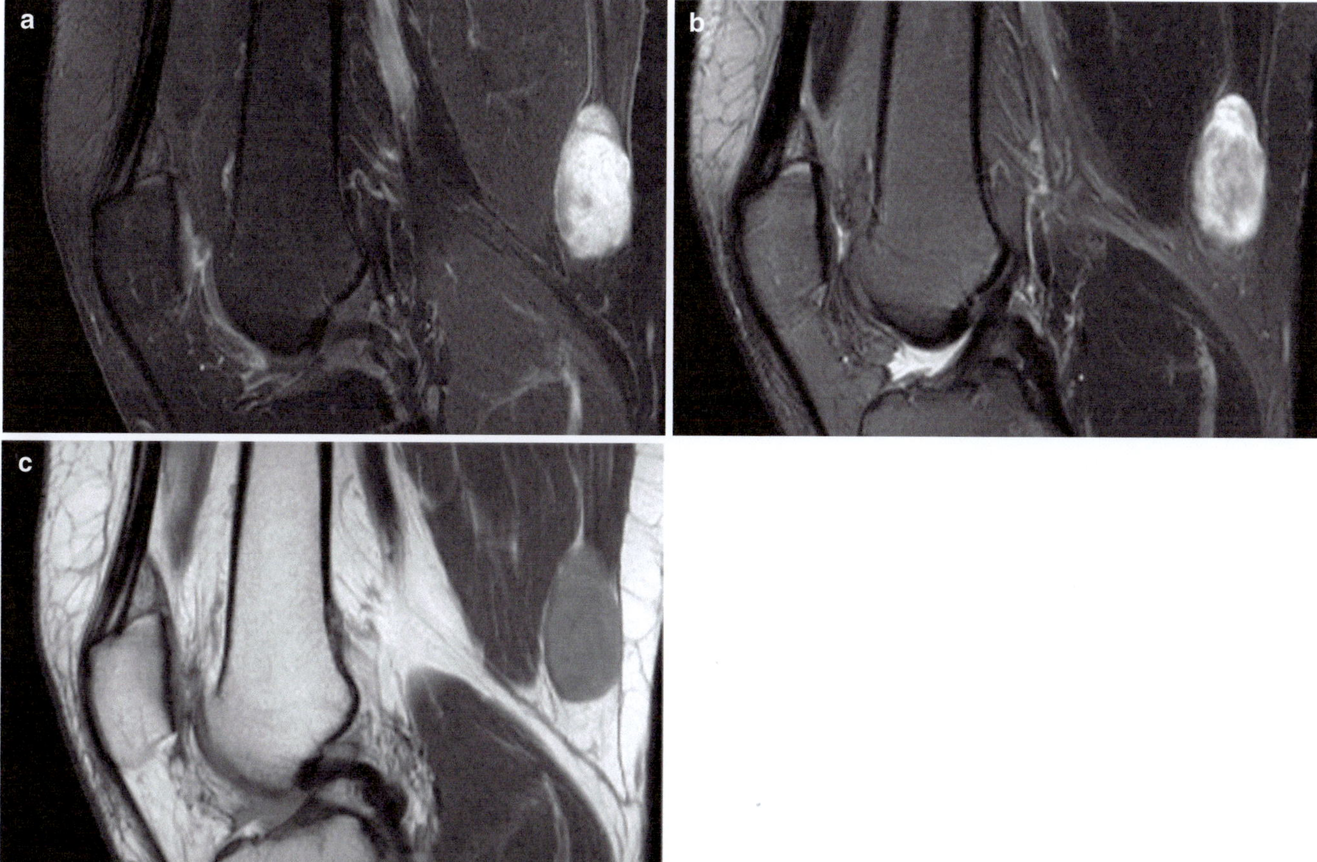

Fig. 10.15 Peripheral nerve sheath tumor: A pathologically confirmed peripheral nerve sheath tumor on this sagittal knee MRI demonstrates a fusiform shape with splitting of the adjacent fat. The lesion demonstrates enhancement on the T1 postcontrast enhancement images (**a**), T2 hyperintensity (**b**), and intermediate signal on proton density images (**c**)

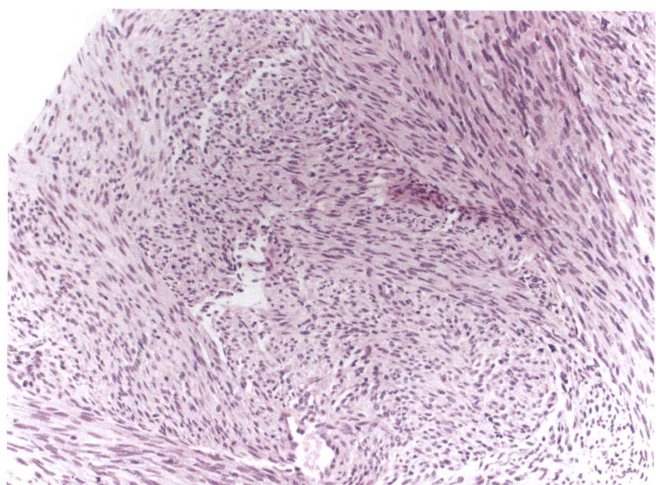

Fig. 10.16 Malignant peripheral nerve sheath tumors. Short intersecting fascicles of hyperchromatic uniform spindle cells are characteristic. Scattered mitotic activity is seen in this resected specimen

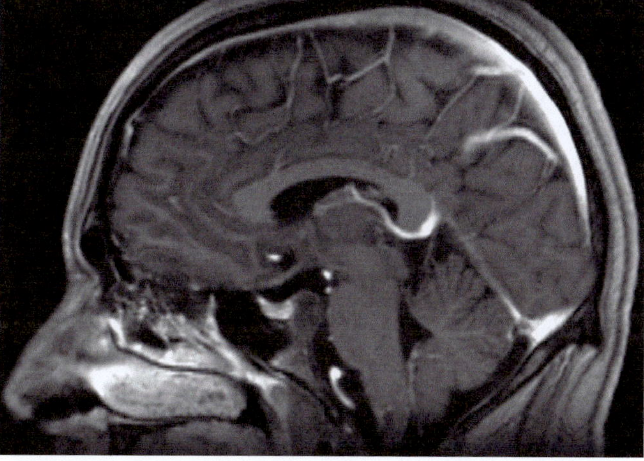

Fig. 10.17 Chordoma. Sagittal T1 postcontrast MRI demonstrates a hypointense soft-tissue lesion in the midline clivus involving both intraosseous and extraosseous prepontine compartments; this is characteristic of chordoma

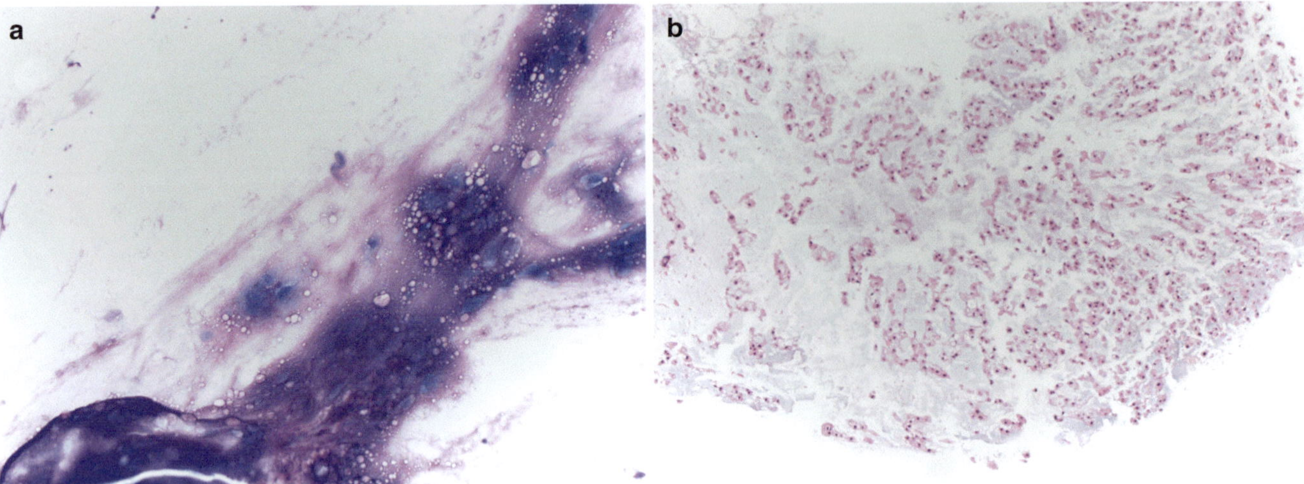

Fig. 10.18 Chordoma. (**a**) Numerous spindled to epithelioid cells with abundant vacuolated cytoplasm are seen within magenta chondromyxoid stroma in an aspirate specimen. (**b**) Lobules composed of cords of bland epithelioid cells with vacuolated cytoplasm are seen in this core biopsy. Abundant pale chondromyxoid stroma is seen in the background

Plain Radiograph

- Findings are nonspecific, but radiographs may demonstrate a soft-tissue mass with peripheral calcification [45].

Magnetic Resonance Imaging

- Usually, synovial sarcoma is a heterogeneous nonspecific mass as seen on MRI.
- The majority are multilocular, with internal septa and well-defined margins.

Fine Needle Aspiration

- Aspirates are typically cellular and contain numerous bland spindle cells with scant cytoplasm and bland comma-shaped hyperchromatic nuclei. Cytologic monotony is usually pronounced. Cellular fragments usually display prominent blood vessels. In cases of biphasic synovial sarcoma, an epithelial component consisting of clusters of glandular cells is present [46].

Core Biopsy

- In contrast to most forms of sarcoma, synovial sarcoma often contains both an epithelial and a mesenchymal component.
  - The epithelial component is usually glandular or occasionally squamous, forming glands, nests, and cords.
  - The mesenchymal component is composed of monotonous spindle cells with inconspicuous cytoplasm typically forming sweeping fascicles. Background collagen production is variably conspicuous, as is vascularity (Fig. 10.19).
- In cases of poorly differentiated synovial sarcoma, mitotic activity is brisk, and the mesenchymal component may adopt a round-cell morphology

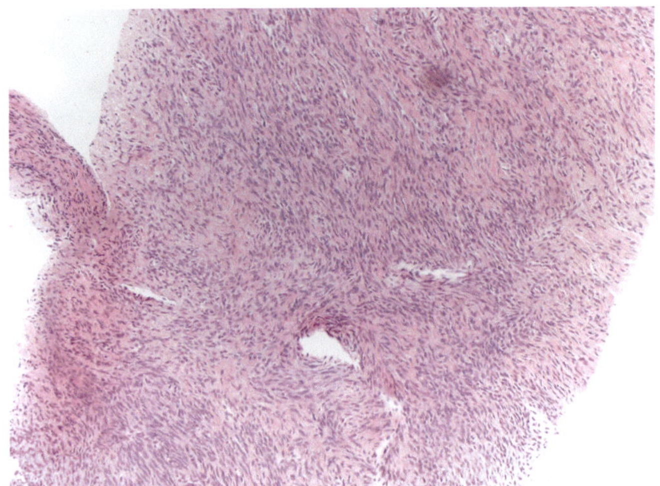

Fig. 10.19 Synovial sarcoma. Core biopsy of a cellular lesion made up of bland spindle cells in an eosinophilic fibroblastic background. Scattered compressed vascular channels are seen

References

1. Kamide T, Nakada M, Hayashi Y, Uchiyama N, Hamada J. Intraparenchymal pneumocephalus caused by ethmoid sinus osteoma. J Clin Neurosci. 2009;16:1487–9.
2. Davies AM. Primary bone tumors. Philadelphia: WB Saunders; 2008.
3. Zhang Y, Rosenberg AE. Bone-forming tumors. Surg Pathol Clin. 2017;10:513–35.
4. Levine SM, Lambiase RE, Petchprapa CN. Cortical lesions of the tibia: characteristic appearances at conventional radiography. Radiographics. 2003;23:157–77.
5. Rosenthal DI, Hornicek FJ, Torriani M, Gebhardt MC, Mankin HJ. Osteoid osteoma: percutaneous treatment with radiofrequency energy. Radiology. 2003;229:171–5.
6. Miller SL, Hoffer FA. Malignant and benign bone tumors. Radiol Clin N Am. 2001;39:673–99.

7. Woertler K. Benign bone tumors and tumor-like lesions: value of cross-sectional imaging. Eur Radiol. 2003;13:1820–35.
8. Wilde GE, Gakhal MS. Radiological reasoning: imaging of a talar mass. Am J Roentgenol. 2011;196:WS47–52.
9. Venugopal SB, Prasad S. Cytological diagnosis of osteoblastoma of cervical spine: a case report with review of literature. Diagn Cytopathol. 2015;43:218–21.
10. Rosenberg ZS, Lev S, Schmahmann S, Steiner GC, Beltran J, Present D. Osteosarcoma: subtle, rare, and misleading plain film features. Am J Roentgenol. 1995;165:1209–14.
11. Yarmish G, Klein MJ, Landa J, Lefkowitz RA, Hwang S. Imaging characteristics of primary osteosarcoma: nonconventional subtypes. Radiographics. 2010;30:1653–72.
12. Sathiyamoorthy S, Ali SZ. Osteoblastic osteosarcoma: cytomorphologic characteristics and differential diagnosis on fine-needle aspiration. Acta Cytol. 2012;56:481–6.
13. VandenBussche CJ, Sathiyamoorthy S, Wakely PE, Ali SZ. Chondroblastic osteosarcoma: Cytomorphologic characteristics and differential diagnosis on FNA. Cancer Cytopathol. 2016;124:493–500.
14. Lee KC, Davies AM, Cassar-Pullicino VN. Imaging the complications of osteochondromas. Clin Radiol. 2002;57:18–28.
15. Ilaslan H, Sundaram M. Advances in musculoskeletal tumor imaging. Orthop Clin North Am. 2006;37:375–91.. vii
16. Bernard SA, Murphey MD, Flemming DJ, Kransdorf MJ. Improved differentiation of benign osteochondromas from secondary chondrosarcomas with standardized measurement of cartilage cap at CT and MR imaging. Radiology. 2010;255:857–65.
17. Eisenberg RL. Bubbly lesions of bone. Am J Roentgenol. 2009;193:W79–94.
18. Rybak LD, Rosenthal DI, Wittig JC. Chondroblastoma: radiofrequency ablation—alternative to surgical resection in selected cases. Radiology. 2009;251:599–604.
19. Kennedy N, Demos TC, Lomasney LM. Radiologic case study. Chondroblastoma with geographic bone destruction and a sclerotic rim. Orthopedics. 2009;32:542.
20. Papaioannou G, Sebire NJ, McHugh K. Imaging of the unusual pediatric 'blastomas'. Cancer Imaging. 2009;9:1–11.
21. Fanning CV, Sneige NS, Carrasco CH, Ayala AG, Murray JA, Raymond AK. Fine needle aspiration cytology of chondroblastoma of bone. Cancer. 1990;65:1847–63.
22. Littrell LA, Wenger DE, Wold LE, Unni KK, White LM, et al. Radiographic, CT, and MR imaging features of dedifferentiated chondrosarcomas: a retrospective review of 174 de novo cases. Radiographics. 2004;24:1397–409.
23. Dodd LG. Fine-needle aspiration of chondrosarcoma. Diagn Cytopathol. 2006;34:413–8.
24. Koplas MC, Lefkowitz RA, Bauer TW, Joyce MJ, Ilaslan H, Landa J, et al. Imaging findings, prevalence and outcome of de novo and secondary malignant fibrous histiocytoma of bone. Skelet Radiol. 2010;39:791–8.
25. Hanrahan CJ, Christensen CR, Crim JR. Current concepts in the evaluation of multiple myeloma with MR imaging and FDG PET/CT. Radiographics. 2010;30:127–42.
26. Dimopoulos M, Terpos E, Comenzo RL, Bruno B, San Miguel J, Pérez-Simon JA, et al. International myeloma working group consensus statement and guidelines regarding the current role of imaging techniques in the diagnosis and monitoring of multiple myeloma. Leukemia. 2009;23:1545–56.
27. Mahnken AH, Wildberger JE, Gehbauer G, Bruno B, San Miguel J, Pérez-Simon JA, et al. Multidetector CT of the spine in multiple myeloma: comparison with MR imaging and radiography. Am J Roentgenol. 2002;178:1429–36.
28. Angtuaco EJ, Fassas AB, Walker R, Sethi R, Barlogie B. Multiple myeloma: clinical review and diagnostic imaging. Radiology. 2004;231:11–23.
29. Taira AV, Herfkens RJ, Gambhir SS, Quon A. Detection of bone metastases: assessment of integrated FDG PET/CT imaging. Radiology. 2007;243:204–11.
30. Algra PR, Bloem JL, Tissing H, Falke TH, Arndt JW, Verboom LJ. Detection of vertebral metastases: comparison between MR imaging and bone scintigraphy. Radiographics. 1991;11:219–32.
31. Taoka T, Mayr NA, Lee HJ, Simonson TM, Rezai K, et al. Factors influencing visualization of vertebral metastases on MR imaging versus bone scintigraphy. Am J Roentgenol. 2001;176:1525–30.
32. Vanel D, Dromain C, Tardivon A. MRI of bone marrow disorders. Eur Radiol. 2000;10:224–9.
33. Propeck T, Bullard MA, Lin J, Doi K, Martel W. Radiologic-pathologic correlation of intraosseous lipomas. Am J Roentgenol. 2000;175:673–8.
34. Kind M, Stock N, Coindre JM. Histology and imaging of soft tissue sarcomas. Eur J Radiol. 2009;72:6–15.
35. Ohguri T, Aoki T, Hisaoka M, Watanabe H, Nakamura K, Hashimoto H, et al. Differential diagnosis of benign peripheral lipoma from well-differentiated liposarcoma on MR imaging: is comparison of margins and internal characteristics useful? Am J Roentgenol. 2003;180:1689–94.
36. Klijanienko J, Caillaud JM, Lagacé R. Fine-needle aspiration in liposarcoma: cytohistologic correlative study including well-differentiated, myxoid, and pleomorphic variants. Diagn Cytopathol. 2004;30:307–12.
37. Dodd LG, Sara Jiang X, Rao K, Bui MM. Pleomorphic liposarcoma: a cytologic study of five cases. Diagn Cytopathol. 2015;43:138–43.
38. Abreu E, Aubert S, Wavreille G, Gheno R, Canella C, Cotten A. Peripheral tumor and tumor-like neurogenic lesions. Eur J Radiol. 2013;82:38–50.
39. Domanski HA, Akerman M, Engellau J, Gustafson P, Mertens F, Rydholm A. Fine-needle aspiration of neurilemoma (schwannoma). A clinicocytopathologic study of 116 patients. Diagn Cytopathol. 2006;34:403–12.
40. Gupta K, Dey P, Vashisht R. Fine-needle aspiration cytology of malignant peripheral nerve sheath tumors. Diagn Cytopathol. 2004;31:1–4.
41. Nishiguchi T, Mochizuki K, Ohsawa M, Inoue T, Kageyama K, Suzuki A, et al. Differentiating benign notochordal cell tumors from chordomas: radiographic features on MRI, CT, and tomography. Am J Roentgenol. 2011;196:644–50.
42. Farsad K, Kattapuram SV, Sacknoff R, Ono J, Nielsen GP. Sacral chordoma. Radiographics. 2009;29:1525–30.
43. Crapanzano JP, Ali SZ, Ginsberg MS, Zakowski MF. Chordoma: a cytologic study with histologic and radiologic correlation. Cancer. 2001;93:40–51.
44. Siegel HJ, Sessions W, Casillas MA, Said-Al-Naief N, Lander PH, Lopez-Ben R. Synovial sarcoma: clinicopathologic features, treatment, and prognosis. Orthopedics. 2007;30:1020–5; quiz 6–7.
45. O'Sullivan PJ, Harris AC, Munk PL. Radiological features of synovial cell sarcoma. Br J Radiol. 2008;81:346–56.
46. Ewing CA, Zakowski MF, Lin O. Monophasic synovial sarcoma: a cytologic spectrum. Diagn Cytopathol. 2004;30:19–23.

11 The Breast

Elizabeth Morency, Luis Z. Blanco Jr, and Lilian C. Wang

While the role of fine needle aspiration (FNA) currently is not as prominent in the diagnosis of conditions of the breast as in other organ sites, it is still a useful diagnostic modality in the setting of a palpable breast mass, especially in conjunction with radiologic findings. On the benign end of the spectrum, aspiration of non-neoplastic breast conditions such as fibrocystic changes and gynecomastia in men or inflammatory/reactive conditions like mastitis or fat necrosis, the results of FNA can quickly and efficiently reassure patients and clinicians alike by ruling out a more dangerous process. In terms of benign fibroepithelial neoplasms such as fibroadenoma and neoplasms of uncertain malignant potential such as phyllodes tumor, the presence of characteristic cytomorphologic features lends itself to diagnosis via FNA as well. Papillary neoplasms may also be sampled and can alert clinicians to the need for excision in order to rule out the presence of concurrent atypical duct hyperplasia (ADH) or ductal carcinoma in situ (DCIS). Finally, on the malignant end of the spectrum, although core biopsy has come to predominate in the diagnosis of primary breast carcinoma, given its higher yield of material not only for diagnosis but also for any necessary ancillary studies, FNA still plays an important diagnostic role in the setting of lymph node metastasis or in answering the clinical question of recurrence versus florid scar tissue with nodules that may arise adjacent to a previous site of resection. FNA is also useful in the diagnosis of metastatic disease and involvement of the breast by lymphoproliferative processes [1, 2].

E. Morency (✉)
Department of Pathology, Northwestern Memorial Hospital, Feinberg School of Medicine, Chicago, IL, USA
e-mail: Elizabeth.morency@northwestern.edu

L. Z. Blanco Jr
Department of Pathology, Northwestern Memorial Hospital, Northwestern University Feinberg School of Medicine, Chicago, IL, USA

L. C. Wang
Department of Radiology, Prentice Women's Hospital, Chicago, IL, USA

Normal Findings

Benign Ductal Epithelial Cells and Adipose Tissue

These findings can be seen in the background of aspirates for palpable abnormalities; however, non-neoplastic breast tissue generally yields hypocellular specimens because it is predominantly composed of fibrous stromal tissue and fat, which do not aspirate well.

Benign Conditions

Fibrocystic Changes

Clinical

- Most common breast disorder.
- Can include a combination of cysts, apocrine metaplasia, stromal fibrosis, glandular proliferation, or adenosis and ductal hyperplasia.
- Can present as palpable, occasionally painful, masses [3].

Radiology

Mammography

- Generally shows oval, circumscribed, isodense masses (Fig. 11.1a).

Ultrasound (US)

- Anechoic oval circumscribed masses consistent with cysts and clusters of cysts (Fig. 11.1b–d) [4].

Fine Needle Aspiration (FNA)

- Aspirates can show variable cytomorphology, depending on the proportion of fibrous tissue to cystic spaces.
- Cyst contents: Characterized by macrophages, inflammatory cells, and proteinaceous material (Fig. 11.2a).
- Adipose tissue (Fig. 11.2b).
- Clusters of small ductal cells and apocrine metaplastic cells.

R. Nayar et al. (eds.), *Atlas of Cytopathology and Radiology*, https://doi.org/10.1007/978-3-030-24756-0_11

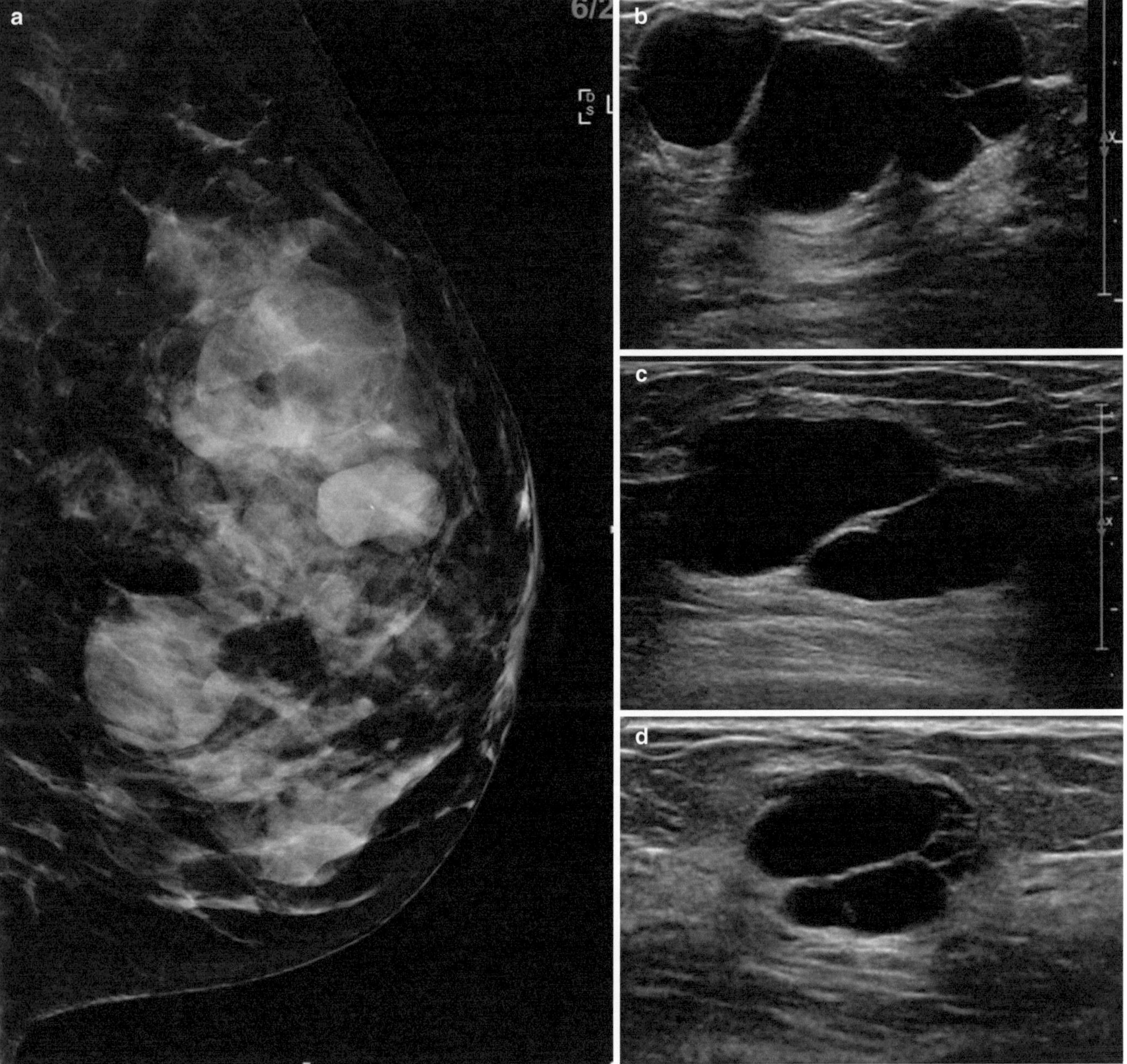

Fig. 11.1 Fibrocystic changes. (**a**) Left mediolateral oblique (MLO) view shows numerous scattered oval circumscribed masses. (**b**, **c**) Ultrasound images of the left breast demonstrate corresponding cysts and clusters of cysts. (**d**) Ultrasound image of the contralateral right breast also demonstrates a cluster of cysts consistent with fibrocystic change

Core Biopsy

- Dilated cysts lined by apocrine metaplastic cells with abundant granular eosinophilic cytoplasm, round nuclei, and prominent nucleoli. Intervening fibrotic stroma and adipose tissue (Fig. 11.2c).

Fat Necrosis

Clinical

- May mimic carcinoma both clinically and mammographically as a mass-forming lesion, typically in patients following trauma or previous surgery.
- Can also be seen in male patients [3].

Radiology

Mammography

- Lucent or fat density mass with or without rim calcification, spiculated or irregular mass/asymmetry, isolated calcifications (Fig. 11.3) [4].

Ultrasound

- Variable appearance from oval circumscribed hypoechoic mass to irregular hypoechoic mass with angular margins and echogenic rim (Fig. 11.4).

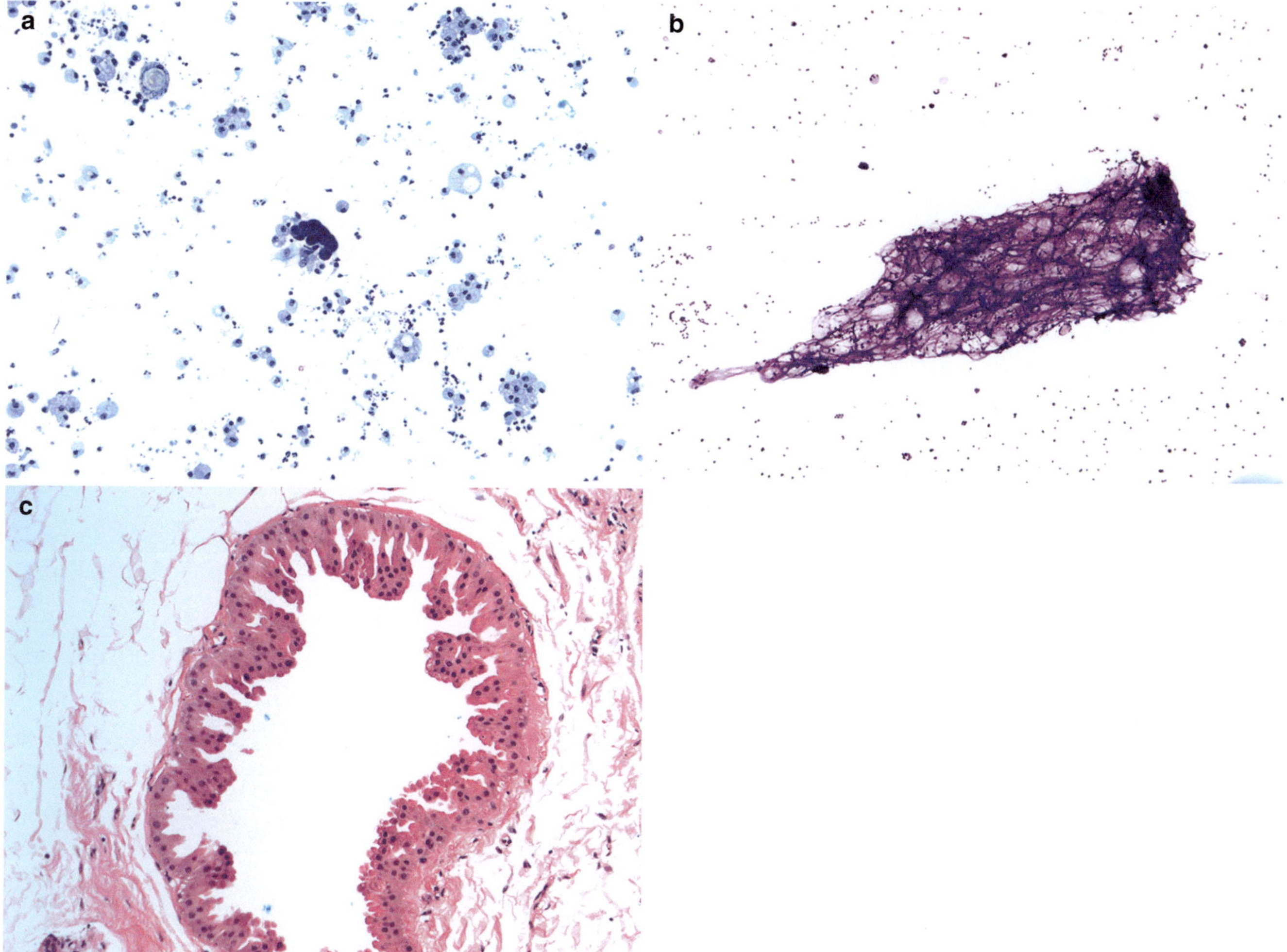

Fig. 11.2 Fibrocystic changes. (**a**) Aspirates can be quite variable, depending on the proportion of fibrous tissue to cystic spaces. This aspirate is predominantly characterized by cyst contents with numerous macrophages with abundant foamy cytoplasm and ovoid to kidney bean-shaped nuclei. Scattered inflammatory cells are usually also present; few neutrophils and lymphocytes are seen (Papanicolaou stain, 200×). (**b**) Scattered clusters of mature adipose tissue can also be seen in aspirates of fibrocystic changes, as displayed in this case (DiffQuik stain, 100). (**c**) Fibrocystic changes. Cyst with apocrine metaplasia. Dilated cyst lined by epithelial cells with round nuclei, variably prominent nucleoli, and abundant eosinophilic cytoplasm with apical snouting and supranuclear eosinophilic granules (hematoxylin and eosin stain [H&E], 200×)

Magnetic Resonance Imaging

- Rim enhancing masses with central fat intensity on non-fat-suppressed T1-weighted images (Fig. 11.5a, b).
- Irregular, heterogeneously enhancing masses (Fig. 11.5c, d).

Fine Needle Aspiration

- Usually hypocellular specimens (can see fatty droplets on slide at time of aspiration).
- Predominantly composed of foamy macrophages, degenerated adipose tissue, acellular debris, and inflammatory cells (Fig. 11.6a).
- May see cholesterol crystals or chunky, dystrophic calcifications (Fig. 11.6b).

Core Biopsy

- Degenerated adipose tissue with loss of nuclei. Foamy macrophages seen scattered between adipocytes (Fig. 11.6c).

Mastitis

Clinical

- Acute: Red, swollen, tender lesion in breast, commonly seen in postpartum period. Secondary to bacteria invading the breast through small defects in the skin of the nipple of a lactating woman.
- Chronic: May occur over time if acute infection is not eradicated or can occur de novo and form a mass lesion composed of lymphoplasmacytic inflammation of large and intermediate sized ducts of unknown etiology.
- Granulomatous: May arise in a patient with tuberculosis or with a fungal infection or less commonly may be idiopathic in young parous women [1].

Radiology

Mammography

- Diffuse skin thickening and trabecular thickening (Fig. 11.7a) [4].

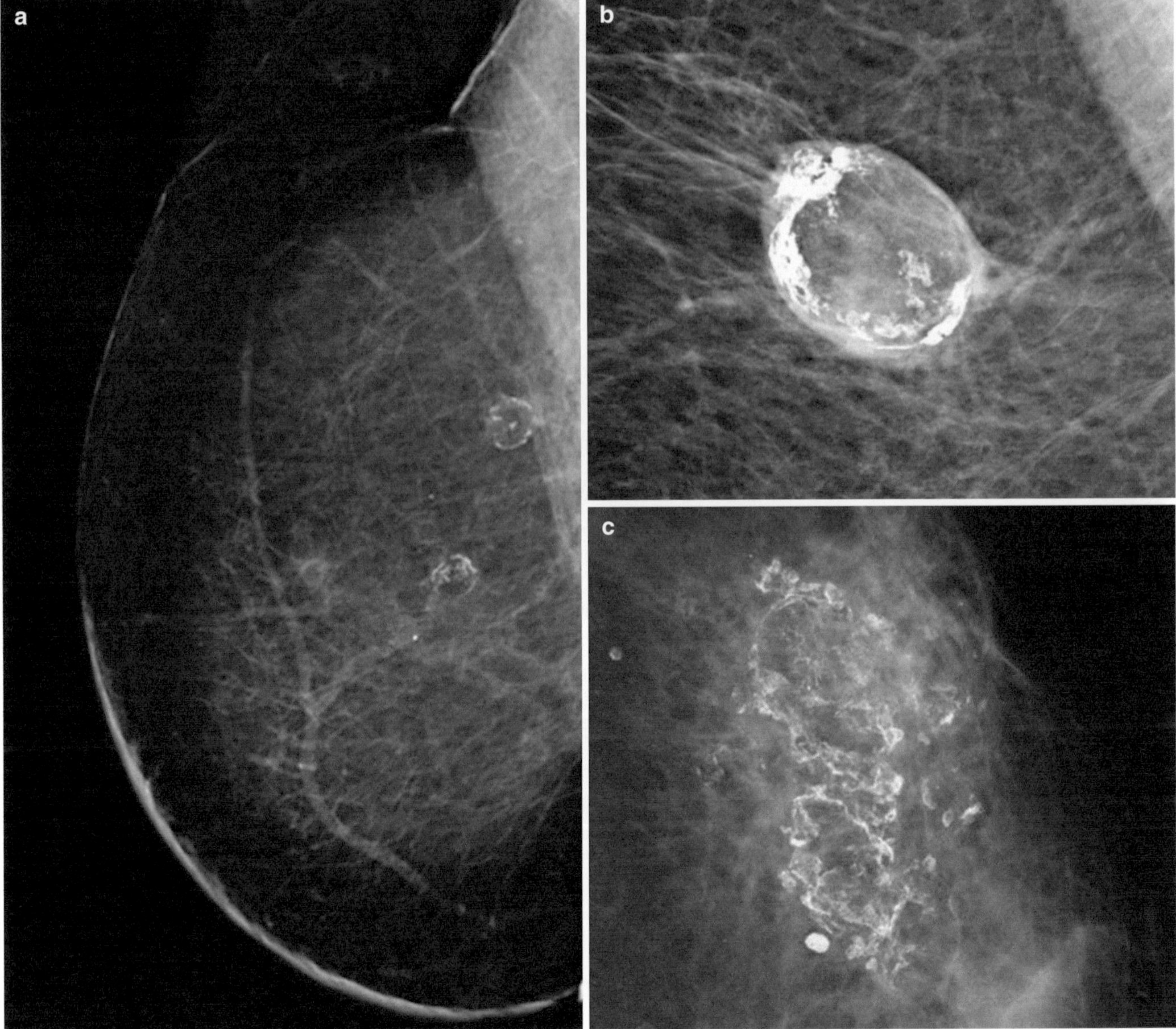

Fig. 11.3 Fat necrosis. (**a**) Right MLO digital mammogram image from patient with history of mastectomy and transverse rectus abdominis muscle (TRAM) flap reconstruction shows rim-calcified lucent masses in the upper breast consistent with fat necrosis. (**b**) Spot magnification view demonstrates an oval, circumscribed, rim-calcified mass consistent with an oil cyst from fat necrosis. (**c**) Left MLO digital mammogram demonstrates coarse dystrophic calcifications with associated lucency characteristic of fat necrosis

Ultrasound

- Skin thickening and subcutaneous edema (Fig. 11.7b).
- Granulomatous mastitis: irregular hypoechoic mass that extends to the skin (Fig. 11.7c).

Fine Needle Aspiration

- Acute: Numerous neutrophils; may see clusters of reactive ductal cells (Fig. 11.8a).
- Chronic: Lymphocytes, plasma cells, and amorphous, inspissated debris corresponding to secretions from ectatic ducts.
- Granulomatous: Epithelioid histiocytes, multinucleated giant cells, lymphocytes, plasma cells, and eosinophils.

Core Biopsy

- Acute: sheets of neutrophils infiltrating breast tissue; bacteria may be seen as well.
- Chronic: lymphoplasmacytic inflammation associated with ducts (Fig. 11.8b).
- Granulomatous: granulomas, giant cells, and lymphoplasmacytic chronic inflammation.

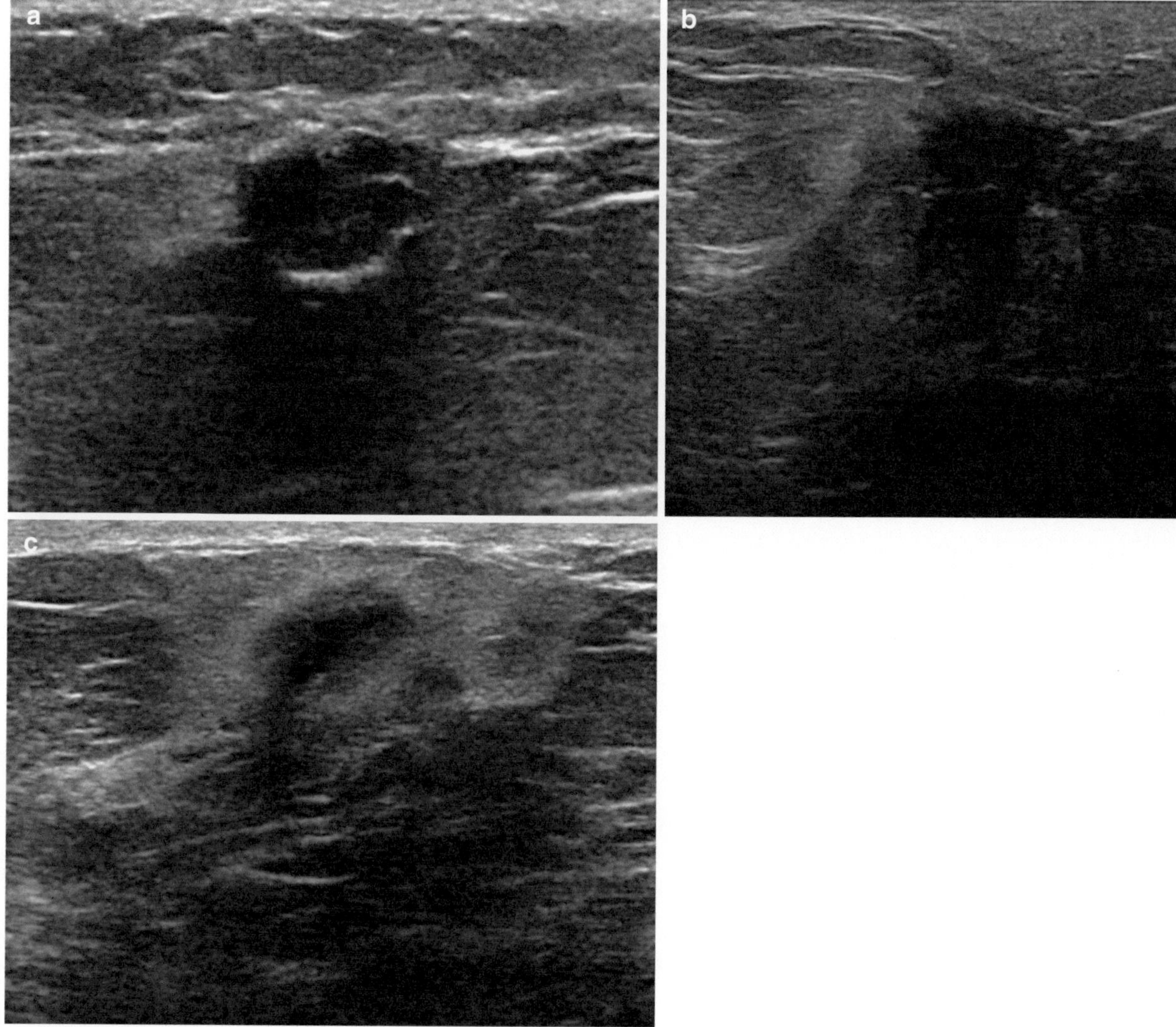

Fig. 11.4 Fat necrosis. (**a**) Oval circumscribed hypoechoic mass with posterior acoustic shadowing. Corresponding mammography demonstrated a lucent mass consistent with an oil cyst. (**b**) Irregular hypoechoic mass with angular and indistinct margins and posterior acoustic shadowing. (**c**) Irregular hypoechoic mass with antiparallel orientation and echogenic halo

Subareolar Abscess

Clinical

- Painful nodule arising in the subareolar region; can be recurrent.
- Aspiration could be performed for microbiology analysis to tailor antibiotic therapy.
- Complete excision recommended to prevent chronic infection and development of sinus tracts [3].

Radiology

Ultrasound

- Complex fluid collection (Fig. 11.9a–c).
- Hypoechoic mass in subareolar breast with extension into adjacent parenchyma or nipple (Fig. 11.9b).
- Overlying skin thickening and edema (Fig. 11.9c) [4].

Fine Needle Aspiration

- Numerous neutrophils and sheets of anucleated squamous cells (Fig. 11.10).
- Histiocytes and giant cells.
- Clusters of reactive ductal cells.

Gynecomastia

Clinical

- Most common abnormality of the breast in men.
- Enlargement of the breast can be diffuse or nodular and frequently is bilateral.
- Can be caused by a number of factors, including low testosterone levels, liver failure, hyperthyroidism, aging, and certain medications, among other less common causes.

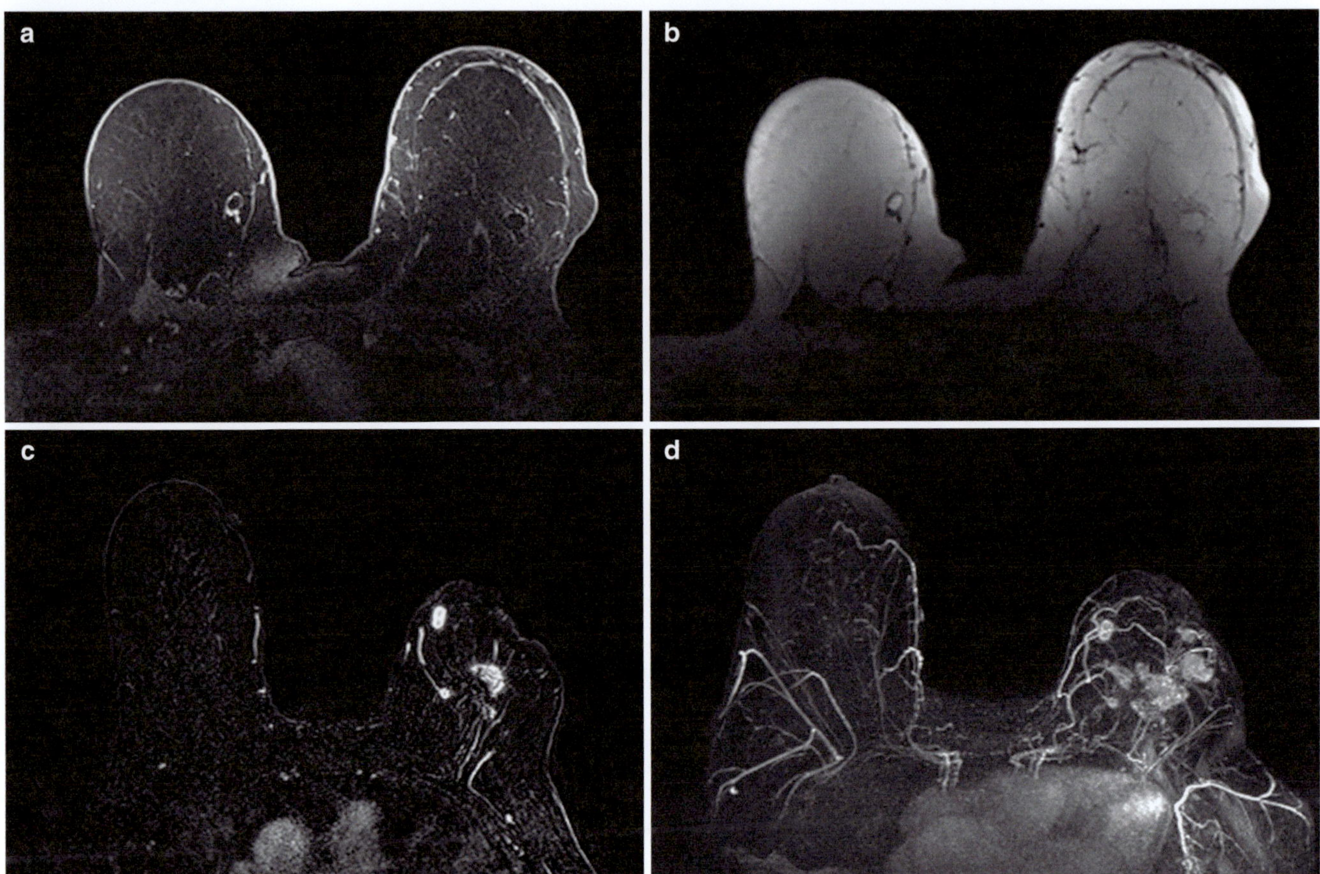

Fig. 11.5 Fat necrosis. (**a**) Axial T1 fat-suppressed postcontrast image demonstrates two oval rim-enhancing masses in the medial right breast and one in the lateral left breast. (**b**) Corresponding axial T1 non–fat-suppressed image shows central fat intensity within the masses consistent with fat necrosis. (**c**) Axial postcontrast T1-weighted MR image demonstrates irregular enhancing masses within the left breast in a patient with history of a left lumpectomy. (**d**) Corresponding maximal intensity projection (MIP) MR image demonstrates multiple additional irregular enhancing masses within the left breast, biopsy proven fat necrosis

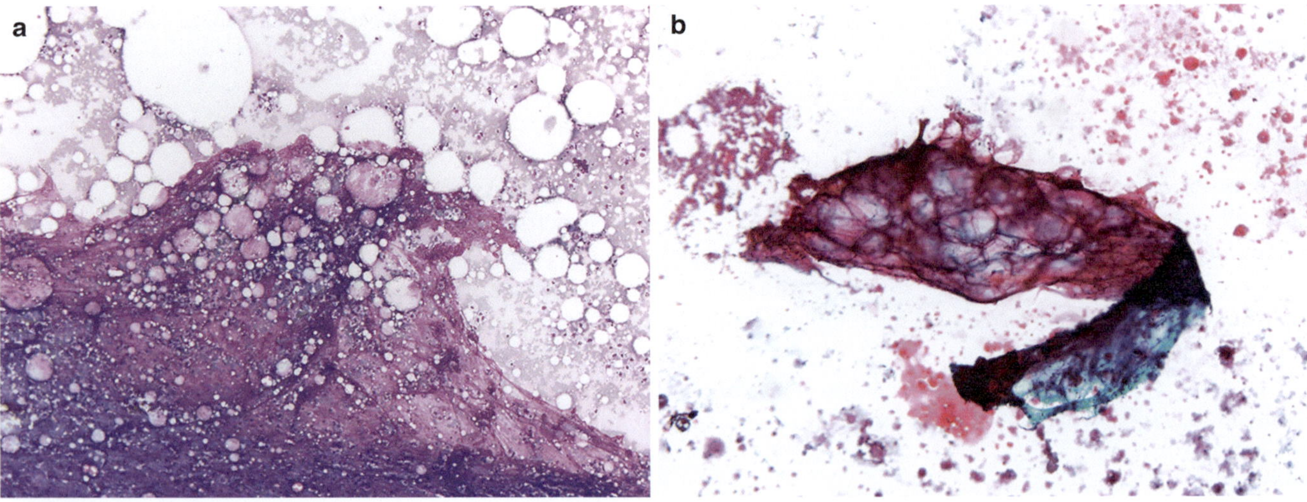

Fig. 11.6 Fat necrosis. (**a**) Usually hypocellular specimens with numerous macrophages and scattered multinucleated giant cells. Clusters of degenerated adipose tissue, background acellular debris, inflammatory cells, and occasional crystals can also be seen (DiffQuik stain, 100×). (**b**) Degenerated, necrotic adipose tissue and focal calcifications. These calcifications can sometimes be seen radiologically, and if they arise adjacent to a prior resection site or scar tissue they can raise a concern for malignancy (DiffQuik stain, 100×). (**c**) The adipose tissue is degenerated, with the majority lacking viable nuclei. Numerous macrophages are scattered between the adipocytes (H&E, 200×)

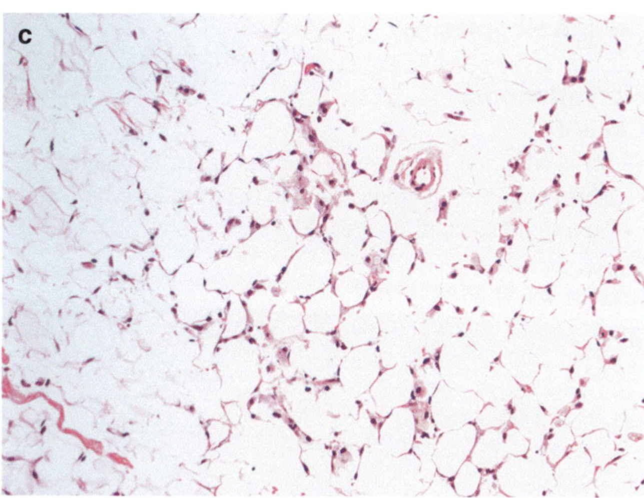

Fig. 11.6 (continued)

Radiology

Mammography

- Fan- or flame-shaped density emanating from nipple, usually asymmetric (Fig. 11.11a).

Ultrasound

- Small, subareolar hypoechoic mass or prominent subareolar ducts in early nodular or late dendritic phase (Fig. 11.12a)
- Similar to normal female breast tissue echogenicity in diffuse glandular pattern (Fig. 11.12b) [4].

Fine Needle Aspiration

- Variable cellularity aspirates.
- Flat sheets of benign ductal cells with small oval nuclei and scant cytoplasm (Fig. 11.13a).

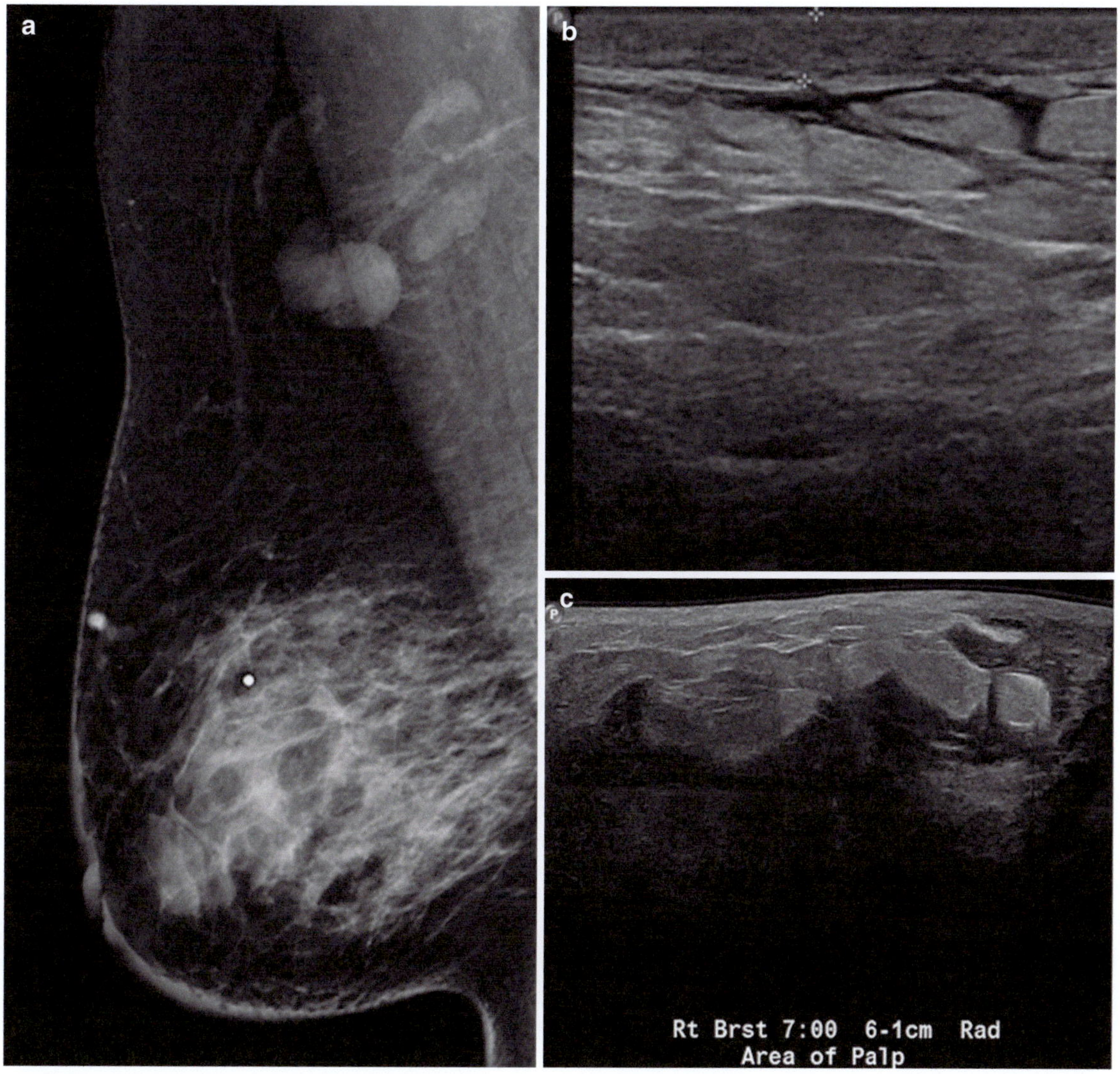

Fig. 11.7 Mastitis. (**a**) Right MLO view demonstrating diffuse skin thickening and trabecular thickening as well as an enlarged right axillary lymph node (reactive). (**b**) US image of the left breast in an area of erythema demonstrates skin thickening and subcutaneous edema without focal fluid collection to suggest abscess. (**c**) US image demonstrates an irregular hypoechoic mass extending to the skin. Biopsy revealed granulomatous mastitis

- Background naked; ovoid to spindled myoepithelial cell nuclei.

Core Biopsy

- Breast tissue with increased number of ducts with loose, cellular, and vascular periductal stroma.
- Hyperplastic epithelium with tapering tufts of cytoplasm into the lumen (Fig. 11.13b).

Benign Neoplasms

Fibroadenoma

Clinical

- Most common benign tumor of the breast in women.
- More common in young women (teens to 30s) but can be seen in patients of all ages [3].

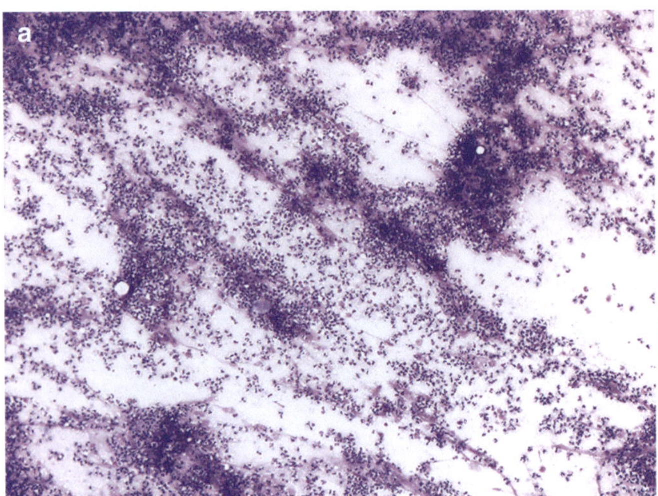

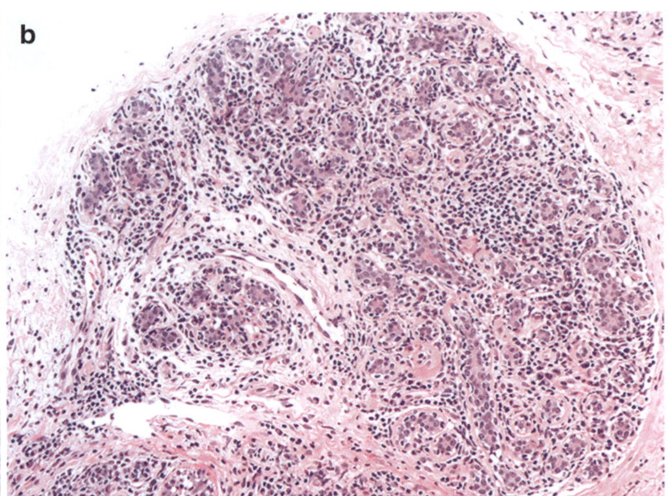

Fig. 11.8 Mastitis. (**a**) Characterized by sheets of neutrophils. Clusters of ductal epithelium may also be present, but care must be taken not to overinterpret reactive atypia as neoplasia in this particular setting (DiffQuik stain, 100×). (**b**) Mastitis, chronic lobular type. Breast lobule with abundant infiltrate consisting of lymphocytes and plasma cells (H&E, 200×)

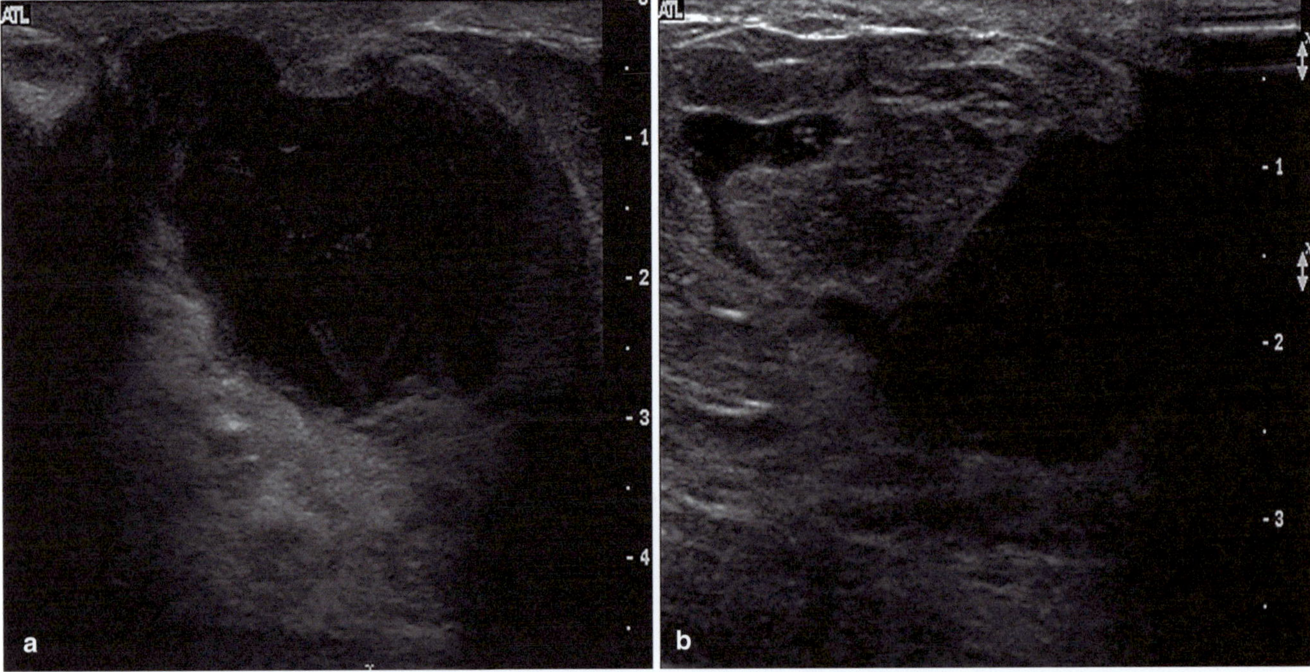

Fig. 11.9 Subareolar abscess. (**a**) US image of the right breast demonstrates a complex fluid collection at 6:00 in the subareolar breast, corresponding to a palpable abnormality with associated erythema. (**b**) US image demonstrates a hypoechoic mass in the subareolar breast with infiltration into the adjacent parenchyma. (**c**) US image demonstrates an irregular hypoechoic mass with extension to the nipple in a patient with symptoms of infection. Overlying skin thickening and edema are also noted

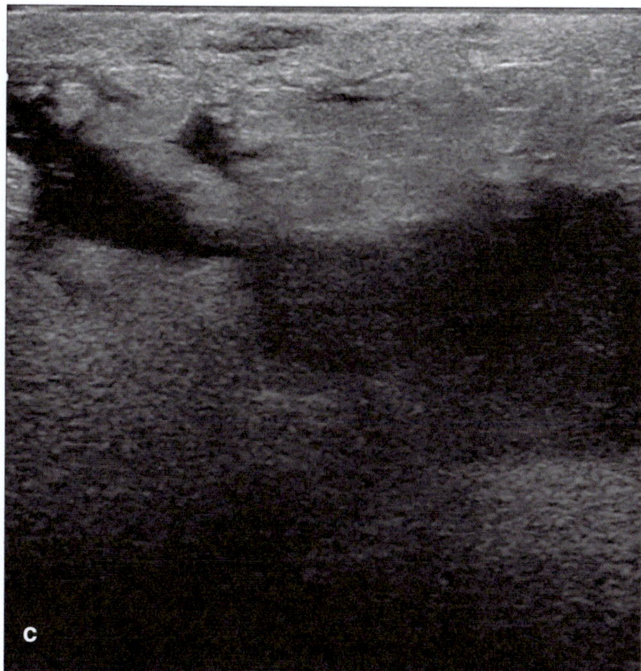

Fig. 11.9 (continued)

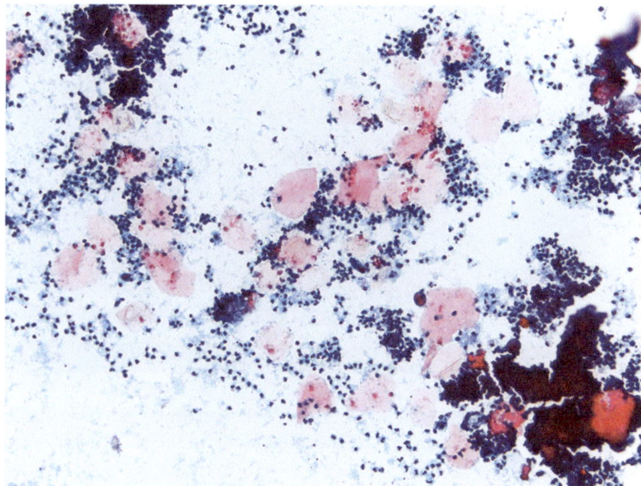

Fig. 11.10 Subareolar abscess. As the name suggests, this lesion is characterized by a usually painful nodule in the subareolar region of the breast. Two main components are present on cytology: numerous neutrophils and sheets of anucleated squamous cells. This condition arises as a consequence of squamous metaplasia and subsequent plugging of the lactiferous ducts. Stasis of normal breast secretions creates a nidus for infection, and over time a red, tender nodule can form (Papanicolaou stain, 200×)

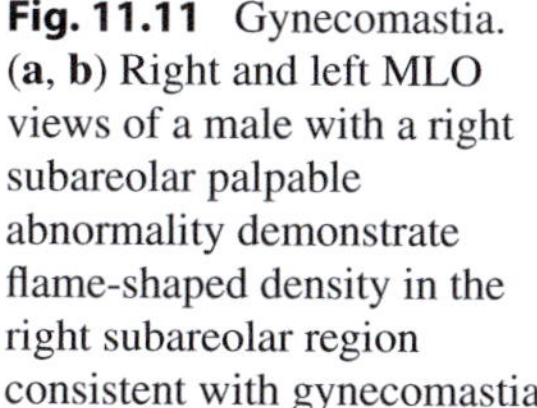

Fig. 11.11 Gynecomastia. (**a**, **b**) Right and left MLO views of a male with a right subareolar palpable abnormality demonstrate flame-shaped density in the right subareolar region consistent with gynecomastia

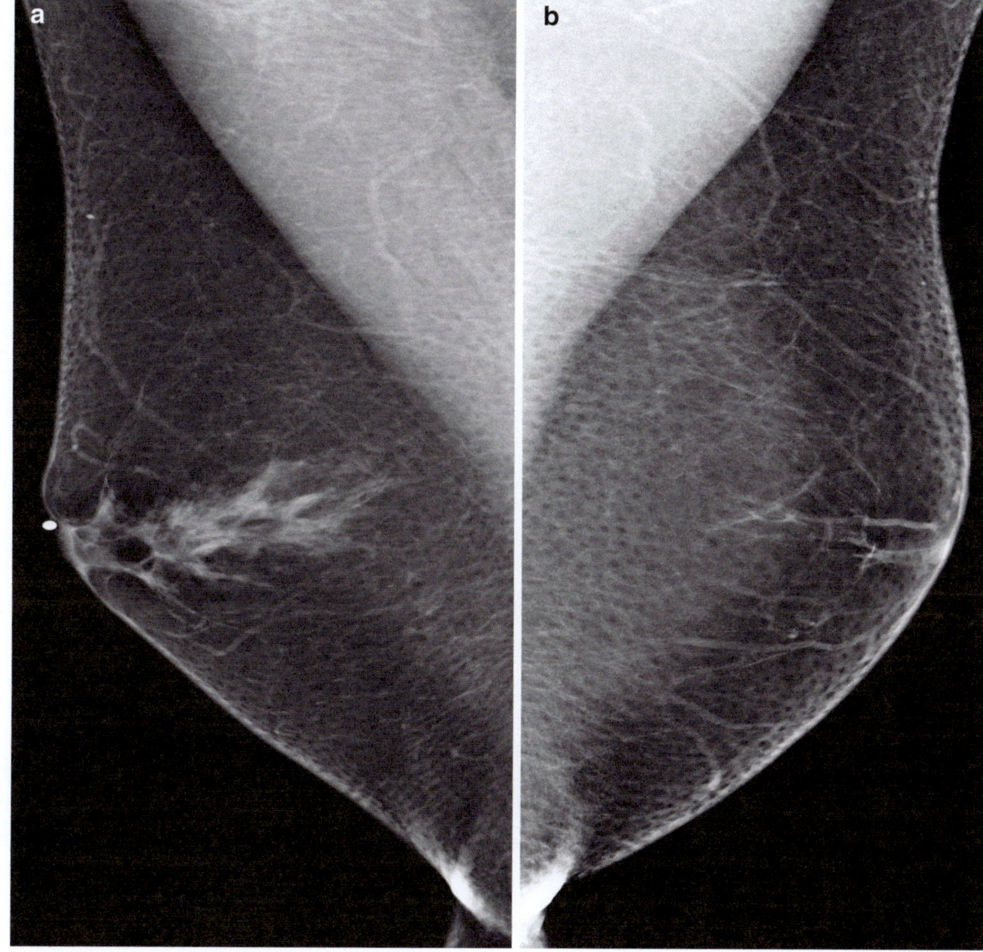

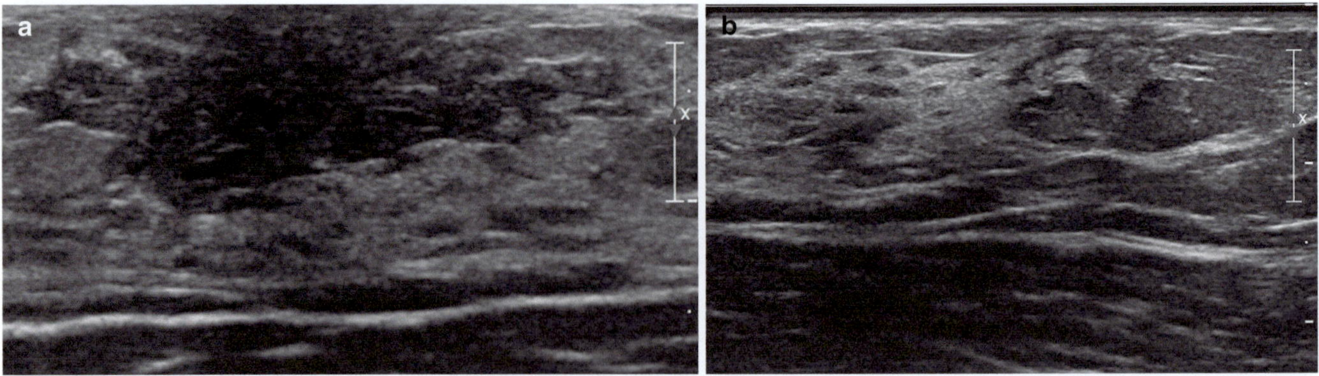

Fig. 11.12 Gynecomastia. (**a**) US image demonstrates a hypoechoic mass with microlobulated margins in the subareolar region. (**b**) US image demonstrates normal parenchymal echogenicity in the subareolar region as seen in the diffuse glandular pattern

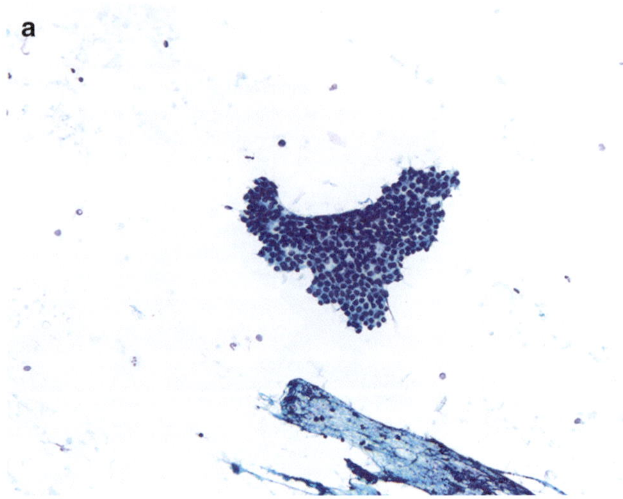

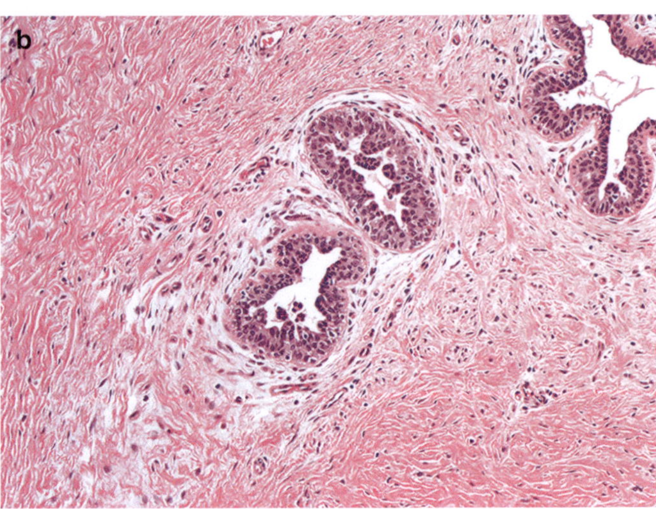

Fig. 11.13 Gynecomastia. (**a**) Findings in gynecomastia are similar to those found in aspirates of fibrocystic changes in women, except that they are instead found in men. Cytologic features include flat sheets of benign ductal cells, macrophages, and even apocrine metaplastic cells (Papanicolaou stain, 200×). (**b**) Gynecomastia, early stage. Increased numbers of ducts with loose, cellular, and vascular periductal stroma. The epithelium is hyperplastic with characteristic tapering tufts of epithelium protruding into the lumen (H&E, 200×)

- Presents as well-circumscribed, freely mobile, rubbery masses.

Radiology

Mammography

- Oval, circumscribed mass; may occasionally have coarse calcifications.

Ultrasound

- Oval, circumscribed hypoechoic mass with homogeneous internal echoes and parallel orientation to the skin (Fig. 11.14a).

Magnetic Resonance Imaging

- Oval, circumscribed T2-hyperintense enhancing mass, occasionally with nonenhancing internal septations (Fig. 11.14b) [4].

Fine Needle Aspiration

- Usually cellular aspirates.
- Large sheets and three-dimensional clusters of bland ductal cells, background naked; ovoid to spindled myoepithelial cell nuclei (Fig. 11.15a).

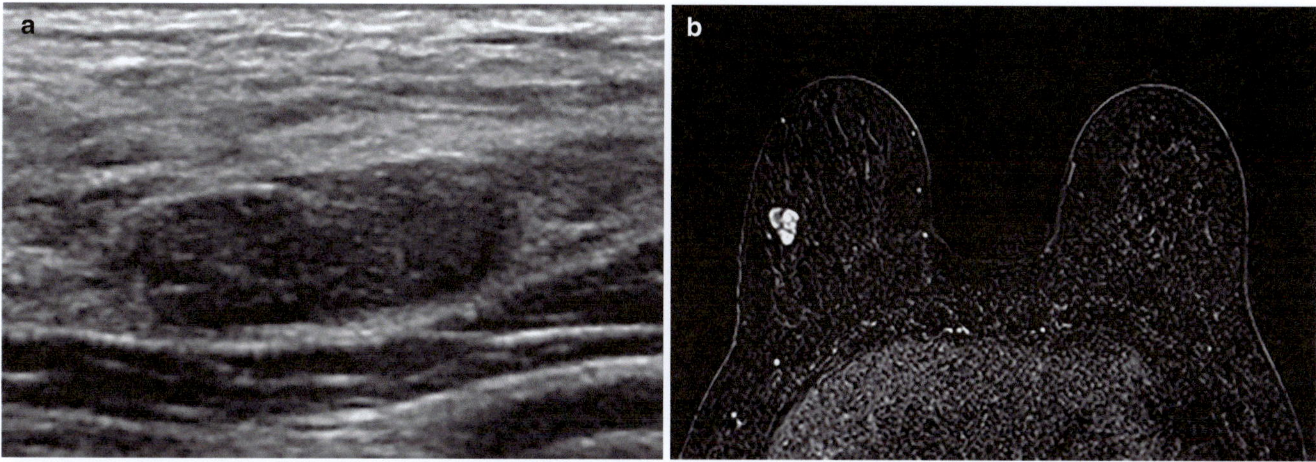

Fig. 11.14 Fibroadenoma. (**a**) US image demonstrates an oval, circumscribed, hypoechoic mass with parallel orientation to the skin. (**b**) Axial postcontrast subtraction MRI image demonstrates an oval circumscribed enhancing mass with nonenhancing internal septations in the outer right breast

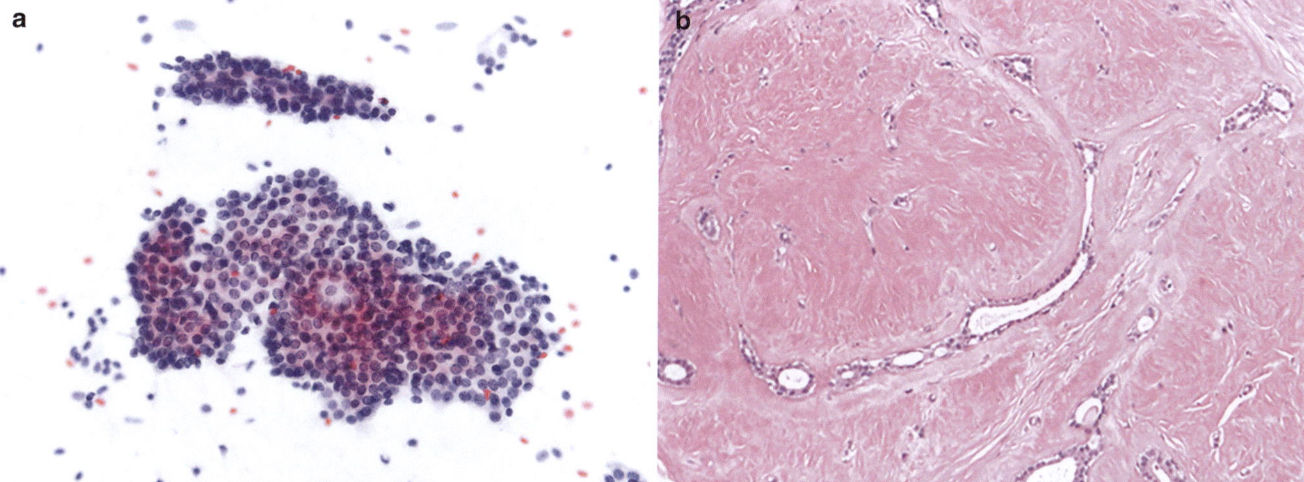

Fig. 11.15 Fibroadenoma. (**a**) These fibroepithelial tumors represent the most common benign tumor of the female breast. Clinically these tumors tend to appear in younger patients, predominantly in those in their late teens and twenties, although they may arise in any age group. They are well-circumscribed, freely mobile, rubbery tumors with a characteristic cytomorphology. Aspirates are characterized by flat sheets of bland ductal cells with staghorn or antler-like contours and numerous background dispersed myoepithelial cells, as seen in this low-power image (Papanicolaou stain, 100×). (**b**) Well-circumscribed proliferation of both benign stromal and benign epithelial elements. In this example, the stroma is fibrous, while the epithelia form glands with open lumina and have the dual outer myoepithelial and inner epithelial layer (H&E, 100×)

Core Biopsy

- Characterized by proliferation of benign stromal and epithelial elements. Abundant fibrous stroma and inner ductal epithelium arranged in glands with open lumina and outer myoepithelial layer (Fig. 11.15b).

Neoplasms of Uncertain Malignant Potential

Papillary Lesions

Clinical

- Usually solid retroareolar tumors, but they can occur anywhere in the breast.
- Central papillary lesions may present with bloody discharge.
- Large papillary lesions can appear as mass lesions, amenable to superficial FNA or FNA under imaging guidance [1].

Radiology

Ultrasound

- Intraductal mass (Figs. 11.16a and 11.17b), complex cystic and solid mass (Fig. 11.16b).

Ductogram

- Intraductal filling defect (Fig. 11.17a) [4].

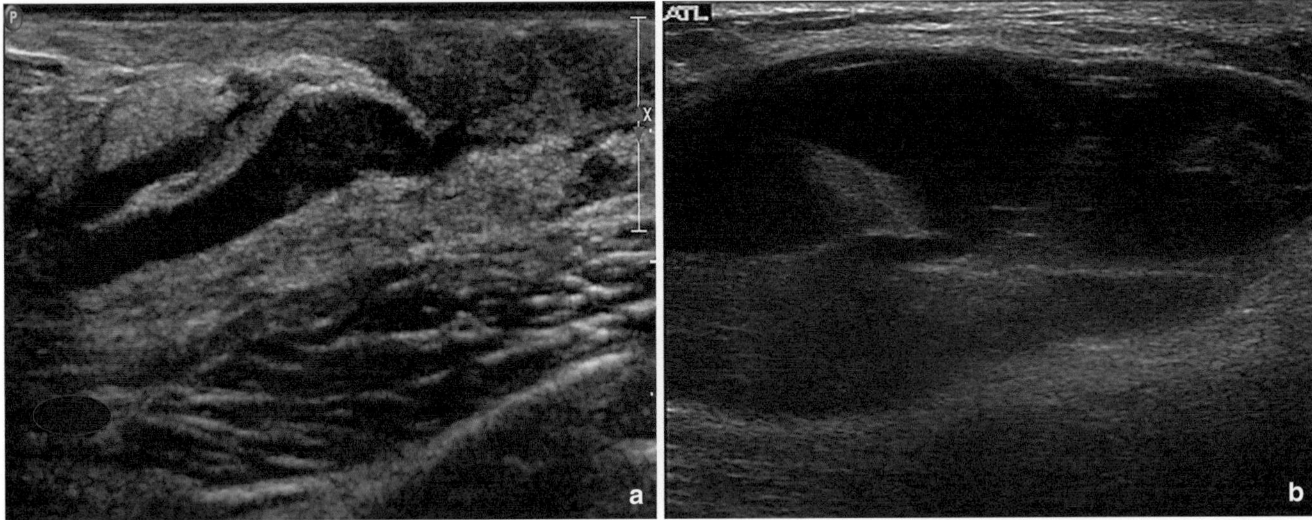

Fig. 11.16 Papillary lesion. (**a**) US image demonstrates an intraductal mass in the subareolar region of a patient with bloody nipple discharge; this is a biopsy-proven papilloma. (**b**) US image in a woman with a left breast palpable abnormality demonstrates a complex cystic and solid mass. Biopsy revealed an encapsulated papillary carcinoma

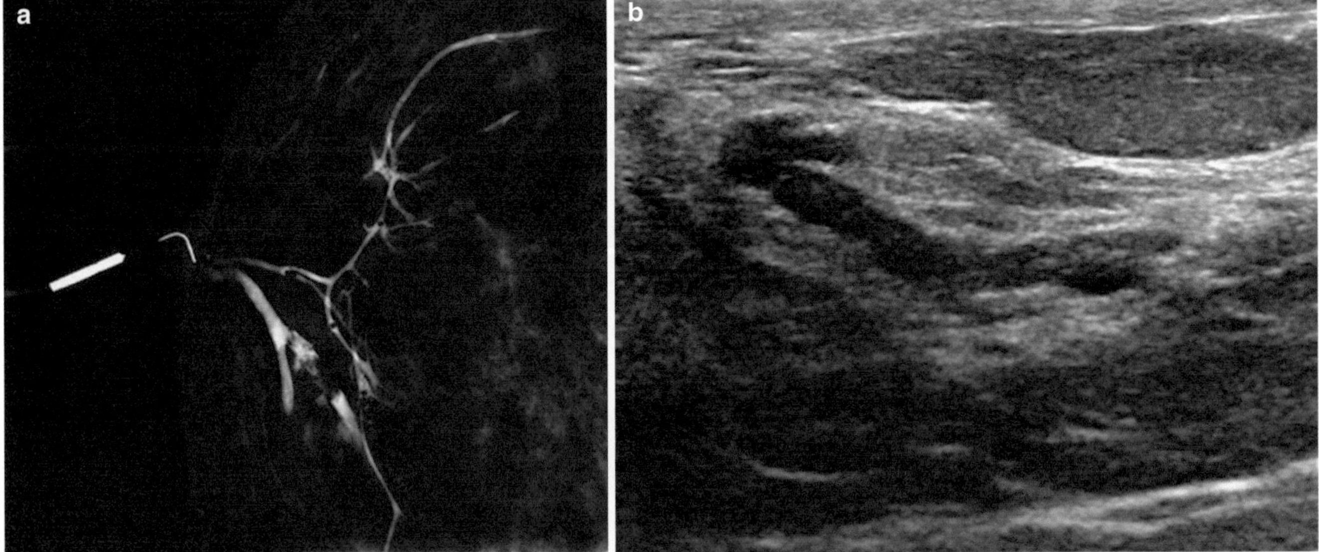

Fig. 11.17 Papillary lesion. (**a**) Right craniocaudal (CC) view from a ductogram in a patient with a right bloody nipple discharge demonstrates an intraductal filling defect with corresponding intraductal mass on US (**b**); biopsy-proven papilloma

Fine Needle Aspiration

- Variable cellularity.
- Three-dimensional papillary groups with fibrovascular cores (Fig. 11.18a).
- Flat sheets of ductal cells with anywhere from mild to marked atypia.
- Background naked; ovoid to spindled myoepithelial cell nuclei.
- Ductal cells may be short and cuboidal or more elongated and tall and columnar in shape.
- Background macrophages and/or blood.

Core Biopsy

- Intraductal proliferation forming papillary structures lined by myoepithelial cells and ductal cells (Fig. 11.18b).

Phyllodes Tumor

Clinical

- Presentation similar to that of fibroadenoma but occurs far less commonly, accounting for only about 1% of all breast tumors.
- Tends to progress more quickly and grow to larger sizes than fibroadenomas. Also generally occurs in a slightly older age group [3].

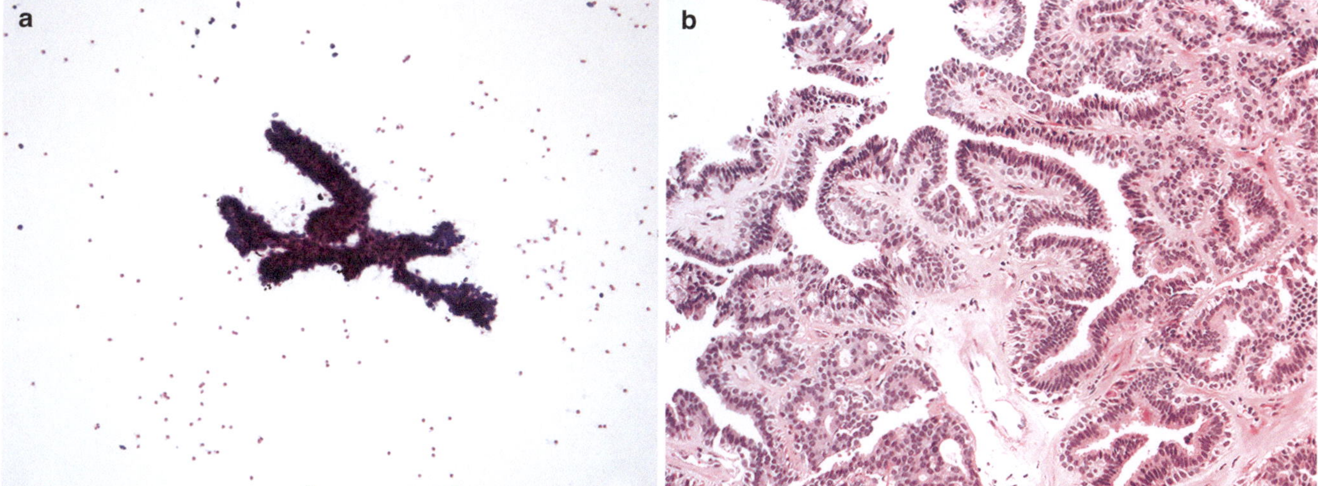

Fig. 11.18 Papillary lesion. (**a**) Less commonly, as in this 32-year-old patient, papillary tumors can present as palpable or radiologically apparent masses that can be targeted by FNA. Cytology shows three-dimensional papillary groups with fibrovascular cores or flat sheets. Cellularity can be moderate to markedly hypercellular, with more cellular smears being a soft sign for possible malignancy. Background myoepithelial cells, macrophages, and blood may also be seen (Papanicolaou stain, 200×). (**b**) Intraductal proliferation forming papillary structures that consist of fibrovascular cores lined by an inner layer of myoepithelial cells and an outer layer of ductal epithelial cells. In this example, the myoepithelial cells are paler with round nuclei, while the ductal epithelial cells are more hyperchromatic with columnar nuclei (H&E, 200×)

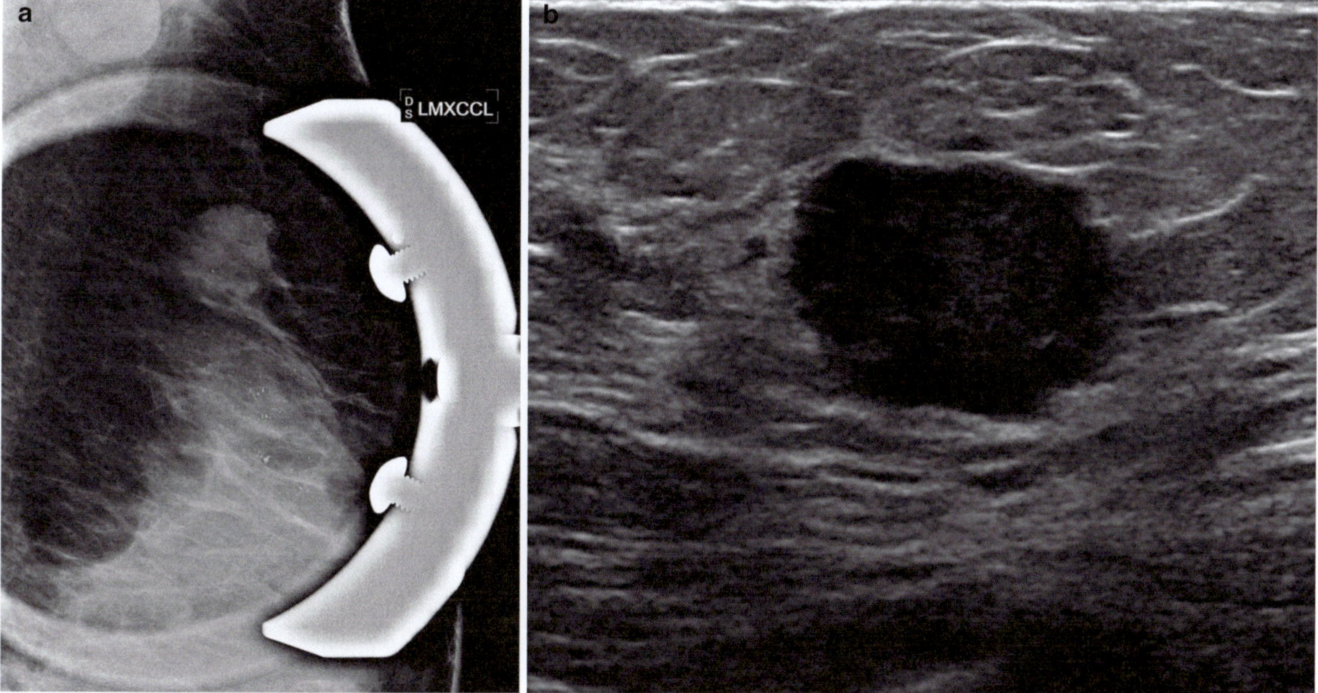

Fig. 11.19 Phyllodes tumor. (**a**) Spot magnification view of the left breast demonstrates a round mass with microlobulated and indistinct margins. (**b**) Corresponding US image demonstrates a round hypoechoic mass with microlobulated and angular margins

Radiology

Mammography

- Oval to round dense mass with circumscribed or lobulated margins, calcifications rare (Fig. 11.19a)

Ultrasound

- Solid, oval or round, circumscribed hypoechoic mass, can have partially non-circumscribed margins or intracystic spaces (Fig. 11.19b)

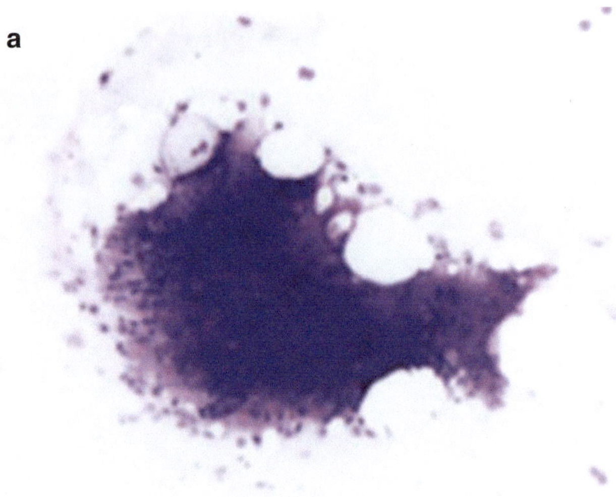

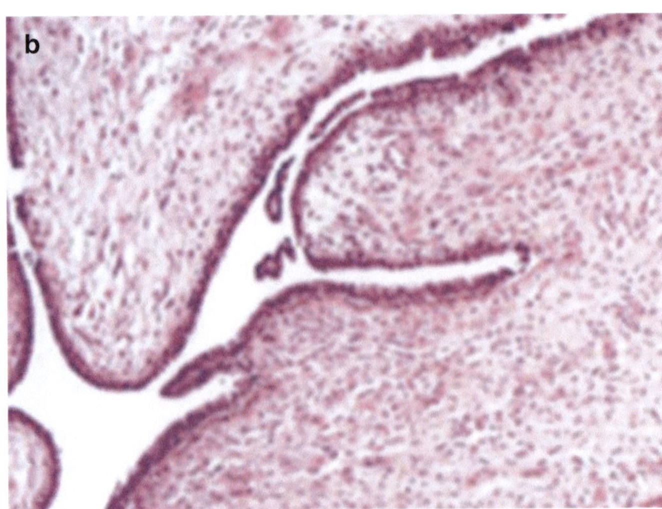

Fig. 11.20 Phyllodes tumor. (**a**) These tumors are also fibroepithelial lesions that share cytomorphologic characteristics with fibroadenoma. However, they tend to occur in a slightly older age group and grow to be quite large in a relatively short period of time. While the epithelial component is essentially identical to that of fibroadenomas with flat clusters of ductal cells, the diagnostic material is a sampling of the stromal component. These cellular stromal fragments are usually flat with angulated margins with embedded spindled nuclei. With Diff-Quik staining, stromal fragments tend to have an intense magenta color, as seen in this image (DiffQuik stain, 400×). (**b**) Phyllodes tumor, benign. Proliferation of atypical stromal cells lined by benign epithelia that together form large clefts and leaf-like architecture. In this example, the stromal component is hypercellular and consists of mildly atypical cells with variably prominent nuclei that are more concentrated near the epithelium (H&E, 200×)

Magnetic Resonance Imaging

- Rapidly enhancing oval or round mass with non-enhancing internal septations, cystic spaces, and increased T2 signal in slit-like spaces [5].

Fine Needle Aspiration

- The major diagnostic feature is stromal fragments. These tend to be cellular, with numerous elongated spindled nuclei with indistinct cytoplasm and variable atypia (Fig. 11.20a).
- Large sheets and three-dimensional clusters of bland ductal cells, similar to what is seen in fibroadenomas.

Core Biopsy

- Proliferation of atypical stromal cells lined by benign epithelium that form large clefts and leaf-like architecture. Increased stromal cellularity adjacent to epithelium is typical (Fig. 11.20b).

Malignant Neoplasms

Breast Carcinoma

Clinical

- Present as palpable firm masses or radiologic abnormalities on imaging.
- Invasive ductal carcinoma is by far the most common malignant tumor of the breast, accounting for anywhere from 40% to 75% of all breast cancers [1].
- Invasive lobular carcinoma is the second-most common type, accounting for 5–15% of cases [6].
- Metaplastic carcinoma is far less common (<1% of all breast cancers) and encompasses a heterogeneous group of tumors with variable components of sarcomatoid (spindle cell), squamous, and poorly differentiated carcinoma [7]

Radiology

Mammography

- Calcifications (Fig. 11.21a, b):
  - Morphology: Fine linear or fine linear branching, fine pleomorphic, coarse heterogeneous, amorphous
  - Distribution: Segmental, linear, grouped, regional
- Masses (most often irregular in shape with non-circumscribed margins), focal asymmetries, or areas of architectural distortion (Figs. 11.22a, b and 11.23a).

Ultrasound

- Most characteristically an irregular hypoechoic mass with non-circumscribed margins, antiparallel orientation, hypoechoic echopattern, and posterior acoustic shadowing (Figs. 11.23b and 11.24).

Magnetic Resonance Imaging

- Irregular, heterogeneously enhancing mass with non-circumscribed margins and suspicious enhancement kinetics (Fig 11.25a)
- Non-mass enhancement in a focal, linear, regional, or segmental distribution with heterogeneous, clumped, or clustered ring internal enhancement pattern (Fig. 11.25b) [4, 5, 8].

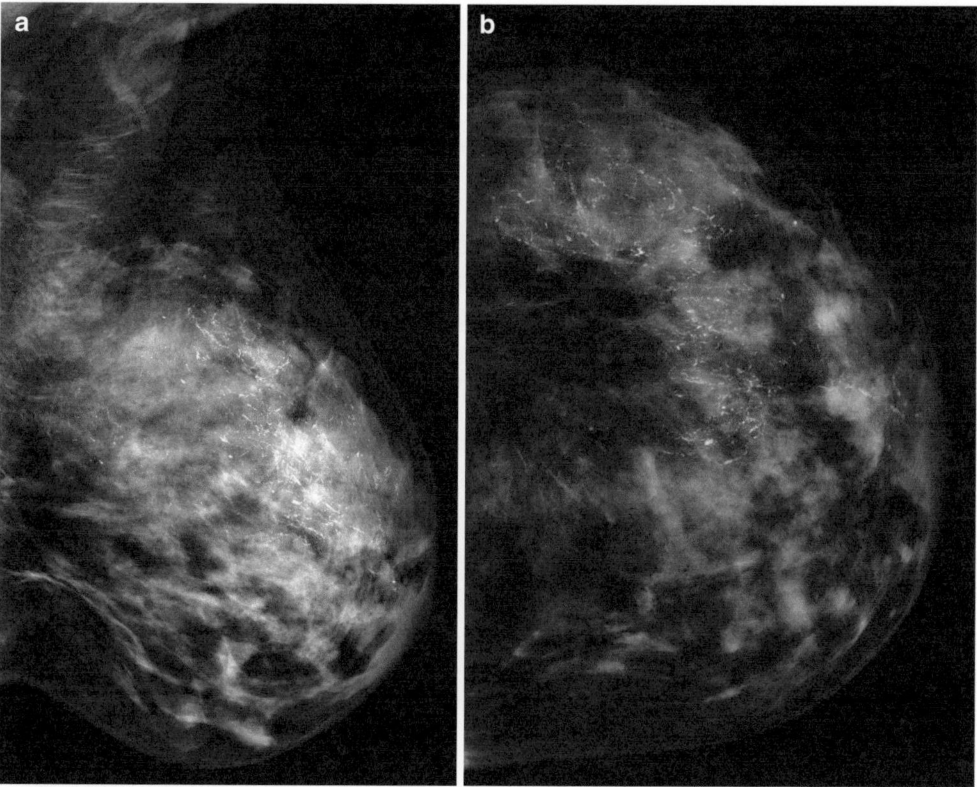

Fig. 11.21 Breast carcinoma. (**a**, **b**) Left MLO and CC views demonstrating extensive segmental pleomorphic and linear branching calcifications in the superior lateral breast. Stereotactic biopsy revealed DCIS

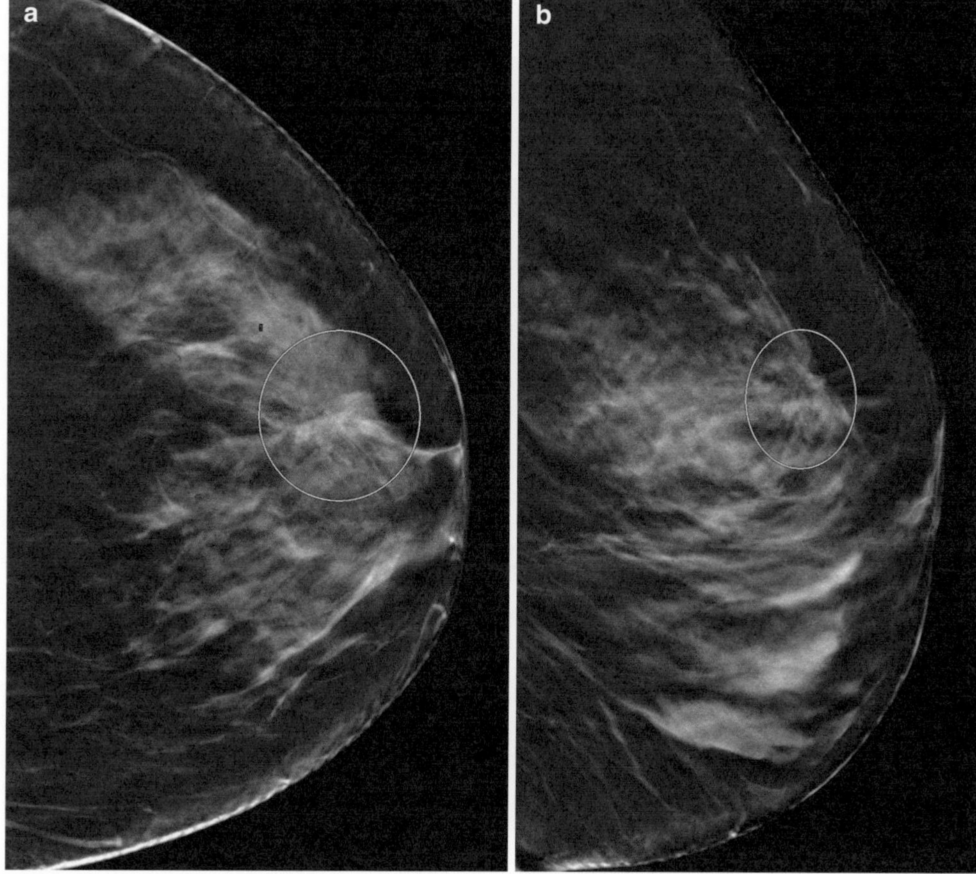

Fig. 11.22 Breast carcinoma. (**a**, **b**) Left CC and lateral tomosynthesis images demonstrate an area of architectural distortion in the upper outer left breast. Biopsy revealed DCIS

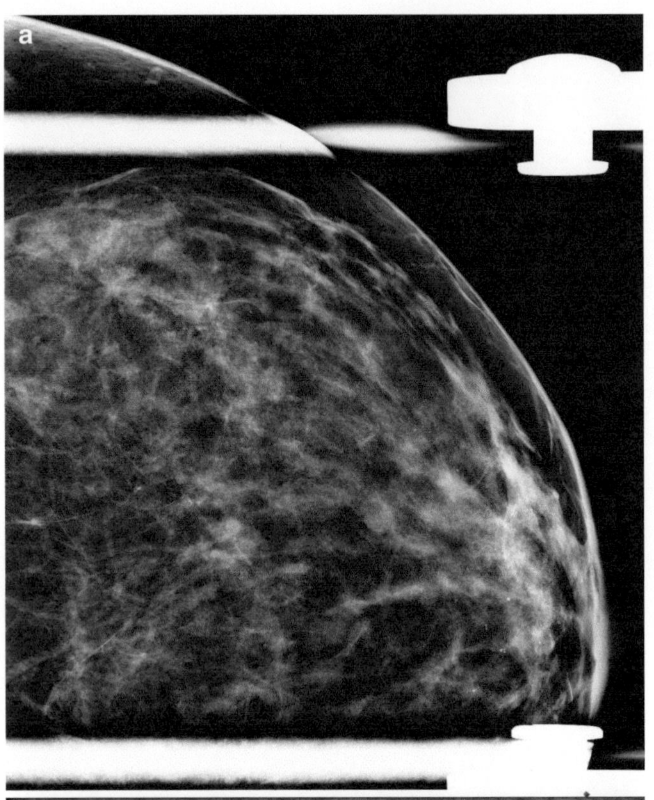

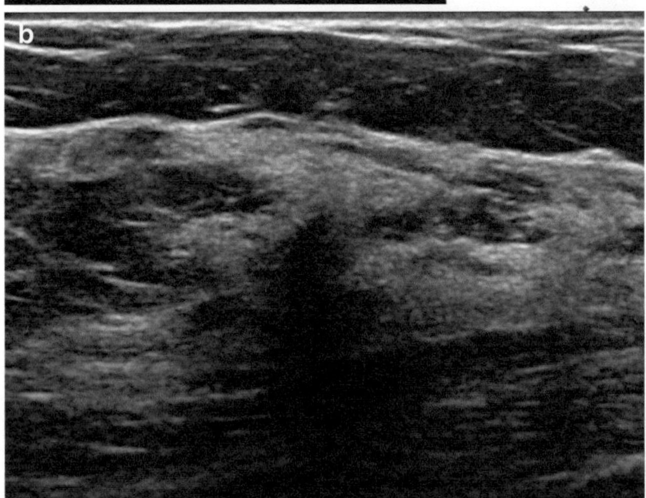

Fig. 11.23 Breast carcinoma. (**a**) Left CC spot compression view demonstrates an irregular spiculated mass in the outer posterior breast with associated distortion. (**b**) US image shows an irregular hypoechoic mass with antiparallel orientation. Biopsy revealed invasive lobular carcinoma

Fine Needle Aspiration

- Ductal carcinoma
  - Hypercellular smears.
  - Individual tumor cells and crowded clusters of cells (Fig. 11.26a).
  - Tumor cells with irregular eccentric pleomorphic prominent nuclei (Fig. 11.26b).
- Lobular carcinoma
  - Not as cellular as aspirates from ductal carcinoma.
  - Intracytoplasmic lumina with mucin droplets (can also be seen in ductal carcinoma but more prominent in lobular carcinoma) (Fig. 11.27a).
  - Fibrous stromal fragments [6].
- Metaplastic carcinoma
  - Variably low to moderately cellular.
  - Spindle cell/sarcomatoid carcinoma: moderate to markedly atypical spindle cells.
  - Squamous cell carcinoma: malignant squamous cells with dense keratinized cytoplasmic and hyperchromatic nuclei.
  - Poorly differentiated carcinoma: malignant epithelioid cells devoid of keratinization [7].

Core Biopsy

- Haphazard glands and disorganized clusters of malignant cells infiltrating through breast stroma with surrounding desmoplastic response (Fig. 11.27b).

Lymphoma

Clinical

- Primary non-Hodgkin lymphoma of the breast is rare and represents approximately 0.5% of all breast cancers.
- Non-Hodgkin lymphoma can involve the breast primarily or secondary to systemic disease.
- The majority of cases are B-cell lymphomas, and the most common subtypes are diffuse large B-cell lymphoma, follicular lymphoma, and lymphomas of mucosal-associated lymphoid tissue (MALT).
- They can present as mass lesions in the breast with or without corresponding axillary lymphadenopathy [9].

Radiology

Mammography

- Solitary or multiple circumscribed to ill-defined mass(es) without spiculation or calcifications
- Infiltrative type: diffuse increased density, trabecular, and skin thickening may be present (Fig. 11.28).
- Axillary lymphadenopathy

Ultrasound

- Partially circumscribed oval or irregular mass with variable posterior acoustic features and mixed echogenicity (Fig. 11.29); can be mostly hyperechoic.

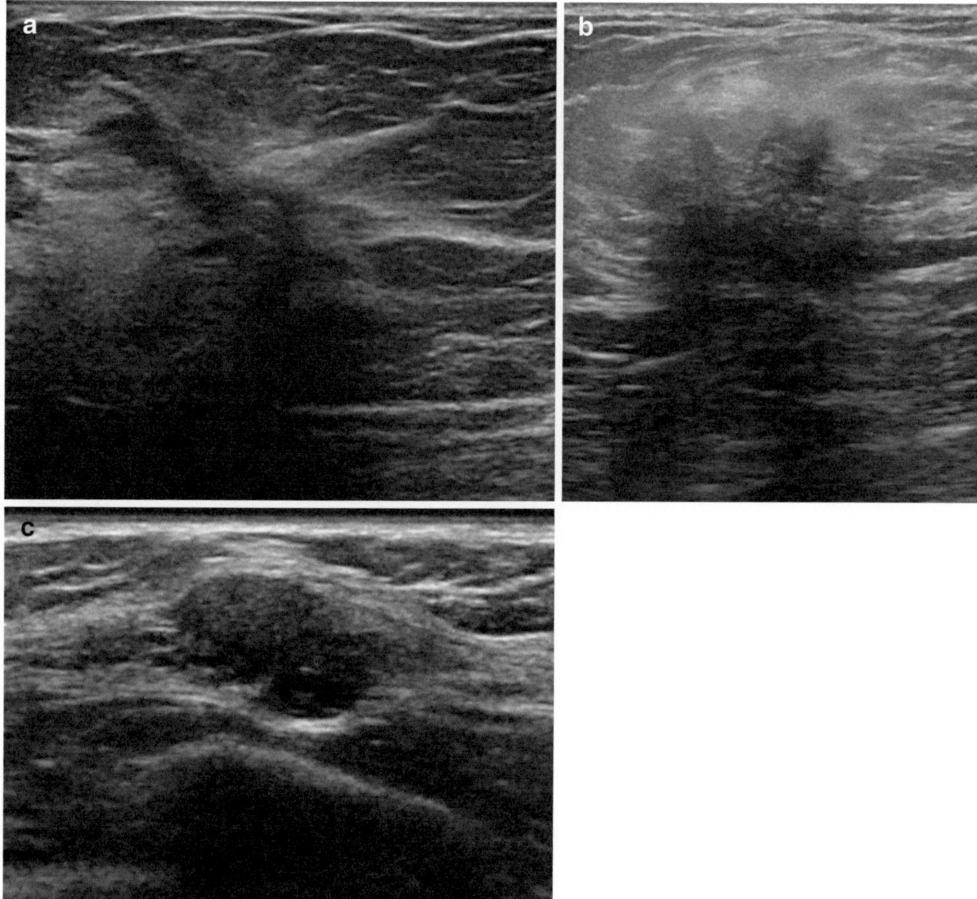

Fig. 11.24 Breast carcinoma. (**a**) Irregular hypoechoic mass with antiparallel orientation and posterior acoustic shadowing, biopsy proven invasive lobular carcinoma. (**b**) Irregular hypoechoic mass with angular margins, associated calcifications, echogenic halo, and posterior acoustic shadowing. Biopsy revealed invasive ductal carcinoma. (**c**) Oval hypoechoic mass with microlobulated and indistinct margins and parallel orientation, biopsy proven invasive ductal carcinoma

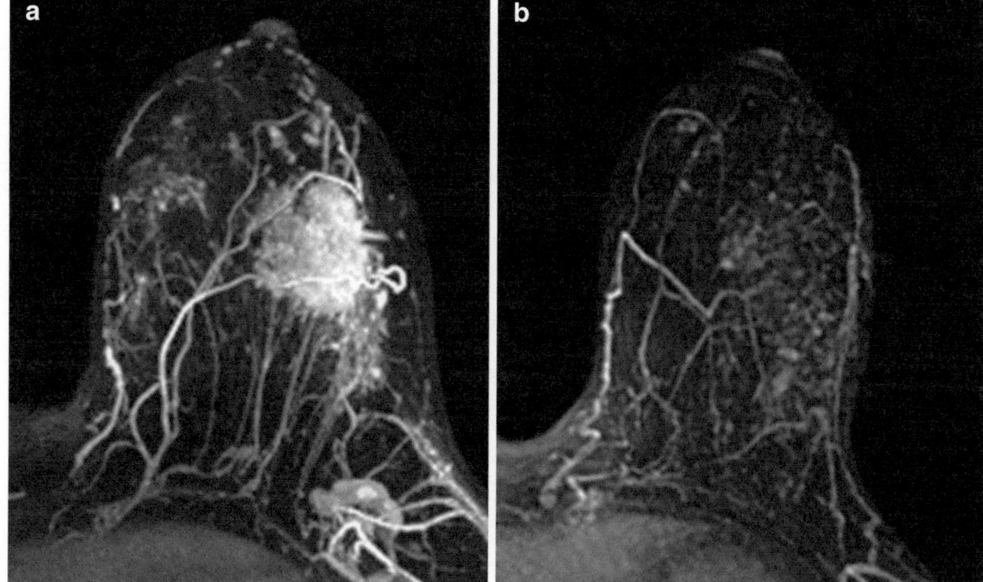

Fig. 11.25 Breast carcinoma. (**a**) MIP MR image of the left breast demonstrates an irregular, heterogeneously enhancing mass with irregular margins and surrounding non-mass enhancement in the outer breast as well as left axillary lymphadenopathy consistent with biopsy proven invasive ductal carcinoma with associated DCIS and axillary metastases. (**b**) MIP MR image of the left breast demonstrates segmental clumped non-mass enhancement in the outer left breast consistent with biopsy proven DCIS

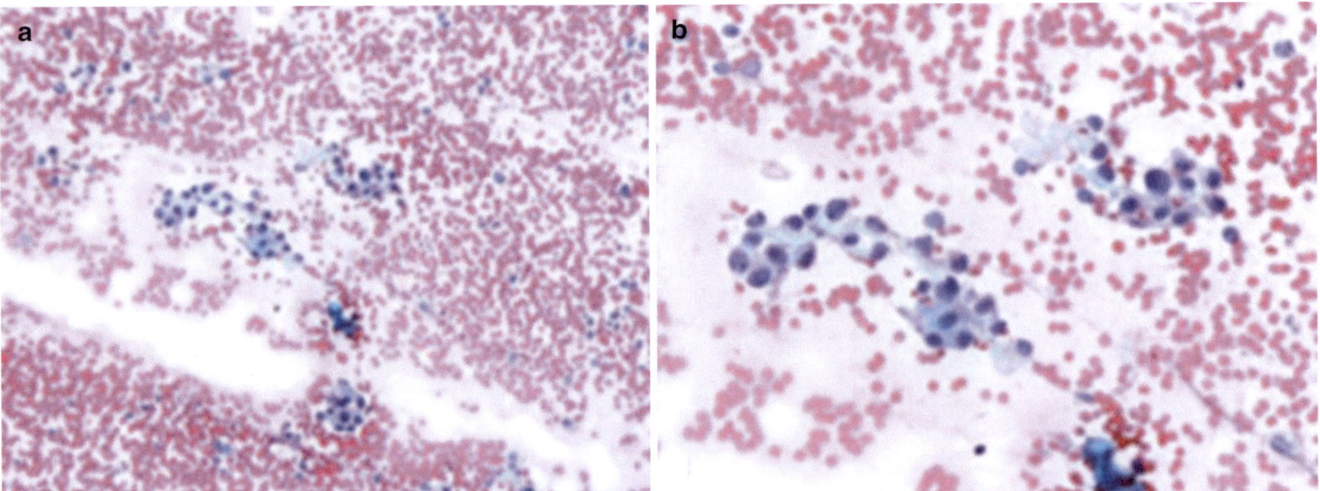

Fig. 11.26 Breast carcinoma. (**a**) Invasive ductal carcinoma is the most common malignant tumor of the breast. It is characterized by hypercellular aspirates of cells with variable degrees of atypia, depending on the grade of the tumor. This 2.5 cm spiculated mass was found in the upper outer quadrant of the right breast in a 53-year-old woman. Medium-power view shows crowded clusters of tumor cells with scant delicate cytoplasm and hyperchromatic enlarged nuclei in a bloody background (Papanicolaou stain, 200×). (**b**) At higher magnification, the nuclear irregularities are more apparent. The nuclei vary in size and have clumped coarse chromatin and prominent red nucleoli (Papanicolaou stain, 400×)

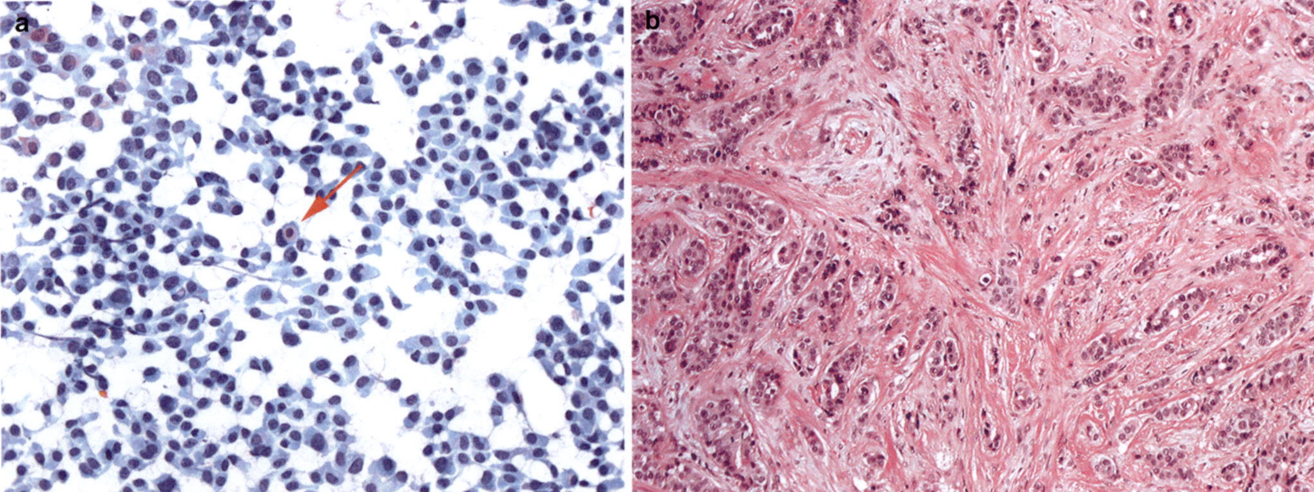

Fig. 11.27 Breast carcinoma. (**a**) This can also present as sheets of plasmacytoid tumor cells with characteristic intracytoplasmic lumina (*arrow*), as seen in this example (Papanicolaou stain, 400×). (**b**) Invasive ductal carcinoma. Haphazard gland and solid clusters of atypical epithelial cells infiltrating through the breast stroma. A pale desmoplastic response is evident surrounding the invading tumor cells (H&E stain, 200×)

Fine Needle Aspiration

- Discohesive lymphoid cells (Figs. 11.30a).
- Background lymphoglandular bodies.
- Tumors cells can vary from monotonous to pleomorphic, depending on subtype of lymphoma.

Core Biopsy

- Sheets of monotonous small round blue discohesive lymphocytes replacing breast tissue (Fig. 11.30b).

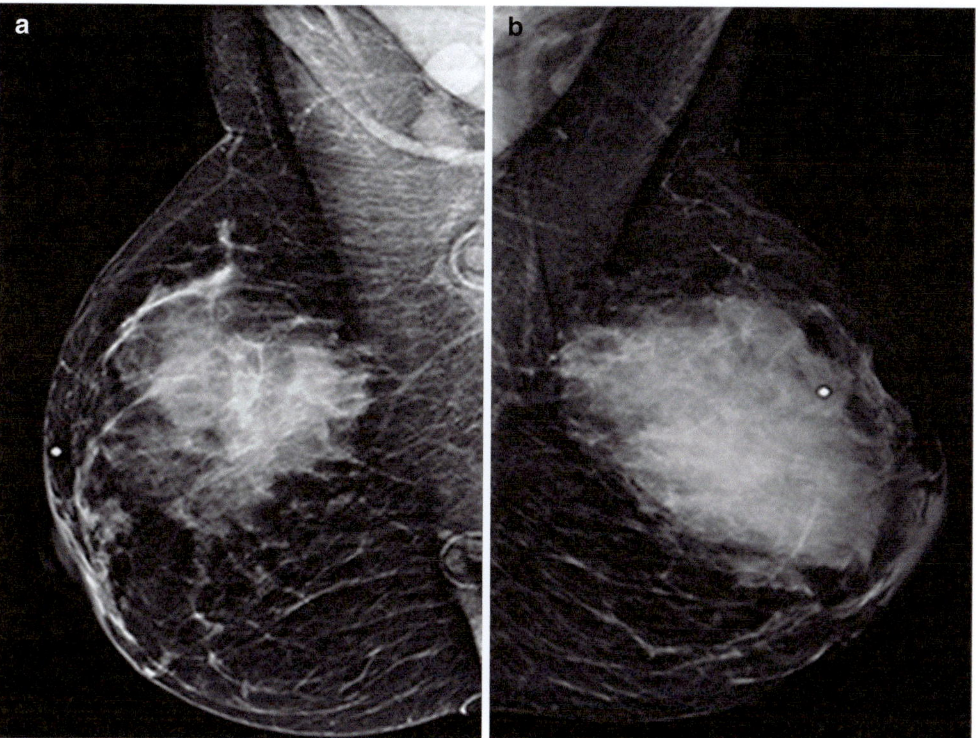

Fig. 11.28 Lymphoma. (**a**, **b**) Right and left MLO views demonstrate large ill-defined masses corresponding to palpable abnormalities in the upper aspects of both breasts

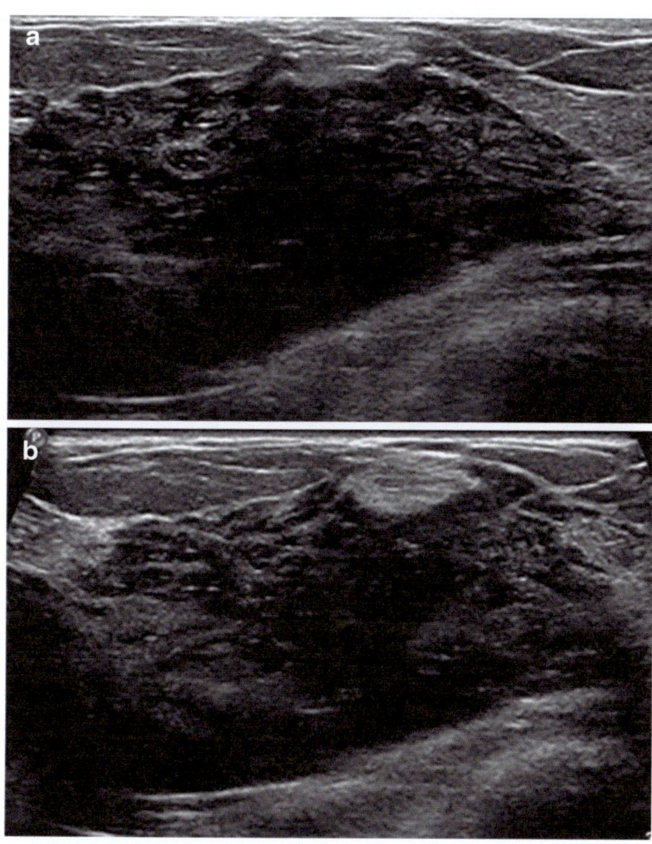

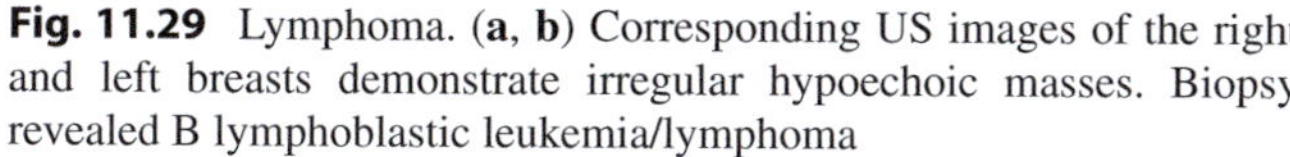

Fig. 11.29 Lymphoma. (**a**, **b**) Corresponding US images of the right and left breasts demonstrate irregular hypoechoic masses. Biopsy revealed B lymphoblastic leukemia/lymphoma

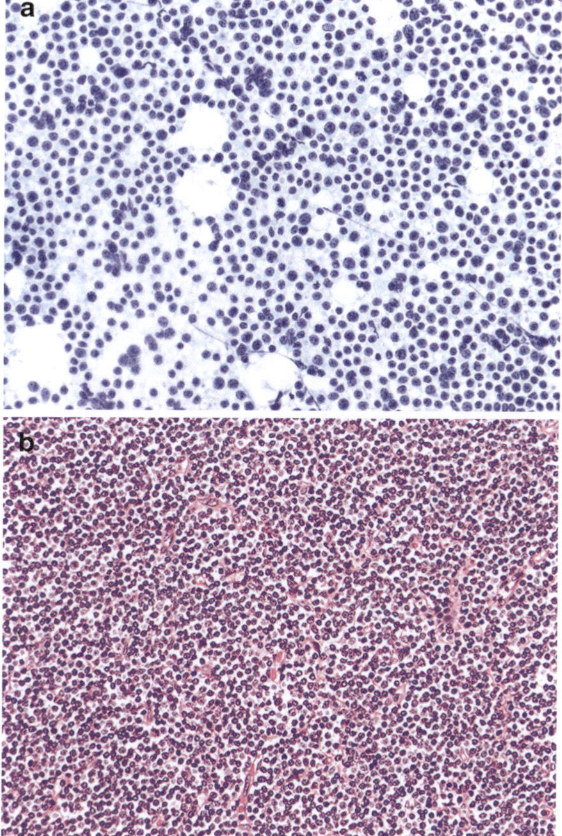

Fig. 11.30 Lymphoma. (**a**) Medium-power view of an ill-defined mass in the upper outer quadrant of a 65-year-old patient with a history of lymphoma shows sheets of monotonous, discohesive lymphoid cells (Papanicolaou stain, 200×). (**b**) Sheets of monotonous, small, round, blue, discohesive lymphocytes replacing the breast tissue (H&E stain, 200×)

References

1. Ducatman B, Wang H. Breast. In: Cibas E, Ducatman B, editors. Cytology: diagnostic principles and clinical correlates. 4th ed. Philadelphia: Elsevier Saunders; 2014. p. 233–65.
2. DeMay R. The art and science of cytopathology, Superficial aspiration cytology, vol. 2. 2nd ed. Chicago: ASCP Press; 2012. p. 1051–143.
3. Guray M, Aysegul S. Benign breast diseases: classification, diagnosis and management. Oncologist. 2006;11:435–49.
4. Fiorica JV. Breast cancer screening, mammography, and other modalities. Clin Obstet Gynecol. 2016;59:688–709.
5. Hongna T, Zhang S, Liu H, Peng W, Li R, Gu Y, et al. Imaging findings in phyllodes tumors of the breast. Eur J Radiol. 2012;81:e62–9.
6. Menet E, Becette V, Briffod M. Cytologic diagnosis of lobular carcinoma of the breast: experience with 555 patients in the Rene Huguenin Cancer Center. Cancer Cytopathol. 2008;114:111–7.
7. Lui P, Tse G, Tan P, Jayaram G, Putti T, Chaiwun B, et al. Fine-needle aspiration cytology of metaplastic carcinoma of the breast. J Clin Pathol. 2007;60:529–33.
8. Guo R, Lu G, Qin B, Fei B. Ultrasound imaging technologies for breast cancer detection and management: a review. Ultrasound Med Biol. 2018;44:37–70.
9. Jain M, Khandekar S, Mahadani J, Raut W. Report of a case of primary breast lymphoma highlighting the importance of fine needle aspiration cytology as an initial diagnostic tool. J Cytol. 2015;32:127–9.

Index

R. Nayar et al. (eds.), *Atlas of Cytopathology and Radiology*, https://doi.org/10.1007/978-3-030-24756-0

M

R